U0484539

Radiotherapy in Managing Brain Metastases A Case-Based Approach

脑转移瘤放射治疗学 基于病例的研究

原著 [美] Yoshiya Yamada
　　 [美] Eric Chang
　　 [美] John B. Fiveash
　　 [美] Jonathan Knisely
主译　周蓉蓉　周　琴

中国科学技术出版社
·北京·

图书在版编目（CIP）数据

脑转移瘤放射治疗学：基于病例的研究 /（美）山田吉屋（Yoshiya Yamada）等原著；周蓉蓉，周琴主译 . — 北京：中国科学技术出版社，2022.4

书名原文：Radiotherapy in Managing Brain Metastases: A Case-Based Approach

ISBN 978-7-5046-9454-6

Ⅰ . ①脑… Ⅱ . ①山… ②周… ③周… Ⅲ . ①脑肿瘤 — 放射治疗学 — 研究 Ⅳ . ① R739.41

中国版本图书馆 CIP 数据核字 (2022) 第 035907 号

著作权合同登记号：01-2022-1361

First published in English under the title
Radiotherapy in Managing Brain Metastases: A Case-Based Approach
edited by Yoshiya Yamada, Eric Chang, John B. Fiveash, Jonathan Knisely
Copyright © Springer International Publishing AG, part of Springer Nature 2020
This edition has been translated and published under licence from Springer Nature Switzerland AG.
All rights reserved.

策划编辑	靳　婷　孙　超
责任编辑	靳　婷
文字编辑	郭仕薪
装帧设计	佳木水轩
责任印制	徐　飞

出　　版	中国科学技术出版社
发　　行	中国科学技术出版社有限公司发行部
地　　址	北京市海淀区中关村南大街 16 号
邮　　编	100081
发行电话	010-62173865
传　　真	010-62179148
网　　址	http://www.cspbooks.com.cn

开　　本	889mm×1194mm　1/16
字　　数	551 千字
印　　张	20.5
版　　次	2022 年 4 月第 1 版
印　　次	2022 年 4 月第 1 次印刷
印　　刷	天津翔远印刷有限公司
书　　号	ISBN 978-7-5046-9454-6 / R・2835
定　　价	268.00 元

（凡购买本社图书，如有缺页、倒页、脱页者，本社发行部负责调换）

译者名单

主　译　周蓉蓉　周　琴

副主译　伍海军　杨　振　张莹莹　张子健

译校者（以姓氏笔画为序）

凡　丹　王翰宇　井　笛　邓　俍　龙艺文
吕知平　朱　红　伍海军　刘铮铮　刘渊渊
李书舟　杨　振　杨晓喻　张　静　张子健
张莹莹　邵其刚　周　雪　周　琴　周蓉蓉
周扬莹　胡永梅　段和新　唐　杜　曹　瑛
梁　瞻　曾　瑜　谭兆华

内容提要

本书引进自世界知名的 Springer 出版社，由脑转移瘤放射治疗领域的国际顶级专家 Yoshiya Yamada、Eric Chang、John B. Fiveash 和 Jonathan Knisely 博士共同编写。著者采用个案分析的形式，从放射肿瘤学家的视角系统解读了脑转移瘤的现代治疗模式。各章均从临床病例出发，详细阐明了相关临床知识点，章末则对本章的关键要点进行了归纳，同时对未来的发展趋势予以展望。本书内容实用、图文并茂，非常适合脑转移瘤多学科诊疗团队的医生阅读参考。

主要译者简介

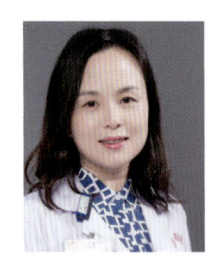

周蓉蓉
- 主任医师,二级教授,博士研究生导师。中南大学湘雅医院肿瘤放射治疗科主任兼肿瘤科副主任,湘雅医院脑转移癌疑难病会诊团队组长。
- 中国毒理学会特种医学毒理专业委员会副主任委员,湖南省医学会放射肿瘤学专业委员会副主任委员,湖南省抗癌协会脑转移癌专业委员会副主任委员。

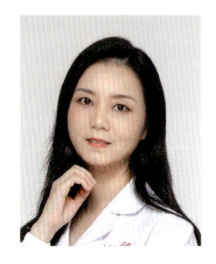

周 琴
- 副主任医师,中南大学湘雅医院肿瘤科。
- 中华医学会放射肿瘤学专业委员会青年委员,中国医师协会放疗分会头颈学组委员,湖南省抗癌协会脑转移癌转移委员会秘书,湖南省医学会放射肿瘤学专业委员会秘书。

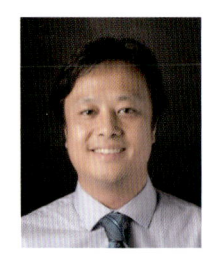

伍海军
- 副主任医师,硕士研究生导师,美国 MD Anderson 癌症中心访问学者,中南大学湘雅医院肿瘤科教研室副主任,头颈病房负责人。
- 中华医学会放射肿瘤治疗学分会头颈肿瘤学组委员,中华医学会放射肿瘤治疗学分会放射生物学组委员,中国临床肿瘤学会(CSCO)头颈肿瘤专家委员会委员。

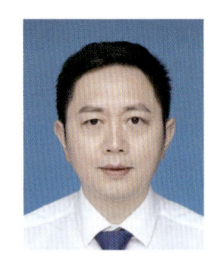

杨 振
- 副教授,中南大学湘雅医院首席放疗物理师,湘雅医院肿瘤放疗技术中心主任。
- 中华医学会医学工程学分会青委,中国生物医学工程学会精确放疗分会物理学组常委,湖南省放射肿瘤专业委员会物理学组副组长,湖南省医学会放射医学与防护专业委员会副主任委员。

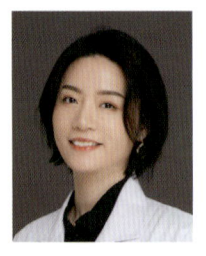

张莹莹
- 副主任医师,美国哈佛大学附属麻省总院博士后,日本大阪医科大学访问学者。
- 中国医师协会放射肿瘤治疗医师分会委员会放射生物免疫学组委员,中日医学科技交流协会肿瘤粒子治疗技术专业委员会副秘书长,湖南省抗癌协会肺癌专业委员会委员会委员,湖南省医学会放射肿瘤治疗委员会胸部肿瘤学组副组长。

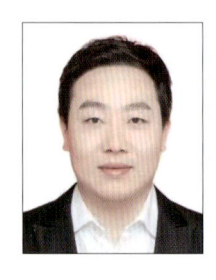

张子健
- 美国 MD Anderson 癌症中心访问学者,中南大学湘雅医院肿瘤放疗中心资深物理师。
- 中国生物医学工程学会精确放疗技术委员会青年委员,中国医药教育协会放射肿瘤专业委员会学会秘书,湖南省医学会放射肿瘤专业委员会胸部肿瘤学组秘书。

中文版序

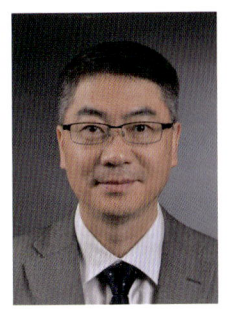

脑部是容易发生肿瘤转移的部位。在靶向药物问世前，传统的抗癌药物对脑转移瘤的治疗效果较差，除少数患者可进行手术治疗外，多数患者需要采用放射治疗。由于脑转移瘤的患者预后很差，加之人们对临床诊断和治疗方面重视不够，各学科交流合作较少，所以目前的处理流程较为粗放。各科医生面对脑转移瘤患者，往往习惯仅从自身学科角度去解决问题，导致患者需要辗转多个科室寻求诊疗。

随着神经肿瘤外科立体定向活检技术和组织病理、分子病理的进步，以及放射外科的发展，靶向药物和免疫检查点抑制药等多种治疗方式的出现，脑转移瘤的诊断和治疗呈现出多学科、综合性和精细化的特征，并且需要多个学科通力合作，因此多学科合作的机制和模式应运而生，脑转移瘤的疗效也显著改善。

湘雅医院脑转移瘤多学科诊疗团队（multi-disciplinary team，MDT）是由来自肿瘤放疗科、肿瘤内科、神经外科、神经内科、病理科、影像科、呼吸科等多个科室组成的诊疗团队，针对同一疾病，采取每周定期会诊的形式，为患者提供最佳的临床路径和治疗方案。这一模式不仅明显缩短了患者就医和等候时间，而且提高了脑转移瘤的诊疗水平。周蓉蓉教授牵头成立的湘雅医院脑转移瘤多学科诊疗团队在高质量临床工作的基础上，开展了高水平的研究和教学工作，成效显著，已成为在国内外影响力较大的脑转移瘤医教研中心。

周教授牵头翻译的这部专著，是在介绍现代脑转移瘤综合诊疗模式的基础上，重点聚焦立体定向放射外科，采用新颖实用的病例教学法，分析和阐明了放射外科在脑转移瘤综合治疗模式中的地位、作用和使用方法。放射外科（尤其是伽马刀）在进入我国的早期阶段，曾引起一些争议；在实际应用中，也存在一些需要澄清的问题；这些问题在本书中都可以找到答案。我深信本书的出版发行，一定会提高我国脑转移瘤放射外科治疗的技术水平和规范化程度，为医者解惑，使患者受益。

中山大学肿瘤防治中心放疗科

原书序

伽利略和米开朗基罗、希波克拉底和披头士乐队,既有科学,又有艺术。当艺术家与科学家的身份交叠,就是最完美的组合,而本书亦如是。著者将科学和艺术交融在一起,聚焦在当今发展最快的肿瘤学领域——脑转移瘤,话题本身已经超越了任何一种类型的癌症。

过去,人们对这一领域缺乏足够的认知,导致脑转移瘤患者预后非常差。而如今,临床医生已经认识到脑转移瘤异质性明显,使得治疗模式不再局限于针对脑转移灶的局部控制,而是通过排兵布阵来调整全身治疗和局部治疗的顺序和强度。"吹尽狂沙始到金",随着对治疗主线的逐步厘清,我们看到了破晓后的曙光。

这部著作非常全面,每一章都以病例为基础来展示内容,不仅为读者提供了最好的实践指南和管理策略,而且还对这一新兴领域未来的发展趋势进行了指引。本书著者是脑转移瘤放射治疗领域的国际知名专家,在此衷心祝贺这部著作的出版发行。我很荣幸为本书作序,我深信,该领域的医学生会发现本书将成为未来医学岁月中最精髓的参考资料。

Paul W. Sperduto, MD, MPP, FASTRO
Minneapolis, MN, USA

译者前言

2020年年末，当中国科学技术出版社第一次询问是否愿意翻译本书时，笔者注意到为本书原著作序的Paul W. Sperduto博士及原著者Yoshiya Yamada、Eric Chang、John B. Fiveash、Jonathan Knisely博士，他们都是国际脑转移瘤放射治疗领域的顶级专家。翻阅书中具体内容，发现著者采用个案分析方法，从放射肿瘤学家的角度来解读脑转移瘤的现代治疗模式。各章均从临床病例出发阐明相关临床知识点，各章末尾还对关键要点进行了归纳，对这个新兴领域未来的发展趋势进行了指引。笔者认为这些对国内放射治疗医师有非常实用的参考价值，联想此前我们刚申请的中南大学研究生教学案例库"脑转移癌MDT教学案例库"建设项目，与本书有异曲同工之处，于是欣然接受了中国科学技术出版社的翻译邀请。

放射治疗应用于脑转移瘤的历史非常悠久，即使是多发脑转移瘤，放射治疗仍旧是一种能够改善生活质量、精准有效的治疗方式。即使靶向治疗等系统性治疗的开启逐渐改变了部分脑转移瘤患者的治疗模式；然而，不管是全脑放射治疗还是不同分割模式的立体定向放射外科治疗，仍然是脑转移瘤最重要的辅助治疗手段。选择哪种放射治疗方式，如何才能更好地将其与系统性治疗结合起来是我们一直在探索的问题。根据脑转移瘤多年的诊治经验来看，许多在日常工作中常被提及的问题都能在书中找到答案。本书从一个个看似简单的病例分析出发，结合预后模型、影像学特点及循证医学证据等，站在放射肿瘤学家的视角，以放射治疗为中心，从临床应用和放疗技术等多方面，深入浅出地阐述了脑转移瘤的综合治疗模式，并围绕各章论点抽丝剥茧展开论述，提炼出各章关键要点，指导性和实用性强。

本书译者均为中南大学湘雅医院肿瘤科长期从事临床一线工作的医师和物理师，而且大部分译者都在国外著名肿瘤医院进行过为期1~2年的放射治疗进修，他们在充实的临床工作之余，辛苦编译，为本书早日与广大读者见面付出了巨大的努力和辛勤的汗水。同时，河北医科大学第四医院放疗科王军教授和耶鲁大学医学院光发达物理师对本书翻译内容给予了积极的建议和指导，我院放射科李浪教授、孟莉教授也对书中的部分专业词汇给予了指正，在此一并表示衷心的感谢。

由于书中所述内容并非译者亲身体验，加之中外语言表达习惯有所差别，虽然翻译过程中我们反复斟酌以求尽可能表达出原著者的本意，但中文译本中仍可能存在一些疏漏之处，望各位读者和同道们不吝赐教！

中南大学湘雅医院肿瘤科 周菁

原书前言

如果有人问"放射肿瘤学最有效的治疗方法是什么？"答案很可能是立体定向放射外科治疗。如果通过权衡潜在的获益和危害来评估一种治疗脑转移瘤的方法，毫无疑问，立体定向放射外科治疗是最有效安全的选择。

如果脑转移瘤无法得到控制，往往会带来非常严重的后果。即使是多发脑转移瘤，放射外科治疗也是一种能够维持患者生活质量，最大限度减少神经认知功能下降风险、无痛、微创、精准有效的治疗方式。

图像引导的精准放射治疗时代已经来临，先进的神经成像技术和复杂精细的放射治疗计划系统地发展，使适形放射治疗与图像引导技术相互结合，成为一个强大且安全有效地解决临床复杂问题的工具。随着放射治疗技术的发展和我们对脑转移性疾病生物学的深入理解，放射外科治疗将继续适应现代综合治疗模式，成为包括靶向治疗和免疫检查点抑制药治疗等系统性治疗的重要辅助治疗手段。

本书实用性强，采用个案分析方法，从放射肿瘤学家的角度来解读脑转移瘤的现代治疗模式。每章均从临床病例出发阐明相关临床知识点，各章末尾均对关键要点进行了归纳。

最后，我们还要将本书献给我们的家人，没有他们的支持，就没有这本书的出版。

Eric Chang
Los Angeles, CA, USA

John B. Fiveash
Birmingham, AL, USA

Jonathan Knisely & Yoshiya Yamada
New York, NY, USA

目 录

绪 篇

第 1 章 脑转移瘤的临床概况 ··· 002

临床篇 脑转移瘤

第 2 章 脑转移瘤概述 ··· 006
 一、病例介绍 ·· 006
 二、流行病学 ·· 007
 三、病理生理学 ··· 008
 四、临床特征 ·· 008
 五、诊断 ·· 009
 六、预后因素 ·· 010
 七、展望和未来 ··· 013
 八、结论 ·· 015

第 3 章 立体定向放射外科的放射生物学 ··· 018
 一、立体定向放射外科中的放射生物学 ··· 018
 二、SBRT 对于微血管的影响 ·· 018
 三、立体定向放射治疗的免疫调节作用 ··· 020
 四、放射治疗反应的生物学基础及其在立体定向放射外科的适用性：4R 理论 ···· 022
 五、细胞周期再分布或重排列 ··· 023
 六、再氧合 ··· 023
 七、再增殖 ··· 023
 八、亚致死损伤修复 ··· 024
 九、结论 ·· 024

第 4 章 脑转移瘤患者及其治疗并发症的对症支持处理 ······································· 027
 一、临床关注 ·· 027
 二、循证基础 ·· 028
 三、脑水肿：对于 VEGF 通路的抑制 ·· 030
 四、脑水肿：实验性治疗策略 ··· 031
 五、治疗后放射性脑坏死 ··· 033

i

六、放射性脑坏死的临床管理 033
　　七、癫痫发作 035
　　八、抗癫痫药物概述 035
　　九、头痛 037
　　十、认知障碍 038
　　十一、不确定的领域和未来发展方向 038
　　十二、结论与建议 039
　　十三、病例介绍 040

第 5 章　脑转移瘤的神经影像学诊断 046
　　一、大脑成像概述 046
　　二、神经解剖学 046
　　三、脑转移瘤成像 051
　　四、特殊情况 052
　　五、结论 054

第 6 章　手术和放射外科联合治疗的进展 056
　　一、病例介绍 056
　　二、概述 059
　　三、循证基础 060
　　四、诊断和治疗 064
　　五、争议及未来发展方向 068

第 7 章　激光间质热疗在脑转移瘤中的应用 073
　　一、病例介绍 073
　　二、概述 074
　　三、手术中的应用 077
　　四、诊断与治疗 078
　　五、循证基础 078
　　六、LITT 治疗脑转移瘤的不确定领域 078
　　七、LITT 的并发症 079

第 8 章　脑转移瘤的系统性治疗 082
　　一、概述 082
　　二、循证基础 082
　　三、研究概述 082
　　四、细胞毒性药物 083
　　五、分子靶向药物 084
　　六、病例介绍 085
　　七、不确定的领域和未来的方向 088

八、结论与建议 090

第 9 章 立体定向放射外科治疗多发脑转移瘤的指征 094
一、病例介绍 094
二、概述 095
三、循证基础 095
四、诊断 103
五、管理和指导方针 104
六、不确定领域及未来研究方向 106
七、结论与建议 107
八、未来发展方向 107

第 10 章 脑转移瘤的大分割立体定向放射外科治疗 110
一、概述 110
二、单次放射外科治疗的局限性 110
三、大分割的放射生物学及理论基础 111
四、大分割 SRS 的临床经验 112
五、最佳大分割 SRS 方案 112
六、大病灶的手术适应证（对比放射外科治疗） 116
七、结论与展望 116
八、病例介绍 117

第 11 章 脑转移放射外科治疗（含术后瘤腔）的靶区勾画 124
一、病例介绍 124
二、概述 124
三、脑转移 CT 及 MRI 影像学特点 125
四、BM 管理的进展 127
五、SRS 的患者选择 129
六、患者体位固定 129
七、模拟及必要的预处理成像 130
八、有 MRI 禁忌证的情况 131
九、BM 的靶区勾画（GTV、CTV） 132
十、OAR 的勾画 135
十一、并发症及缓解策略 136
十二、随访 138
十三、不确定性领域 138
十四、现行指南 138

第 12 章 全脑放疗的指征 143
一、病例介绍 143

二、概述 143
三、患者选择 144
四、全脑放疗的分割方式 146
五、术后全脑放疗 146
六、全脑放疗后的再程放疗 147
七、立体定向外科治疗后的挽救性全脑放疗 148
八、软脑膜病变 148
九、预防性头部放疗 149
十、1～3 个脑转移瘤：WBRT ± SRS 150
十一、1～4 个脑转移瘤：SRS ± WBRT 150
十二、未来研究方向：4 个以上的脑转移瘤 151
十三、具有中枢神经系统活性的系统治疗在脑转移中的作用 152
十四、神经毒性和避免照射海马的全脑放疗（HA-WBRT） 153

第 13 章 粒子治疗在脑转移瘤治疗中的应用 161
一、病例介绍 161
二、质子的基本特点 162
三、质子立体定向放射外科技术 165
四、剂量学注意事项 166
五、临床应用 167
六、重离子 SRS 在脑转移瘤中的应用 167
七、讨论 167

第 14 章 特殊类型脑转移瘤的治疗 172
一、颅底转移瘤 172
二、脉络膜转移瘤 174
三、脑干转移瘤 178
四、硬脑膜转移瘤 181
五、软脑膜病 183

第 15 章 补救治疗 / 再放疗 / 再治疗 188
一、病例介绍 188
二、概述 189
三、循证基础 190
四、诊断与治疗 191
五、治疗的不确定性 193
六、未来研究方向 193
七、治疗指南 194
八、结论与建议 195

技术篇　治疗计划与实施技术

第 16 章　常用的放射外科技术 ··········· 198
 一、病例介绍 ··········· 198
 二、主要技术概述 ··········· 198
 三、循证基础 ··········· 201
 四、治疗计划考量 ··········· 201
 五、小野剂量学 ··········· 204
 六、定位精度 ··········· 205
 七、不确定性领域和发展趋势 ··········· 207
 八、指南 ··········· 209

第 17 章　多发性脑转移瘤的单中心治疗计划 ··········· 213
 一、多发性脑转移瘤治疗的研究背景及历史 ··········· 213
 二、多发性脑转移瘤的单中心治疗技术 ··········· 213
 三、IMRS ··········· 219
 四、VMAT ··········· 219
 五、VMAT 计划中其他该考虑的情况 ··········· 221
 六、单中心动态适形弧计划 ··········· 222
 七、多发性转移瘤自动治疗计划方案 ··········· 224
 八、病例介绍 ··········· 227

第 18 章　脑转移瘤治疗中的耐受剂量 ··········· 241
 一、概述 ··········· 241
 二、循证基础 ··········· 242
 三、中枢神经系统的正常组织剂量限制 ··········· 242
 四、全身系统治疗联合脑照射 ··········· 245
 五、再程照射 ··········· 246
 六、不确定性领域 ··········· 246
 七、结论与建议 ··········· 247
 八、病例介绍 ··········· 248

第 19 章　放射外科计划的质量评估 ··········· 255
 一、背景 ··········· 255
 二、剂量 – 体积度量 ··········· 255
 三、病例介绍 ··········· 262
 四、建议 ··········· 264

第 20 章　无头架放射外科的图像引导技术（包括体表成像） ··········· 267
 一、病例介绍 ··········· 267

二、背景和动机 ··· 268

三、图像引导无头架式放射治疗 ··· 269

四、图像引导放射治疗中的几何不确定性 ··· 272

五、员工培训和资格认证 ·· 274

六、建议和未来展望 ·· 274

第 21 章　放射外科治疗的安全程序和检查清单 ·· 277

一、概述 ··· 277

二、减少风险的概念 ·· 278

三、病例介绍 ··· 280

四、主要建议 ··· 283

五、未来及展望 ··· 285

第 22 章　小野放疗的质量保证 ·· 288

一、概述 ··· 288

二、相对剂量学 ··· 289

三、探测器类型 ··· 290

四、病例介绍 ··· 292

五、特定患者的质量保证 ·· 294

六、未来及展望 ··· 295

第 23 章　保护海马的全脑放疗技术 ·· 297

一、病例介绍 ··· 297

二、概述 ··· 298

三、早期探索 ··· 298

四、WBRT 临床实验评估 ·· 299

五、技术、剂量及分次数的演变 ··· 299

六、当代 WBRT 实践 ··· 301

七、危及器官的保护 ·· 306

八、不确定性问题及展望 ·· 310

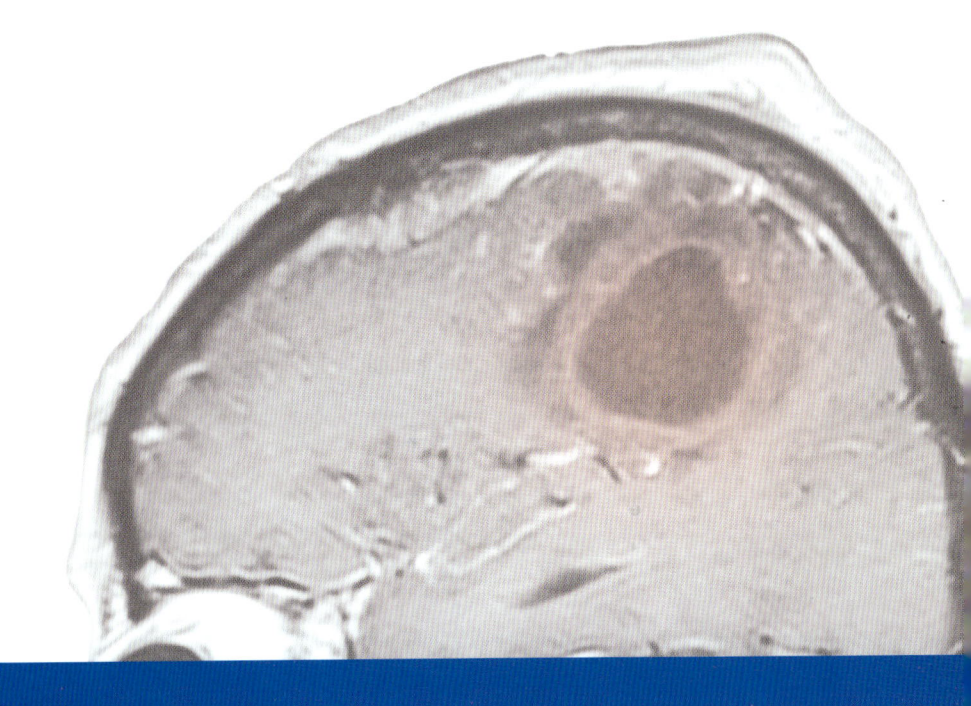

绪 篇
Overview

第 1 章　脑转移瘤的临床概况 ………………………………………………… 002

第 1 章 脑转移瘤的临床概况
Introduction

Eric Chang　John B.Fiveash　Jonathan Knisely　Yoshiya Yamada　著
周　琴　译
张莹莹　校

毫无疑问，医疗技术的进步以及对疾病生物学认知的增加已经改变了目前脑转移瘤的治疗模式。即使合并脑转移，Ⅳ期癌症患者经过系统治疗仍可获得长期生存。目前脑转移瘤管理的基本原则是通过对治疗的排兵布阵使肿瘤得到良好控制的同时把对生活质量的影响降到最低。

从词的来源上讲，"stereotactic"一词来源于希腊语"stereos"，意思是立体的，而拉丁语中"tactic"的意思是触摸。17世纪，伟大的法国数学家勒内·笛卡尔奠定了立体定向放射外科的数学基础，促进了笛卡尔几何学的发展。基于此，大脑内肿瘤可以被精准地绘制出来。

1908 年，笛卡尔几何坐标系作为 Horsley-Clarke 仪器工作的基础首次被提出。这篇开创性的论文描述了一种用来固定电极并且根据笛卡尔坐标明确病变位置进行电刺激或者消融治疗的装置。他们创造了短语"立体定向"[1]。Robert H Clarke，英国神经生理学家和解剖学家，首次提出将笛卡尔几何坐标应用于大脑；Sir Victor Horsley，一位杰出的外科医生和神经生理学家，首次在术中使用电刺激来发现人类癫痫灶（图 1-1）。1905 年，第一个 Horsley-Clarke 装置在伦敦面世，其组成成分为黄铜，通过将其连接到猫和猴子的头骨探测和绘制大脑结构。1918 年，加拿大麦吉尔大学（McGill University）的神经解剖学家 Abrey Mussen 改良了 Horsley-Clarke 装置，制造出第一个能在人体应用的立体定向装置。他的同事 Clarke 提出镭可以立体定向植入脑肿瘤并发挥治疗作用[2]。不同版本的固定框架被神经生理学家和解剖学家用来制作猴子和其他哺乳动物的大脑图谱。20 世纪 30 年代，立体定向脑电图和诱发电位的研究实现了里程碑式的突破并展示出其应用前景[3]。1933 年，德国外科医生马丁·科施纳（Martin Kirschner），急诊医学的先驱者，首次将该设备用于人体。"K"丝也被描述为一种立体定向的方法，以定向电凝三叉神经节来治疗三叉神经痛的患者[4]。1947 年，Spiegel 和 Wycisto 也描述了一种类似的设备，将脑电图摄影术与局部定位系统结合，制作癫痫患者的脑电图，这是第一个图像引导的神经导航在人类中的应用尝试。Lars Leksell，伽马刀放射外科之父，开发了一种用钉子固定在颅骨上的弧形电极载体，该电弧的位置是可调的，电极指向感兴趣的目标，无须考虑入射角度，将弧形的旋转中心放置在目标内即可[5]。1948 年，立体定向瘤内注射放射性磷的装置首次用于治疗颅咽管瘤。他继续采用立体定向的方式，使用高能质子束进行动物实验[6]。由于利用同步回旋加速器生产高能质子束的技术烦琐，Leksell 决定用 ^{60}Co 作为辐射源，并于 1967 年在卡罗林斯卡学院首次投入使用。该设备的初衷是提供高精准度高剂量的辐射以无创的方式治疗病变。例如原本需采用丘脑切除术治疗的帕金森病，通过这种治疗可以避免手术及其并发症。第一代装置的成功促进了第二代装置的研发，179 个 ^{60}Co 放射源以近似半圆顶状进行排列，全部瞄准一个中心点，在中心点产生球形损毁病变。于是，一种名为"伽马刀"配有 201 个放射源的新型机器开始在全世界普及，现在全世界每年有 7 万多患者接受伽马刀放射外科治疗。

Godfrey Hounsfield，计算机断层扫描（computed Tomography，CT）之父，率先在人脑标本上进行 CT 扫描。1971 年 10 月，首次在患者身体上使用 CT 来诊断右额叶囊肿[7]。CT 扫描可以在三维空间中成像和记录，直接提供脑肿瘤的确切位置，从而淘汰了脑电图摄影，同时开创了立体定向放射外科作为神经肿瘤一种治疗工具的新时代。CT 成像还提供了精确辐射剂量计算所需的电子密度图，从而通过附着在颅骨上的基准框架使用立体定位进行精确放射治疗，并在 CT 定义的空间内进行高度精确的剂量计算。磁共振成像的引入进一步提高了准确识别和勾画大脑内肿瘤的能力，并迅速被纳入立体定向放射外科的工作流程。

在伽马刀快速发展的同时，直线加速器也得到了发展。加速电子束打击钨合金等致密靶产生的 X 线可以形成单一辐射束，并能从任何角度准确地靶向中心点。1953 年，直线加速器在伦敦 Hammersmith 医院首次用于治疗患者[8]。神经外科医生 Osvaldo Betti 和工程师 Victor Derechinsky 对用于放射外科的直线加速器进行了改良，并在

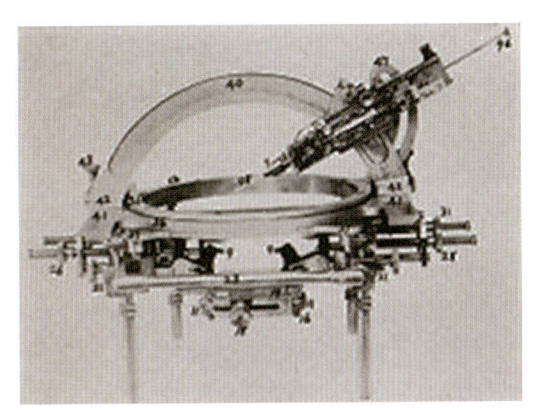

版图三十

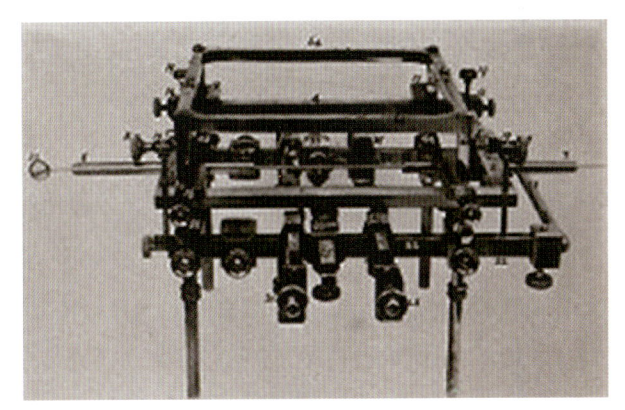

版图三十二

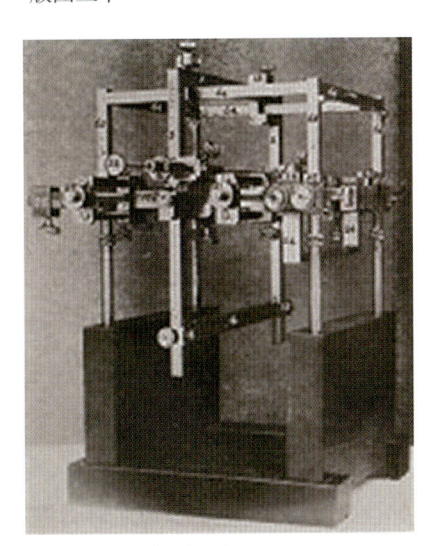

版图三十一

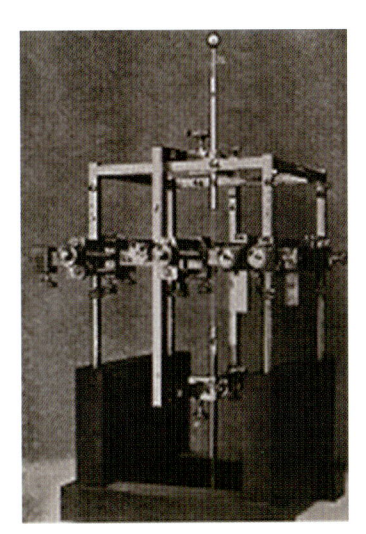

版图三十三

▲ 图 1-1 **Horsley–Clarke** 框架照片
经许可转载，引自 Pereira 等[14]

1982年治疗了第一位患者[9]。20世纪80年代后期，盖恩斯维尔、蒙特利尔、波士顿和海德堡的研究中心开始发表他们的初步经验。到20世纪90年代，能达到必需精度的机械实现了商业化，直线加速器立体定向放射外科得到广泛应用。原始系统使用不同直径的圆柱形准直器来产生球形靶区，使靶区在三维方向接近肿瘤形状。在20世纪90年代中期，更先进的微型多叶准直器问世，它是一种装在辐射束路径上的装置，可使辐射束精确地适形肿瘤的轮廓，而不是依赖多球体云去接近肿瘤的三维特征[10]。这个装置后来被用来调整治疗区域内的辐射强度，并获得更好的适形度。斯坦福大学的神经外科医生John Adler开发了一种便携式直线加速器装置，安装在机器人手臂上，使用正交X线成像而不是等中心的方式来引导脑肿瘤的治疗。这种便携式直线加速器最终发展成为射波（Cyber）刀，并在2001年获得了FDA的批准。

认识到固定颅骨对于放射外科安全和精度的重要性，神经外科医生应用立体定向框架固定颅骨，并作为立体定向导航的坐标参考系统。1986年，首次提出了一种以颅骨作为基准参考的无框架模式来实施放射外科治疗[11]。在20世纪90年代早期，X线立体摄影测量技术或正交千伏级定位系统被引入，提供基于X线影像的立体显示法来帮助验证放射外科的定位[12]。2003年，Yenice等在立体定向放射外科治疗中，使用CT成像提供容积数据[13]。容积图像引导的立体定向放射外科，或无框放射外科，目前在伽马刀或直线加速器的平台应用。

虽然立体定向放射外科起源于17世纪，但它通过不断的技术创新发展成为当今最有效、最安全的癌症治疗方法之一。以下章节将以病例为基础，介绍21世纪立体定向放射外科和其他形式的放射治疗方法在脑转移治疗中的应用。这本书为大家提供来自放射治疗领域公认的顶级专家最为实用的指导。我们真诚地感谢他们愿意奉献和牺牲自己的时间来分享他们的专业知识。没有他们，就没有这本书。

参考文献

[1] Horsley V, Clarke RH. The structure and functions of the cerebellum examined by a new method. Brain. 1908;31(1):45–124.

[2] Jensen RL, Stone JL, Hayne RA. Introduction of the human Horsley-Clarke stereotactic frame. Neurosurgery. 1996;38:563–7.

[3] Gerard RW, Marshall WH, Saul IJ. Electrical activity of the cat's brain. Arch Neurol Psychiatr. 1936;36:675–738.

[4] Dick W. Martin Kirschner: 1879–1942—a surgeon in prehospital care. Resuscitation. 2006;68(3):319–21.

[5] Gildenberg P. The history of stereotactic neurosurgery. Neurosurg Clin N Am. 1990;1:765–80.

[6] Lozano AL, Gildenberg PL, Tasker RR. Textbook of stereotactic functional neurosurgery. 2nd ed. Berlin Heidelberg: Springer-Verlag; 2009. p. 67.

[7] Beckmann EC. CT scanning the early days. Br J Radiol. 2006;79(937):5–8.

[8] Thwaites DI, Tuohy JB. Back to the future: the history and development of the clinical linear accelerator. Phys Med Biol. 2006;51:R343–62.

[9] Betti OO, Derechinsky YE. Irradiations stereotaxiques multifaisceaux. Neurochirurgie. 1982;28:55–6.

[10] Schlegel W, Pastry O, Bortfeld T, et al. Computer systems and mechanical tools for stereotactically guided conformation therapy with linear accelerators. Int J Radiat Oncol Biol Phys. 1992;24:781–7.

[11] Roberts DW, Strohbehn JW, Hatch JF, et al. A frameless stereotaxic integration of computerized tomographic imaging and the operating microscope. J Neurosurg. 1986;64:545–9.

[12] Selvik G. Roentgen stereophotogrammetric analysis. Acta Radiol. 1990;31:113–26.

[13] Yenice KM, Lovelock DM, Hunt MA, et al. CT image-guided intensity modulated therapy for paraspinal tumors using stereotactic immobilization. Int J Radiat Oncol Biol Phys. 2003;55:583–93.

[14] Pereira EAC, Green AL, Nandi D, Aziz TZ. History of stereotactic surgery in Great Britain. In: Lozano AL, Gildenberg PL, Tasker RR, editors. Textbook of stereotactic functional neurosurgery. 2nd ed. Berlin Heidelberg: Springer-Verlag; 2009. p. 67.

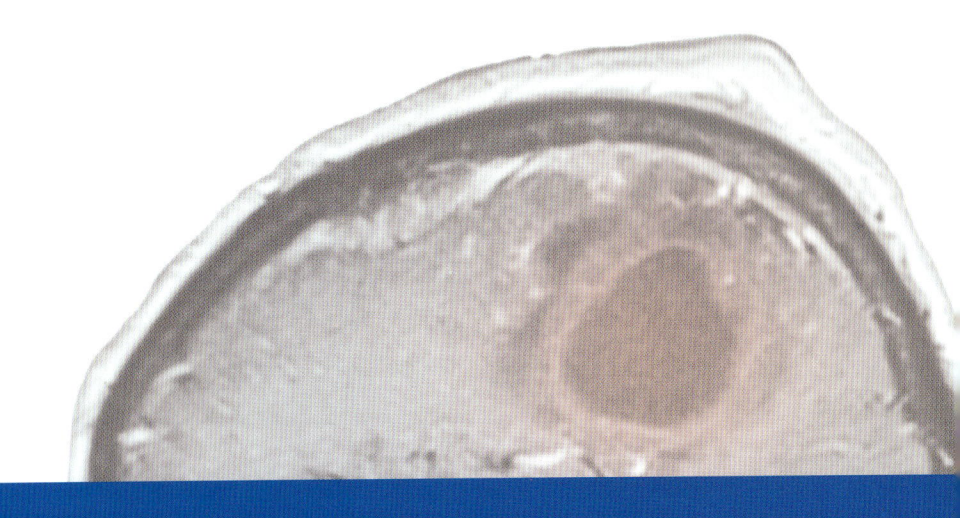

临床篇
脑转移瘤
Clinical Overview : Brain Metastases

第 2 章	脑转移瘤概述	006
第 3 章	立体定向放射外科的放射生物学	018
第 4 章	脑转移瘤患者及其治疗并发症的对症支持处理	027
第 5 章	脑转移瘤的神经影像学诊断	046
第 6 章	手术和放射外科联合治疗的进展	056
第 7 章	激光间质热疗在脑转移瘤中的应用	073
第 8 章	脑转移瘤的系统性治疗	082
第 9 章	立体定向放射外科治疗多发脑转移瘤的指征	094
第 10 章	脑转移瘤的大分割立体定向放射外科治疗	110
第 11 章	脑转移放射外科治疗（含术后瘤腔）的靶区勾画	124
第 12 章	全脑放疗的指征	143
第 13 章	粒子治疗在脑转移瘤治疗中的应用	161
第 14 章	特殊类型脑转移瘤的治疗	172
第 15 章	补救治疗 / 再放疗 / 再治疗	188

第 2 章 脑转移瘤概述
Brain Metastases: Introduction

Mihir Naik Joycelin F. Canavan Samuel T. Chao 著
段和新 译
张莹莹 校

一、病例介绍

患者，女，54 岁，既往有左侧乳腺癌病史，初诊分期为 $T_{1c}N_2M_0$，在乳腺癌治疗 4 年后出现头晕和步态不稳。其原发灶组织病理检测雌激素受体（estrogen receptor，ER）表达阳性，孕激素受体（progesterone receptor，PR）表达阳性，人表皮生长因子受体 2（human epidermal receptor-2，HER2）基因扩增。当时接受了化疗，乳腺癌改良根治术和重建，以及术后胸壁放射治疗，此外还接受了 1 年的曲妥珠单抗靶向治疗。最初，头晕和步态不稳患者以为是高血压所致，后因症状逐渐加重至急诊室就诊。完善 CT 检查显示右侧小脑有较大的占位性肿块，磁共振（magnatic resonance imageing，MRI）检查如图 2-1 所示。随后患者接受颅内占位切除术，术后病理确认为转移性腺癌，但 ER、PR、TTF-1（thyroid transcription factor-1）均为阴性。复查 CT 未发现其他颅外病灶。

根据该患者最初的乳腺癌组织学结果，使用诊断 - 特异性分级预后评估系统（diagnosis-specific graded prognostic assessment，DS-GPA）预测的中位生存期为 25.3 个月。考虑到患者脑转移瘤病理的 ER、PR 表达均为阴性，中位生存期缩短至 15.1 个月。我们讨论了患者脑转移瘤切除术后的处理，是选择对术腔行立体定向放射治疗（stereotactic radiosurgery，SRS）还是全脑放射治疗（whole-brain radiation，WBRT）。患者选择接受 WBRT，放疗总剂量为 37.5Gy/15 次。放疗后患者出现了面部肿胀、浆液性耳炎、脱发等不良反应；除了轻度失衡、轻度间歇性疲劳、轻度短期记忆和识词困难外，没有严重的晚期后遗症。之后患者服用了阿那曲唑，脑转移治疗后 7 年，患者仍然存活且没有全身或颅内进展的证据。图 2-2 为 7 年后随访的 MRI。此时她仍然从事室内设计师的工作。

虽然患者出现脑转移瘤则预示着预后不良，

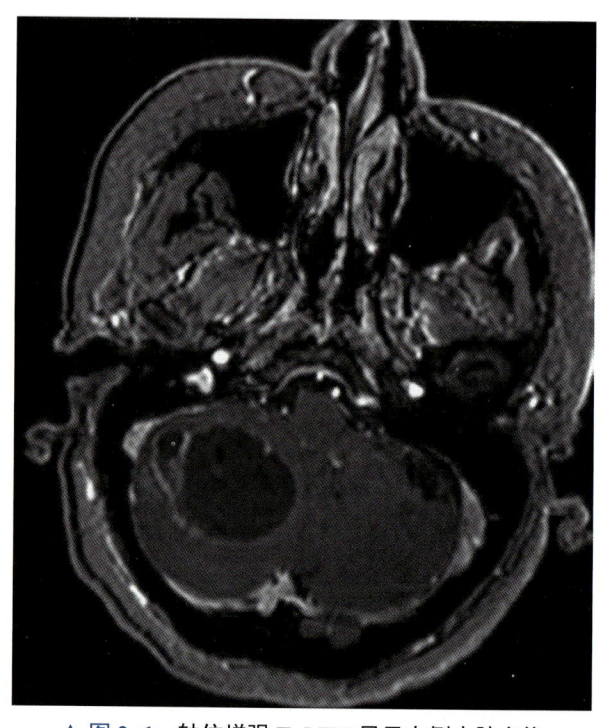

▲ 图 2-1 轴位增强 T_1 MRI 显示右侧小脑占位

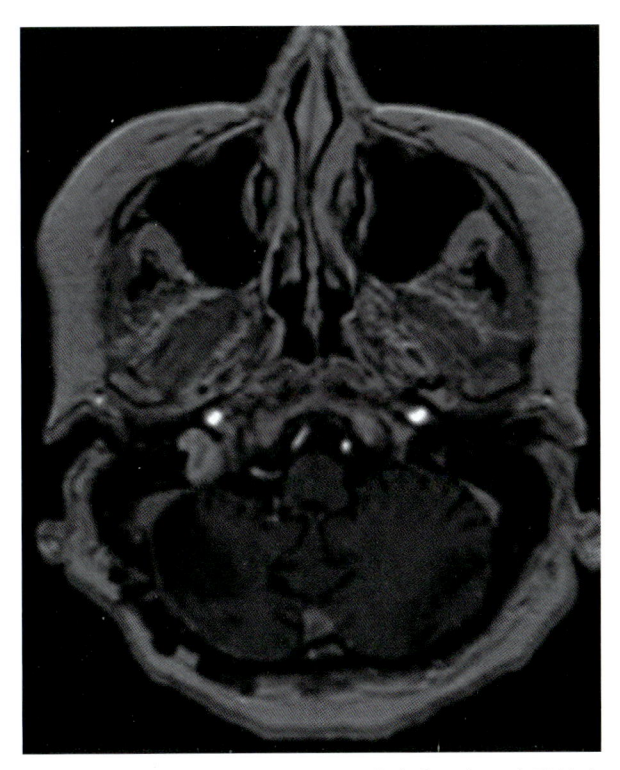

▲ 图 2-2 轴位增强 T_1 MRI 显示在患者开颅和全脑放疗后 7 年术腔病情稳定无复发

且 DS-GPA 预后模型也预测她的生存期最多为几年，但患者却长期存活。尽管这是一个特殊病例，但一般来讲，预后模型能帮助预测哪些患者预后较好，哪些患者可能预后较差，从而协助指导治疗。本章将回顾脑转移瘤的流行病学和预后模型。

二、流行病学

脑转移瘤是成人最常见的颅内肿瘤，大多数是在已知原发灶或转移病灶的情况下发生。在实体瘤患者中，10%~30% 的成人和 3%~13% 的儿童会发生脑转移[1-4]。

由于 MRI 技术不断进步，颅内小的转移瘤可以早期诊断；同时随着系统治疗疗效的提高，颅外疾病得到了更好的控制，因而脑转移瘤的发病率可能会增加[3, 4]。

据估计，脑转移瘤的发病率为（7~14）/10 万，但这个数据来自于基于人群发病率的研究，而这些研究通常低估了真实的发病情况[5]。

危险因素

在成人中，最常导致脑转移的原发肿瘤包括肺癌、乳腺癌、肾癌、结肠直肠癌和黑色素瘤[4]。在儿童中，脑转移瘤最常来源于肉瘤、神经母细胞瘤和生殖细胞肿瘤[3, 6, 7]。

1. 肺癌

肺癌是导致脑转移最常见的原发恶性肿瘤，腺癌占所有脑转移瘤患者的 50% 以上[3, 8]。30%~43% 的患者仅发生脑转移，而没有其他部位受累的证据[9]。一项分析了 975 例 I 期或 II 期非小细胞肺癌（non-small-cell lung cancer，NSCLC）患者的研究发现，脑转移相关的危险因素与年龄较小、肿瘤体积较大、淋巴血管间隙受侵和肺门淋巴结受累相关[8]。

小细胞肺癌（small-cell lung cancer，SCLC）的特点是早期转移，脑是最常见的转移部位，2 年内累积发病率超过 50%[10]。初诊时，MRI 检查发现 15% 的患者存在无症状的脑转移[11]。通过预防性颅脑照射（prophylactic cranial irradiation，PCI），3 年后发生脑转移的风险可以从 59% 下降至 33%，并伴随着生存获益（21% vs. 15%）[10]。

2. 乳腺癌

在女性乳腺癌患者中，肺转移、激素受体阴性和 HER2 过表达患者的脑转移发生率特别高[12, 13]。一项研究显示约 30% 以肺转移为首发转移部位的患者随后发生了脑转移[12]。

另一项包含 1434 名接受保乳治疗加全身化疗的女性的队列研究中，不同乳腺癌亚型的 5 年累积脑转移发生率不同：Luminal A 型为 0.1%，Luminal B 型为 3.3%，Luminal HER2 型为 3.2%，HER2 型为 3.7%，三阴性/基底样亚型为 7.4%[14]。

接受曲妥珠单抗治疗的 IV 期乳腺癌患者中枢神经系统（central nervous system，CNS）转移发生率可高达 34%[15]。目前认为较高的 CNS 事件发生率可能与全身治疗疗效的提高带来的患者存活率增加以及曲妥珠单抗无法渗透到 CNS 有关[16]。

3. 肾细胞癌

复发的肾细胞癌患者中有 2%～10% 发生脑转移，80% 甚至更多的患者伴有脑转移临床症状[3]。肾细胞癌脑转移以伴有瘤内出血为特点。来自纪念斯隆 – 凯特琳癌症中心（Memorial Sloan-Kettering Cancer Center，MSKCC）神经外科的系列研究表明，46% 的肾细胞癌脑转移患者出现瘤内出血[17]。

4. 结直肠癌

有研究表明，转移性结直肠癌的脑转移发生率约为 2.3%[18]。颅内转移通常是晚期表现，绝大多数患者在其他部位（尤其是肺部）合并有转移[18]。尽管肿瘤大多转移到幕上区域，但仍有高达 40% 的患者发生小脑转移，其中 23% 的患者为孤立性的小脑转移[18]。

5. 黑色素瘤

黑色素瘤是脑转移的第三大常见原因，占所有脑转移病灶的 6%～11%[3]。头颈部皮肤黑色素瘤更容易发生脑转移[19]，并且常伴有瘤内出血[19, 20]，比例高达 40%。80% 的黑色素瘤脑转移瘤位于幕上，15% 位于幕下或软脑膜，5% 位于脑干[21]。

三、病理生理学

由于 CNS 缺乏淋巴引流，因此脑转移最常见的途径是血行播散[22]。转移灶通常位于灰/白质交界区域，此处血管的直径缩小，成为肿瘤细胞团块的捕获器[23, 24]。这种类型的扩散称为实质性脑转移，是脑转移最常见的表现。图 2-3 是轴位 MRI 显示的脑实质转移灶。转移灶的分布通常与大脑血供相一致[23]。

- 大脑半球约 80%。
- 小脑 15%。
- 脑干 5%。

脑转移也可能发生在硬脑膜（硬脑膜脑转移瘤）和软脑膜（软脑膜脑转移瘤）。软脑膜脑转移预后很差，治疗选择有限。图 2-4 和图 2-5 分别显示硬脑膜转移和软脑膜疾病患者的轴位 MR 图像。

四、临床特征

尽管出现神经症状或行为异常的任何癌症患者都应该怀疑脑转移，但其他多种原因也可导致上述症状。在一项对 800 多名癌症患者进行神经症状评估的分析中，只有 16% 的患者有脑转移[25]。

最常见的脑转移症状包括头痛（50%）、肢体乏力（40%）、精神状态改变（30%）、癫痫发作（15%）和共济失调（10%）。随着肿瘤的生长和周围水肿对附近结构产生的占位效应，这些症状往往会随着时间的推移而恶化[26]。症状通常在数天或数周内演变。与紧张性头痛相比，32% 的脑肿瘤患者弯腰时头痛更严重，40% 的患者出现恶心或呕吐。增加胸腔内压的动作，如咳嗽、打喷嚏或 Valsalva 动作（深吸气后屏气，再用力做呼气动作）也可能导致头痛恶化，转移瘤合并出血也可导致急性神经系统症状[26, 27]。

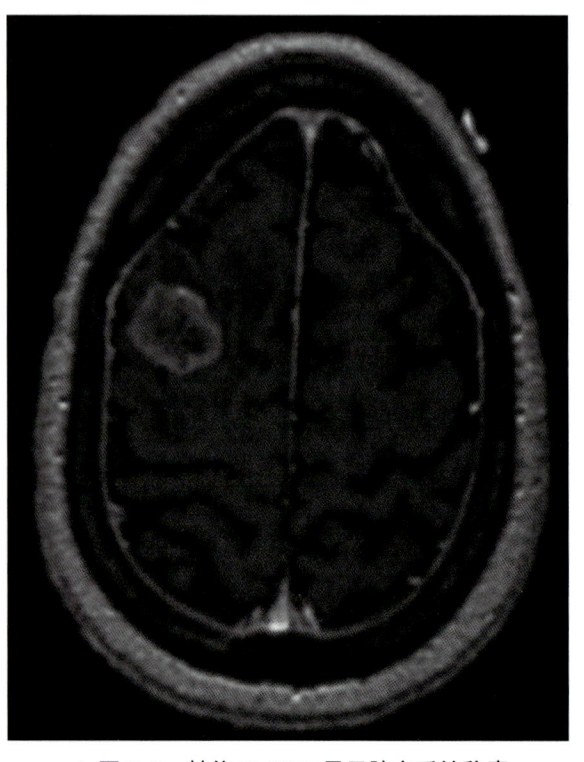

▲ 图 2-3　轴位 T_1 MRI 显示脑实质转移瘤

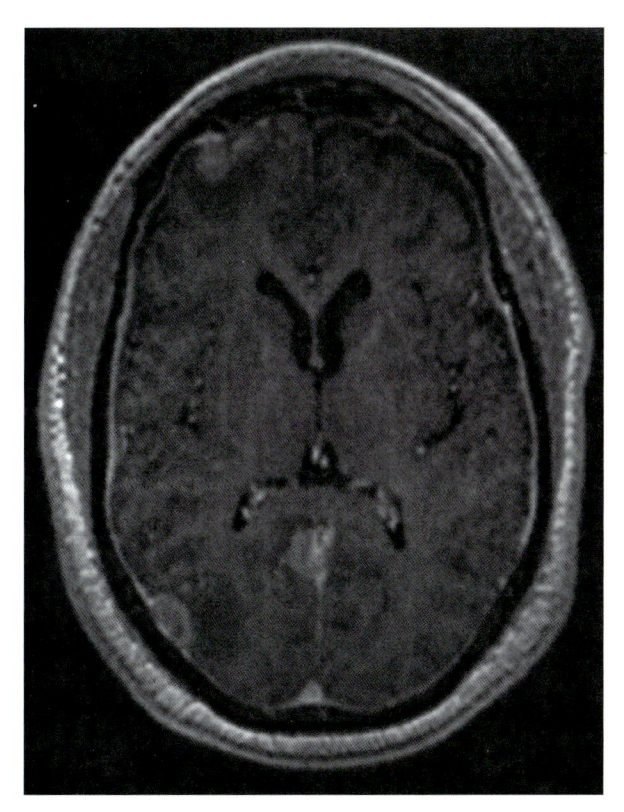

▲ 图 2-4 轴位 T₁ MRI 显示硬脑膜脑转移瘤

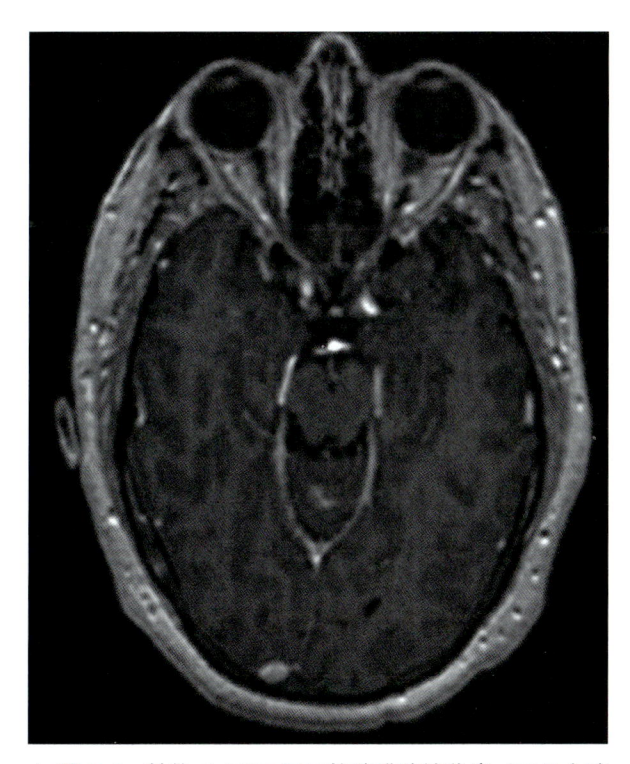

▲ 图 2-5 轴位 T₁ MRI 显示软脑膜脑转移瘤（可见小脑线性增强）

五、诊断

脑转移更常见于已确诊的恶性肿瘤患者。然而，高达 30% 的脑转移是在原发肿瘤发现的同时或之前被诊断出来的[28]。在出现急性神经系统症状时，颅脑 CT 通常被作为初筛方法，而钆增强 MRI 则是脑转移瘤的最佳检查手段。与平扫 CT 中的脑组织相比，转移瘤通常为等密度或低密度，并在增强扫描后强化[29]。急性出血可导致平扫 CT 检查信号增强[29]。但最常见的 CT 表现为实性或边缘强化，伴有中央囊性非强化区。囊性区域可能是由鳞癌中的角蛋白沉积、坏死或腺癌中的黏蛋白分泌所致[26]。

有助于区分脑转移瘤与其他 CNS 病变的影像学特征包括许多方面，如多发病变、病变位于灰质和白质交界处、边界清楚、环状强化伴显著的瘤周水肿[28]。

T₁ 平扫 MRI 图像可发现亚急性出血，表现为明显的高信号。黑色素、脂肪和蛋白质也可在非对比 T₁ 加权图像上显示高信号[29]。T₂ 加权序列可以检测出血或黑色素，表现为信号减低，有时也是黑色素瘤脑转移在 MRI 上看到的唯一异常信号[29]。T₂ 加权图像能更好地评估瘤周水肿，特别是液体衰减反转恢复（fluid-attenuated inversion recovery，FLAIR）序列，脑脊液信号被抑制，从而更好地显示脑室和脑沟附近的高信号。

磁敏感加权成像是一种高分辨率的梯度回波序列，能更好地发现出血和观察静脉结构，目前正在探索该技术识别脑肿瘤其他内部特征的能力[28, 29]。

当对脑转移的诊断有疑问时，应该进行组织活检进一步确认，特别是对于孤立性病灶。正电子发射断层扫描（positron emission tomography，PET）在这些患者中也可能有用，可以识别原发肿瘤或其他更容易活检的转移性病灶。先进的 MRI 序列，如弥散加权成像、灌注成像和磁共振波谱，也可以提供补充信息，有助于鉴别转移瘤与原发性脑瘤或其他非肿瘤性疾病，如脓肿、缺血和放射性坏死[28]。

六、预后因素

虽然脑转移瘤的发生很常见，但脑转移患者的预后存在很大的异质性。有研究者为临床医生和患者设计并改进了几种预后模型，以更好地了解患者预后，并帮助临床试验对患者进行选择和分层[30]。

脑转移患者的最早预后分析模型之一是递归分区分析（recursive partitioning analysis，RPA）。该研究回顾性分析了 1979—1993 年美国肿瘤放射治疗协作组织（radiation therapy oncology group，RTOG）开展的 3 个研究，包括 1200 例患者，使用卡诺夫斯基评分（Karnofsky performance status，KPS）、年龄、原发肿瘤的控制情况和是否存在颅外转移来预测总生存率（表 2-1）[31]。患者被分为三类：Ⅰ类包括 KPS 评分 ≥ 70 分、年龄 < 65 岁、原发肿瘤控制良好、无颅外转移（extracranial metastases，ECM）的患者；Ⅲ类包括 KPS 评分 < 70 分的患者；Ⅱ类包括除Ⅰ类、Ⅲ类外的其他患者。患者占比分别为 20%、65% 和 15%。值得注意的是，虽然纳入分析的研究对象没有包括 SCLC 患者，但随后的分析证实 RPA 在这类患者中依然有用[32]。但是，RPA 在预测预后方面仍存在一些局限性，包括对Ⅲ类患者的定义为所有 KPS < 70 分的患者，没有考虑到患者特征的不同，包括全身疾病的状态、脑转移瘤的数量和不同的组织学分类。

表 2-1 递归分区分析（RPA）系统

	RPA 分类标准
Ⅰ类	年龄 < 65 岁 KPS 评分 ≥ 70 分 原发肿瘤已控制 没有颅外转移
Ⅱ类	不属于Ⅰ类或Ⅲ类的所有患者
Ⅲ类	KPS 评分 < 70 分

经 Elsevier 许可转载，引自 Sperduto 等[37]

为了更好地了解 SRS 治疗脑转移瘤患者的预后因素，有研究者建立了放射外科评分指数（score index for radiosurgery，SIR）。SIR 是年龄、KPS、颅外疾病状态、脑转移瘤数量和脑转移瘤最大体积这 5 个预后因素得分的总和（总分 0～2 分）[33]。然而，评估全身性疾病所需的详细检查限制了该预测模型的广泛应用[34]。Lorenzoni 等发表了另一种预后模型，称为脑转移基本评分（basic score for brain metastases，BSBM），旨在简化评分系统。BSBM 只包括 3 个预后因素，即 KPS、原发肿瘤的控制情况和是否存在颅外转移病灶[35]。

然而，RPA、SIR 和 BSBM 在判断脑转移瘤预后方面有几个局限性，不能给出更简易和客观的预后判断。例如，RPA 和 BSBM 没有考虑转移的数量，而 RPA、BSBM 和 SIR 需要对全身疾病的控制进行评估，这种评估结果可能会不一致。此外，SIR 需要考虑放疗时最大病灶体积等治疗因素，这使得在做出任何治疗决定之前很难使用预后指标来预测结果。与此同时，旨在评估全脑放疗后接受 SRS 推量治疗的随机试验 RTOG 9508 的结果公布，脑转移瘤的数量对患者的生存有预测作用[36]。

因此，2008 年，Sperduto 等发表了一种称为分级预后评估（graded prognostic assessment，GPA）的新预后模型，该模型可以消除其他预后因素中的主观成分，如颅外疾病的控制，并考虑到转移灶的数量对脑转移瘤患者总生存期的预后影响[36, 37]。GPA 使用了来自五项随机试验 1960 名脑转移患者的数据，并发现 GPA 比其他模型更能预测预后。GPA 使用了影响脑转移瘤预后的四个因素，包括年龄、KPS、转移瘤数量和颅外转移情况。每个因素的得分为 0 分、0.5 分或 1.0 分，GPA 是根据四个因素的累积得分计算的。GPA 根据得分分为四个组，即 GPA 0～1 分，中位生存时间为 2.6 个月；GPA 1.5～2.5 分，中位生存时间为 3.8 个月；GPA 3.0 分，平均生存期为 6.9 个月；GPA 3.5～4.0 分，平均生存期为 11 个月。因主观性小，易于使用，GPA 成为临床实践中常用的预后模型（表 2-2）。

表 2-2 分级预后评估（GPA）系统

预后因素	GPA 评分标准		
	0	0.5	1.0
年龄（岁）	> 60	50～60	< 50
KPS 评分（分）	< 70	70～80	90～100
颅外转移	存在	—	不存在
脑转移瘤数量（个）	> 3	2～3	1

GPA 评分	中位生存期（个月）
0～1.0	2.6
1.5～2.5	3.8
3.0	6.9
3.5～4.0	11.0

经 Elsevier 许可转载，引自 Sperduto 等[37]

有研究者认为不同原发肿瘤预后不同，应该开发针对特定原发部位的预后模型[38]。一项纳入 11 个机构的患者进行的多中心回顾性研究观察了 1985—2007 年 4259 名接受脑转移治疗的患者，目的是确定疾病特异性预后因素[39]。研究成果促进了诊断特异性分级预后评估系统（diagnosis-specific graded prognostic assessment，DS-GPA）的发展（表 2-3 和表 2-4）。它表明总体存活率的预后因素也因原发病而不同。例如，NSCLC 和 SCLC 的预后因素包括 KPS 评分、年龄、颅外转移和脑转移瘤的数量。对于黑色素瘤和肾癌，有意义的预后因素则是 KPS 评分和脑转移瘤的数量。对于乳腺癌和胃肠癌，唯一重要的预后因素是 KPS 评分。

为了更好地预测不同原发肿瘤脑转移患者的预后，研究者们开展了进一步研究。如具有某些组织学亚型（如 HER2 扩增和 ER 阴性）的乳腺癌患者更容易发生脑转移[40-42]。虽然最初的 DS-GPA 只发现 KPS 评分是乳腺癌患者的预后因素，但通过分析包括 HER2 和 ER/PR 表达状态在内的更大样本的患者，形成了改良预测模型：乳腺癌特异性 GPA 指标（breast cancer-specific GPA Index，Breast-GPA）[43]。这项研究的重要意义在于发现乳腺癌的分子病理亚型对乳腺癌患者的预后有重要影响。三阴性（ER/PR 阴性和 HER2 阴性）乳腺癌患者的生存期最短，而 Luminal B 型

表 2-3 新诊断脑转移患者 DS-GPA 指标的定义

	预后因素	DS-GPA 评分标准				
		0	0.5	1.0		
非小细胞肺癌/小细胞肺癌	年龄（岁）	> 60	50～60	< 50	—	—
	KPS 评分（分）	< 70	70～80	90～100	—	—
	颅外转移	存在	—	不存在		
	脑转移瘤数量（个）	> 3	2～3	1		
		0	1	2		
黑色素瘤/肾细胞癌	KPS 评分（分）	< 70	70～80	90～100	—	—
	脑转移瘤数量（个）	> 3	2～3	1		
		0	1	2	3	4
乳腺癌/胃肠道癌	KPS 评分（分）	< 70	70	80	90	100

经 Elsevier 许可转载，引自 Sperduto 等[39]

表 2-4 新诊断脑转移患者按诊断和 DS-GPA 评分分层的中位生存期

诊断	DS-GPA 中位生存期（个月）			
	总体	0~1.0	1.5~2.5	3.0	3.5~4.0
非小细胞肺癌	7.0	3.0	6.5	11.3	14.8
小细胞肺癌	4.9	2.8	5.3	9.6	17.1
黑色素瘤	6.7	3.4	4.7	8.8	13.2
肾细胞癌	9.6	3.3	7.3	11.3	14.8
乳腺癌	11.9	6.1	9.4	16.9	18.7
胃肠道癌	5.4	3.1	4.4	6.9	13.5

经 Elsevier 许可转载，引自 Sperduto 等 [39]

表 2-5 女性乳腺癌脑转移患者的分级预后评估（Breast-GPA）系统

预后因素	Breast-GPA 评分标准				
	0.0	0.5	1.0	1.5	2.0
KPS 评分（分）	≤50	60	70~80	90~100	—
分子亚型	三阴性	—	Luminal A 型	HER2 型	Luminal B 型
年龄（岁）	≥60	<60	—	—	—

Breast-GPA 评分	中位生存期（个月）
0~1.0	3.4
1.5~2.0	7.7
2.5~3.0	15.1
3.5~4.0	25.3

经 Elsevier 许可转载，引自 Sperduto 等 [43]

(ER/PR 阳性和 HER2 阳性)患者的生存时间最长。本研究清晰地表明乳腺癌脑转移患者不同亚组的预后差异。Breast-GPA 评分为 0.5~1.0 分患者，中位生存期仅为 3.4 个月，而 Breast-GPA 评分为 3.5~4.0 分患者，中位生存期为 25.3 个月。此外，在 Breast-GPA 预后模型中，ECM 和脑转移瘤数目与乳腺癌预后依然无关（表 2-5）[43]。后续临床试验也显示了全身治疗在脑转移瘤治疗中的有效性，如 LANDSCAPE 试验结果显示，在放疗前使用拉帕替尼和卡培他滨作为一线治疗时，颅内反应率可达 66%[44]。此外，其他研究正在关注 T-DM1 在 HER2 阳性乳腺癌中的活性，为临床医生在治疗乳腺癌脑转移患者时提供更多的选择[45]。

鉴于 NSCLC 脑转移发生率很高，且许多研究表明存在表皮生长因子受体（epidermal growth factor receptor, EGFR）和间变性淋巴瘤激酶（anaplastic lymphoma kinase, ALK）基因突变患者的存活率显著提高，进一步改进此类脑转移患者的预后模型显得尤为重要[46-48]。Sperduto 等发表了应用分子标记的肺癌分级预后的评估系统（graded prognostic assessment for lung cancer using molecular markers, Lung-molGPA）[49]。由于考虑了 EGFR 和 ALK 基因改变对非小细胞肺癌和脑转移患者生存的影响，这种新的 Lung-molGPA 与 RTOG RPA 和原来的 DS-GPA 相比，预后能力都有所改善。虽然该研究中只有 4% 的患者 Lung-molGPA 评分为 3.5~4.0 分，但该组患者的中位生存期却接近 4 年（表 2-6）。在不同患者群体的其他大数据样本研究中，也验证 Lung-molGPA 的结果[50]。此外，对 EGFR 突变阳性和 ALK+ 的 NSCLC 给予更好的靶向治疗有望改善这部分脑转移瘤患者的预后。例如，第一代 EGFR 酪氨酸激酶抑制药（tyrosine kinase inhibitors, TKI）在脑转移瘤具有中等疗效，但第二代、第三代的 EGFR 抑制药如阿法替尼和奥希替尼在脑转移瘤患者中显示出更高的疗效，且降低了 CNS 转移的风险[51]。在最近的一项Ⅲ期研究中，奥希替尼在 CNS 疗效可评估的患者中，CNS 的客观有效率可达 70%；且在 T790M 阳性的晚期非小细胞肺癌患者中，奥希替尼相较于化疗（培美曲塞联合铂类）在 CNS 中显示出更好的疗效[52]。其他研究表明，在 ALK+ NSCLC 患者中，ALK 抑制药对未治疗和治疗过的脑转移患者均有效。在一线接受 ALK 抑制药治疗的患者中，总的颅内缓解率为 39.2%，颅内疾病控制率为 70.3%。随着靶向治疗对 CNS 反应率的提高，甚至有研究者提出用这些靶向药物代替放疗来治疗脑转移瘤[53]。

表 2-6 分子标记的肺癌分级预后的评估（Lung-molGPA）系统

预后因素	Lung-molGPA 评分标准		
	0	0.5	1.0
年龄（岁）	≥ 70	< 70	NA
KPS 评分（分）	< 70	80	90～100
颅外转移	存在		不存在
脑转移瘤数量（个）	> 4	1～4	NA
基因状态	EGFR 且 ALK 阴性/未知	NA	EGFR/ALK 阳性

GPA 评分	腺癌中位生存期（个月）	非腺癌中位生存期（个月）
0～1.0	6.9	5.3
1.5～2.0	13.7	9.8
2.5～3.0	26.5	12.8
3.5～4.0	46.8	

引自 Sperduto 等[49]。EGFR. 表皮生长因子受体；ALK. 间变性淋巴瘤激酶

为了继续改善不同组织亚型脑转移患者预后的预测，研究者对 711 例肾细胞癌（renal cell carcinoma，RCC）患者进行了一项多中心回顾性研究，以寻找临床参数指导医生为患者选择更加合适的护理模式和靶向治疗。正如在 DS-GPA 系统中指出一致，RCC 脑转移患者的预后只和 KPS 评分和脑转移瘤数目有关[43]。这项研究表明，虽然现在的肾细胞癌分级评分系统中 KPS 评分和脑转移瘤数量的预后作用得到了确认，但在这个更新的队列研究中，还发现了其他预后因素，包括年龄、ECM 和血红蛋白。

另一种脑转移瘤发生率较高的常见恶性肿瘤是恶性黑色素瘤。诊断为黑色素瘤的患者一生中发生转移的概率可能超过 50%[54]。一项针对各种突变（包括 BRAF、C-KIT 和 NRAS 突变）在恶性黑色素瘤中预后价值的研究表明，BRAF 阳性的患者比 BRAF 阴性的患者存活时间更长，并且相较于 1985—2005 年治疗的患者，2006—2015 年患者的总体生存期明显改善[55]。最初的黑色素瘤–GPA 模型显示，只有 KPS 评分和脑转移瘤数目是影响生存的预后因素[39]，更新的黑色素瘤分级预后评估（graded prognostic assessment for melanoma using molecular markers，Melanoma-molGPA）显示，有五个显著影响生存的预后因素，包括年龄、KPS 评分、ECM、脑转移瘤数目和 BRAF 基因突变状态（表 2-7）[56]。该研究表明，两个不同治疗时期的患者（1985—2005 年 vs. 2006—2015 年），中位生存期从 6.7 个月提高到 9.8 个月，黑色素瘤患者的中位生存期因 Melanoma-molGPA 评分差异显著不同。例如，Melanoma-molGPA 评分为 0～1.0 分的患者中位生存期只有 4.9 个月，而 Melanoma-molGPA 评分为 3.5～4 分的患者，中位生存期接近 34.1 个月。此外，近 50% 的转移性黑色素瘤患者 BRAF V600 呈阳性，这是预后提高的重要指标，因为新的 BRAF 抑制药（如维莫非尼和达拉非尼），有助于改善颅内反应率，并与放射治疗协同改善临床预后[57,58]。

考虑到评估脑转移患者预后的复杂性和多样性，一个用户易于使用的软件可以在 www.brainmetgpa.com 网站在线使用，也可以作为智能手机应用程序直接被使用，为临床医生准确地评估和预测患者的预后提供一个有用的工具。随着我们对脑转移生物学机制认识的不断提高，同时有更好地透过血脑屏障新型药物的不断研发，预后评估系统将继续得到完善，脑转移瘤患者的生存也会持续得到提高。

七、展望和未来

如前所述，分子病理类型是预测脑转移瘤患者生存的重要因素。EGFR、ALK 和 BRAF 基因

表 2-7 分子标记的黑色素瘤的分级预后评估（Melanoma-molGPA）系统

预后因素	Melanoma-molGPA 评分标准		
	0	0.5	1.0
年龄（岁）	≥70	<70	
KPS 评分（分）	≤70	80	90～100
颅外转移	存在		不存在
脑转移瘤数量（个）	>4	2～4	1
BRAF 基因状态	阴性/未知	阳性	

GPA 评分	中位生存期（个月）
0～1.0	4.9
1.5～2.0	8.3
2.5～3.0	15.8
3.5～4.0	34.1

经 Elsevier 许可转载，引自 Sperduto 等[56]

突变的患者可以接受靶向药物治疗，从而改善全身和颅内疾病控制效果，延长总生存。随着更多分子靶点的确定和靶向药物的研发，这些预后评分系统将需要不断修订和完善。例如，使用 TKI 药物可提高总生存率，但如果联合使用，可能会增加药物毒性[59]。因此，预后评估将继续成为研究的主要方向之一，既往的研究成果将指引我们继续前进。

同样，在后续章节讨论中，我们需要了解如何使用这些预后模型和分子因素来优化我们对脑转移瘤患者的管理。尽管对预后差的患者可以基本上都采取支持性护理治疗和 WBRT，但对于预后好的患者管理我们还需要更加精细化，包括全身治疗及对传统手术、SRS 和 WBRT 的综合选择[59]。我们除了需要考虑生存，还要考虑疾病的自然转归，包括局部复发和远处转移。Ayala-Peacock 及其同事开发了一个 Nomogram 模型来预测新发脑转移（distant brain failure, DBF）的可能[60]。发现 DBF 对临床决策选择 WBRT 还是 SRS 特别重要，我们可能对 DBF 风险较高的患者进行 WBRT。有趣的是，在 Ayala-Peacock 等的研究中，预测 DBF 风险不仅要考虑脑转移瘤的数量、组织学、颅外疾病的状态和肿瘤负荷，还要考虑边缘剂量。而且脑转移瘤的总体体积比脑转移瘤的数量更具预测性。Routman 等研究都很好地证明了这一点[61]。这些结果表明，治疗决策不应该像我们过去那样只考虑脑转移瘤数量，而应该考虑颅内的肿瘤负荷。

此外，患者的疾病表现也可能影响他们的预后。例如，同时性脑转移患者与异时性脑转移患者的预后可能不同。同时被诊断的脑转移瘤可能预示肿瘤更具侵袭性。Woody 和同事专门研究了 NSCLC 中同时出现脑转移的患者，并证实了 DS-GPA 系统在这组患者中的有效性[62]。我们需要确认是否其他组织学类型的肿瘤也具有相似性。

最后，预后可能不仅需要关注疾病的自然转归，特别是总体生存率和复发，还应关注治疗的毒性反应，包括神经认知障碍和放射性坏死。Miller 等在对 1939 名患者（5747 个病灶）的研究中发现分子病理学可以预测放射性坏死的风险。*HER2* 扩增、*BRAF* 600+ 突变、肺腺癌和 *ALK* 重排，这些与生存率的提高相关的因素同时也是放射性坏死的预测因子[63]。因此，除了总体存活率和肿瘤控制之外，预期毒性反应也会影响治疗的选择。

Kotecha 及其同事建议，对于直径 <0.5cm 的脑转移瘤，放疗剂量可以较 RTOG 规定的 24Gy 处方剂量有所降低。具体来说，降低剂量对 *EGFR* 突变的 NSCLC、Luminal A 型乳腺癌和 *BRAF* 突变黑色素瘤在局控率方面可能没有太大的影响。这表明，这些预后因素除了影响治疗方式的选择，同时也对放疗剂量的选择产生影响。放射基因组学和机器学习是这方面研究的前沿内容[64]，未来我们可能会利用这一手段来个性化定制患者的放疗剂量，并进一步提高脑转移患者的总生存率和降低毒性反应。虽然少见，但脑转移患者存活 10 年甚至是更长的时间确实是有

可能的[65]。

预后模型提示我们除了考虑标准的临床因素，还需要考虑分子病理学、脑转移瘤的总体积和治疗因素（包括系统治疗和放疗剂量）。随着预测模型的不断完善，我们将进入一个个体化的医疗时代。

八、结论

脑转移是恶性肿瘤最常见的神经系统并发症。随着 MRI 检查技术在分期诊断中的常规应用，以及癌症患者的生存期不断延长，其发病率正在不断增加。在过去，预后一直侧重于关注临床特征，现在则需要结合分子特征和治疗因素综合考虑。预后模型还需要不断地更新和完善。

> **要 点**
> - 脑转移瘤是成人最常见的颅内肿瘤。
> - MRI 是诊断脑转移瘤最佳的影像技术。
> - DS-GPA 系统正在纳入分子病理学因素综合分析脑转移瘤的预后，特别是乳腺癌、NSCLC 以及黑色素瘤。
> - 预后模型将继续通过纳入其他临床数据、治疗因素（包括全身性药物的使用）和分子病理信息来获得不断完善。

参考文献

[1] Jyoti B, Alam A, Hofer S, Brada M. Brain metastases. In: Lisak R, Truong D, Carroll W, Bhidarasiri R, eds. International neurology. 2nd ed. Hoboken, NJ: Wiley; 2016.

[2] Stelzer KJ. Epidemiology and prognosis of brain metastases. Surg Neurol Int. 2013;4(Suppl 4):S192–202.

[3] Nayak L, Lee EQ, Wen P. Epidemiology of brain metastases. Curr Oncol Rep. 2012;14:48–54.

[4] Tabouret E, Chinot O, Metellus P, et al. Recent trends in epidemiology of brain metastases: an overview. Anticancer Res. 2012;32:4655–62.

[5] Fox BD, Cheung VJ, Patel AJ, Suki D, Rao G. Epidemiology of metastatic brain tumors. Neurosurg Clin N Am. 2011;22:1–6.

[6] Graus F, Walker RW, Allen JC. Brain metastases in children. J Pediatr. 1983;103(4):558.

[7] Bouffet E, Doumi N, Thiesse P, Mottolese C, Jouvet A, Lacroze M, et al. Brain metastases in children with solid tumors. Cancer. 1997;79(2):403–10.

[8] Hubbs JL, Boyd JA, Hollis D, Chino JP, Saynak M, Kelsey CR. Factors associated with the development of brain metastases: analysis of 975 patients with early stage nonsmall cell lung cancer. Cancer. 2010;116(21):5038–46.

[9] Shi AA, Digumarthy SR, Temel JS, Halpern EF, Kuester LB, Aquino SL. Does initial staging or tumor histology better identify asymptomatic brain metastases in patients with non–small cell lung cancer. J Thorac Oncol. 2006;1(3):205–10.

[10] Aupérin A, Arriagada R, Pignon J-P, Le Péchoux C, Gregor A, Stephens RJ, et al. Prophylactic cranial irradiation for patients with small-cell lung cancer in complete remission. Prophylactic Cranial Irradiation Overview Collaborative Group. N Engl J Med. 1999;341(7):476–84.

[11] Hochstenbag M, Twijnstra A, Wilmink J, Wouters E, Ten Velde GPM. Asymptomatic brain metastases (BM) in small cell lung cancer (SCLC): MR-imaging is useful at initial diagnosis. J Neuro-Oncol. 2000;48(3):243–8.

[12] Slimane K, Andre F, Delaloge S, Dunant A, Perez A, Grenier J, et al. Risk factors for brain relapse in patients with metastatic breast cancer. Ann Oncol. 2004;15(11):1640–4.

[13] Crivellari D, Pagani O, Veronesi A, Lombardi D, Nole F, Thurlimann B, et al. High incidence of central nervous system involvement in patients with metastatic or locally advanced breast cancer treated with epirubicin and docetaxel. Ann Oncol. 2001;12(3):353–6.

[14] Arvold ND, Oh KS, Niemierko A, Taghian AG, Lin NU, Abi-Raad RF, et al. Brain metastases after breast-conserving therapy and systemic therapy: incidence and characteristics by biologic subtype. Breast Cancer Res Treat. 2012;136(1):153–60.

[15] Pestalozzi BC, Zahrieh D, Price KN, Holmberg SB, Lindtner J, Collins J, et al. Identifying breast cancer patients at risk for central nervous system (CNS) metastases in trials of the International Breast Cancer Study Group (IBCSG). Ann Oncol. 2006;17(6):935–44.

[16] Lin NU, Winer EP. Brain metastases: the HER2 paradigm. Clin Cancer Res. 2007;13(6):1648–55.

[17] Wronski M, Arbit E, Russo P, Galicich JH. Surgical resection of brain metastases from renal cell carcinoma in 50 patients. Urology. 1996;47(2):187–93.

[18] Mongan JP, Fadul CE, Cole BF, Zaki BI, Suriawinata AA, Ripple GH, et al. Brain metastases from colorectal cancer: risk factors, incidence, and the possible role of chemokines. Clin Colorectal Cancer. 2009;8(2):100–5.

[19] Daryanani D, Plukker JT, de Jong MA, Haaxma-Reiche H, Nap R, Kuiper H, et al. Increased incidence of brain metastases in cutaneous head and neck melanoma. Melanoma Res. 2005;15(2):119–24.

[20] Wronski M, Arbit E. Surgical treatment of brain metastases from melanoma: a retrospective study of 91 patients. J Neurosurg. 2000;93(1):9–18.

[21] Sloan AE, Nock CJ, Einstein DB. Diagnosis and treatment of melanoma brain metastasis: a literature review. Cancer Control. 2009;16(3):248–55.

[22] Gavrilovic IT, Posner JB. Brain metastases: epidemiology and pathophysiology. J Neuro-Oncol. 2005;75(1):5–14.

[23] Delattre JY, Krol G, Thaler HT, Posner JB. Distribution of brain metastases. Arch Neurol. 1988;45(7):741–4.

[24] Hwang TL, Close TP, Grego JM, Brannon WL, Gonzales F. Predilection of brain metastasis in gray and white matter junction and vascular border zones. Cancer. 1996;77(8):1551–5.

[25] Clouston PD, DeAngelis LM, Posner JB. The spectrum of neurological disease in patients with systemic cancer. Ann Neurol. 1992;31(3):268–73.

[26] Sneed PK, Kased N, Huang K, Rubenstein JL. Chapter 52: brain metastases and neoplastic meningitis. In: Abeloff MD, Armitage JO, Niederhuber JE, Kastan MB, WG MK, editors. Clinical oncology. Philadelphia: Churchill Livingstone; 2008. p. 827–41.

[27] Forsyth PA, Posner JB. Headaches in patients with brain tumors: a study of 111 patients. Neurology. 1993;43(9):1678–83.

[28] Nowosielski M, Radbruch A. The emerging role of advanced neuroimaging techniques for brain metastases. Chin Clin Oncol. 2015;4(2):23.

[29] Bashour SI, William WN, Patel S, Rao G, Strom E, McAleer MF, et al. Brain metastasis from solid tumors. In: Brain Metastases from Primary Tumors: Epidemiology, Biology, and Therapy. Vol. 2. Cambridge, MA: Elsevier; 2015.

[30] Venur VA, Ahluwalia MS. Prognostic scores for brain metastasis patients: use in clinical practice and trial design. Chin Clin Oncol. 2015;4(2):18.

[31] Gaspar L, Scott C, Rotman M, Asbell S, Phillips T, Wasserman T, et al. Recursive partitioning analysis (RPA) of prognostic factors in three Radiation Therapy Oncology Group (RTOG) brain metastases trials. Int J Radiat Oncol Biol Phys. 1997;37(4):745–51.

[32] Videtic GM, Adelstein DJ, Mekhail TM, Rice TW, Stevens GH, Lee SY, et al. Validation of the RTOG recursive partitioning analysis (RPA) classification for small-cell lung cancer-only brain metastases. Int J Radiat Oncol Biol Phys. 2007;67(1):240–3.

[33] Weltman E, Salvajoli JV, Brandt RA, de Morais Hanriot R, Prisco FE, Cruz JC, et al. Radiosurgery for brain metastases: a score index for predicting prognosis. Int J Radiat Oncol Biol Phys. 2000;46(5):1155–61.

[34] Nieder C, Mehta MP. Prognostic indices for brain metastases–usefulness and challenges. Radiat Oncol. 2009;4:10.

[35] Lorenzoni J, Devriendt D, Massager N, David P, Ruiz S, Vanderlinden B, et al. Radiosurgery for treatment of brain metastases: estimation of patient eligibility using three stratification systems. Int J Radiat Oncol Biol Phys. 2004;60(1):218–24.

[36] Andrews DW, Scott CB, Sperduto PW, Flanders AE, Gaspar LE, Schell MC, et al. Whole brain radiation therapy with or without stereotactic radiosurgery boost for patients with one to three brain metastases: phase III results of the RTOG 9508 randomised trial. Lancet. 2004;363(9422):1665–72.

[37] Sperduto PW, Berkey B, Gaspar LE, Mehta M, Curran W. A new prognostic index and comparison to three other indices for patients with brain metastases: an analysis of 1,960 patients in the RTOG database. Int J Radiat Oncol Biol Phys. 2008;70(2):510–4.

[38] Golden DW, Lamborn KR, McDermott MW, Kunwar S, Wara WM, Nakamura JL, et al. Prognostic factors and grading systems for overall survival in patients treated with radiosurgery for brain metastases: variation by primary site. J Neurosurg. 2008;109(Suppl):77–86.

[39] Sperduto PW, Chao ST, Sneed PK, Luo X, Suh J, Roberge D, et al. Diagnosis-specific prognostic factors, indexes, and treatment outcomes for patients with newly diagnosed brain metastases: a multi-institutional analysis of 4,259 patients. Int J Radiat Oncol Biol Phys. 2010;77(3):655–61.

[40] Bendell JC, Domchek SM, Burstein HJ, Harris L, Younger J, Kuter I, et al. Central nervous system metastases in women who receive trastuzumab-based therapy for metastatic breast carcinoma. Cancer. 2003;97(12):2972–7.

[41] Gabos Z, Sinha R, Hanson J, Chauhan N, Hugh J, Mackey JR, et al. Prognostic significance of human epidermal growth factor receptor positivity for the development of brain metastasis after newly diagnosed breast cancer. J Clin Oncol. 2006;24(36):5658–63.

[42] Tham YL, Sexton K, Kramer R, Hilsenbeck S, Elledge RJC. Primary breast cancer phenotypes associated with propensity for central nervous system metastases. Cancer. 2006;107(4):696–704.

[43] Sperduto PW, Kased N, Roberge D, Xu Z, Shanley R, Luo X, et al. Effect of tumor subtype on survival and the graded prognostic assessment for patients with breast cancer and brain metastases. Int J Radiat Oncol Biol Phys. 2012;82(5):2111–7.

[44] Bachelot T, Romieu G, Campone M, Dieras V, Cropet C, Dalenc F, et al. Lapatinib plus capecitabine in patients with previously untreated brain metastases from HER2-positive metastatic breast cancer (LANDSCAPE): a single-group phase 2 study. Lancet Oncol. 2013;14(1):64–71.

[45] Bartsch R, Berghoff AS, Vogl U, Rudas M, Bergen E, Dubsky P, et al. Activity of T-DM1 in Her2-positive breast cancer brain metastases. Clin Exp Metastasis. 2015;32(7):729–37.

[46] Sperduto PW, Yang TJ, Beal K, Pan H, Brown PD, Bangdiwala A, et al. The effect of gene alterations and tyrosine kinase inhibition on survival and cause of death in patients with adenocarcinoma of the lung and brain metastases. Int J Radiat Oncol Biol Phys. 2016;96(2):406–13.

[47] Barnholtz-Sloan JS, Sloan AE, Davis FG, Vigneau FD, Lai P, Sawaya RE. Incidence proportions of brain metastases in patients diagnosed (1973 to 2001) in the Metropolitan Detroit Cancer Surveillance System. J Clin Oncol. 2004;22(14):2865–72.

[48] Schouten LJ, Rutten J, Huveneers HA, Twijnstra A. Incidence of brain metastases in a cohort of patients with carcinoma of the breast, colon, kidney, and lung and melanoma. Cancer. 2002;94(10):2698–705.

[49] Sperduto PW, Yang TJ, Beal K, Pan H, Brown PD, Bangdiwala A, et al. Estimating survival in patients with lung cancer and brain metastases: an update of the graded prognostic assessment for lung cancer using molecular markers (Lung-molGPA). JAMA Oncol. 2017;3(6):827–31.

[50] Nieder C, Hintz M, Oehlke O, Bilger A, Grosu AL. Validation of the graded prognostic assessment for lung cancer with brain metastases using molecular markers (Lung-molGPA). Radiat Oncol. 2017;12(1):107.

[51] Hochmair M. Medical treatment options for patients with epidermal growth factor receptor mutation-positive non-small cell lung cancer suffering from brain metastases and/or leptomeningeal disease. Target Oncol. 2018;13(3):269–85.

[52] Wu YL, Ahn MJ, Garassino MC, Han JY, Katakami N, Kim HR, et al. CNS efficacy of osimertinib in patients with T790M-positive advanced non-small-cell lung cancer: data from a randomized phase III trial (AURA3). J Clin Oncol. 2018;36(26):2702–9.

[53] Martinez P, Mak RH, Oxnard GR. Targeted therapy as an alternative to whole-brain radiotherapy in EGFR-mutant or ALK-positive non-small-cell lung cancer with brain metastases. JAMA Oncol. 2017;3(9):1274–5.

[54] Davies MA, Liu P, McIntyre S, Kim KB, Papadopoulos N, Hwu WJ, et al. Prognostic factors for survival in melanoma patients with brain metastases. Cancer. 2011;117(8):1687–96.

[55] Sperduto PW, Jiang W, Brown PD, Braunstein S, Sneed P, Wattson DA, et al. The prognostic value of BRAF, C-KIT, and NRAS mutations in melanoma patients with brain metastases. Int J Radiat Oncol Biol Phys. 2017;98(5):1069–77.

[56] Sperduto PW, Jiang W, Brown PD, Braunstein S, Sneed P, Wattson DA, et al. Estimating survival in melanoma patients with brain metastases: an update of the graded prognostic assessment for melanoma using molecular markers (MelanomamolGPA). Int J Radiat Oncol Biol Phys. 2017;99(4):812–6.

[57] Long GV, Margolin KA. Multidisciplinary approach to brain metastasis from melanoma: the emerging role of systemic therapies. Am Soc Clin Oncol Educ Book. 2013;33(1):393–8.

[58] Wolf A, Zia S, Verma R, Pavlick A, Wilson M, Golfinos JG, et al. Impact on overall survival of the combination of BRAF inhibitors and stereotactic radiosurgery in patients with melanoma brain metastases. J Neuro-Oncol. 2016;127(3):607–15.

[59] Juloori A, Miller JA, Parsai S, Kotecha R, Ahluwalia MS, Mohammadi AM, et al. Overall survival and response to radiation and targeted therapies among patients with renal cell carcinoma brain metastases. J Neurosurg. 2019;1(aop):1–9.

[60] Ayala-Peacock DN, Attia A, Braunstein SE, Ahluwalia MS, Hepel J, Chung C, et al. Prediction of new brain metastases after radiosurgery: validation and analysis of performance of a multi-institutional nomogram. J Neuro-Oncol. 2017;135(2):403–11.

[61] Routman DM, Bian SX, Diao K, Liu JL, Yu C, Ye J, et al. The growing importance of lesion volume as a prognostic factor in patients with multiple brain metastases treated with stereotactic radiosurgery. Cancer Med. 2018;7(3):757–64.

[62] Woody NM, Greer MD, Reddy CA, Videtic GMM, Chao ST, Murphy ES, et al. Validation of the disease-specific GPA for patients with 1 to 3 synchronous brain metastases in newly diagnosed NSCLC. Clin Lung Cancer. 2018;19(1):e141–e7.

[63] Miller JA, Bennett EE, Xiao R, Kotecha R, Chao ST, Vogelbaum MA, et al. Association between radiation necrosis and tumor biology after stereotactic radiosurgery for brain metastasis. Int J Radiat Oncol Biol Phys. 2016;96(5):1060–9.

[64] Kang J, Rancati T, Lee S, Oh JH, Kerns SL, Scott JG, et al. Machine learning and radiogenomics: lessons learned and future directions. Front Oncol. 2018;8:228.

[65] Kotecha R, Vogel S, Suh JH, Barnett GH, Murphy ES, Reddy CA, et al. A cure is possible: a study of 10-year survivors of brain metastases. J Neuro-Oncol. 2016;129(3):545–55.

第3章 立体定向放射外科的放射生物学
Radiobiology of Stereotactic Radiosurgery

Anuradha Thiagarajan　Yoshiya Yamada　著
谭兆华　译
张莹莹　校

一、立体定向放射外科中的放射生物学

立体定向放射外科（stereotactic radiosurgery，SRS）的出现使肿瘤放射治疗有了革命性的发展，特别是在脑转移瘤的治疗领域。立体定向放射外科具有三个主要特点：分次剂量高（单次通常为6Gy以上）；大剂量低分割（1～5次）；高精准度。放射治疗技术的发展对高精准度起到了促进作用。其中，调强放射治疗技术（intensity-modulated radiation therapy，IMRT）可使肿瘤和功能区之间生成陡峭的剂量梯度，而精密图像引导系统的发展实现了患者摆位过程中失误的最小化。

相较于全脑放射治疗较低的局部控制率，特别是对于放射抵抗的肿瘤类型，立体定向放射外科的疗效不受原发肿瘤组织学类型的影响，一些放疗相对抵抗的肿瘤如肾细胞癌、结肠癌和黑色素瘤与乳腺癌这类对放疗敏感的肿瘤相比，立体定向放射外科的控制率相当。针对放疗抵抗的肿瘤进行立体定向放射外科显示良好的疗效，12个月的局部控制率为70%～90%[1-4]。

然而，立体定向放射外科中的放射生物学还有很多未知领域，立体定向放射治疗（stereotactic body radiation therapy，SBRT）中治疗效应的放射生物学靶点仍存在争议。我们推测立体定向放射外科较高的局部控制率并不仅仅因为其较大的等效生物学剂量（biologically equivalent dose，BED），其他生物学因素和（或）细胞通路也与立体定向放射外科的病理生理学反应相关。下面的章节将对以上内容进行详细论述。

二、SBRT对于微血管的影响

Fuks等的实验室研究数据显示，当>8～10Gy时，酸性鞘磷脂酶通路的活化能够刺激肿瘤内皮细胞凋亡，干扰肿瘤血管生成，增加肿瘤细胞的死亡率[5]。图3-1描述了这一系列过程。在内皮细胞中，这种酶的分泌形式即酸性鞘磷脂酶（acid sphingomyelinase，ASMase）浓度要远高于体内其他细胞（约为20倍），从而导致内皮细胞通过酸性鞘磷脂酶途径对辐射诱导的细胞凋亡极其敏感，>8Gy的高剂量辐射会引起酸性鞘磷脂酶从细胞质迅速移动至细胞膜富含鞘糖脂和胆固醇的脂筏中。鞘磷脂水解产生促凋亡的神经酰胺，而神经酰胺反过来作为第二信使，刺激促凋亡的BAX通路，最后，线粒体释放出细胞色素C，发生线粒体介导的凋亡反应。此外，通过生成膜筏，神经酰胺能够改变细胞内外的信号通路。Garcia-Barros等以移植黑色素瘤和纤维肉瘤细胞系为对象的实验数据显示，在接受单次15～20Gy[6,7]大剂量放疗之后的1～6h内，肿瘤内皮细胞会发生神经酰胺介导的细胞凋亡。而在另一个实验中，老鼠体内的酸性鞘磷脂酶和BAX

被敲除，就未观察到细胞凋亡发生。激活酸性鞘磷脂酶通路的放射治疗剂量的阈值为8～10Gy，增至20～25Gy仍可观察到剂量-效应关系。微血管功能障碍能够调控辐射诱导的肿瘤细胞DNA损伤过程，将肿瘤细胞内亚致死损伤转化为致死损伤。但在研究发表之时，这一原理尚未被阐明。有趣的是，Fuks等近期的实验显示，在接受单次大剂量照射的1h内，在肿瘤细胞内会发生大量神经酰胺介导的局部缺血/再灌损伤，进而内皮细胞凋亡产生活性氧自由基，造成DNA损伤[8]。从机制上来看，活性氧自由基能够激活保守的小分子泛素样修饰蛋白（small ubiquitin modifer，SUMO）产生应激反应，消耗尚未结合的染色质SUMO3。在多介质同源性修复的活化过程中，SUMO3这一修饰蛋白是关键成分。染色质SUMO3的消耗会导致同源重组整体失活，致死染色体核型异常，肿瘤克隆原细胞死亡，进而局部肿瘤被治愈。

虽然低剂量（1.8～3Gy）的常规分割放疗也会造成内皮细胞损伤，但因为内皮细胞凋亡反应受到了同时激活的肿瘤细胞乏氧诱导因子1（hypoxia-inducible factor 1，HIF-1）的抑制，低剂量放射引起的内皮细胞凋亡和微血管功能障碍并未使肿瘤细胞的死亡明显增加。分次低剂量辐照后，在反复乏氧/再氧合过程中产生的活性氧自由基导致储存在乏氧肿瘤细胞内特殊的细胞质应激颗粒中的HIF-1信使核糖核酸（mRNA）进行转录。HIF-1产生血管内皮生长因子（vascular endothelial growth factor，VEGF）和其他促血管生成因子，对抗并抑制辐射诱导的内皮细胞凋亡。

Oh等研究了辐射对于肿瘤组织和正常乳腺组织内皮细胞在血管新生及其相关分子通路方面的影响[9]。他们证明了正常组织源性的内皮细胞

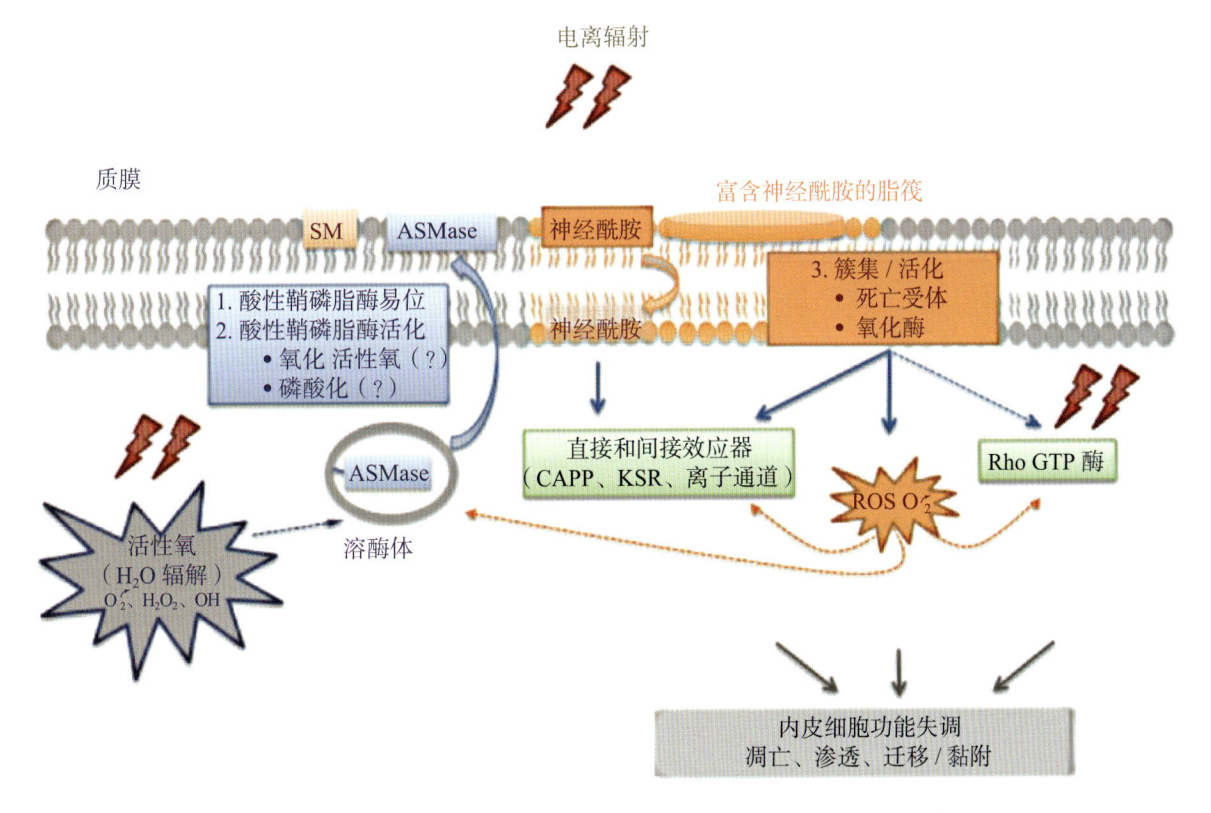

▲ 图 3-1 立体定向消融放射治疗激活内皮细胞中细胞膜信号通路

ASMase. 酸性鞘磷脂酶；CAPP. 神经酰胺活化的蛋白磷酸酶；KSR. 激酶抑制因子；NOX. 氧化酶；ROS. 活性氧；SM. 鞘磷脂；GTP. 三磷酸鸟苷（引自 Corre 等[48]，开放信息源）

和肿瘤源性内皮细胞对辐射的反应存在明显差异。重要的是，他们观察到与正常组织内皮细胞相比，肿瘤组织内皮细胞对辐射的敏感程度明显更高。也就是说，肿瘤血管和正常组织血管的辐射反应差别不仅归因于内皮细胞辐射敏感度的内在差异，还与肿瘤组织和正常组织的毛细血管结构差异有关。肿瘤毛细血管的内膜通常由连接不良的内皮细胞组成，且支撑的基底膜由于周细胞覆盖稀疏而不完整，因此易发生渗漏。此外，肿瘤微血管常常弯曲，分枝末端坏死，分布不均，杂乱无章。当血液流经狭窄、尚未成熟的毛细血管时，流动缓慢且经常间断，辐射之后，内皮细胞通常会发生肿胀，这对血液流动进一步产生干扰。不成熟肿瘤毛细血管的结构缺陷使其极易受到外部压力的影响，增强了大剂量辐射诱导的内皮细胞凋亡[10,11]。

然而最近，内皮细胞凋亡理论的准确性遭到了质疑，因为这些数据尚未得到其他实验室的证实。大部分发表的论文表明，在辐射后，尽管肿瘤内皮细胞逐渐消失，但血管系统仅有轻微的变化。目前流行的理论认为酸性鞘磷脂酶通路和内皮细胞凋亡是定向放射外科治疗杀伤肿瘤的关键因素，但 Moding 等的实验数据质疑了这一观点。由于使用移植的肿瘤模型并不能完全模拟原始肿瘤的血管系统和免疫监视功能，Moding 利用基因工程小鼠模型进行研究，在具有天然免疫活性的实验鼠体内培养肿瘤，以求更真实地再造人类癌症的肿瘤间质和微环境[12]。利用双重组酶技术，定向突变肿瘤细胞和内皮细胞基因，在小鼠体内培养原发性肉瘤。并通过选择性突变促凋亡基因 *BAX* 或者 DNA 损伤反应基因 *ATM*，调控内皮细胞的辐射敏感性，使血管系统对于辐射诱导的细胞死亡反应敏感，或者保护血管不受由膜损伤引发的细胞凋亡影响。有趣的是，在单次剂量 20Gy 的放疗之后，Moding 并未在小鼠原发性肉瘤模型中观察到内皮细胞凋亡的快速波动。同样，他们还观察到内皮细胞 *BAX* 基因的缺失并不会影响辐射诱发的内皮细胞死亡或肉瘤对于放射治疗的反应。而放射治疗 24h 后，内皮细胞中 *ATM* 缺失加速了内皮细胞死亡并延缓肿瘤再生，但这种效应并未转化为肿瘤清除。重要的是，在补充实验中，他们证实肿瘤细胞的 *ATM* 缺失增强了放射治疗的疗效，据此提出不同的观点，认为并非内皮细胞，肿瘤细胞才是放射治疗清除肉瘤的关键靶点。Moding 最后指出其研究主要集中于软组织肉瘤，需要进一步实验证实内皮细胞凋亡对于其他类型肿瘤辐射反应的作用。

三、立体定向放射治疗的免疫调节作用

除了酸性鞘磷脂酶途径以外，人们逐渐认识到一直在肿瘤监视和抑制过程中起关键作用的免疫系统，也是立体定向放射治疗反应的重要组成部分。传统的分次放疗被认为是具有免疫抑制作用的，因为体积较大的正常组织，如白细胞循环血液池和骨髓造血细胞（由辐射敏感的淋巴细胞组成）受到了不可避免的照射。然而越来越多的证据表明，利用立体定向放射外科对肿瘤进行高剂量辐射，可以形成原位瘤苗，诱发并增强抗肿瘤免疫反应。极低分割的立体定向放射外科能够增强诸如组织相容复合体、黏附分子、热休克蛋白、细胞因子等免疫调节分子的表达，并增加肿瘤表面死亡受体的表达。此外，立体定向外科的直接毒性释放了大量肿瘤特异性抗原，导致 CD8 阳性 T 细胞激活及其介导的免疫反应，进一步增强肿瘤细胞死亡（图 3-2）[13]。

Lugade 等发现 B_{16} 黑色素瘤小鼠接受单次剂量 15Gy 的放疗后，通过促进引流淋巴结内抗原递呈和抗肿瘤 T 细胞激活，抗肿瘤免疫效应细胞显著增加[74]。此外，辐射改善了效应 T 细胞进入肿瘤的迁移过程。与单次剂量 15Gy 相比，每日 1 次共 5 次的分割放疗的疗效不佳，强调了分割剂量大小在诱发抗肿瘤免疫反应方面的重要性，但对于最佳的分割剂量仍存在争议。在另一乳腺癌临床前小鼠模型研究中，将小鼠随机分

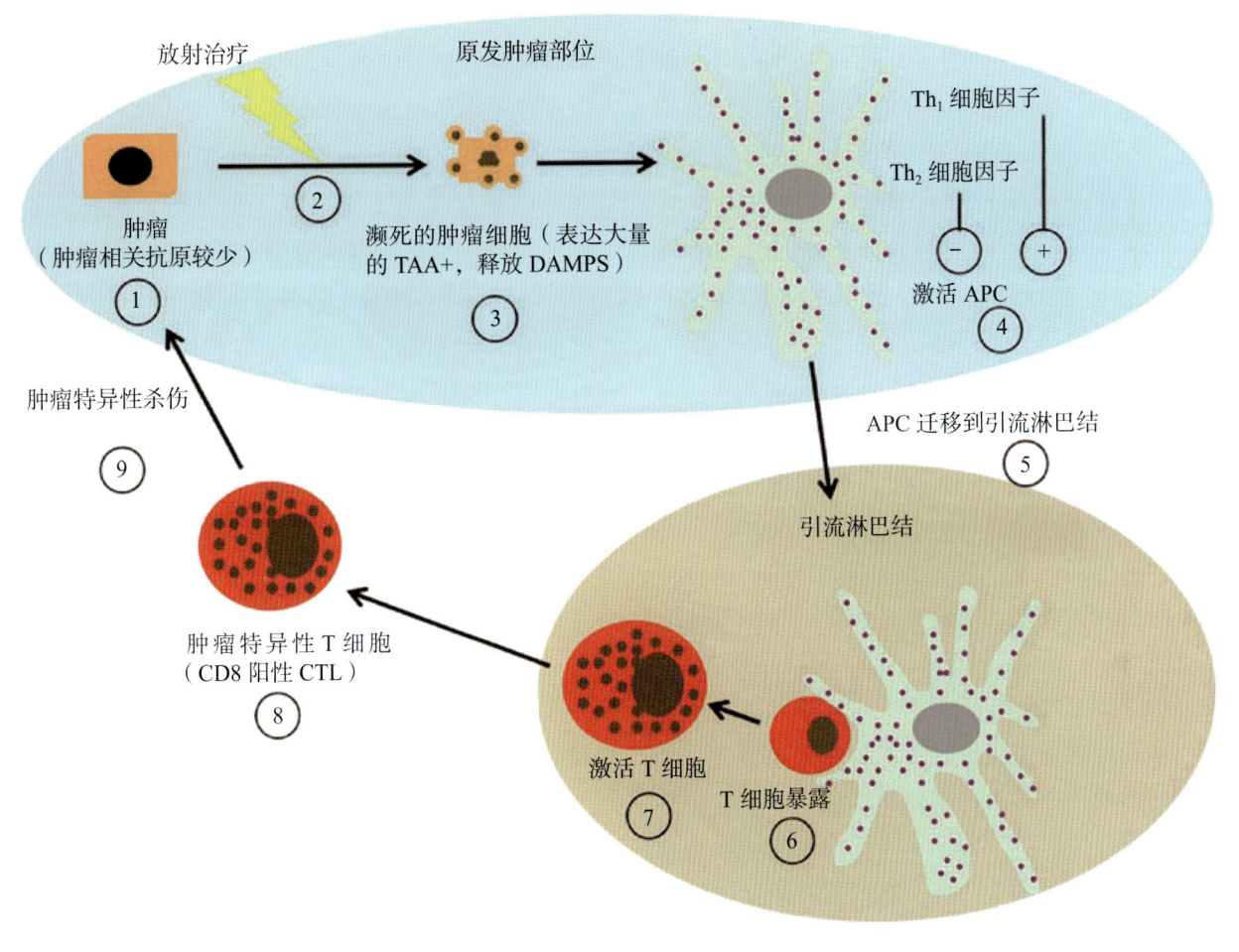

▲ 图 3-2 立体定向放射治疗引起的抗肿瘤免疫调节机制

A. 在原发肿瘤微环境内（蓝色区域），治疗前肿瘤表达有限的辐照肿瘤相关抗原（TAA）；B. 辐射暴露诱发；C. 濒死的肿瘤细胞在表面表达大量肿瘤相关抗原，释放损伤相关危险信号（DAMPS）；D. 肿瘤相关抗原和 DAMPS 被抗原递呈细胞提取，引起抗原呈递细胞活化。Th1 细胞因子可增强抗原递呈细胞活化，而 Th2 细胞因子则抑制其活化；E. 活化的抗原呈递细胞迁移至引流淋巴结（DLN：灰色区域）；F. 在引流淋巴结内，T 细胞通过与活化的抗原递呈细胞直接接触而暴露；G. 活化的 T 细胞的增大变圆；H. 活化的肿瘤特异性 T 细胞（CD8 阳性 CTL）自引流淋巴结迁移至肿瘤微环境中；I. 在肿瘤微环境中，CD8⁺CTL 进行肿瘤特异性杀伤（引自 Kaur 和 Asea[13]，开放信息源）

成 8 组，不接受或分别接受三种不同的放射治疗（20Gy/1 次，8Gy/3 次，6Gy/5 次），并分别联合或者不联合单克隆抗体细胞毒 T 淋巴细胞相关抗原 4（CTLA-4），随后监测原发病灶和转移病灶处肿瘤的生长和消退情况，发现抗 CTLA-4 抗体和任一分割放疗相结合时，原发病灶处的抗肿瘤反应增强。不仅如此，远隔效应，即放疗区域外显著的肿瘤生长抑制，仅在接受免疫和分次放疗联合治疗的小鼠中出现，其中以 8Gy/3 次的分割方案组疗效最佳。

Lee 等通过检测黑色素瘤实验鼠模型中消融放射治疗剂量的效应，进一步证实了立体定向放射外科抗肿瘤免疫的增强作用[16]。在小鼠接受极低分割 – 单次 20Gy 的辐射治疗 1～2 周后，对其肿瘤微环境和淋巴组织的病理学检查发现肿瘤消退和 T 细胞进入。而在缺乏 T 细胞的无胸腺小鼠组，肿瘤体积并未明显减小。另外利用 CD8 阳性抗体消耗 CD8 阳性 T 细胞后的野生型 B_{16} 肿瘤小鼠重复上述实验也发现消融放射的效应减低。综上，这些实验表明 CD8 阳性 T 细胞对于消融放射治疗后辐射诱导的抗肿瘤免疫反应至关重要。

尽管这些临床前研究表明，免疫系统对于

SBRT后肿瘤清除不可或缺，然而，相对于剂量递增使肿瘤细胞死亡增加，免疫应答相对于放疗剂量增加在SBRT总体疗效的贡献程度仍有待确定。值得注意的是，如前所述，继发性肿瘤细胞死亡通常发生在定向消融放疗后的1~3天内，而辐射诱导的肿瘤特异性免疫反应通常需要1~2周。此外，即使在人纤维肉瘤细胞（HT-1080）移植瘤的免疫缺陷小鼠中，单次20Gy的辐射2~3天后，也出现了继发肿瘤细胞死亡[17]。综上所述，可以推测出高剂量低分割放射治疗能够引发直接或间接的消融性细胞死亡，释放大量肿瘤抗原，从而提高抗肿瘤免疫反应。而且，众所周知高剂量放疗引发的细胞损伤能够释放各种各样的促氧化剂和炎症因子，如肿瘤坏死因子（tumor necrosis factor，TNF）、白细胞介素（interleukin-1，IL-1）以及释放危险信号的黏附分子，从而增强免疫反应。这类炎症介质促进抗原递呈细胞的抗原摄取，激发抗原递呈细胞成熟并迁移至引流淋巴结。随后，产生的效应细胞被趋化因子募集回肿瘤中，攻击辐射后存活下来的肿瘤细胞。在肿瘤放射治疗后1~2周，抗肿瘤免疫应答达到高峰，尽管可能不会参与引起第二波肿瘤细胞死亡，但可以抑制存活下来的肿瘤细胞增殖，从而抑制复发和转移。

立体定向放射治疗部分克服了肿瘤诱导的免疫抑制，除此以外，更值得关注的是，SBRT可以与免疫治疗产生协同作用，以抗原加工的各个步骤为靶点，生成效应细胞并将其转运至肿瘤中[18, 19]。一些旨在激活免疫系统的临床疗法，如细胞因子治疗，已经被应用于肿瘤治疗中。虽然少数出现反应的患者出现了强烈且持久的肿瘤缓解，但是这些方法整体的临床反应率较低。近期，越来越多的证据表明，利用细胞毒T淋巴细胞相关抗原4（cytotoxic T lymphocyte assicated protein4，CTLA-4）抗体和程序化细胞死亡因子（PD-1）/PD-L$_1$，免疫检查点抑制药是激发抗肿瘤免疫更为有效的手段[15, 20-22]。此外，多个临床前研究表明免疫检查点抑制药和放射治疗相辅相成、协同作用。因此，最近在进行的多个临床试验尝试将立体定向放射治疗与各种免疫疗法相结合。其早期的结果十分可喜，接受免疫检查点抑制药和SBRT联合治疗的患者，观察到在放射区域外的病灶出现远隔效应。在一项Ⅰ期临床研究中，转移黑色素瘤或肾细胞癌患者SBRT治疗（分1~3次共20Gy）后接受高剂量的IL-2，一种促进免疫T细胞生成的细胞因子。与接受单独SBRT的患者相比，同时接受SBRT和IL-2的患者外周血内CD4$^+$T细胞的增殖水平以及早反应效应记忆细胞表型的表达水平要高得多[23]。在Postow等个案报道，使用SBRT（3次共28.5Gy）与免疫检查点抑制药伊匹木单抗相结合治疗转移性黑素瘤，观察到了远隔效应[24]。然而，激活免疫系统最佳的分割方案，以及免疫治疗与放射治疗结合的最佳时机还有待更多的临床研究来确定。

四、放射治疗反应的生物学基础及其在立体定向放射外科的适用性：4R理论

4R理论—细胞周期再分布（redistribution），亚致死细胞损伤的再修复（repair），细胞的再氧合（reoxygeneration）和再增殖（repopulation），这是常规分割放射治疗后肿瘤产生的生物学反应的重要组成部分[25]。这些因素是否有利于肿瘤清除取决于特定的疾病状况以及应用对象是肿瘤细胞还是正常组织。传统的放射肿瘤增敏疗法以及延长治疗窗口期就是基于对这些因素的考虑。接下来我们将探讨4R理论在立体定向放射外科治疗反应中的作用。

生物等效剂量（BED）是基于线性平方模型（linear-quadratic model，L-Q模型），便于比较不同剂量方案的生物学效应。这一模型假设辐射诱发的克隆原性细胞死亡主要是因为DNA双链断裂，且在分次放疗的间隔期间，乏氧细胞可以完全再氧合，亚致死损伤得到完全修复。虽然

这一模型准确描述了单次低剂量的传统分割放疗产生的效用，但其在立体定向外科消融剂量范围（如单次≥8~10Gy）的辐射生物效应准确性尚存争议，许多研究者对此进行了精细的检验[26-31]。Park等利用结合了L-Q模型和多靶模型的通用生存曲线（universal survival curve，USC）模型描述了极低分割放疗的生物效应。总的来说，Park发现L-Q模型严重高估了消融剂量范围的辐射效应，在更广的剂量区间内，USC模型比L-Q模型更好地反映了测量数据。而其他研究则发现，在较大的单次照射剂量范围内（单次可达20Gy），急性反应和晚反应组织的体内研究终点与L-Q模型具有很好的关联性[32-34]。另外，Mehta等最近开展的一项研究对接受传统分割放疗或SBRT的早期非小细胞肺癌患者的局控率进行分析，发现临床数据并不能区分L-Q和USC模型[35]。L-Q模型的支持者也提出质疑：这些用于阐明高剂量特异性肿瘤杀伤机制的替代模型是否真的更适合实验和临床数据的统计分析值得探讨；有没有令人信服的证据能证实增加更多可调参数能够提供更佳的临床终点预测[31, 36]。

五、细胞周期再分布或重排列

细胞周期影响细胞的辐射敏感性，在增殖期（S-phase）具有更强的抗辐射性。辐照使细胞周期检查点被激活后出现短暂的细胞周期停滞，随后，由于幸存的肿瘤细胞随着细胞周期进展到辐射敏感性更强的阶段，其对辐射变得更为敏感，这一过程被称为细胞周期再分布。虽然在立体定向放射外科，这一现象的生物学意义（若存在）尚且未知，整体治疗时间的缩短阻止了肿瘤细胞通过再分布进入辐射敏感性更高的细胞周期却是肯定的。

六、再氧合

众所周知，乏氧肿瘤细胞是抗电离辐射杀伤的[37-38]。与处在生理性氧环境的细胞相比，对于乏氧细胞群，需要约三倍剂量的辐射才能达到同等的杀伤效果。在人类大部分癌症中均可观察到不同程度的乏氧现象：约90%的实体瘤氧浓度<40~60mmHg，这是正常组织的常见数值，乏氧细胞通常占肿瘤的10%~20%[39, 40]。传统观点认为由于分次放疗可以减弱肿瘤乏氧的保护作用。这是由再氧合现象引起的，在这一过程中，乏氧肿瘤细胞在特定辐射剂量下存活，当肿瘤的氧气供应增加（血流量波动）或氧气消耗需求减少时，乏氧肿瘤细胞发生再氧合，在下一次辐射前变为含氧细胞[41, 42]。考虑到肿瘤内大范围血管破坏是立体定向放射反应的基础，在接受高剂量低分割立体定向放疗后，乏氧肿瘤细胞不太可能出现再氧合现象。即便如此，大量肿瘤细胞死亡后，氧气消耗也会显著减少，因此，存活的乏氧肿瘤细胞也可能发生再氧合。立体定向放射之后肿瘤细胞内氧合状态的变化尚待进一步阐明。

有证据表明，与传统分次放疗相比，肿瘤乏氧对于立体定向放射外科/立体定向放射治疗的不利影响更大。Fowler等的临床前研究评估了在不同剂量分割方案下（包括大剂量在内）引起相同皮肤反应的剂量对移植鼠乳腺肿瘤的控制率，发现与分次放疗相比，单次大剂量放疗的肿瘤控制率较差，若使用乏氧细胞放疗增敏剂米索硝唑对小鼠进行预处理，消除乏氧肿瘤细胞的抗辐射性，则可克服这一劣势[43]。

同样，近期Brenner等一项关于单次或低分割立体定向放射治疗脑转移瘤的肿瘤控制率分析显示，在生物等效剂量相同的情况下，与分次立体定向放疗相比，单次放疗的肿瘤控制率较低，因此作者推测观察到的结果与单次放疗时肿瘤乏氧对于肿瘤局部控制成负相关[44]。

七、再增殖

在肿瘤和正常组织内，电离辐射造成的细胞损耗会引发细胞补偿性再增殖。众所周知，在传统分次放疗中，放射治疗 3～4 周后肿瘤细胞会出现再增殖[45]。可以预见，利用立体定向放射的消融剂量，肿瘤细胞再增殖会更早出现。然而，由于 SRS 和 SBRT 的治疗周期较短，通常在 2 周之内，因此肿瘤再增殖没有实际临床意义。

八、亚致死损伤修复

有报道显示哺乳动物细胞的亚致死辐射损伤修复的半衰期约为 30min[17, 46]。这一现象的发生被认为是 SRS 和 SBRT 中剂量递送时间延长的潜在缺陷，射线引起的细胞毒性效应因此降低，不利于肿瘤控制。但通过采用无均整器光子束模式可以大大提高剂量率缩短照射时间，从而很大程度上缓解上述缺陷。

立体定向放射外科治疗后，血管损伤引发的肿瘤内微环境恶化是如何影响亚致死辐射损伤修复尚不清楚。因此，高剂量下 L-Q 模型的普适性也经常遭到质疑：高剂量下修复是否会饱和。然而大量证据显示事实并非如此。首先，如前文所述，至少 20Gy 之内，早期和晚期组织的剂量反应曲线均与 L-Q 模型相符；其次，1Gy（γ-H2AX 试验测定）和 80Gy（脉冲凝胶电泳测定）照射后，细胞双链断裂修复的速率和程度相当[47]。因此，关于高分次剂量下修复饱和的担忧可能并无必要。

九、结论

随着放射治疗和图像引导技术的迅速进展，立体定向放射治疗越来越广泛应用于颅内和颅外肿瘤病灶的治疗。然而，立体定向放射外科治疗的生物学机制尚不清楚。越来越多的证据提示，单次剂量 > 8～10Gy 的立体定向放射治疗可以诱发严重的肿瘤血管损伤，继而引起继发性或间接性肿瘤细胞死亡。由此导致的肿瘤细胞降解引发肿瘤特异性抗原大量释放，激活抗肿瘤免疫反应，从而抑制肿瘤复发和转移。从机制上了解介导立体定向放射治疗效应的关键分子对设计辐射增敏靶向药物必要性，可以进一步增强立体定向放疗效率，提高治愈比率。4R 理论的作用和 L-Q 模型在描述立体定向放射外科生物学效应的准确性尚存争议。随着我们对极低分割情况下关键分子、细胞和组织效应了解的加深，我们有责任继续积累放射外科对肿瘤及正常组织治疗效应的有意义的临床前及临床实验数据，来开发或完善反映肿瘤控制内在机制的模型，并利用这些模型来提高肿瘤控制疗效。尽管人们对于联合治疗，特别是将立体定向外科与免疫治疗联合的兴趣不断增加，但很大一部分患者对治疗反应很小或完全无反应。因此，加强对复杂的耐药机制、立体定向放射治疗与免疫治疗结合的最佳时机和剂量的理解，同时进一步探索远隔效应受损的机制，对制定最有效并可复制的治疗策略至关重要。

> **要 点**
> - 临床前模型和不断增加的临床数据显示，当辐射 > 8Gy 时，受照肿瘤内皮细胞凋亡是由细胞膜中生成神经酰胺介导，并导致肿瘤细胞内受损的双链断裂重新修复。
> - 单次高剂量放疗后产生的免疫介导效应，可能对于放射外科治疗脑转移瘤的消融作用非常重要。
> - 传统放射生物学认为，高剂量、大分割辐射可在很大程度上导致受照细胞致死性损伤。
> - 立体定向放射外科采用的高剂量辐射，具有常规分割放疗所没有的独特的放射生物学反应机制。

参考文献

[1] Muacevic A, et al. Stereotactic radiosurgery without radiation therapy providing high local tumor control of multiple brain metastases from renal cell carcinoma. Minim Invasive Neurosurg. 2004;47(4):203–8.

[2] Shuto T, et al. Gamma knife surgery for metastatic brain tumors from renal cell carcinoma. J Neurosurg. 2006;105(4):555–60.

[3] Wowra B, et al. Repeated gamma knife surgery for multiple brain metastases from renal cell carcinoma. J Neurosurg. 2002;97(4):785–93.

[4] Auchter RM, et al. A multiinstitutional outcome and prognostic factor analysis of radiosurgery for resectable single brain metastasis. Int J Radiat Oncol Biol Phys. 1996;35(1):27–35.

[5] Kolesnick R, Fuks Z. Radiation and ceramide-induced apoptosis. Oncogene. 2003;22(37):5897–906.

[6] Garcia-Barros M, et al. Host acid sphingomyelinase regulates microvascular function not tumor immunity. Cancer Res. 2004;64(22):8285–91.

[7] Garcia-Barros M, et al. Tumor response to radiotherapy regulated by endothelial cell apoptosis. Science. 2003;300(5622):1155–9.

[8] Bodo S, et al. Single-dose radiotherapy disables tumor cell homologous recombination via ischemia/reperfusion injury. J Clin Invest. 2019;129(2):786–801.

[9] Oh ET, et al. Radiation-induced angiogenic signaling pathway in endothelial cells obtained from normal and cancer tissue of human breast. Oncogene. 2014;33(10):1229–38.

[10] Carmeliet P, Jain RK. Principles and mechanisms of vessel normalization for cancer and other angiogenic diseases. Nat Rev Drug Discov. 2011;10(6):417–27.

[11] Song CW. Modification of blood flow. In: Mools M, Vaupel P, editors. Blood perfusion and microenvironment of human tumors, implications for clinical radio oncology. Berlin: Springer; 1998. p. 194–207.

[12] Moding EJ, et al. Tumor cells, but not endothelial cells, mediate eradication of primary sarcomas by stereotactic body radiation therapy. Sci Transl Med. 2015;7(278):278ra34.

[13] Kaur P, Asea A. Radiation-induced effects and the immune system in cancer. Front Oncol. 2012;2:191.

[14] Lugade AA, et al. Local radiation therapy of B16 melanoma tumors increases the generation of tumor antigen-specific effector cells that traffic to the tumor. J Immunol. 2005;174(12):7516–23.

[15] Dewan MZ, et al. Fractionated but not single-dose radiotherapy induces an immune-mediated abscopal effect when combined with anti-CTLA-4 antibody. Clin Cancer Res. 2009;15(17):5379–88.

[16] Lee Y, et al. Therapeutic effects of ablative radiation on local tumor require CD8+ T cells: changing strategies for cancer treatment. Blood. 2009;114(3):589–95.

[17] Song CW, et al. Is indirect cell death involved in response of tumors to stereotactic radiosurgery and stereotactic body radiation therapy? Int J Radiat Oncol Biol Phys. 2014;89(4):924–5.

[18] Schoenhals JE, et al. Preclinical rationale and clinical considerations for radiotherapy plus immunotherapy: going beyond local control. Cancer J. 2016;22(2):130–7.

[19] Bernstein MB, et al. Immunotherapy and stereotactic ablative radiotherapy (ISABR): a curative approach? Nat Rev Clin Oncol. 2016;13(8):516–24.

[20] Callahan MK, Postow MA, Wolchok JD. CTLA-4 and PD-1 pathway blockade: combinations in the clinic. Front Oncol. 2014;4:385.

[21] Postow MA, Callahan MK, Wolchok JD. Immune checkpoint blockade in cancer therapy. J Clin Oncol. 2015;33(17):1974–82.

[22] Wang X, et al. Suppression of type I IFN signaling in tumors mediates resistance to anti-PD-1 treatment that can be overcome by radiotherapy. Cancer Res. 2017;77(4):839–50.

[23] Seung SK, et al. Phase 1 study of stereotactic body radiotherapy and interleukin-2–tumor and immunological responses. Sci Transl Med. 2012;4(137):137ra74.

[24] Postow MA, et al. Immunologic correlates of the abscopal effect in a patient with melanoma. N Engl J Med. 2012;366(10):925–31.

[25] Steel GG, McMillan TJ, Peacock JH. The 5Rs of radiobiology. Int J Radiat Biol. 1989;56(6):1045–8.

[26] Dutreix J, Cosset JM, Girinsky T. Biological equivalency of high single doses used in intraoperative irradiation. Bull Cancer Radiother. 1990;77(2):125–34.

[27] Park C, et al. Universal survival curve and single fraction equivalent dose: useful tools in understanding potency of ablative radiotherapy. Int J Radiat Oncol Biol Phys. 2008;70(3):847–52.

[28] Hanin LG, Zaider M. Cell-survival probability at large doses: an alternative to the linear-quadratic model. Phys Med Biol. 2010;55(16):4687–702.

[29] Kirkpatrick JP, Meyer JJ, Marks LB. The linear-quadratic model is inappropriate to model high dose per fraction effects in radiosurgery. Semin Radiat Oncol. 2008;18(4):240–3.

[30] Guerrero M, Li XA. Extending the linear-quadratic model for large fraction doses pertinent to stereotactic radiotherapy. Phys Med Biol. 2004;49(20):4825–35.

[31] Brenner DJ. The linear-quadratic model is an appropriate methodology for determining isoeffective doses at large doses per fraction. Semin Radiat Oncol. 2008;18(4):234–9.

[32] van der Kogel AJ. Chronic effects of neutrons and charged particles on spinal cord, lung, and rectum. Radiat Res Suppl. 1985;8:S208–16.

[33] Douglas BG, Fowler JF. The effect of multiple small doses of x

rays on skin reactions in the mouse and a basic interpretation. Radiat Res. 1976;66(2):401–26.

[34] Peck JW, Gibbs FA. Mechanical assay of consequential and primary late radiation effects in murine small intestine: alpha/beta analysis. Radiat Res. 1994;138(2):272–81.

[35] Mehta N, et al. Stereotactic body radiation therapy and 3-dimensional conformal radiotherapy for stage I non-small cell lung cancer: a pooled analysis of biological equivalent dose and local control. Pract Radiat Oncol. 2012;2(4):288–95.

[36] Brown JM, Carlson DJ, Brenner DJ. The tumor radiobiology of SRS and SBRT: are more than the 5 Rs involved? Int J Radiat Oncol Biol Phys. 2014;88(2):254–62.

[37] Brizel DM, et al. Oxygenation of head and neck cancer: changes during radiotherapy and impact on treatment outcome. Radiother Oncol. 1999;53(2):113–7.

[38] Nordsmark M, Overgaard M, Overgaard J. Pretreatment oxygenation predicts radiation response in advanced squamous cell carcinoma of the head and neck. Radiother Oncol. 1996;41(1):31–9.

[39] Gray LH, et al. The concentration of oxygen dissolved in tissues at the time of irradiation as a factor in radiotherapy. Br J Radiol. 1953;26(312):638–48.

[40] Brown JM, Wilson WR. Exploiting tumour hypoxia in cancer treatment. Nat Rev Cancer. 2004;4(6): 437–47.

[41] Kallman RF, Dorie MJ. Tumor oxygenation and reoxygenation during radiation therapy: their importance in predicting tumor response. Int J Radiat Oncol Biol Phys. 1986;12(4):681–5.

[42] Brown JM. Evidence for acutely hypoxic cells in mouse tumours, and a possible mechanism of reoxygenation. Br J Radiol. 1979;52(620):650–6.

[43] Fowler JF, et al. Optimum fractionation of the C3H mouse mammary carcinoma using x-rays, the hypoxic-cell radiosensitizer Ro-07-0582, or fast neutrons. Int J Radiat Oncol Biol Phys. 1976;1(7–8):579–92.

[44] Shuryak I, et al. High-dose and fractionation effects in stereotactic radiation therapy: analysis of tumor control data from 2965 patients. Radiother Oncol. 2015;115(3):327–34.

[45] Bese NS, Hendry J, Jeremic B. Effects of prolongation of overall treatment time due to unplanned interruptions during radiotherapy of different tumor sites and practical methods for compensation. Int J Radiat Oncol Biol Phys. 2007;68(3): 654–61.

[46] Song CW, et al. Radiobiological basis of SBRT and SRS. Int J Clin Oncol. 2014;19(4):570–8.

[47] Rothkamm K, et al. Pathways of DNA double-strand break repair during the mammalian cell cycle. Mol Cell Biol. 2003;23(16):5706–15.

[48] Corre I, Guillonneau M, Paris F. Membrane signaling induced by high doses of ionizing radiation in the endothelial compartment. Relevance in radiation toxicity. Int J Mol Sci. 2013;14(11):22678–96.

第 4 章 脑转移瘤患者及其治疗并发症的对症支持处理
Supportive Medical Management of Brain Metastases Patients Including Treatment Complications

Peter C. Pan　Laura E. Donovan　Rajiv S. Magge　著
张　静　译
张莹莹　校

一、临床关注

据统计，6%～30% 原发恶性肿瘤的患者会发生转移[1, 2]。其中，肺癌脑转移尤其常见，由于脑的容量较大，以及肺癌对于脑转移的偏向性使得在一些研究[3]中肺癌脑转移的发生率高达 50%[3]。此外，黑色素瘤、肾细胞癌和乳腺癌也容易转移至脑部。随着恶性肿瘤患者总体预后的改善，脑转移的患病率持续上升。

大脑各部位均可发生转移。肿瘤细胞以类似于白细胞外渗的方式从血流中迁移出来，在趋化因子的引导下，滚动、黏附，然后穿过血脑屏障[4]。上皮间质转化（epithelial-mesenchymal transition，EMT）是转移的经典模型；然而，最新的研究却支持另一种入侵模型。在入侵模型中，颅内的间充质细胞（如小胶质细胞）既可以充当肿瘤细胞入侵的起始因子，也可以是肿瘤细胞入侵的引导者，肿瘤细胞并不一定需要获得间充质特征就可以实现转移[5, 6]。肿瘤细胞体积大，迁移过程中会导致血管内皮结构不可逆地损伤，同时肿瘤细胞还可以释放血管内皮生长因子（vascular endothelial growth factor，VEGF）、细胞因子和生长因子，进一步增加血管通透性[7-9]。VEGF 不仅可以通过下调紧密连接中的 zonula occluden –1（ZO-1）直接损伤血脑屏障，还能作用于内皮细胞[10]上的 VEGFR2 导致微血管增生。在这种情况下，尽管血脑屏障的完整性丧失，但只会导致屏障功能的部分损害[11]，损害的程度与转移瘤的大小成比例[12]，因而阻碍了化疗药物向肿瘤组织的有效递送[13]。此外，星形胶质细胞通过缝隙连接与肿瘤细胞传递信号以及上调生存基因的表达引起化疗耐药，进一步导致化疗的有效性下降[13, 14]。尽管受到这些影响，在过去的十年中，针对实体肿瘤的靶向和免疫治疗方法仍因为其显著的进展在临床上获得了关注。转移性病变的典型表现是在近皮质的脑实质出现点状或圆形的均匀增强性病变。也可以表现为边缘强化的囊性或大小不均匀的强化病变。

神经肿瘤学脑转移反应评估（Response Assessment in Neuro-Oncology Brain Metastase，RANO-BM）工作组将可测量的病变定义为至少在一个维度上可测量到最小为 10mm 的增强性病变，并且在两个或多个相距 5mm 或更小的轴位切面上可见[15]。但这一标准导致许多病变不能很好地被捕捉到，例如毫米级的病变、主要为囊性的病灶，以及硬脑膜、颅骨或软脑膜病变。但在正电子发射断层扫描（positron emission tomography，PET）中，这些病变的葡萄糖摄取通常是升高的[16]。

尽管这些病变导致的功能障碍通常不像类似

急性血管损伤那样令人典型。但通过标准的定位技术可以准确地预测相应的神经功能损害，如执行功能障碍、精神活动迟缓和人格改变与额叶病变有关，偏侧化运动或感觉缺陷通常出现在丘脑周围。颞顶和枕叶病变可引起同侧视野缺损；幕下病变通常导致延髓体征或共济失调。

瘤周脑水肿会导致受影响组织范围的增大，从而增加了相应部位脑组织的神经功能缺损。瘤周水肿通常在转移灶周围，表现为无强化的 T_2 高信号，可能伴有弥散限制减少。研究表明，虽然水肿普遍存在，但没有水肿并不能排除转移，尤其是对于直径< 1cm 的转移瘤[17]。有趣的是，同一项研究发现，在泌尿生殖系癌症和皮肤癌中，导致水肿形成的肿瘤大小阈值更高，约为 3cm[17]。

虽然过度换气、床头抬高和高渗盐水和甘露醇等渗透疗法在控制颅内压升高方面都有作用[18]，但皮质类固醇是瘤周水肿的首选治疗方法[19]。然而，由于皮质类固醇有许多不良反应，使其长期使用受限。

肿瘤更倾向于转移到近皮质的实质内，这种现象可以解释此类人群癫痫发作风险升高的原因。目前，各个地区对于预防性使用抗癫痫药（antiepileptics，AED）的意见尚不统一，越来越多的证据和最新的指南建议不要预防性使用抗癫痫药。对于有症状的癫痫患者，应仔细选择抗癫痫药物，并注意避免使用可能影响化疗代谢的 CYP_{450} 诱导剂。

虽然脑转移瘤对于放射治疗具有良好的反应，但放射治疗也会导致正常组织的损伤并引起一系列不良反应，包括短期内的疲劳和脑水肿，以及更多的慢性问题，包括白质脑病、认知功能障碍、坏死和血管病变。在儿童恶性肿瘤患者中，这些慢性病变导致的长期并发症尤其令人担忧。

随着疗效的改善和患者寿命的延长，脑转移和治疗相关的神经毒性反应的发生率与日俱增，因此，识别和管理它们就愈发重要。

二、循证基础

1. 瘤周脑水肿

瘤周脑水肿会导致癫痫发作、头痛、脑病，如果体积足够大，还会导致脑疝。与灰质相比，由于脑白质对液体的阻力较低，水肿更容易在白质中积聚[20]。尽管水肿对症状的影响很大，但关于水肿程度是否与肿瘤预后相关，目前研究并未达成一致的结论。在一项对单个脑转移瘤进行手术的研究中，脑水肿的程度是与预后相关的独立因素[21]。而另一项对因脑转移瘤而接受手术切除的患者的研究发现，水肿的中位体积或水肿体积与肿瘤体积之比没有预后价值[22]。另一项研究则支持以下结论，即肿瘤周围水肿与肿瘤体积的比率是总生存率的一个强有力的预测因素，特别是颅后窝转移瘤中水肿的程度在空间受限的颅后窝可能更重要[23]。

2. 皮质类固醇

自 20 世纪 50 年代末以来，皮质类固醇就在临床应用于减轻瘤周脑水肿[24, 25]，并一直是标准治疗[26]。类固醇可以收缩血管[27]，减少白三烯的形成[28]，并通过激活糖皮质激素受体减少 VEGF 的表达[29]，以及促进细胞骨架和紧密连接蛋白恢复使血脑屏障修复来发挥其抗水肿作用[30, 31]。

类固醇的潜在不良反应几乎涉及每个器官系统，包括对胃的刺激、体重增加、糖耐量减低、转氨酶升高、伤口愈合不良、骨质疏松、缺血性坏死、肌病、痤疮、高血压、精神病、肾上腺素减退和青光眼等[20]。长期治疗（持续时间超过 3 周）和低蛋白血症（< 2.5g/dl）与更大的毒性相关[32]。出于这些原因，不建议对无症状的患者使用皮质类固醇，而对于有症状的患者，应使用最低有效剂量来控制症状。

与其他皮质类固醇相比，地塞米松的盐皮质激素活性相对较低，感染和神经精神影响的风险也较低，因此地塞米松在临床上更加受到青睐[27]。为了暂时缓解脑水肿的轻微症状，常规可以使用每天 4~8mg 地塞米松的起始剂量，症状如果较严重，可使用较高的剂量，每天给予 16mg [19, 33, 34]。虽然地塞米松的血浆半衰期为 2h 左右，但其生物半衰期为 36~54h，这使得临床医生可以使用一个方便的给药方案——即每天 1~2 次 [34-36]。从剂量逐渐减少到维持治疗所需的最低剂量，常规来说需要 2 周时间 [37]。由于用药后可能出现肾上腺抑制，即使皮质类固醇治疗只用了两周，在后续治疗中，也需要缓慢减量 [36]。

3. 皮质类固醇：胃肠道预防

对于伴有糖皮质激素的消化性溃疡和上消化道（gastrointestinal，GI）出血的患者，我们通常使用组胺 H_2 受体拮抗药或质子泵抑制药。关于类固醇是否会增加消化道出血风险，早期文献中的一些相关描述不一 [38-41]。Narum 等最近对 3 万多名患者进行了一项大型综述和 Meta 分析，发现仅在住院人群中发现胃肠道出血或穿孔的风险增加 [42]。而在门诊人群中，很少发生此类风险事件（0.13%），尽管有风险比值比（odds ratio，OR 值）增加，但无统计学意义。

日本 Kondo 等进行了一项关于消化性溃疡出血止血后再出血率的研究，接受了泼尼松龙 20mg 或以上（大致相当于地塞米松 3mg 或以上）的患者比使用较少皮质类固醇的患者再出血率更高 [43]。但目前还无法确定每天 3mg 地塞米松是否为胃肠道出血风险的"安全"界限。曾等针对中国台湾地区全民健康保险数据库的大型回顾性分析纳入了近 9000 例住院病例和门诊病例，数据相对令人信服。他们发现即使是短程（7 天）低剂量（甲泼尼龙 4mg 或地塞米松 0.8mg 或更高剂量）的激素治疗，也与消化性溃疡出血风险升高有关。而同时服用阿司匹林或其他非甾体抗炎药 [44] 的患者风险更高，这一发现与早期报道中联合使用风险升高的结果相似 [45]。

除了消化道出血的直接死亡风险之外，皮质类固醇的使用也使癌症患者面临更高的其他风险，比如他们可能已经正在接受深静脉血栓（deep venous thrombus，DVT）或肺栓塞（pulmonary embolism，PE）的抗凝治疗，而在皮质类固醇的使用中通常需要停止这些治疗。即使在胃肠道出血稳定后，医生仍可能会对是否恢复抗凝治疗犹豫不决，迫使他们考虑效果较差的替代方案，如下腔静脉过滤器（这可能会使患者面临更多的并发症，而四肢的凝血负担也不会减轻）。另外，正如前面提到的，皮质类固醇似乎确实会造成胃肠道出血的威胁。Narum 等的数据并没有令人信服的证据来证明糖皮质激素的使用是完全安全的 [42]。而曾等和近藤等的研究都提供了皮质类固醇的使用可以导致损害的证据 [43, 44]。因此在没有确切数据的情况下，临床上默认皮质类固醇有可能增加胃肠道出血的风险，患者应接受预防治疗。由于与组胺 H_2 受体拮抗药和质子泵抑制药的不良反应相比，任何一次胃肠道出血事件的潜在危险和死亡风险都要大得多，对于住院患者中，我们应给予质子泵抑制剂，如泮托拉唑（通常剂量为每天 40mg）静脉给药。对于门诊治疗的患者，尽管总体发生率较低，但还是建议使用组胺 H_2 受体拮抗药或质子泵抑制药进行预防（除非类固醇剂量＜ 0.8mg/d 地塞米松的等效剂量）。

4. 皮质类固醇：机会性感染

长期以来，人们普遍认为皮质类固醇的使用与机会性肺孢子虫感染有关。美国国家综合癌症网络指南建议对于服用泼尼松 20mg/d（或地塞米松 3mg/d）4 周或更长 [46] 的患者进行预防性治疗。这个建议是基于一项对服用地塞米松并患上机会性肺孢子虫肺炎患者的回顾性研究：研究中被感染的患者总地塞米松的中位剂量为 4.5mg/d [47]，但有 25% 感染者服用的地塞米松仅仅为 2.4mg/d。因此，临床应用时我们推荐将地塞米松用量限制在 3mg/d，但这并非是机会性肺孢子虫感染发生的阈值剂量。临床实践中医生的判断是最重要的，针对有免疫缺陷的患者，如人类免疫缺陷病毒（human immunodeficiency viral，HIV）感染、T 细胞计数低或营养不良等，医生应给予更严格的控制。

在预防性治疗时，应当考虑皮质类固醇的生物半衰期，即使对于每天不使用皮质类固醇的患者也应当如此。因为感染的易感期可能会超过皮质类固醇治疗的最后日期。一项研究发现，在发现感染之前的 4 周内，近一半的机会性肺孢子虫肺炎患者间歇（而不是每天）服用类固醇，或者根本没有服用类固醇[48]。如果预防性抗生素耐受性良好，我们建议在皮质类固醇停用后将预防期延长至 2[49]～4 周[48]。典型的预防性抗生素包括甲氧苄啶 - 磺胺甲噁唑（160～800mg）二联片剂（1 片，每周 3 次）、阿托伐醌（1500mg/d）、氨苯砜（100mg/d）。甲氧苄啶 - 磺胺甲噁唑可引起过敏反应、肝肾功能障碍和血细胞减少症，但通常耐受性良好，被视为一线用药；在磺胺过敏的情况下，可以考虑使用阿托伐醌和氨苯砜[50]。

5. 皮质类固醇：与免疫疗法的相互作用

免疫检查点抑制药的出现使得包括非小细胞肺癌、肾细胞癌和黑色素瘤在内的恶性肿瘤患者有了更多的治疗选择。由于这些癌症常发生脑转移，皮质类固醇不仅用于治疗癌周脑水肿，还用于治疗免疫检查点抑制药使用后继发的免疫相关不良反应。因此，皮质类固醇对免疫治疗的影响越来越受到关注。

在 CTLA-4 介导下，幼稚的 T 细胞群对皮质类固醇的暴露特别敏感，而分化的效应记忆 T 细胞则相对不敏感，这表明皮质类固醇的给药时机很重要。因此，在抗肿瘤免疫反应成功产生后再给予皮质类固醇，不太可能降低免疫治疗的疗效[51]。一项大型黑色素瘤临床研究的观察结果支持这一观点，即使用皮质类固醇治疗免疫相关不良事件并不会影响患者对于纳武利尤单抗的应答[52]。

三、脑水肿：对于 *VEGF* 通路的抑制

肿瘤细胞分泌的血管内皮生长因子（*VEGF*）可导致血管通透性增加和脑水肿。靶向血管内皮生长因子通路有助于血管形态正常化和减轻脑水肿。通过 *VEGF* 通路治疗脑水肿的药物包括血管内皮生长因子配体抑制药如贝伐珠单抗、靶向血管内皮生长因子受体拮抗药如西地尼布和雷莫芦单抗，以及多种酪氨酸激酶抑制药如索拉非尼、舒尼替尼和尼达尼布等[53]。与皮质类固醇不同，血管内皮生长因子途径抑制不会导致免疫抑制。这在免疫治疗中是一个优势，许多脑转移瘤患者在接受抗血管靶向治疗的同时也接受了免疫检查点抑制药治疗，这可能使治疗的效应更为长久。

贝伐珠单抗是一种血管内皮生长因子 A（*VEGF*-A）抑制药，是减少脑水肿的最常用的类固醇激素替代药物。贝伐珠单抗剂量为 5～7.5mg/kg，每 2～3 周 1 次，最多 9 个周期，文献中描述该药可在脑水肿治疗中发挥作用，在非适应证的情况下，它的应用可以使皮质类固醇的用量减少，甚至达到避免使用皮质类固醇的效果[54, 55]。

贝伐珠单抗最常见的不良反应是高血压、便秘和疲劳，通常可以保守治疗。最令人关注的不良事件是血栓和出血风险的增加，包括（但不限于）心肌梗死、急性缺血性脑卒中、深静脉血栓形成、肺栓塞、出血和胃肠道出血等。胃肠道穿孔是一种罕见的并发症，发生率 < 1%，但其中大约 1/4 的情况比较严重甚至致命。导致穿孔的原因是多方面的，其中较高的剂量（每周 5mg/kg，而不是每周 2.5mg/kg）是一个危险因素[56]。胃肠穿孔的典型症状包括腹痛、便秘和呕吐[57]，因此对于应用贝伐珠单抗的患者应密切监测，及时治疗便秘。

尽管理论上 *VEGF* 抑制药可导致脑出血风险增加，但大量文献发现颅内出血的风险并没有超过基线水平。Khasraw 等的一项包括胶质母细胞瘤、结肠癌、非小细胞肺癌、卵巢癌和血管肉瘤患者的大型回顾性研究报道了纪念斯隆 - 凯特林癌症中心使用贝伐珠单抗的经验，该研究报道使用和未使用贝伐珠单抗治疗患者的脑出血频率分别为 3.7% 和 3.6%[58]。卡登等和贝塞等在 2008

年和 2010 年对抗血管内皮生长因子的临床研究也分别得出了类似的结论，并报道了使用贝伐珠单抗治疗和未使用患者之间的脑出血发生率均较低且相似[59, 60]。此外，针对贝伐珠单抗在非小细胞肺癌中的安全性的二期 PASSPORT 研究中也没有报道 CNS 出血的病例，但报道出现了两例肺出血事件[61]。

目前对于活动性颅内或颅外出血患者，使用抗血管内皮生长因子治疗是否安全，尚没有很好的研究，需要更多的数据来验证。可能加剧现有出血的风险是临床医生担心的主要原因。在临床实践中，有急性出血是贝伐珠单抗治疗的禁忌证之一。

贝伐珠单抗会干扰伤口愈合。这对于有压疮风险的偏瘫或卧床患者，以及患有糖尿病或外周血管疾病且经常出现伤口不愈合的患者来说，显得尤为重要。在外科患者中，贝伐珠单抗不仅有延迟伤口愈合的风险，还有导致出血和裂开的风险。贝伐珠单抗的半衰期很长，约为 20 天。在手术之前，临床上推荐 4～8 周的洗脱期；而对于术后的患者，推荐至少延迟 28 天待伤口完全愈合后再使用贝伐珠单抗[62]。

限制贝伐珠单抗使用的主要问题是，其不常见但严重的不良反应、对手术时机的影响以及治疗费用的增加。其长期有效性也令人担忧，持续性的 VEGF 阻断可能导致其他替代途径（如碱性成纤维细胞生长因子或基质细胞衍生因子 1-α）激活从而促进血管生成[63]。此外，目前尚不清楚在所有转移性肿瘤亚型中是否都可采用针对 VEGF 的抗水肿策略。神经胶质瘤文献显示 VEGF 表达和抗 VEGF 治疗水肿疗效具有显著的异质性[64, 65]。比较非小细胞肺癌、小细胞肺癌、黑色素瘤、肾细胞癌和结直肠癌脑转移瘤血管生成的组织病理学特征的研究发现，不同肿瘤 VEGF 表达不同，水肿表现不同，对抗 VEGF 治疗的反应也有显著的异质性[64, 65]。其中，肾细胞癌微血管增殖最高，黑色素瘤最低[66]。

四、脑水肿：实验性治疗策略

1. 人促肾上腺皮质激素释放因子（human corticotropin-releasing factor，hCRF）

hCRF，是皮质醇超家族中的一员，由 41 个氨基酸残基组成，这种内源性多肽可以刺激下丘脑 - 垂体轴（hypothalamic-pituitary axis，HPA）。20 世纪 80 年代和 90 年代初的一些文献表明，它可以在各种组织中抑制血管渗漏[67]。一项来自于大鼠胶质瘤模型的临床前研究显示，注射 hCRF 后，MRI 增强相的对比度减弱，肿瘤组织水分含量呈剂量依赖性减少[68]。与此同时，血浆皮质酮水平并没有改变，肾上腺切除术也没有消除 hCRF 的上述作用，因此著者认为这种效应不依赖于肾上腺类固醇的释放，此外，著者发现内皮屏障抗原（endothelial barrier antigen，EBA）水平在 hCRF 处理的动物中表达最高，推测导致 EBA 等血脑屏障特异性蛋白的上调可能是 hCRF 的作用机制之一。

尽管临床前证据显示 hCRF 有良好的应用前景，但临床水平的研究却没有取得令人信服的证据。一项针对 17 例脑转移瘤患者静脉注射 hCRF 的 I 期研究结果表明：hCRF 减轻 MRI 所示脑水肿的疗效并不确定，而注射该药物后可导致包括脸红、头痛、胃肠紊乱和低血压在内的不良反应[69]。一项对 200 例合并有瘤周脑水肿的原发性或继发性恶性肿瘤患者的前瞻性、随机、双盲研究显示，使用醋酸促肾上腺皮质激素（皮下注射的人工合成 hCRF 制剂）与安慰剂对照，没有观察到有统计学意义的地塞米松剂量减少[70, 71]。另一项随机试验中，研究者试图比较在出现亚急性瘤周脑水肿的患者中促肾上腺皮质激素与地塞米松加量（4mg）的疗效，结果显示两组的反应率都很低，促肾上腺皮质激素组为 3/20，地塞米松组为 3/17。该研究最终因招募缓慢而提前终止[72]。

促肾上腺皮质激素的效应似乎很明显[73]，但尚不清楚为什么临床前数据显示的有效性没有转化为临床有效性。但若参考某些反应皮质类固醇负担减少的替代指标，如肌病，促肾上腺皮质激素在上述临床研究的实验组中都表现出一定的减轻皮质类固醇负担的效应，但效应程度不大。虽然目前促肾上腺皮质激素可以考虑作为一种减少皮质类固醇负担的辅助治疗药物，但它取代地塞米松的有效性并没能得到证实。

2. 神经激肽 1 受体拮抗药

神经激肽 1（neurokinin 1，NK1）受体拮抗药还处于研究阶段，可能是治疗脑水肿的一种方法。关于创伤性脑损伤[74, 75]和缺血性脑卒中文献[76]的最新数据表明，血管通透性和脑水肿存在一种由 P 物质和 NK1 受体介导的途径，这两个途径都对 NK1 受体抑制有反应。在小鼠黑色素瘤模型中，研究者试图使用福沙匹坦（阿瑞匹坦的前体药物）来减轻脑水肿，结果显示，福沙匹坦组动物肿瘤中的 P 物质和 NK1 受体表达增加，脑含水量减少，伊文思蓝外渗减少（提示血脑屏障通透性正常化）[77]。

3. 非甾体抗炎药（nonsteroidal antiinflammatory drug, NSAID）

非甾体抗炎药长期以来被认为是皮质类固醇的替代物。然而，迄今为止，并没有出现令人信服的证据[78]。

吲哚美辛是一种非选择性环氧合酶 1 和环氧合酶 2 抑制药，它很容易穿过血脑屏障[79]，减少前列腺素的合成。但吲哚美辛是否能减少脑水肿，证据并不一致[80, 81]。环氧化酶被抑制后，脂氧合酶途径发生转变并产生白三烯，而白三烯又会引起脑水肿，使得水肿并不能减轻[80]。而另一个环氧合酶和脂氧合酶的双重抑制药，甲氯芬酯钠[82]，在一个病例报道中显示出显著的活性，但在随后的使用兔脑瘤的动物模型试验中这种作用未能得到重复[83]。

4. 选择性环氧化酶 –2（cyclooxygenase-2, COX-2）抑制药

众所周知，胶质瘤中的肿瘤浸润性小胶质细胞通过环氧化酶 –2（COX-2）依赖通路产生前列腺素 E_2（prostaglandin E_2，PGE_2），促进肿瘤发生和脑水肿[49, 84, 85]。研究发现多种颅内肿瘤如原发性胶质瘤、脑膜瘤、转移性癌症（肺、乳腺、胃、黑色素瘤）内有前列腺素合成水平升高，而这种升高也被认为与肿瘤更高的分级相关。此外，血栓素 B_2（thromboxane B_2，TXB_2）和前列腺素 E_2（PGE_2）在转移瘤中均显著升高，使得 COX-2 抑制药成为一种有前景的治疗脑水肿的方法[86]。有文献证实，脑出血中环氧合酶 –2（COX-2）被抑制。在临床前期的脑出血大鼠模型中，使用 COX-2 抑制药塞来昔布进行治疗，可以减少前列腺素 E_2（PGE_2）的产生，也减轻了脑水肿（通过脑含水量测量体现），并改善了旋转棒感觉运动的试验结果[87]。随后，同一组研究人员在一项小型、多中心随机开放试验中证实塞来昔布可减少急性颅内出血的周围血肿[88]。此外，临床前证据表明塞来昔布也能抑制 VEGF 的表达[89]，这使得塞来昔布成为脑水肿研究中特别热门的候选药物。

是否能穿透血脑屏障是决定靶向小胶质细胞 COX-2 通路可行性的一个重要因素。脑脊液（cerebrospinal fluid，CSF）中的药物浓度相对容易测量，检测结果可代表脑组织药物浓度。有研究表明环氧合酶 –2 抑制药塞来昔布、罗非昔布和伐地昔布在 CSF 中的浓度普遍比血浆中低两个数量级以上[90]。但罗非昔布和伐地昔布的脑脊液浓度相对较高，超过了 COX-2 抑制浓度的中位数（IC_{50}），而塞来昔布的脑脊液浓度低于 6.3nmol/L，这个数值显著低于其 IC_{50} 值 39.3nmol/L，这表明塞来昔布对脑脊液的渗透不足，无法抑制 COX-2。然而，不同研究报道的浓度差异很大。上述研究之前，另一项临床病例报道了一名颅后窝胶质母细胞瘤患者使用塞来昔布每日 4 次、每次 200mg 的治疗结果，接受治疗后，患者塞来昔布脑脊液浓度达到 40nM，接近 IC_{50} 浓度[91]。

有趣的是，在上述颅后窝胶质母细胞瘤的病例中，使用塞来昔布治疗的患者在辅助治疗期间的两次 MRI 扫描和 2 个月后随访的扫描中都没有出现脑水肿。这导致人们很容易将这种效应归

因于塞来昔布。然而，著者指出，即使没有使用塞来昔布治疗，患者也可能不会出现瘤周水肿。目前，塞来昔布和COX-2抑制药治疗脑水肿有效的临床证据仍然很少，且仅限于病例报道。由于担忧心血管事件风险增加，以及美国食品药品管理局（Food and Drug Administration，FDA）在2005年发布的黑匣子警告[92]，人们对于将选择性COX-2抑制药作为皮质类固醇替代品的热情大大降低了。

5. 乳香

伯克和温克在1997年的一份德语研究初步报道了H_{15}在减少神经胶质瘤患者脑水肿方面的有效性，H_{15}是一种植物治疗制剂，来源于乳香树的树胶树脂（乳香）。从2001年，一项小型研究中报道了在11名神经胶质瘤患者和1名转移性黑色素瘤患者中，H_{15}表现出类似的抗水肿效果，在12名患者中，8名有临床或影像学反应，其中也包括黑色素瘤患者[93]。另一项针对2010年以来接受放射治疗的44名原发性和继发性恶性脑肿瘤患者进行的小型、安慰剂对照的双盲随机对照试验发现，与26%的安慰剂患者相比，60%接受治疗的患者（每天4200mg乳香），脑水肿减轻了75%及以上，唯一的不良反应是轻微的胃肠道不适[94]。据推测乳香的抗水肿作用是脂肪氧合酶抑制的结果[95]。同时服用含脂肪的食物似乎可以提高乳香的生物利用度[96]。虽然乳香的抗水肿疗效需要更大的随机试验来进行验证，但现有关于疗效的数据是可信的，值得进一步研究。

五、治疗后放射性脑坏死

放射治疗后，脑白质毛细血管结构和脑血管通透性可以发生变化，有可能导致治疗后几周内发生急性脑水肿。在MRI上，可表现为无强化的T_2高信号病变，并且可能仅表现为暂时和可逆的急性改变；如果有症状，通常需要使用皮质类固醇治疗[97]。

少突胶质细胞的放射性损伤可导致髓鞘合成的一过性中断，症状通常发生在治疗后数周至3个月的早期延迟反应期[98]。虽然这个过程有时会延长，但随着损伤的恢复，过程表现为自限性。其最常见的临床表现是嗜睡和乏力。

迟发性放射损伤主要是脑白质病变和放射性坏死，通常呈进行性加重且治疗困难。随着放射治疗总剂量、分割剂量和照射体积的增加，迟发性放射损伤的风险增加，即当总剂量超过60Gy和分割大小超过1.8～2Gy时风险更高[99, 100]。

辐射引起的脑坏死有两种模型：血管损伤或神经胶质损伤。在血管模型中，放疗损伤血管内皮细胞，刺激转化生长因子β（transforming growth factor-beta，TGF-β）的释放，导致微血管病变。而进行性血管功能不全导致梗死和坏死，这时将伴随血脑屏障完整性的破坏和炎性T淋巴细胞和巨噬细胞的浸润。在神经胶质损伤模型中，胶质前体的破坏导致脱髓鞘坏死和炎性浸润。浸润的巨噬细胞释放肿瘤坏死因子-α（tumor necrosis factor-alpha，TNF-α）、白细胞介素1α（interleukin-1 alpha，IL-1α）和白细胞介素6（interleukin-6，IL-6）等促炎细胞因子使慢性炎症持续存在，进一步加重内皮细胞和CNS组织的损伤[101]。由于内皮细胞的增殖率较低（长达数月），使晚期放射坏死往往在放射治疗后几个月甚至数年后才出现[102]。

放射外科可用于治疗脑转移瘤，单次剂量达到10Gy或12Gy的脑组织体积大小是放射性脑坏死风险的相关因素[103]。有时放射性脑坏死和肿瘤复发很难区分，确诊需要病理证实。不过，现在一些较为先进的成像技术，如磁共振灌注成像和2-(^{18}F)氟-脱氧-D-葡萄糖[2-(fluorine-18) fluoro-deoxy- D-glucose，FDG]正电子发射断层扫描（PET）可能有助于诊断。

六、放射性脑坏死的临床管理

放射性脑坏死的临床常用治疗模式是皮质类固醇，但现在贝伐珠单抗越来越受到重视。此外，外科手术仍然是重要的治疗方式。这些年来，诸如高压氧治疗和抗凝治疗等其他方式受到关注。但数据仅限于一些小型的随机试验，研究数据质量总体仍然很低[104]。

治疗放射性坏死的最主要方法是手术。它的优点包括快速减瘤，消除占位效应等。但是手术风险很高，受益时间也可能很短暂。因此，放射性脑坏死的显微外科治疗已不再是一线治疗方法，主要用于难治性的病例[105]。

糖皮质激素不仅可以延缓脑水肿，也有助于缓解放射性脑坏死[106, 107]。在糖皮质激素无效的情况下，越来越多的证据表明贝伐珠单抗的有效性，因此贝伐珠单抗得到较广泛的使用。VEGF在放射性坏死的病理生理学中似乎发挥着一定的作用，这也可以用贝伐珠单抗的疗效机制来解释[108]。一项针对8名放射性坏死患者的早期回顾性研究中，2周内接受5mg/kg（或每3周7.5mg/kg）的贝伐珠单抗治疗，所有患者在影像学上均有改善，日平均减少地塞米松用量8.6mg[109]。另一项回顾性研究中表明，90%的症状性放射性坏死的患者在使用贝伐珠单抗治疗后得到改善[110]。最令人信服的数据来自一项随机对照的双盲研究，在该研究中，14名放射性坏死患者每3周接受剂量7.5mg/kg的生理盐水或贝伐珠单抗治疗；在6周时依据神经学或影像学标准进行评估，所有随机接受安慰剂治疗的患者均出现恶化，而所有接受贝伐珠单抗的患者均表现出临床改善和MRI影像改善。研究中采用每3周7.5mg/kg，连续12周（4次剂量）的剂量方案的患者，中位随访10个月后，未观察到放射性脑坏死复发，因此他们建议该方案为一种合理的治疗方案[111]。2013年另一项研究报道[110]，放射性脑坏死患者接受平均剂量为7.4mg/kg和5.4mg/kg贝伐珠单抗治疗后，仍有超过一半的患者复发。随着临床经验的积累，临床医生对于贝伐珠单抗的使用剂量和时间将会越来越清楚。

高压氧疗法（hyperbaric oxygen therapy，HBOT）可以通过改善血管生成和组织灌注促进组织愈合，是一种在临床上受欢迎的用来的替代糖皮质激素和贝伐珠单抗的治疗方法。然而，尽管多年来出现了许多典型的病例报道，却仍然没有获得包括双盲安慰剂对照研究在内的确切可靠数据的证实[112]。1976年的一份报道中，一名患有"放射性脑炎"的患者每天接受两个绝对大气压（atmospheres absolute，ATA）的HBOT治疗2h。在前五次治疗中情况似乎有所恶化，但在血管扩张剂环扁桃酯联合HBOT治疗20次后，患者病情逐渐改善并恢复到可走动状态[113]。后来在1997年的一项研究中，10例发生了放射性脑坏死的儿童患者接受了每天90~120min的2.0~2.4个ATA的HBOT，连续至少20次。研究结果表明所有患者的症状都表现稳定。但由于在HBOT之前、期间和之后都使用了皮质类固醇，尚不清楚有多少效果是由HBOT单独产生的[114]。

一项随机开放标签的临床研究中将依达拉奉（一种由FDA在2017年批准的抗氧化自由基清除剂，用于治疗肌萎缩性侧索硬化）联合皮质类固醇与单用皮质类固醇进行了对比。尽管作者的结论是通过检测非增强型T_2病灶的缩小程度和依据LENT（late effects normal tissue task force）-SOMA（subjective，objective，management，analytic）标准分析，联合依达拉奉治疗组较单纯皮质类固醇组治疗脑坏死的疗效提高。但其数据及解读遭到了质疑，相对于其非常小的效应，T_2病变缩小数据的差异过大，并且两组的置信区间有重叠[115]。

除上述方法外，还有许多其他有效的方法。一些病例报道中描述抗凝可以改善微循环。典型的治疗方案是在急性期使用肝素，然后华法林维持治疗[116]。在软组织放射性坏死的临床前和小规模试点研究表明己酮可可碱，可以通过降低红细胞黏度来促进循环[117]。而己酮可可碱和维生素E联合使用似乎对其他系统器官的放射性坏死也有好处。这些结果启发了2008年的一个小型临床试验——在立体定向放射外科或全脑放射治疗后发生放射性坏死的患者中使用每天2次

400mg 的己酮可可碱和每天 2 次 400U 的维生素 E。通过对水肿的体积测量发现，除一名患者外，其余所有患者均有改善。然而其中大多数患者在急性加重时仍辅助使用了皮质类固醇[118]。激光间质热疗（laser interstitial thermal therapy，LITT）被用于症状快速恶化、皮质类固醇难治以及有贝伐珠单抗禁忌证的局灶性脑放射性坏死，目前已至少有两个成功的病例报道[119,120]。第 7 章将对激光间质热疗进行更深入地探讨。

七、癫痫发作

尽管早期证据表明预防性使用抗癫痫药物对患者有益[121]，但后来的证据并没有很好地支持这一观点。这些研究均针对脑转移性肿瘤，包括两项涉及预防性使用抗癫痫药物的非手术患者的前瞻性随机研究以及三项涉及预防性使用抗癫痫药物的术后患者研究。在针对预防性抗癫痫药物应用于非手术患者的两项研究中，未接受治疗和接受治疗的患者相比，癫痫发作率未发现有统计学差异（第一项研究中，使用药物为苯妥英钠或苯巴比妥[122]，在第二项研究中为丙戊酸钠[123]）。在三项术后预防性使用抗癫痫药物的研究中，有两项是前瞻性随机研究。一项研究显示术后使用 7 天的苯妥英钠未导致 30 天癫痫发作率有统计学意义的降低[124]，另一项研究中，术后使用苯妥英钠或苯巴比妥也未导致早期（< 1 周）或晚期（> 1 周）癫痫发作率有统计学意义的降低[125]。同样，回顾性研究发现，接受预防性抗癫痫药物治疗的患者癫痫发生率也没有降低，其中 50% 以上的患者服用了左乙拉西坦[126]。

2008 年一项 Cochrane 回顾分析发现，已有的证据既不支持也不反对苯妥英钠、苯巴比妥或丙戊酸钠在预防癫痫发作中的作用[127]。在那些预防性使用抗癫痫药物治疗的人中，不良事件的风险似乎更高，但这个结论不能扩展到苯妥英钠、苯巴比妥或丙戊酸钠之外的其他抗癫痫药物。

临床实践模式各不相同，术后使用左乙拉西坦作为临时预防用药很普遍。左乙拉西坦的耐受性优于苯妥英钠、苯巴比妥和丙戊酸钠，且大部分证据表明，后几种药物缺乏疗效，或者不良反应发生率较高，而左乙拉西坦并未发现类似的证据。毫无疑问，左乙拉西坦在抗癫痫治疗中是有效的，在一些脑转移患者中可以预防首次癫痫发作。脑转移患者是癫痫发作风险的高危人群。假设让所有患者根据经验一开始就服用最大治疗剂量的左乙拉西坦，那么可以推论，在那些将会出现症状性癫痫的患者中，至少有一部分可以预防首次发作。然而，很明显，这并不是一个最佳的方案，因为对根本不会发生癫痫的患者来说，不良反应导致的治疗负担很高。经验性降低剂量可能会降低不良反应带来的负担，但研究者不清楚较低的经验性剂量会损失多少治疗效果——因为并不清楚在较高剂量下有多少患者的癫痫发作会得到控制，而在较低剂量下有多少得不到控制。此外，研究者也不知道在此类人群中，什么剂量能使疗效达到最佳获益。因此，目前指南不支持预防性用药。2019 年神经外科医生大会建议无论是在术后还是非手术状态下，不要对无癫痫发作的患者进行预防性治疗[128]。这一观点得到了美国临床肿瘤学会和美国儿科学会的认可[129]，并与美国神经病学会实践指南中采用的立场[130] 相吻合。

八、抗癫痫药物概述

抗癫痫药物（antiepileptics，AED）细胞色素 P_{450} 酶诱导剂通常在化疗中被避免使用，因为它可能会影响化疗药物的代谢，且会以不可预知的方式来影响化疗疗效。非酶诱导的抗癫痫药物如左乙拉西坦通常比酶诱导的药物如苯妥英钠、苯巴比妥和卡马西平在临床上更受欢迎。而酶抑制药的典型药物是丙戊酸盐。

巴比妥是最古老的抗癫痫药物之一。苯巴比妥是一种半衰期相对较长的巴比妥酸盐，可静脉给予，也可口服，它可以延长 γ- 氨基丁酸（γ-aminobutyric acid，GABA）受体的开放时间。虽然在肿瘤相关治疗中的地位下降，但它仍广泛用于苯二氮䓬类难治性癫痫持续状态的急性治疗。镇静、致畸和骨质疏松是其众多不良反应中的一部分，且它属于细胞色素 P_{450} 酶诱导剂，使其仅成为脑肿瘤患者抗癫痫治疗的次要选择[131]。

苯妥英钠，类似于苯巴比妥，也是一种使用历史悠久的抗癫痫药物，临床使用较少。像许多其他的抗癫痫药物一样，苯妥英钠作用于钠通道，干扰高频重复脉冲放电。苯妥英钠不适用脑肿瘤患者，不仅因为它是一种 P_{450} 酶诱导剂，还因为其药代动力学因素及不良反应较大。这两个因素使苯妥英钠的给药复杂化，必须采用缓慢的剂量滴定法。单位剂量增加时，血浆苯妥英钠浓度的上升并非是线性增加：在较低血药浓度时，苯妥英钠浓度上升幅度较小，而在较高血药浓度时，苯妥英钠浓度上升幅度较大[132]。一旦患者接近治疗浓度，建议小幅增加剂量。苯妥英钠还与蛋白质高度亲和。在低白蛋白血症患者（老年人、孕妇、营养不良、恶性肿瘤）中，仅关注苯妥英钠的总水平将会低估苯妥英钠游离部分的药理活性。如果患者在服用其他蛋白质结合药物（如丙戊酸钠），其对蛋白质的竞争性结合将使整个方案调整更加复杂化[133]。苯妥英钠中毒的典型表现是垂直眼震和共济失调。苯妥英钠对镇静的作用小于苯巴比妥，但致畸性是一个令人担忧的问题。长期使用苯妥英钠会导致一系列不良反应，包括小脑萎缩、牙龈增生和骨质疏松。紫色手套综合征是一种罕见的严重并发症，在注射部位表现为疼痛、水肿和变色。苯妥英钠的前药磷苯妥因（Fospenytoin）可静脉注射给药，由于不会导致紫手套综合征，已取代苯妥因用于治疗癫痫持续状态[134]。

卡马西平是一种与苯妥英钠和拉莫三嗪类似的钠通道阻滞药，也是一种与苯妥英钠和苯巴比妥相似的细胞色素 P_{450} 酶诱导剂。卡马西平诱导自身的代谢，即用药数周后，需要增加剂量以维持血浆药物水平。怀孕期间的女性也会发生半衰期缩短，同样需要增加剂量。卡马西平的不良反应包括低钠血症、史 – 约综合征（Stevens-Johnson 综合征）和中毒性表皮坏死松解。携带 HLA-B1502 等位基因的患者发生中毒性表皮坏死松解的风险增加，常见于亚洲人群，因此亚洲人在开始用药前应进行此基因检测[135]。奥卡西平是卡马西平的衍生物，对细胞色素 P_{450} 酶的抑制作用不强，但常与低钠血症有关，由于半衰期较短，通常需要每日 3 次给药。艾司利卡西平是奥卡西平活性形式的前体药物，半衰期较长，允许每日 1 次给药，不良反应类似奥卡西平。

拉莫三嗪是一种有效的钠通道阻滞药，耐受性好，因此常被作为脑肿瘤患者的用药选择之一。它另一个被熟知的原因是，如果静脉滴注速度太快，有导致史 – 约综合征和毒性表皮坏死松解症的风险。使用拉莫三嗪时，应从低剂量开始，以缓慢的速率滴定，使其非常有效的同时具有良好的耐受性。相比其他 AED，它具有广谱活性，疲劳率和认知不良反应更低，以及致畸性最低的优点，还有稳定情绪的作用。此外，它每日 1 次用药方便，且不会显著干扰细胞色素 P_{450} 酶。然而，值得注意的是，像卡马西平一样，怀孕期间拉莫三嗪血药浓度可能会下降[136]。口服避孕药期间，拉莫三嗪的血药浓度也会降低[137]，需要监测。

丙戊酸钠是细胞色素 P_{450} 系统抑制药。高致畸性限制了它在育龄女性中的使用。在上述人群之外，丙戊酸钠是一种非常有效的抗癫痫药物。目前仍在癫痫患者中广泛使用，治疗浓度范围通常为 $50\sim100\mu g/ml$[138]，主要不良反应包括疲劳、胃刺激、肝毒性、高氨血症和体重增加。该药物具有口服和静脉两种剂型，由于它是一种较老的药物，价格便宜。与拉莫三嗪类似，丙戊酸钠具有稳定情绪的作用，在预防偏头痛方面有一定疗效。

托吡酯是一种口服广谱抗癫痫药物，对 α- 氨基 –3– 羟基 –5– 甲基异噁唑 –4– 本体酸（α-amino-3-hydroxy-5-methylisoxazole-4-proprionic acid,

AMPA）/红藻酸受体、GABA 和碳酸酐酶均有活性。其不良反应包括肾结石风险增加、体重减轻和严重的认知影响。托吡酯还被用作偏头痛的预防药物，以及丛集性头痛和特发性震颤。也有数据表明它还可用作情绪稳定剂[139]。除了可以控制癫痫，这些作用对于经常头痛、伴有姿势运动性震颤或情绪障碍的患者可能具有额外的优势。

唑尼沙胺是一种广谱抗癫痫药物，作用于钠通道、T 型钙通道，并像托吡酯一样作用于碳酸酐酶[140]。它的不良反应与托吡酯相似。唑尼沙胺的一个独特优势是其半衰期较长（超过 48h），从而减轻了偶尔错过服药的影响。

左乙拉西坦是应用最广泛的抗癫痫药物，它可与 SV2A（突触囊泡蛋白）结合，是一种广谱抗癫痫药物。它价格便宜、与蛋白质亲和力不高、对细胞色素 P_{450} 系统也没有明显的影响，并且可以静脉注射和口服，是大多数患者的首选。该药物不通过肝脏代谢，没有直接肾毒性。但有严重肾脏疾病时，左乙拉西坦的清除可能受阻，因此需要减少剂量。它的主要不良反应包括疲劳、易怒和抑郁，且在高剂量时更常见。布瓦西坦是左乙拉西坦的第二代衍生物，与 SV2A 的亲和力更高，进入大脑的渗透性也更好[141]。与左乙拉西坦相比，它引起的精神不良反应更少[142]。

拉考沙胺是左乙拉西坦的一种替代药物，使用广泛且耐受性良好。它与苯妥英钠、卡马西平、拉莫三嗪等药物机制类似，作用于钠通道。不同的是，拉莫三嗪并不影响钠通道的快速失活，而是增强了缓慢失活[143]。其不良反应包括恶心、疲劳和剂量依赖性的 PR 间期延长。

氯硝西泮和氯巴安定都是长效苯二氮䓬类药物，作用于 GABA 受体，它可增加氯通道打开的频率，主要的不良反应是镇静和构音障碍。

其他抗癫痫药物

吡仑帕奈是一种 AMPA 受体拮抗药，但由于有可供选择的替代药物，并不常用。由于其对行为的不良影响，是一种被警示的药物。加巴喷丁和普瑞巴林是钙通道调节药，活性不高，很少作为单一疗法使用，常用于辅助治疗。非氨基甲酸酯是一种 N-甲基–D-天冬氨酸（N-methyl-D-aspartate，NMDA）受体拮抗药，由于有引起再生障碍性贫血和肝脏毒性的风险，仅作为严重癫痫的保留用药[144]。替加宾和氨己烯酸分别是 GABA 再吸收和降解的抑制药，是抗癫痫药物的辅助药物，但因其潜在的严重不良反应而不被推荐。鲁非胺和乙氧昔胺在局灶性癫痫发作中有有限的活性，在伴有症状性癫痫的脑转移患者中亦效应不大。

九、头痛

头痛是脑转移瘤患者的常见症状。如果出现神经功能缺损、体位性头痛、恶心、呕吐和脑膜炎等症状，提示应进一步评估具体原因。头痛可能与疾病进展、脑水肿、颅内压升高、脑出血、脑积水和伤口感染或脑膜炎有关。第一步应该是确定和解决直接原因。为了缓解症状，对乙酰氨基酚可以用作一线治疗。如果对乙酰氨基酚无效，非甾体抗炎药（NSAID）可作为二线药物使用。对于化疗后骨髓抑制或出血的患者应考虑到非甾体抗炎药的血小板抑制作用。当这些相对保守的措施对于疼痛无效时，可使用阿片类药物。脑转移患者的难治性头痛往往需要疼痛或头痛专家的帮助。

我们还需要特别关注患者是否有过度用药相关性头疼，过度并长期使用镇痛剂（包括对乙酰氨基酚和非甾体抗炎药）可以诱发头疼，特别是那些每周使用镇痛剂超过 2 天，持续数周或数月以上的患者风险更大。过度用药导致的头痛与先前的头痛具有不同的特征，它表现为新发的或进行性恶化的头痛，往往在用药数月内发生并逐渐恶化，进一步使用止痛剂又会反过来加剧病情发展。日常预防性药物（如三环类抗抑郁药、选择性抗抑郁药和 β 受体拮抗药）可减轻头痛发作频率，从而减少镇痛剂的使用，起到预防过度用药引起的相关头痛的作用。虽然预防性使用药物的数据主要集中在偏头痛和紧张性头痛的文献中，但对于经常性头痛并排除了其他原因的脑转移患者也可以考虑使用。尽早发现并对有相关风险的患者进行教育很重要，这样可能使患者避免陷入困境。

十、认知障碍

长期以来，放射治疗后的认知障碍一直是令人担忧的问题，随着癌症患者寿命的延长，这一问题变得越来越重要。这种认知障碍通常涉及更高级的功能，如注意力或记忆，这可能是白质束损伤的结果，并与参与更高级认知的大脑皮质区域的萎缩有关[145]。放射治疗剂量和体积的增加似乎与认知能力下降的风险增加有关。

在保留海马齿状回亚颗粒区神经干细胞方面研究的进展，促使临床开展了对海马保护的适形放射治疗技术的研究。一项多中心Ⅱ期临床研究（RTOG 0933）中，研究者将2个月、4个月和6个月的结果与历史对照进行了比较，结果提示海马保护改善了认知功能[146]。尽管该研究结果富有前景，仍需更大规模的临床试验来证实。此外，或许更重要的是，认知功能不仅依赖于海马体，还依赖于帕佩兹回路的完整性，但很显然，这些结构在放疗时无法避开。放疗后大脑皮质下脑白质病变的严重程度也可能限制海马保护带来的获益。毫无疑问，这个问题还有待更多的探索研究。

目前还没有有效的药物可以预防或治疗放疗相关的认知障碍。多奈哌齐（一种抗胆碱酯酶）以及美金刚（一种N-甲基-D-天冬氨酸受体拮抗药）已经开始被研究用于治疗和预防放疗相关的认知障碍。

2015年启动的一项Ⅲ期安慰剂对照随机试验发现，在接受部分或全脑照射的患者中，使用多奈哌齐（5mg，6周，随后10mg，18周）的患者在24周时记忆和运动功能有了显著改善，特别是在那些治疗前认知障碍更严重的患者中改善更为明显[147]。然而，患者的综合得分并没有显著提高。2006年的一项更早的Ⅱ期研究发现，在24周时，患者的情绪及健康相关的生活质量评估也有改善，且药物毒性极小[148]。

2013年启动的一项大型Ⅲ期随机安慰剂对照临床试验，在全脑放疗开始后3天内给患者服用美金刚（每天20mg，24周），结果显示，在第8周、16周和24周时，实验组和安慰剂组的大多数认知评估得分中位值没有统计学差异，但发现实验组至出现第一次失败的神经认知测试的时间有显著延长[149]。美金刚耐受性良好，更多将美金刚用于正在接受全脑放疗的患者中的Ⅲ期临床试验正在进行中，这种药物在降低神经认知毒性方面是否有效有待相关结果证实。

十一、不确定的领域和未来发展方向

虽然糖皮质激素仍然是瘤周水肿、放疗相关水肿和放射性坏死的主要治疗手段，但学术界对其不良反应和疗效的异质性仍很关注，并正在推动研究以找寻更好的治疗方法。未来研究的方向应集中在提高对肿瘤病理生理学和放射生物学内在机制的理解。对生物学功能和靶点优化的更深入理解，将有助于找到更有效的治疗手段。

幸运的是，目前已有较多治疗脑转移患者癫痫发作的药物可供选择。通过影像学或电生理检测来优化癫痫发作的风险分层可能有助于确定哪些患者最有可能发生癫痫，从而受益于预防性治疗。

遗憾的是，头痛和认知障碍的治疗选择仍非常有限。对于头痛，特别是偏头痛的潜在机制，虽然我们在分子水平上的理解和认识获得了较大进展，但这些新进展是否能转化为更好的治疗手段还有待观察。

十二、结论与建议

脑转移患者的治疗复杂，依赖于多学科协作的模式。脑水肿的加重，无论与肿瘤相关还是与治疗相关，都是导致临床症状的根源。以症状控制所需最低剂量的糖皮质激素进行治疗，是目前疗效最好的方法。贝伐珠单抗虽然在减少脑水肿和处理对类固醇无效的放射性坏死有效，但可能会导致手术时机复杂化，并有一些少见但可能致命的不良反应。左乙拉西坦是治疗癫痫最常用的药物，但也有一些有效和可靠的替代药物供选择。虽然个体的风险需要考虑，但对于癫痫的预防性治疗目前尚没有统一的建议。因此，需要进一步研究以建立有证据支持的头痛和认知功能障碍管理指南。另外，头痛也可能是某种潜在问题的警告信号。镇痛药的使用期间必须进行适当监测，特别要注意可能出现用药过度相关的头痛。美金刚和多奈哌齐的应用虽然缺乏大规模临床试验的疗效证据，但耐受性良好，可尝试用于预防和治疗放疗后神经认知障碍。

要 点

- 对症状性脑水肿使用地塞米松，开始2mg/d，早晨给药，必要时增加剂量以改善症状。
- 考虑在所有使用地塞米松的患者中使用质子泵抑制剂（PPI）或组胺 H_2 受体拮抗药进行胃肠道不良反应的预防。在大型回顾性研究中，即使地塞米松剂量低至 0.8mg/d，持续用药超过 7 天就会增加消化性溃疡出血风险。
- 对所有使用地塞米松 $\geq$ 3mg/d，并超过 4 周或更长时间的患者进行肺孢子虫病预防。对于高危患者（艾滋病病毒感染、T 细胞计数低、营养不良），在更低糖皮质激素治疗剂量时就要考虑进行肺孢子虫病预防。
- 放射性损伤分为急性反应、早期迟发反应和晚期迟发反应，其中晚期迟发反应包括放射性坏死和进行性脑白质病变。
- 用地塞米松治疗放射性坏死。如果为难治性的，考虑每3周使用 7.5 mg/kg 贝伐珠单抗治疗，若有效继续使用 4 次以延长有效期。如果有手术机会且症状发展迅速，在某些病例中手术可能比贝伐珠单抗更合适。
- 不建议对无癫痫发作的脑转移患者进行癫痫的预防性处理。但在使用苯妥英钠和苯巴比妥进行癫痫预防的研究中，其所报道的不良反应严重影响了最终的数据和结论。因此，对于癫痫发作风险高的患者，可以考虑使用左乙拉西坦和其他现代抗癫痫药物进行预防治疗。
- 症状性癫痫患者，除非有特殊禁忌证，一线使用左乙拉西坦。拉考沙胺是一种有效但价格昂贵的替代品。丙戊酸钠有效，临床应用时间较长，且较为便宜，但在育龄女性中有使用禁忌，且并不是所有患者都耐受良好。拉莫三嗪的耐受性特别好，但必须缓慢滴注以避免皮疹。
- 托吡酯和丙戊酸钠对偏头痛有预防作用。
- 拉莫三嗪、托吡酯和丙戊酸钠有稳定情绪的作用。
- 多奈哌齐的数据有限，但该药耐受性良好，开始5mg/d，6 周后增加到 10mg/d，在 24 周时似乎改善了记忆、运动功能、情绪和健康相关的生活质量指标。
- 美金刚的数据有限。但它的耐受性很好，如果从放射治疗开始时使用，20mg/d，持续 24 周，可能有助于延迟和减缓认知能力的下降。

十三、病例介绍

（一）病例1：癫痫发作

问：亚洲男性，59岁，作家，既往患有高血压、高脂血症、阵发性室上性心动过速和控制良好的双相情感障碍。他被诊断为转移性黑色素瘤，检查中发现脑皮质有三个毫米级的增强病变，分别位于右侧额叶、右侧顶叶和左侧顶叶，周围水肿轻微，临床怀疑为转移。患者没有任何症状，神经系统体征也不明显。既往没有癫痫发作的个人或家族史。是否应该开始癫痫预防？

答：不建议对癫痫进行预防。

问：上述患者的三个病灶均接受立体定向放射治疗。肿瘤科医生给了予伊匹木单抗和纳武利尤单抗联合治疗。患者耐受良好，但是在治疗四个月后出现了第一次癫痫发作。同时没有颅内进展的证据。可以给予什么抗癫痫药物治疗？

答：左乙拉西坦通常是首选，但在双相障碍患者中可能不是最佳选择。拉考沙胺可导致PR间期延长，也不是心律失常患者的最佳选择。托吡酯的认知损害可能会过多地干扰他的工作，应该避免。丙戊酸钠和拉莫三嗪均有稳定情绪的作用，均为合理的选择。然而，鉴于血管风险，拉莫三嗪更好，同时也避免了与丙戊酸钠相关的体重增加。拉莫三嗪使用时应注意从低剂量（25mg/d）开始给药并缓慢滴注（每2周可增量25~50mg/d）。

（二）病例2：放射性坏死

问：一位64岁的白种人男性，既往不吸烟，患有高血压和2型糖尿病，诊断为非小细胞肺癌，基因检测为 *EML4-ALK* 融合突变，正在接受克唑替尼治疗。检查发现孤立性左侧Rolandic区转移灶，采用立体定向放射治疗。治疗3个月后，患者表现为头痛加重，右侧肢体无力加重，在放射治疗部位可见边界不清的不均匀增强病变并伴有周围水肿。该患者没有发现其他部位的病变，怀疑是放射性脑坏死。怎么治疗？

答：首先应该尝试皮质类固醇。考虑到症状程度如头痛加剧，右侧无力，建议服用地塞米松，剂量从4mg起始，每日两次。

问：患者的头痛和恶心有所改善，但即使增加地塞米松剂量，右侧无力仍继续进展，下一步治疗可以考虑哪些选择？

答：在这种情况下，可以考虑贝伐珠单抗，每3周给药7.5mg/kg。在Levin等的研究中，所有接受4剂（12周）治疗的患者都有持久的反应。对于类固醇治疗后仍进展的患者，若病变可切除，也可以考虑手术或LITT治疗来代替贝伐珠单抗。

参考文献

[1] Davis FG, Dolecek TA, McCarthy BJ, Villano JL. Toward determining the lifetime occurrence of metastatic brain tumors estimated from 2007 United States cancer incidence data. Neuro-Oncology. 2012;14(9):1171–7.

[2] Noh T, Walbert T. Brain metastasis: clinical manifestations, symptom management, and palliative care. In: Handbook of clinical neurology [Internet]. Elsevier; 2018 [cited 2019 Apr 13]. p. 75–88. Available from: https://linkinghub.elsevier.com/retrieve/pii/B9780128111611000062.

[3] Nayak L, Lee EQ, Wen PY. Epidemiology of brain metastases. Curr Oncol Rep. 2012;14(1):48–54.

[4] Strell C, Entschladen F. Extravasation of leukocytes in comparison to tumor cells. Cell Commun Signal [Internet]. 2008 [cited 2019 Apr 13];6(1). Available from: https://biosignal.biomedcentral.com/articles/10.1186/1478-811X-6-10.

[5] Pukrop T, Dehghani F, Chuang HN, Lohaus R, Bayanga K, Heermann S, et al. Microglia promote colonization of brain tissue by breast cancer cells in a Wnt-dependent way: microglia promote brain metastasis. Glia. 2010;58(12):1477–89.

[6] Nguyen DX, Chiang AC, Zhang XH-F, Kim JY, Kris MG, Ladanyi M, et al. WNT/TCF signaling through LEF1 and HOXB9 mediates lung adenocarcinoma metastasis. Cell.

2009;138(1):51–62.

[7] Senger DR, Van De Water L, Brown LF, Nagy JA, Yeo K-T, Yeo T-K, et al. Vascular permeability factor (VPF, VEGF) in tumor biology. Cancer Metastasis Rev. 1993;12(3–4):303–24.

[8] Persidsky Y, Ramirez SH, Haorah J, Kanmogne GD. Blood–brain barrier: structural components and function under physiologic and pathologic conditions. J Neuroimmune Pharmacol. 2006;1(3):223–36.

[9] Dobrogowska DH, Lossinsky AS, Tarnawski M, Vorbrodt AW. Increased blood–brain barrier permeability and endothelial abnormalities induced by vascular endothelial growth factor. J Neurocytol. 1998;27(3):163–73.

[10] da Fonseca ACC, Matias D, Garcia C, Amaral R, Geraldo LH, Freitas C, et al. The impact of microglial activation on blood-brain barrier in brain diseases. Front Cell Neurosci [Internet]. 2014 [cited 2019 Apr 13];8. Available from: http://journal.frontiersin.org/article/10.3389/fncel.2014.00362/abstract.

[11] Lockman PR, Mittapalli RK, Taskar KS, Rudraraju V, Gril B, Bohn KA, et al. Heterogeneous blood-tumor barrier permeability determines drug efficacy in experimental brain metastases of breast cancer. Clin Cancer Res. 2010;16(23):5664–78.

[12] Fidler IJ. The biology of brain metastasis. Cancer J. 2015;21(4):10.

[13] Lowery FJ, Yu D. Brain metastasis: unique challenges and open opportunities. Biochim Biophys Acta Rev Cancer. 2017;1867(1):49–57.

[14] Kim S-J, Kim J-S, Park ES, Lee J-S, Lin Q, Langley RR, et al. Astrocytes upregulate survival genes in tumor cells and induce protection from chemotherapy. Neoplasia. 2011;13(3):286–98.

[15] Lin NU, Lee EQ, Aoyama H, Barani IJ, Barboriak DP, Baumert BG, et al. Response assessment criteria for brain metastases: proposal from the RANO group. Lancet Oncol. 2015;16(6):e270–8.

[16] Galldiks N, Langen K-J, Albert NL, Chamberlain M, Soffietti R, Kim MM, et al. PET imaging in patients with brain metastasis—report of the RANO/PET group. Neuro-Oncology [Internet]. 2019 [cited 2019 Apr 13]; Available from: https://academic.oup.com/neuro-oncology/advance-article/doi/10.1093/neuonc/noz003/5274178.

[17] Schneider T, Kuhne JF, Bittrich P, Schroeder J, Magnus T, Mohme M, et al. Edema is not a reliable diagnostic sign to exclude small brain metastases. Ahmad A, editor. PLOS ONE. 2017;12(5):e0177217.

[18] Walcott BP, Kahle KT, Simard JM. Novel treatment targets for cerebral edema. Neurotherapeutics. 2012;9(1):65–72.

[19] Wen PY, Schiff D, Kesari S, Drappatz J, Gigas DC, Doherty L. Medical management of patients with brain tumors. J Neuro-Oncol. 2006;80(3):313–32.

[20] Bebawy JF. Perioperative steroids for peritumoral intracranial edema: a review of mechanisms, efficacy, and side effects. J Neurosurg Anesthesiol. 2012;24(3):5.

[21] Spanberger T, Berghoff AS, Dinhof C, Ilhan-Mutlu A, Magerle M, Hutterer M, et al. Extent of peritumoral brain edema correlates with prognosis, tumoral growth pattern, HIF1a expression and angiogenic activity in patients with single brain metastases. Clin Exp Metastasis. 2013;30(4):357–68.

[22] Kerschbaumer J, Bauer M, Popovscaia M, Grams AE, Thomé C, Freyschlag CF. Correlation of tumor and peritumoral edema volumes with survival in patients with cerebral metastases. Anticancer Res. 2017;37(2):871–6.

[23] Calluaud G, Terrier L-M, Mathon B, Destrieux C, Velut S, François P, et al. Peritumoral edema/tumor volume ratio: a strong survival predictor for posterior fossa metastases. Neurosurgery [Internet]. 2018 [cited 2019 Apr 13]; Available from: https://academic.oup.com/neurosurgery/advance-article/doi/10.1093/neuros/nyy222/5035747.

[24] McClelland S, Long DM. Genesis of the use of corticosteroids in the treatment and prevention of brain edema. Neurosurgery. 2008;62(4):965–8.

[25] Galicich JH, French LA, Melby JC. Use of dexamethasone in treatment of cerebral edema associated with brain tumors. J Lancet. 1961;81:46–53.

[26] Ryken TC, Kuo JS, Prabhu RS, Sherman JH, Kalkanis SN, Olson JJ. Congress of Neurological Surgeons systematic review and evidence-based guidelines on the role of steroids in the treatment of adults with metastatic brain tumors. Neurosurgery. 2019;84(3):E189–91.

[27] Batchelor T, DeAngelis LM. Medical Management of Cerebral Metastases. Neurosurg Clin N Am. 1996;7(3):435–46.

[28] Black KL, Hoff JT, McGillicuddy JE, Gebarski SS. Increased leukotriene C4 and vasogenic edema surrounding brain tumors in humans. Ann Neurol. 1986;19(6):592–5.

[29] Michinaga S, Koyama Y. Pathogenesis of brain edema and investigation into anti-edema drugs. Int J Mol Sci. 2015;16(12):9949–75.

[30] Papadopoulos MC, Saadoun S, Binder DK, Manley GT, Krishna S, Verkman AS. Molecular mechanisms of brain tumor edema. Neuroscience. 2004;129(4):1009–18.

[31] Murayi R, Chittiboina P. Glucocorticoids in the management of peritumoral brain edema: a review of molecular mechanisms. Childs Nerv Syst. 2016;32(12):2293–302.

[32] Weissman DE, Dufer D, Vogel V, Abeloff MD. Corticosteroid toxicity in neuro-oncology patients. J Neuro-Oncol. 1987;5(2):125–8.

[33] Ryken TC, McDermott M, Robinson PD, Ammirati M, Andrews DW, Asher AL, et al. The role of steroids in the management of brain metastases: a systematic review and evidence-based clinical practice guideline. J Neuro-Oncol. 2010;96(1):103–14.

[34] Vecht CJ, Hovestadt A, Verbiest HBC, van Vliet JJ, van Putten WLJ. Dose-effect relationship of dexamethasone on Karnofsky performance in metastatic brain tumors: a randomized study of doses of 4, 8, and 16 mg per day. Neurology. 1994;44(4):675.

[35] Weissman DE, Janjan NA, Erickson B, Wilson FJ, Greenberg M, Ritch PS, et al. Twice-daily tapering dexamethasone

treatment during cranial radiation for newly diagnosed brain metastases. J NeuroOncol. 1991;11(3):235–9.

[36] Ryan R, Booth S, Price S. Corticosteroid-use in primary and secondary brain tumour patients: a review. J Neuro-Oncol. 2012;106(3):449–59.

[37] Hempen C, Weiss E, Hess CF. Dexamethasone treatment in patients with brain metastases and primary brain tumors: do the benefits outweigh the sideeffects? Support Care Cancer. 2002;10(4):322–8.

[38] Conn HO, Blitzer BL. Nonassociation of adrenocorticosteroid therapy and peptic ulcer. N Engl J Med. 1976;294(9):473–9.

[39] Messer J, Reitman D, Sacks HS, Smith H, Chalmers TC. Association of adrenocorticosteroid therapy and peptic-ulcer disease. N Engl J Med. 1983;309(1):21–4.

[40] Conn HO, Poynard T. Adrenocorticosteroid administration and peptic ulcer: a critical analysis. J Chronic Dis. 1985;38(6):457–68.

[41] Gøtzsche PC. Steroids and peptic ulcer: an end to the controversy? J Intern Med. 1994;236(6):599–601.

[42] Narum S, Westergren T, Klemp M. Corticosteroids and risk of gastrointestinal bleeding: a systematic review and meta-analysis. BMJ Open. 2014;4(5):e004587.

[43] Kondo Y, Hatta W, Koike T, Takahashi Y, Saito M, Kanno T, et al. The use of higher dose steroids increases the risk of rebleeding after endoscopic hemostasis for peptic ulcer bleeding. Dig Dis Sci. 2018;63(11):3033–40.

[44] Tseng C-L, Chen Y-T, Huang C-J, Luo J-C, Peng Y-L, Huang D-F, et al. Short-term use of glucocorticoids and risk of peptic ulcer bleeding: a nationwide population-based case-crossover study. Aliment Pharmacol Ther. 2015;42(5):599–606.

[45] Piper JM. Corticosteroid use and peptic ulcer disease: role of nonsteroidal anti-inflammatory drugs. Ann Intern Med. 1991;114(9):735.

[46] Baden LR, Swaminathan S, Angarone M, Blouin G, Camins BC, Casper C, et al. Prevention and treatment of cancer-related infections, version 2.2016, NCCN clinical practice guidelines in oncology. J Natl Compr Cancer Netw. 2016;14(7):882–913.

[47] Yale SH, Limper AH. Pneumocystis carinii pneumonia in patients without acquired immunodeficiency syndrome: associated illnesses and prior corticosteroid therapy. Mayo Clin Proc. 1996;71(1):5–13.

[48] Calero-Bernal ML, Martin-Garrido I, DonazarEzcurra M, Limper AH, Carmona EM. Intermittent courses of corticosteroids also present a risk for Pneumocystis pneumonia in non-HIV patients. Can Respir J. 2016;2016:1–7.

[49] Wick W, Küker W. Brain edema in neurooncology: radiological assessment and management. Oncol Res Treat. 2004;27(3):261–6.

[50] LoPiccolo J, Mehta SA, Lipson EJ. Corticosteroid use and pneumocystis pneumonia prophylaxis: a teachable moment. JAMA Intern Med. 2018;178(8):1106.

[51] Giles AJ, Hutchinson M-KND, Sonnemann HM, Jung J, Fecci PE, Ratnam NM, et al. Dexamethasoneinduced immunosuppression: mechanisms and implications for immunotherapy. J Immunother Cancer [Internet]. 2018 [cited 2019 Apr 13];6(1). Available from: https://jitc.biomedcentral.com/articles/10.1186/s40425-018-0371-5.

[52] Weber JS, Hodi FS, Wolchok JD, Topalian SL, Schadendorf D, Larkin J, et al. Safety profile of nivolumab monotherapy: a pooled analysis of patients with advanced melanoma. J Clin Oncol. 2017;35(7):785–92.

[53] Berghoff AS, Preusser M. Anti-angiogenic therapies in brain metastases. memo – Mag Eur Med Oncol. 2018;11(1):14–7.

[54] Banks PD, Lasocki A, Lau PKH, Sandhu S, McArthur G, Shackleton M. Bevacizumab as a steroid-sparing agent during immunotherapy for melanoma brain metastases: a case series. Health Sci Rep. 2019;2(3):e115.

[55] Wang Y, Wang E, Pan L, Dai J, Zhang N, Wang X, et al. A new strategy of CyberKnife treatment system based radiosurgery followed by early use of adjuvant bevacizumab treatment for brain metastasis with extensive cerebral edema. J Neuro-Oncol. 2014;119(2):369–76.

[56] Hapani S, Chu D, Wu S. Risk of gastrointestinal perforation in patients with cancer treated with bevacizumab: a meta-analysis. Lancet Oncol. 2009;10(6):559–68.

[57] Saif MW, Elfiky A, Salem RR. Gastrointestinal perforation due to bevacizumab in colorectal cancer. Ann Surg Oncol. 2007;14(6):1860–9.

[58] Khasraw M, Holodny A, Goldlust SA, DeAngelis LM. Intracranial hemorrhage in patients with cancer treated with bevacizumab: the memorial Sloan-Kettering experience. Ann Oncol. 2012;23(2):458–63.

[59] Carden CP, Larkin JMG, Rosenthal MA. What is the risk of intracranial bleeding during anti-VEGF therapy? Neuro-Oncology. 2008;10(4):624–30.

[60] Besse B, Lasserre SF, Compton P, Huang J, Augustus S, Rohr U-P. Bevacizumab safety in patients with central nervous system metastases. Clin Cancer Res. 2010;16(1):269–78.

[61] Socinski MA, Langer CJ, Huang JE, Kolb MM, Compton P, Wang L, et al. Safety of bevacizumab in patients with non–small-cell lung cancer and brain metastases. J Clin Oncol. 2009;27(31):5255–61.

[62] Gordon CR, Rojavin Y, Patel M, Zins JE, Grana G, Kann B, et al. A review on bevacizumab and surgical wound healing: an important warning to all surgeons. Ann Plast Surg. 2009;62(6):707–9.

[63] Gerstner ER, Duda DG, di Tomaso E, Ryg PA, Loeffler JS, Sorensen AG, et al. VEGF inhibitors in the treatment of cerebral edema in patients with brain cancer. Nat Rev Clin Oncol. 2009;6(4):229–36.

[64] Eichler AF, Loeffler JS. Multidisciplinary management of brain metastases. Oncologist. 2007; 12(7):884–98.

[65] Pope WB, Lai A, Nghiemphu P, Mischel P, Cloughesy TF. MRI in patients with high-grade gliomas treated with bevacizumab and chemotherapy. Neurology. 2006;66(8):1258–60.

[66] Berghoff AS, Ilhan-Mutlu A, Dinhof C, Magerle M, Hackl

[66] M, Widhalm G, et al. Differential role of angiogenesis and tumour cell proliferation in brain metastases according to primary tumour type: analysis of 639 cases. Neuropathol Appl Neurobiol. 2015;41(2):e41–55.

[67] Wei ET, Gao GC. Corticotropin-releasing factor: an inhibitor of vascular leakage in rat skeletal muscle and brain cortex after injury. Regul Pept. 1991;33(2):93–104.

[68] Tjuvajev J, Uehara H, Desai R, Beattie B, Matei C, Zhou Y, et al. Corticotropin-releasing factor decreases vasogenic brain edema. Cancer Res. 1996;56(6):1352–60.

[69] Villalona-Calero MA, Eckardt J, Burris H, Kraynak M, Fields-Jones S, Bazan C, et al. A phase I trial of human corticotropin-releasing factor (hCRF) in patients with peritumoral brain edema. Ann Oncol. 1998;9(1):71–7.

[70] Recht L, Mechtler LL, Wong ET, O'Connor PC, Rodda BE. Steroid-sparing effect of corticorelin acetate in peritumoral cerebral edema is associated with improvement in steroid-induced myopathy. J Clin Oncol. 2013;31(9):1182–7.

[71] Recht LD, Mechtler L, Phuphanich S, Hormigo A, Hines V, Milsted R, et al. A placebo-controlled study investigating the dexamethasone-sparing effects of corticorelin acetate in patients with primary or metastatic brain tumors and peritumoral edema. J Clin Oncol. 2009;27(15_suppl):2078.

[72] Shapiro WR, Mechtler L, Cher L, Wheeler H, Hines V, Milsted R, et al. A randomized, double-blind study comparing corticorelin acetate with dexamethasone in patients with primary malignant glioma who require increased dexamethasone doses to control symptoms of peritumoral brain edema. J Clin Oncol. 2009;27(15_suppl):2080.

[73] Mechtler L, Wong ET, Hormigo A, Pannullo S, Hines V, Milsted R, et al. A long-term open-label extension study examining the steroid-sparing effects of corticorelin acetate in patients with cerebral tumors. J Clin Oncol. 2009;27(15_suppl):2079.

[74] Donkin JJ, Nimmo AJ, Cernak I, Blumbergs PC, Vink R. Substance P is associated with the development of brain edema and functional deficits after traumatic brain injury. J Cereb Blood Flow Metab. 2009;29(8):1388–98.

[75] Gabrielian L, Helps SC, Thornton E, Turner RJ, Leonard AV, Vink R. Substance P antagonists as a novel intervention for brain edema and raised intracranial pressure. In: Katayama Y, Maeda T, Kuroiwa T, editors. Brain edema XV [Internet]. Vienna: Springer Vienna; 2013 [cited 2019 Apr 16]. p. 201–4. Available from: http://link.springer.com/10.1007/978-3-7091-1434-6_37.

[76] Turner RJ, Helps SC, Thornton E, Vink R. A substance P antagonist improves outcome when administered 4 h after onset of ischaemic stroke. Brain Res. 2011;1393:84–90.

[77] Harford-Wright E, Lewis KM, Ghabriel MN, Vink R. Treatment with the NK1 antagonist emend reduces blood brain barrier dysfunction and edema formation in an experimental model of brain tumors. Alonso MM, editor. PLoS ONE. 2014;9(5):e97002.

[78] Rutz HP. Effects of corticosteroid use on treatment of solid tumours. Lancet. 2002;360(9349):1969–70.

[79] Bannwarth B, Netter P, Lapicque F, Péré P, Thomas P, Gaucher A. Plasma and cerebrospinal fluid concentrations of indomethacin in humans: relationship to analgesic activity. Eur J Clin Pharmacol. 1990;38(4):343–6.

[80] Cotev S, Shapira Y, Davidson E, Wiedenfeld Y, Icu ES. Indomethacin reduces cerebral prostaglandin synthesis but not edema after experimental head injury. Crit Care Med. 1987;15(4):370.

[81] Deluga KS, Plötz FB, Betz AL. Effect of indomethacin on edema following single and repetitive cerebral ischemia in the gerbil. Stroke. 1991;22(10):1259–64.

[82] Ambrus JL, Halpern J, Baerwald H, Johnson RJ. Cyclo-oxygenase and lipo-oxygenase inhibitors may substitute for steroid treatment in brain oedema. Lancet. 1985;2(8447):148–9.

[83] Weissman DE, Stewart C. Experimental drug therapy of peritumoral brain edema. J NeuroOncol [Internet]. 1988 [cited 2019 Apr 17];6(4). Available from: http://link.springer.com/10.1007/BF00177429.

[84] Nathoo N. The eicosanoid cascade: possible role in gliomas and meningiomas. J Clin Pathol. 2004;57(1):6–13.

[85] Badie B, Schartner JM, Hagar AR, Prabakaran S, Peebles TR, Bartley B, et al. Microglia cyclooxygenase-2 activity in experimental gliomas: possible role in cerebral edema formation. Clin Cancer Res. 2003;9(2):872–7.

[86] Castelli MG, Chiabrando C, Fanelli R, Martelli L, Butti G, Gaetani P, et al. Prostaglandin and thromboxane synthesis by human intracranial tumors. Cancer Res. 1989;49(6):1505–8.

[87] Chu K, Jeong S-W, Jung K-H, Han S-Y, Lee S-T, Kim M, et al. Celecoxib induces functional recovery after intracerebral hemorrhage with reduction of brain edema and perihematomal cell death. J Cereb Blood Flow Metab. 2004;24(8):926–33.

[88] Lee S-H, Park H-K, Ryu W-S, Lee J-S, Bae H-J, Han M-K, et al. Effects of celecoxib on hematoma and edema volumes in primary intracerebral hemorrhage: a multicenter randomized controlled trial. Eur J Neurol. 2013;20(8):1161–9.

[89] Wei D, Wang L, He Y, Xiong HQ, Abbruzzese JL, Xie K. Celecoxib inhibits vascular endothelial growth factor expression in and reduces angiogenesis and metastasis of human pancreatic cancer via suppression of Sp1 transcription factor activity. Cancer Res. 2004;64(6):2030–8.

[90] Dembo G, Park SB, Kharasch ED. Central nervous system concentrations of cyclooxygenase-2 inhibitors in humans. Anesthesiology. 2005;102(2):409–15.

[91] Rutz HP, Hofer S, Peghini PE, Gutteck-Amsler U, Rentsch K, Meier-Abt PJ, et al. Avoiding glucocorticoid administration in a neurooncological case. Cancer Biol Ther. 2005;4(11):1186–9.

[92] Lenzer J. FDA advisers warn: COX 2 inhibitors increase risk of heart attack and stroke. BMJ. 2005;330(7489):440.

[93] Streffer JR, Bitzer M, Schabet M, Dichgans J, Weller M. Response of radiochemotherapy-associated cerebral edema

to a phytotherapeutic agent, H15. Neurology. 2001;56(9): 1219–21.
[94] Kirste S, Treier M, Wehrle SJ, Becker G, AbdelTawab M, Gerbeth K, et al. Boswellia serrata acts on cerebral edema in patients irradiated for brain tumors: a prospective, randomized, placebo-controlled, double-blind pilot trial. Cancer. 2011;117(16):3788–95.
[95] Glaser T, Winter S, Groscurth P, Safayhi H, Sailer E-R, Ammon HPT, et al. Boswellic acids and malignant glioma: induction of apoptosis but no modulation of drug sensitivity. Br J Cancer. 1999;80(5–6):756–65.
[96] Sterk V, Büchele B, Simmet T. Effect of food intake on the bioavailability of boswellic acids from a herbal preparation in healthy volunteers. Planta Med. 2004;70(12):1155–60.
[97] Burger PC, Mahaley MS, Dudka L, Vogel FS. The morphologic effects of radiation administered therapeutically for intracranial gliomas. A Postmortem study of 25 cases. Cancer. 1979;44(4):1256–72.
[98] Fink J, Born D, Chamberlain MC. Radiation necrosis: relevance with respect to treatment of primary and secondary brain tumors. Curr Neurol Neurosci Rep. 2012;12(3):276–85.
[99] Constine LS, Konski A, Ekholm S, McDonald S, Rubin P. Adverse effects of brain irradiation correlated with MR and CT imaging. Int J Radiat Oncol Biol Phys. 1988;15(2):319–30.
[100] Shah R, Vattoth S, Jacob R, Manzil FFP, O'Malley JP, Borghei P, et al. Radiation necrosis in the brain: imaging features and differentiation from tumor recurrence. Radiographics. 2012;32(5):13 43–59.
[101] Eissner G, Kohlhuber F, Grell M, Ueffing M, Scheurich P, Hieke A. Critical involvement of transmembrane tumor necrosis factor-cu in endothelial programmed cell death mediated by ionizing radiation and bacterial endotoxin. Blood. 1995;86(11):4184–93.
[102] Yoshii Y. Pathological review of late cerebral radionecrosis. Brain Tumor Pathol. 2008;25(2):51–8.
[103] Lawrence YR, Li XA, el Naqa I, Hahn CA, Marks LB, Merchant TE, et al. Radiation dose–volume effects in the brain. Int J Radiat Oncol Biol Phys. 2010;76(3 Suppl):S20–7.
[104] Chung C, Bryant A, Brown PD. Interventions for the treatment of brain radionecrosis after radiotherapy or radiosurgery. Cochrane Gynaecological, Neuro-oncology and Orphan Cancer Group, editor. Cochrane Database Syst Rev [Internet]. 2018 [cited 2019 Apr 13]; Available from: http://doi.wiley. com/10.1002/14651858.CD011492.pub2.
[105] McPherson CM, Warnick RE. Results of contemporary surgical management of radiation necrosis using frameless stereotaxis and intraoperative magnetic resonance imaging. J Neuro-Oncol. 2004;68(1):41–7.
[106] Eyster EF, Nielsen SL, Sheline GE, Wilson CB. Cerebral radiation necrosis simulating a brain tumor. J Neurosurg. 1974;40(2):267–71.
[107] Shaw PJ, Bates D. Conservative treatment of delayed cerebral radiation necrosis. J Neurol Neurosurg Psychiatry. 1984;47(12):1338–41.
[108] Furuse M, Nonoguchi N, Kawabata S, Miyatake S-I, Kuroiwa T. Delayed brain radiation necrosis: pathological review and new molecular targets for treatment. Med Mol Morphol. 2015;48(4):183–90.
[109] Gonzalez J, Kumar AJ, Conrad CA, Levin VA. Effect of bevacizumab on radiation necrosis of the brain. Int J Radiat Oncol Biol Phys. 2007;67(2): 323–6.
[110] Deibert CP, Ahluwalia MS, Sheehan JP, Link MJ, Hasegawa T, Yomo S, et al. Bevacizumab for refractory adverse radiation effects after stereotactic radiosurgery. J Neuro-Oncol. 2013;115(2):217–23.
[111] Levin VA, Bidaut L, Hou P, Kumar AJ, Wefel JS, Bekele BN, et al. Randomized double-blind placebocontrolled trial of bevacizumab therapy for radiation necrosis of the central nervous system. Int J Radiat Oncol Biol Phys. 2011;79(5):1487–95.
[112] Bennett MH, Feldmeier J, Hampson NB, Smee R, Milross C. Hyperbaric oxygen therapy for late radiation tissue injury. Cochrane Gynaecological, Neuro-oncology and Orphan Cancer Group, editor. Cochrane Database Syst Rev [Internet]. 2016 [cited 2019 Apr 13]; Available from: http://doi.wiley. com/10.1002/14651858.CD005005.pub4.
[113] Hary GB, Mainous EG. The treatment of radiation necrosis with hyperbaric oxygen (OHP). Cancer. 1976;37(6):2580–5.
[114] Chuba PJ, Aronin P, Bhambhani K, Eichenhorn M, Zamarano L, Cianci P, et al. Hyperbaric oxygen therapy for radiation-induced brain injury in children. Cancer. 1997;80(10): 2005–12.
[115] Tang Y, Rong X, Hu W, Li G, Yang X, Yang J, et al. Effect of edaravone on radiation-induced brain necrosis in patients with nasopharyngeal carcinoma after radiotherapy: a randomized controlled trial. J Neuro-Oncol. 2014;120(2):441–7.
[116] Rizzoli HV, Pagnanelli DM. Treatment of delayed radiation necrosis of the brain. J Neurosurg. 1984;60(3):589–94.
[117] Dion MW, Hussey DH, Doornbos JF, Vigliotti AP, Wen B-C, Anderson B. Preliminary results of a pilot study of pentoxifylline in the treatment of late radiation soft tissue necrosis. Int J Radiat Oncol Biol Phys. 1990;19(2):401–7.
[118] Williamson R, Kondziolka D, Kanaan H, Lunsford LD, Flickinger JC. Adverse radiation effects after radiosurgery may benefit from oral vitamin E and pentoxifylline therapy: a pilot study. Stereotact Funct Neurosurg. 2008;86(6):359–66.
[119] Rahmathulla G, Recinos PF, Valerio JE, Chao S, Barnett GH. Laser interstitial thermal therapy for focal cerebral radiation necrosis: a case report and literature review. Stereotact Funct Neurosurg. 2012;90(3):192–200.
[120] Fabiano AJ, Alberico RA. Laser-interstitial thermal therapy for refractory cerebral edema from post-radiosurgery metastasis. World Neurosurg. 2014;81(3–4):652.e1–4.
[121] North JB, Hanieh A, Challen Robert G, Penhall Robert K, Hann Christopher S, Frewin DB. Postoperative epilepsy: a double-blind trial of phenytoin after craniotomy. Lancet.

[122] Forsyth PA, Weaver S, Fulton D, Brasher PMA, Sutherland G, Stewart D, et al. Prophylactic anticonvulsants in patients with brain tumour. Can J Neurol Sci. 2003;30(02):106–12.

[123] Glantz MJ, Cole BF, Friedberg MH, Lathi E, Choy H, Furie K, et al. A randomized, blinded, placebo- controlled trial of divalproex sodium prophylaxis in adults with newly diagnosed brain tumors. Neurology. 1996;46(4):985–91.

[124] Wu AS, Trinh VT, Suki D, Graham S, Forman A, Weinberg JS, et al. A prospective randomized trial of perioperative seizure prophylaxis in patients with intraparenchymal brain tumors. J Neurosurg. 2013;118(4):873–83.

[125] Franceschetti S, Binelli S, Casazza M, Lodrini S, Panzica F, Pluchino F, et al. Influence of surgery and antiepileptic drugs on seizures symptomatic of cerebral tumours. Acta Neurochir. 1990;103(1–2): 47–51.

[126] Ansari SF, Bohnstedt BN, Perkins SM, Althouse SK, Miller JC. Efficacy of postoperative seizure prophylaxis in intra-axial brain tumor resections. J NeuroOncol. 2014;118(1):117–22.

[127] Tremont-Lukats IW, Ratilal BO, Armstrong T, Gilbert MR. Antiepileptic drugs for preventing seizures in people with brain tumors. Cochrane Database Syst Rev [Internet]. 2008 [cited 2019 Apr 20];(2). Available from: https://www.cochranelibrary.com/cdsr/doi/10.1002/14651858.CD004424.pub2/abstract.

[128] Chen CC, Rennert RC, Olson JJ. Congress of Neurological Surgeons systematic review and evidence-based guidelines on the role of prophylactic anticonvulsants in the treatment of adults with metastatic brain tumors. Neurosurgery. 2019;84(3):E195–7.

[129] Chang SM, Messersmith H, Ahluwalia M, Andrews D, Brastianos PK, Gaspar LE, et al. Anticonvulsant prophylaxis and steroid use in adults with metastatic brain tumors: summary of SNO and ASCO endorsement of the Congress of Neurological Surgeons guidelines. Neuro-Oncology. 2019;21(4):424–7.

[130] Glantz MJ, Cole BF, Forsyth PA, Recht LD, Wen PY, Chamberlain MC, et al. Practice parameter: anticonvulsant prophylaxis in patients with newly diagnosed brain tumors: report of the quality standards Subcommittee of the American Academy of Neurology. Neurology. 2000;54(10):1886–93.

[131] Waxman DJ, Azaroff L. Phenobarbital induction of cytochrome P-450 gene expression. Biochem J. 1992; 281(3):577–92.

[132] Jusko WJ, Koup JR, Alván G. Nonlinear assessment of phenytoin bioavailability. J Pharmacokinet Biopharm. 1976;4(4):327–36.

[133] Monks A, Boobis S, Wadsworth J, Richens A. Plasma protein binding interaction between phenytoin and valproic acid in vitro. Br J Clin Pharmacol. 1978;6(6):487–92.

[134] Chokshi R, Openshaw J, Mehta NN, Mohler E. Purple glove syndrome following intravenous phenytoin administration. Vasc Med. 2007;12(1): 29–31.

[135] Ferrell PB, McLeod HL. Carbamazepine, HLAB*1502 and risk of Stevens–Johnson syndrome and toxic epidermal necrolysis: US FDA recommendations. Pharmacogenomics. 2008;9(10):1543–6.

[136] Tran TA, Leppik IE, Blesi K, Sathanandan ST, Remmel R. Lamotrigine clearance during pregnancy. Neurology. 2002;59(2):251–5.

[137] Sabers A, Buchholt JM, Uldall P, Hansen EL. Lamotrigine plasma levels reduced by oral contraceptives. Epilepsy Res. 2001;47(1–2):151–4.

[138] Turnbull DM, Rawlins MD, Weightman D, Chadwick DW. Plasma concentrations of sodium valproate: their clinical value. Ann Neurol. 1983;14(1):38–42.

[139] Marcotte D. Use of topiramate, a new antiepileptic as a mood stabilizer. J Affect Disord. 1998;50(2–3):245–51.

[140] Leppik IE. Zonisamide: chemistry, mechanism of action, and pharmacokinetics. Seizure. 2004;13:S5–9.

[141] Rosenstiel P. Brivaracetam (UCB 34714). Neurotherapeutics. 2007;4(1):84–7.

[142] Biton V, Berkovic SF, Abou-Khalil B, Sperling MR, Johnson ME, Lu S. Brivaracetam as adjunctive treatment for uncontrolled partial epilepsy in adults: a phase III randomized, double-blind, placebocontrolled trial. Epilepsia. 2014;55(1):57–66.

[143] Doty P, Rudd GD, Stoehr T, Thomas D. Lacosamide. Neurotherapeutics. 2007;4(1):145–8.

[144] Kaufman DW, Kelly JP, Anderson T, Harmon DC, Shapiro S. Evaluation of case reports of aplastic anemia among patients treated with felbamate. Epilepsia. 1997;38(12):1265–9.

[145] Seibert TM, Karunamuni R, Kaifi S, Burkeen J, Connor M, Krishnan AP, et al. Cerebral cortex regions selectively vulnerable to radiation dosedependent atrophy. Int J Radiat Oncol Biol Phys. 2017;97(5):910–8.

[146] Gondi V, Pugh SL, Tome WA, Caine C, Corn B, Kanner A, et al. Preservation of memory with conformal avoidance of the hippocampal neural stemcell compartment during whole-brain radiotherapy for brain metastases (RTOG 0933): a phase II multiinstitutional trial. J Clin Oncol. 2014;32(34):3810–6.

[147] Rapp SR, Case LD, Peiffer A, Naughton MM, Chan MD, Stieber VW, et al. Donepezil for irradiated brain tumor survivors: a phase III randomized placebo-controlled clinical trial. J Clin Oncol. 2015;33(15):1653–9.

[148] Shaw EG, Rosdhal R, D'Agostino RB, Lovato J, Naughton MJ, Robbins ME, et al. Phase II study of donepezil in irradiated brain tumor patients: effect on cognitive function, mood, and quality of life. J Clin Oncol. 2006;24(9):1415–20.

[149] Brown PD, Pugh S, Laack NN, Wefel JS, Khuntia D, Meyers C, et al. Memantine for the prevention of cognitive dysfunction in patients receiving whole-brain radiotherapy: a randomized, doubleblind, placebo-controlled trial. Neuro-Oncology. 2013;15(10):1429–37.

第 5 章 脑转移瘤的神经影像学诊断
Neuroimaging of Brain Metastases

Mira A. Patel　Eric Lis　Yoshiya Yamada　著
谭兆华　译
周　琴　校

一、大脑成像概述

采用钆对比剂的头部增强 MRI 检查是评估脑转移瘤最有效的成像方式。与 CT 相比，MRI 的优势在于它能够区分 CNS 组织，并且具有更高的软组织分辨能力。T_1（纵向弛豫时间）和 T_2（横向弛豫时间）加权成像是评价脑转移瘤的标准 MR 序列。

T_1 加权像可以检测正常脑组织中的异常信号。在 T_1 加权像上，灰质表现为低信号，白质表现为较高信号。CSF 在 T_1 加权像表现为低信号，钆对比剂增强 MRI 中血管增强明显，通常呈高信号，而脑转移瘤常常表现为类球形结构，随钆的累积而增强。如果转移瘤中心没有钆对比剂的灌注，则会表现为环形强化。值得注意的是，炎症或水肿在 T_1 像上表现为低信号[1]。

T_2 加权像是评估肿瘤相关血管源性脑水肿程度的理想选择。CSF 在 T_2 加权像上特征性地表现为高信号，白质表现为低信号，而灰质表现为较高信号。水肿在 T_2 像表现为高信号，磁共振成像液体衰减反转恢复序列（fluid attenuated inversion recovery，FLAIR）与 T_2 加权成像类似，不同之处是在 FLAIR 上，CSF 信号受到抑制。由于这种特性，FLAIR 序列能更好地识别脑室周围强化病灶，并将血管源性水肿与脑脊液分辨开来。

脑转移瘤通常位于灰质与白质的交界处，且边界清楚，对周围脑组织有压迫效应。脑转移瘤是否合并出血，或者伴有明显水肿带均取决于原发肿瘤的组织学类型。

二、神经解剖学

大脑从前往后被一条深沟分为左右两个半球。中央沟是界定大脑额叶和顶叶的边界[2]（图 5-1）。中央沟是一条走行在脑断面外缘一直延伸至顶点的中线，在轴位成像上像极了 Ω 标志，这两种标志都可以用于辨别中央前回和中央后回（图 5-1）。此外，中央前回（运动区）不被脑沟分割。额叶的上矢状窦沟终止于运动区前方，从不横切运动区。外侧裂将顶叶和额叶与颞叶分开，大脑中动脉走行在外侧裂中。顶叶和枕叶被顶枕沟分隔。

（一）额叶和顶叶

额叶负责执行功能并且控制包括判断力、推理力、创造力和抑制能力在内的联想行为。运动皮层是额叶皮质最后面的一个区域，位于中央沟的前部[3,4]。

嗅束位于额叶的眶面。顶叶位于额叶的后部以及枕叶的前面。顶叶重要的皮质结构包括中央后回的感觉皮质，它紧靠中央沟的后面。

临床相关性

如果额叶脑转移瘤累及中央前回或引起该

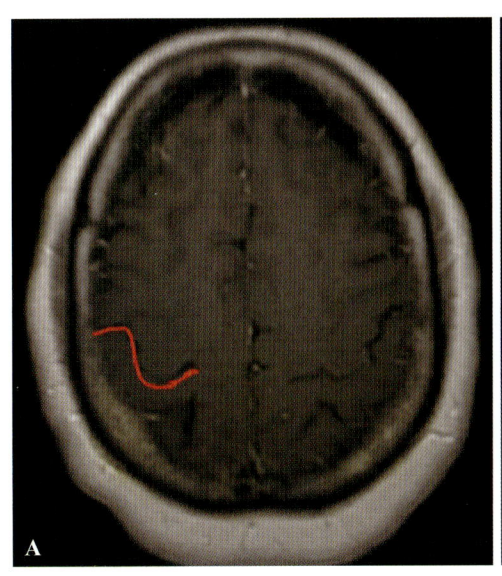

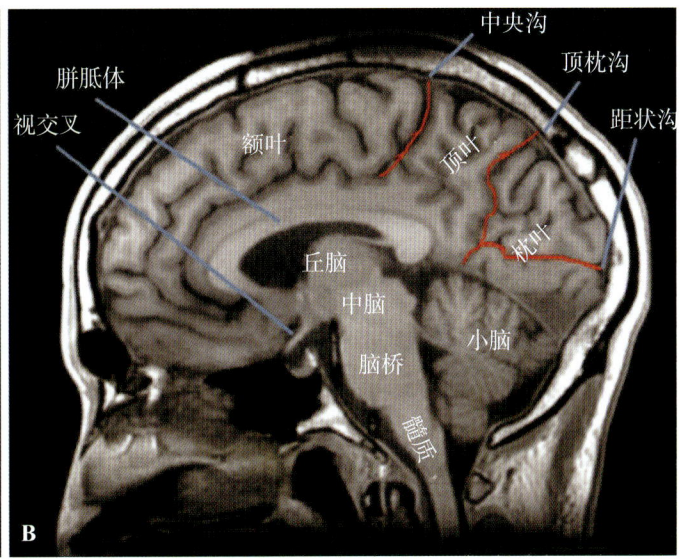

▲ 图 5-1　A. 轴位 T_1 加权图像，红色线呈 Ω 形，用来代表分离额叶和顶叶的中央沟。B. 矢状位 T_1 加权图像显示正常脑解剖，红色表示主脑沟

部位出现明显的血管源性水肿，肿瘤可能导致运动功能障碍。布罗卡区位于额叶前下，是额叶一个重要的语言产生中枢，如果受到影响可能会导致表达性失语症。额叶前部的脑转移瘤通常不会导致明显的行为抑制或认知功能障碍，但是额叶脑转移瘤过大可能会导致对侧中线移位（图 5-2）。

顶叶病变通常不表现为病理性神经学缺陷，但如果累及中央后回，则可能与感觉障碍有关。就像额叶一样，顶叶的大体积脑转移瘤伴随血管源性水肿可能导致中线移位或颅内压增加（increased intracranial pressure，ICP），引起头痛、恶心、呕吐，甚至在少数情况下引起小脑扁桃体疝。

（二）颞叶

颞叶位于额叶和顶叶下方，是大脑重要的语言和记忆中心。左侧颞叶后部包括韦尼克区，是掌管语言理解的区域。海马位于内侧颞叶，在冠状位成像上可见[5]（图 5-3）。海马体是边缘系统的重要结构，主要负责长期记忆和调节情绪。

临床相关性

根据肿瘤所处位置的不同，位于颞叶的脑转移瘤可能表现为语言障碍或记忆缺陷。患者通常有语言理解障碍，并且表现出接受性失语症。癫痫发作最常见于颞叶转移的患者。颞叶的微小转移可能不会出现任何症状。

（三）间脑和基底神经节大脑皮质

间脑由丘脑和下丘脑所组成。双侧丘脑传递感觉信息大脑皮质，并介导视听反射[6]。下丘脑调节内分泌功能，并通过垂体柄与脑垂体进行信息交流。基底神经节包括内囊、屏状核、苍白球、尾状核、杏仁核和壳核，负责情绪、认知功能，以及运动和感觉信息的整合[7, 8]（图 5-4）。岛叶也是边缘系统的一部分，负责情感体验；同样是大脑皮质的一部分，折叠在大脑外侧裂内（图 5-4）。

临床相关性

如果间脑和基底神经节的脑转移瘤体积很大，可能会阻碍脑脊液的流动，导致脑积水和相关症状。丘脑或内囊的转移瘤会引起明显的水肿，进而破坏外侧和皮质的信息传递，导致躯体感觉障碍。

（四）小脑

小脑位于大脑下方的颅后窝，分为四个部

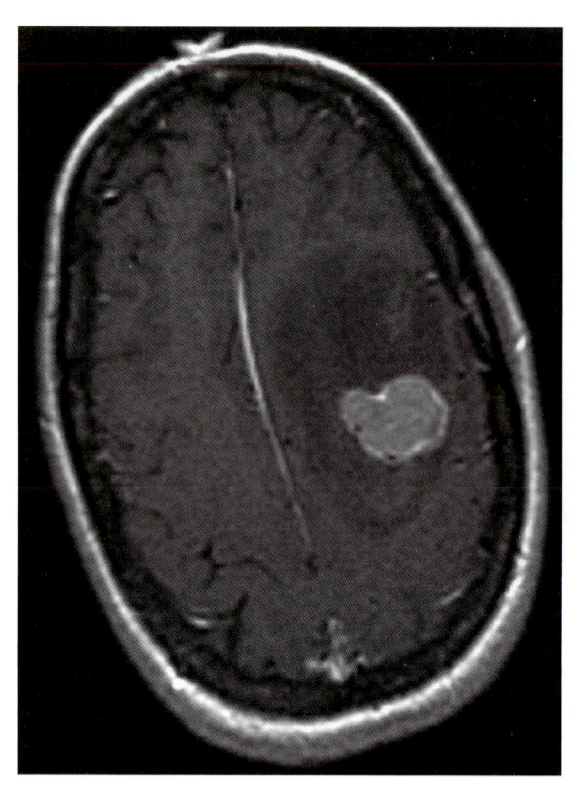

▲ 图 5-2 轴位 T_1 增强加权图像显示左额叶脑转移瘤明显增强，伴随周围低信号血管源性水肿，导致右侧中线偏移

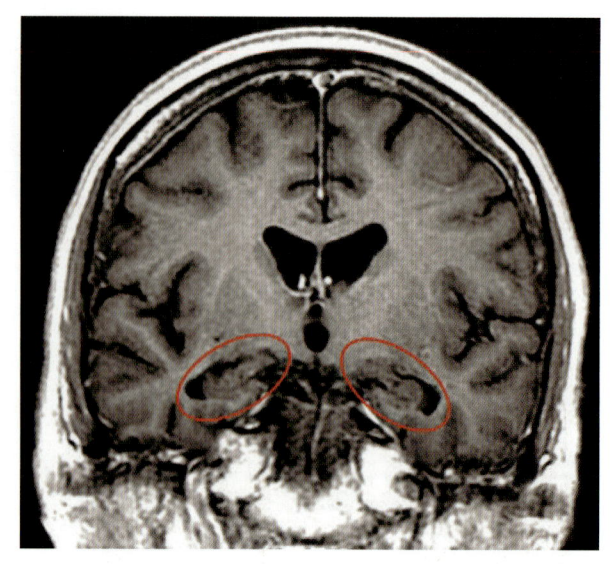

▲ 图 5-3 冠状位 T_1 加权像显示双侧海马位于颞叶内侧，用红色椭圆形表示

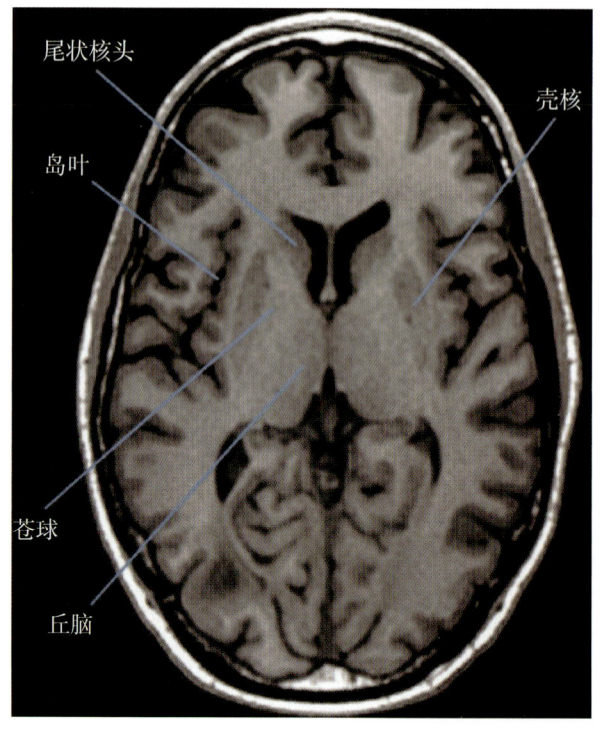

▲ 图 5-4 轴位 T_1 加权图像显示基底神经节

分，即绒球小结叶、小脑蚓部、小脑前叶和后叶。小脑通过蚓部、绒球小结叶和前庭系统的相互作用来调节平衡和运动。小脑扁桃体是小脑半球内侧下方的一对小凸起（图 5-5）。如果怀疑有软脑膜疾病，需要采用 T_1 增强 MRI 对患者的小脑和颅后窝进行仔细检查。

临床相关性

位于颅后窝的脑瘤患者出现症状较快，特别是毗邻如脑干和中脑导水管等重要结构时，会迅速引起颅后窝局部占位效应（图 5-5）。

小脑转移瘤可表现为步态共济失调或平衡、协调能力障碍。如果第四脑室或中脑导水管受到肿瘤压迫，可引起颅内压升高，患者表现为头痛，患者抱怨通过仰卧、恶心或呕吐可缓解头痛症状。

在颅内压发生显著或急性变化时（如体积大的脑肿瘤伴脑水肿）小脑扁桃体可能通过枕骨大孔向下膨出形成脑疝。这样的临床表现预示着医疗紧急情况，减轻颅内压必须尽快执行。

（五）视觉通路和蝶鞍

视觉通路的前半部分由眼眶、视神经和视交叉组成。眼外肌和泪器在眼眶内。眼球的重要结构包括角膜、晶状体、巩膜和视网膜[9]。视神经

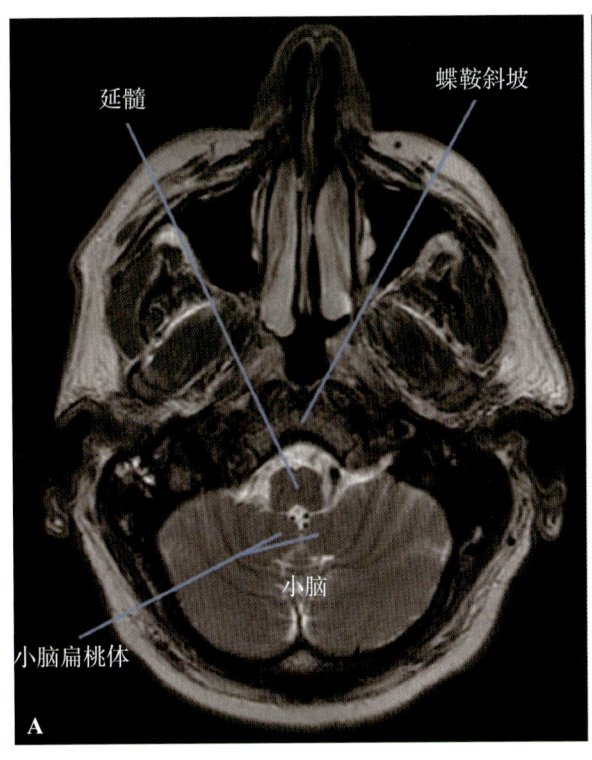

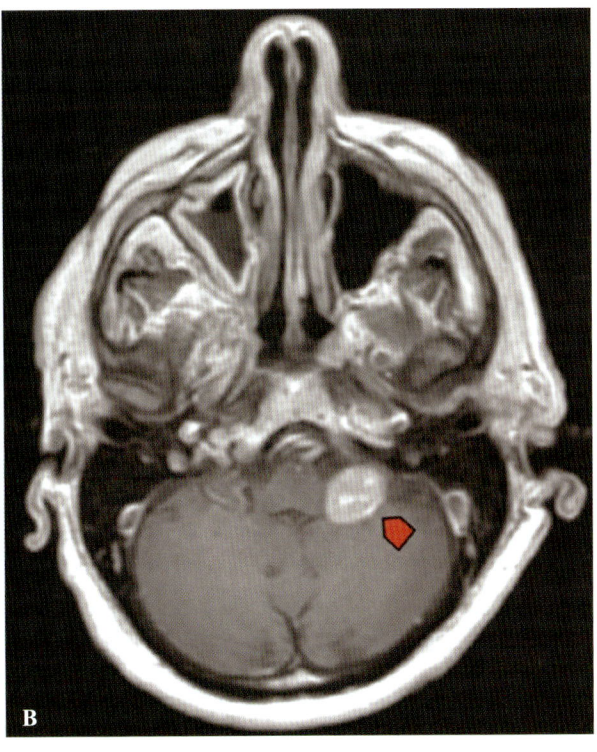

▲ 图 5-5　A. 轴位 T$_2$ 加权图像显示颅后窝的关键结构；B. 轴位 T$_1$ 加权增强图像显示左侧小脑转移瘤强化（红箭）；注意延髓基部

在视交叉处交汇，在 T$_2$ 加权轴位成像上最容易看到（图 5-6）。视交叉位于垂体和蝶鞍的上方，垂体柄、第三脑室和乳头体的前方，通过轴位 T$_2$ 成像、交叉参考矢状面和冠状面成像，最容易识别视交叉（图 5-6）。当在轴位成像上勾画视交叉时，除非成像平面与交叉平面平行，否则将在多个轴位切面上予以勾画。视网膜上的神经纤维投射到外侧膝状核，然后到达初级视觉皮质的所在地距状沟。距状沟从枕极附近开始，向前延伸到脑胼胝体压部，在那里与顶枕叶裂的内侧部分相接，形成锐角（图 5-1）。

垂体柄起源于第三脑室的漏斗隐窝，向上形成位于蝶鞍的垂体。垂体前叶在 T$_1$ 和 T$_2$ 加权像上呈等信号，而垂体后叶在 T$_1$ 像上呈高信号。脑垂体负责分泌调节机体的生长发育、体液平衡、新陈代谢和性功能的多种激素。

临床相关性

肿瘤转移到视觉结构并不常见，但是肿瘤的占位效应局部压迫视觉器官可以引起视觉障碍，这取决于病变的位置。如果肿瘤压迫近端视交叉，可导致双侧视野缺损，如果肿瘤压迫远端视交叉或视神经，可导致单侧视野缺损（图 5-6）。距状沟的病变也可能引起复杂的视觉障碍。当在距状沟附近进行放射外科治疗时，医师应注意治疗带来的潜在后遗症，如放射性坏死及对视力的潜在影响。这在治疗邻近双侧距状沟的脑转移瘤时尤为重要。

脑垂体转移瘤可能表现为内分泌失调，但更常见的是由于压迫视交叉，导致双颞侧偏盲。

（六）脑干

脑干由三部分组成，即中脑、脑桥和延髓，它负责维持生命的基本功能，包括呼吸和心跳（图 5-1）[10]。中脑连接间脑与脑桥，轴位显像呈 W 形。第Ⅳ对脑神经从中脑出脑。脑桥位于中脑和延髓之间，腹侧面向前凸起，分隔大脑半球。第Ⅴ、第Ⅵ、第Ⅶ、第Ⅷ对脑神经的神经核位于脑桥。脑桥的后面是第四脑室的顶部。延髓位于脑

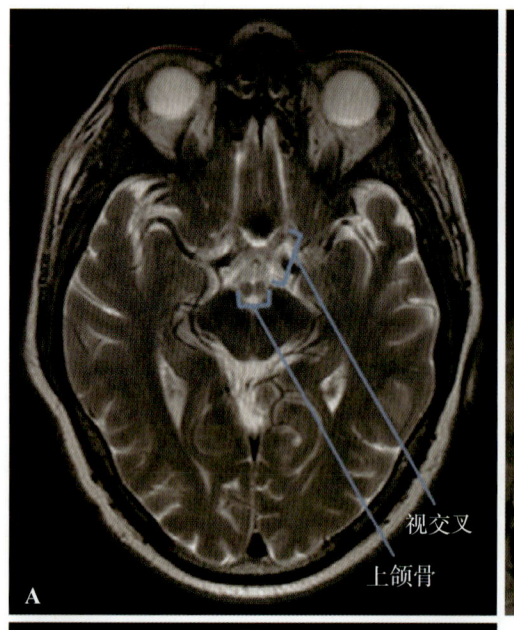

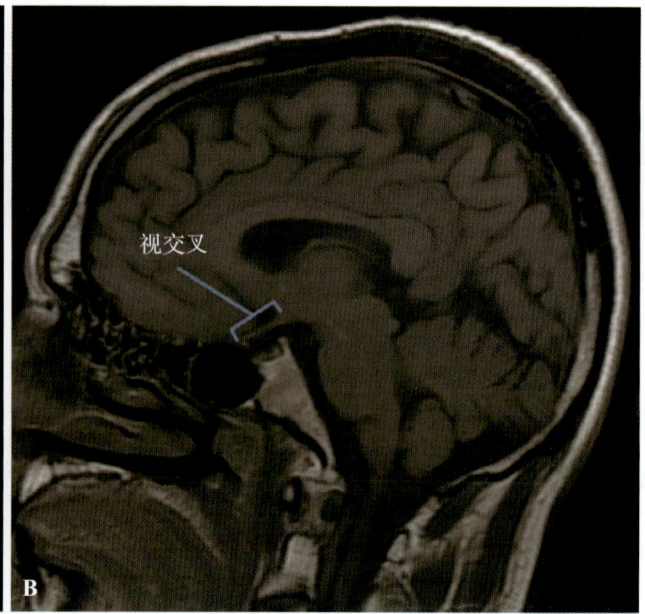

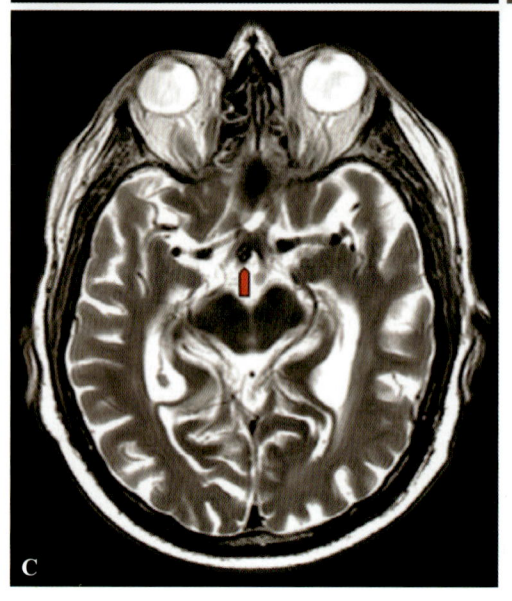

▲ 图 5-6 A. 轴位 T_2 加权 MR 图像显示视交叉和后方的乳头体；B. 矢状位 T_1 加权 MR 图像显示视交叉的位置；C. 轴位 T_2 加权 MR 图像显示右侧视交叉处有转移（红箭）

该患者表现为视力模糊、头痛、恶心和右侧同向偏盲

桥和脊髓之间。第Ⅸ、Ⅹ、Ⅺ和Ⅻ对脑神经从延髓发出。勾画脑干时，脑干的上界起自中脑导水管层面，下界为 C_1 神经根或者枕骨大孔。

临床相关性

脑转移瘤很少发生在脑干。患者可能没有症状，或者出现与脑神经核或脑室系统附近局部水肿相关的症状；也可能表现为脑神经病变或与颅内压升高相关的头痛。

（七）颅底：颅中窝

海绵窦是一个硬脑膜静脉窦，毗邻颞骨和蝶骨，位于脑垂体的外侧[11]。它包含许多重要的结构，如第Ⅲ、Ⅳ、Ⅶ、Ⅷ、Ⅳ对脑神经及颈内动脉。在轴位成像中，注意不要将海绵窦的脉管系统勾画成视交叉。海绵窦位于视交叉的下方，在轴位成像上，当双侧颈内动脉向前穿过海绵窦可以被识别（图 5-7）。

梅克尔（Meckel）腔，又称为三叉神经腔，是另一个重要的神经解剖学结构，因为它是第Ⅴ对脑神经将疾病传播到颅外部分的途径。Meckel 腔是颅中窝的一个硬脑膜囊，位于海绵窦的外侧（图 5-7）。实际上，它看起来像是截断的三个手

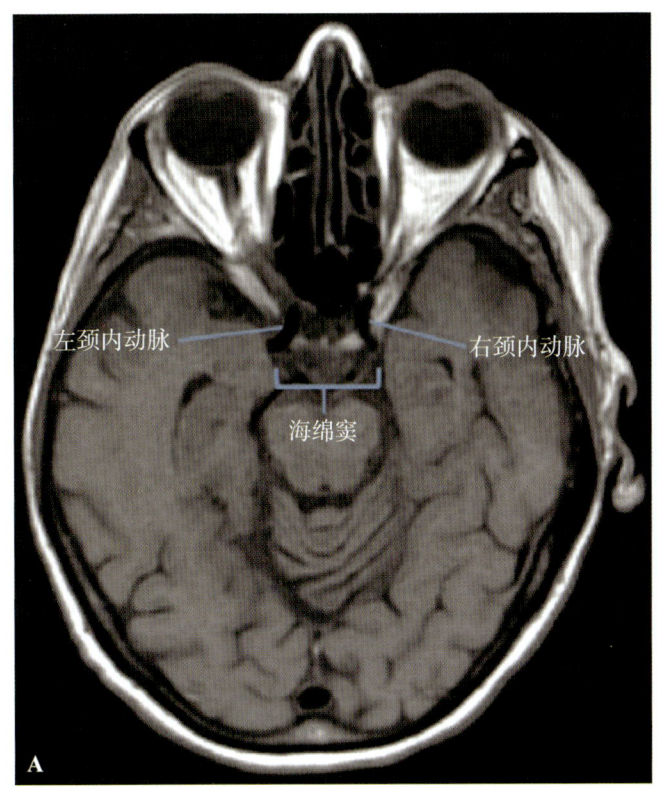

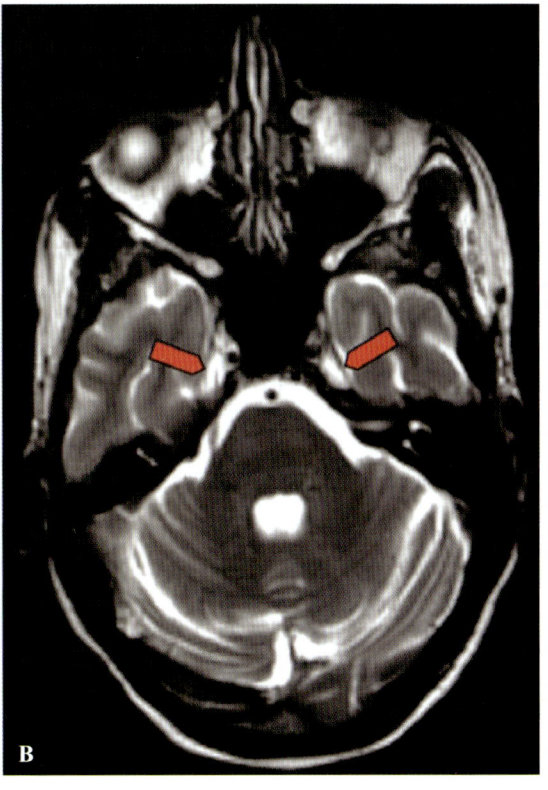

▲ 图 5-7 A. 轴位 T_1 加权 MR 图像显示左右颈内动脉及海绵窦；B. 轴位 T_2 加权 MR 图像显示双侧 Meckel 腔（三叉神经腔）（红箭）

指套，"手指"伸向前方，并包含第 V 对脑神经的分支[12]。

在脑转移瘤的放射治疗过程中，耳蜗是一个需要识别并进行保护的重要结构。在 T_2 序列上耳蜗可以清楚显示，它位于小脑和颞叶之间的颅中窝，在脑干的外侧（图 5-8）。如果耳蜗受损，患者可能会出现永久性听觉障碍和（或）耳鸣。在骨窗显示的 CT 扫描图像中耳蜗也很容易被识别。

临床相关性

海绵窦是个高风险病变结构，虽然它比较小，但包含了几个重要的结构，海绵窦血栓发病率高，并且可能危及生命。患者可表现为视力下降、眼球突出、单侧或双侧眶周水肿、畏光、眼外运动麻痹、面部麻木和头痛等。

三、脑转移瘤成像

脑实质转移瘤很容易在 MRI 增强像上识别，增强对比相对于鉴别小病变非常重要。增强 MRI 薄层（2mm 层厚）扰相梯度回波序列（spoiled gradient recalled echo，SPGR）对识别脑转移瘤尤其有用。3D 薄层应用于颅骨放射外科计划。脑转移瘤最常见的部位是白质/灰质交界处，通常是边界清楚的强化病变，可能是不均匀强化。尽管脑转移瘤周围没有完整的囊膜，但很多确实形成了假包膜，并且没有浸润到肿瘤增强边缘以外的脑实质。很多脑转移瘤，甚至是小的病变，都伴有血管源性水肿的增加，FLAIR 成像常表现为高信号。然而，如果是实体瘤的脑转移，周围的水肿带不包含肿瘤细胞，为了勾画和制订放疗计划，造影增强的病变定义为肿瘤大体体积和临床靶体积。血管丰富的转移瘤，如黑色素瘤、甲状腺癌或肾细胞癌，也可表现为出血性。近期或亚急性出血在 T_1 加权序列 MRI 上通常是明亮的，在没有静脉对比剂的情况下，出血性病变表现为增强。另外，在磁敏感加权成像 SWI 序列上可以

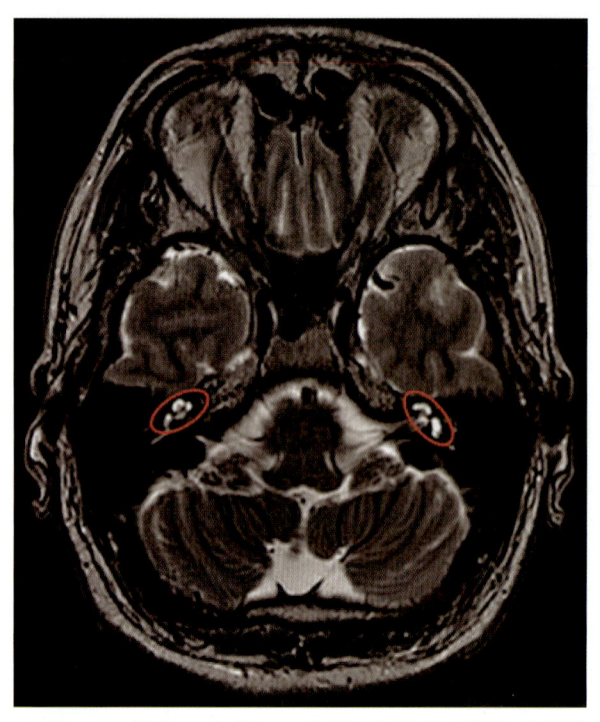

▲ 图 5-8 轴位 T_2 加权 MR 图像显示双侧耳蜗信号增强（红色椭圆形）

看到未增强的转移瘤，这一序列对血红蛋白中铁的存在非常敏感（图 5-9）。

在癌症患者中，高达 11% 的颅内肿块病变不是转移瘤[13]。原发性脑肿瘤可能被误诊为转移瘤。非恶性占位性病变可能伪装成脑转移瘤，如脓肿、肉芽肿，甚至有相关旅行史的患者的寄生虫感染。急性脱髓鞘疾病和血管内血栓形成也可以类似脑转移瘤。

先前接受过放射治疗的患者，放射性坏死很难与存在活性的恶性肿瘤区分开。MR 灌注成像有助于区分有活性的癌症和放射性坏死。灌注成像是在静脉注射对比剂进行灌注成像，同时从感兴趣区域（ROI）取样采集信号。在动态对比剂增强（dynamic contrast enhancement，DCE）的情况下，使用 T_1 加权序列。由于脑转移瘤通常是血管源性，一个有用的灌注指标是相对脑血容量或血浆容量。这是通过比较肿瘤中的血容量与正常的大脑区域的血容量计算出来的，该计算是基于对脑各感兴趣区进行参数对比。血容量和毛细血管渗透率的估计值可以被计算出来。在放射性坏死的情况下，血容量会受到限制，而毛细血管的渗透性可能会升高（图 5-10）。在转移瘤有活性的情况下，血浆容量应该很高。

四、特殊情况

软脑膜病（leptomeningeal disease，LMD），即软脑膜癌，是实体瘤播散至蛛网膜下腔、蛛网膜和软脑膜的种植转移。脑膜转移发生在 5%~8% 的实体瘤患者中，由于治疗此类继发性疾病的能力有限，预后往往很差。在 MR 成像中，LMD 在对比后的 T_1 加权图像上显示最清楚，而软脑膜沉积物在脑实质表面呈不规则结节样增强，在脑沟表现最明显[14]（图 5-11）。受累的脑沟 T_1 FLAIR 信号增强也可能伴随有脑膜转移。在弥漫性软脑膜转移的病例中，受累的脑沟亮度增强，在钆增强 T_1 加权像上看起来如在 T_2 加权图像中的脑脊液一样亮。临床上，LMD 可能表现出非特异性的体征和症状，如混合性脑神经病变，颅内压升高或脑膜刺激征。最常见的受累脑神经是第Ⅵ、第Ⅶ和第Ⅷ对脑神经，患者可以表现为视觉障碍，面部无力和听力问题，还可能出现头痛、恶心或呕吐。

硬脑膜疾病是肿瘤累及硬脑膜，常表现为硬脑膜增厚[15]。患者可以表现为体位性头痛、脑膜刺激或无症状。重要的是不要混淆硬脑膜疾病和软脑膜疾病，因为它们涉及不同层次的脑膜。

脑脊液流动受阻时会发生脑积水。正常情况下，脑脊液由脉络丛产生，从侧脑室流出，经室间孔（Monroe 孔）流向第三脑室，再经中脑导水管（Sylvius 导水管）进入第四脑室，经中间孔（Magendie 孔）和外侧孔（Luschka 孔）到蛛网膜下腔，在整个由脑膜界定的空间（包括脑和脊髓表面）中循环，并被蛛网膜绒毛重新吸收，与硬脑膜窦中的静脉血融合。沿此路径的任何外部或内部的梗阻，包括肿瘤、出血或软脑膜沉积物，都可能导致脑室扩张和颅内压升高的临床症

第 5 章 脑转移瘤的神经影像学诊断
Neuroimaging of Brain Metastases

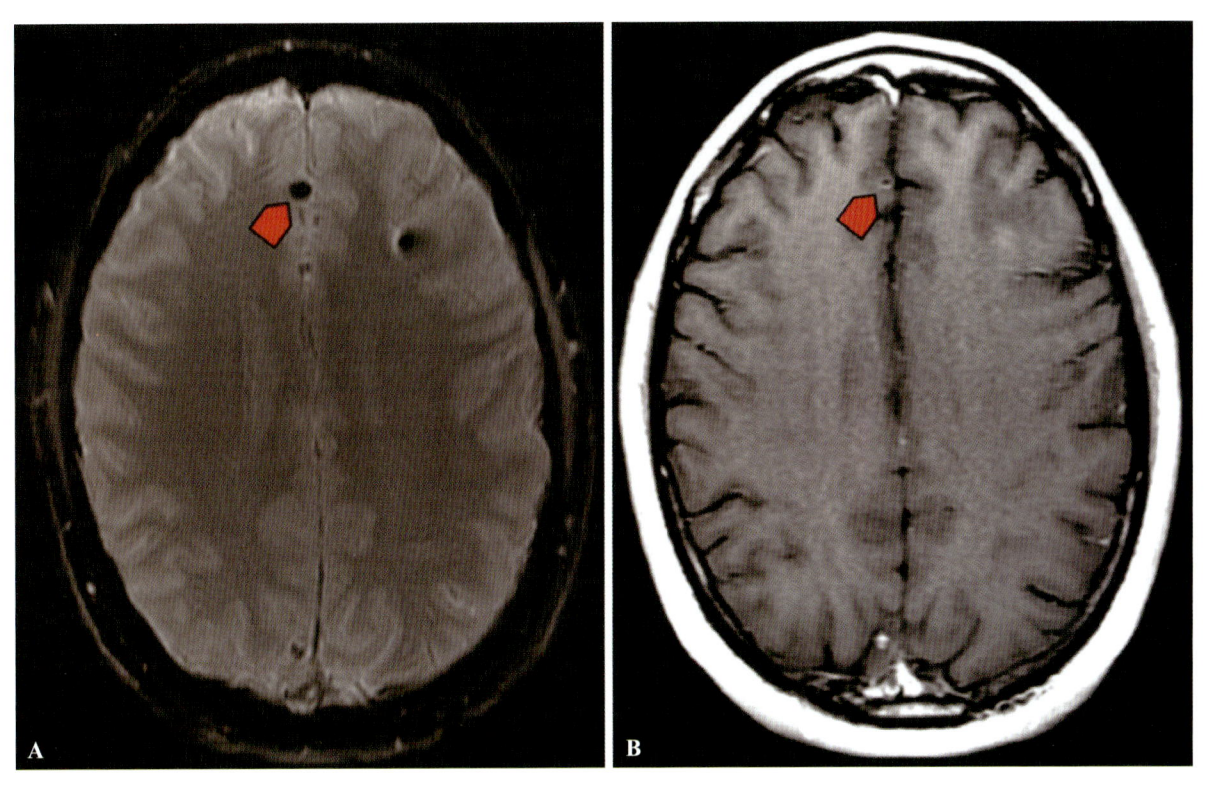

▲ 图 5-9 右额叶转移患者，磁敏感加权成像（SWI）（A）显示转移部位信号增强，而 T_1 增强后成像（B）并未显示同一转移瘤的对比增强；病变在两个影像上均以箭表示

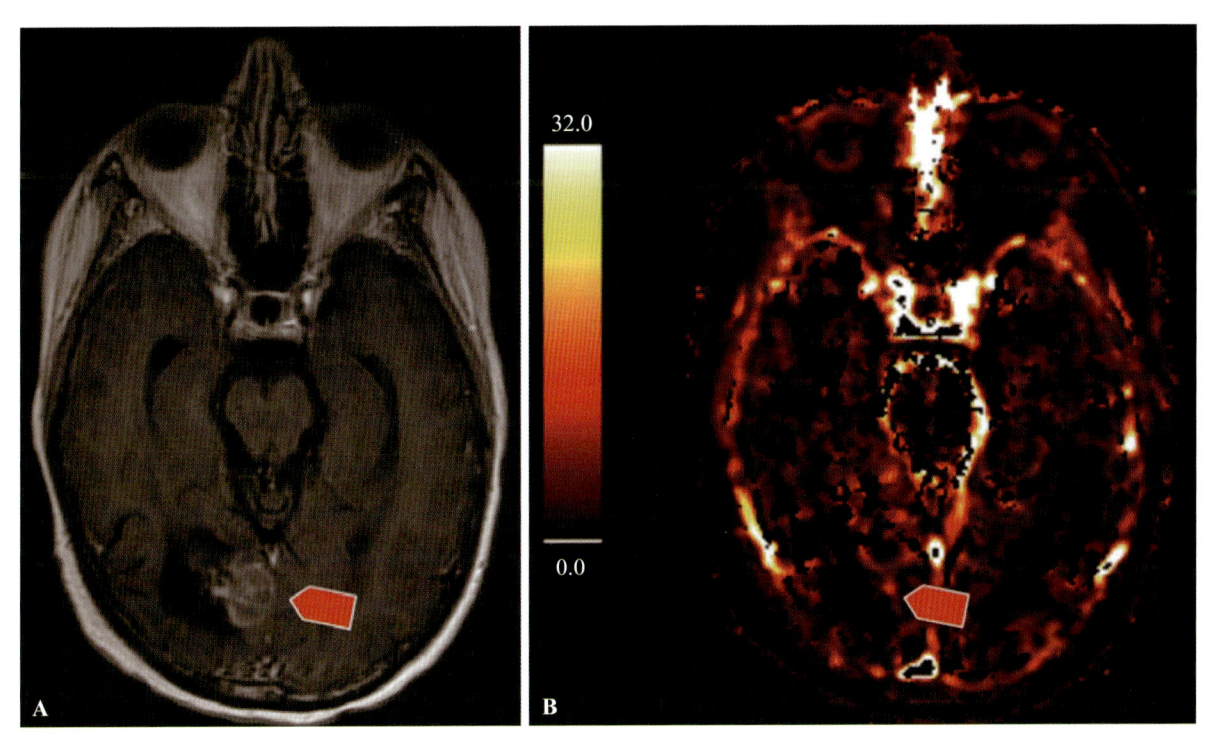

▲ 图 5-10 A. T_1 加权造影后成像显示右侧枕叶病变增强；B. 灌注成像上不表现为高的灌注和血容量，推测为放射性坏死；箭指示增强部位

053

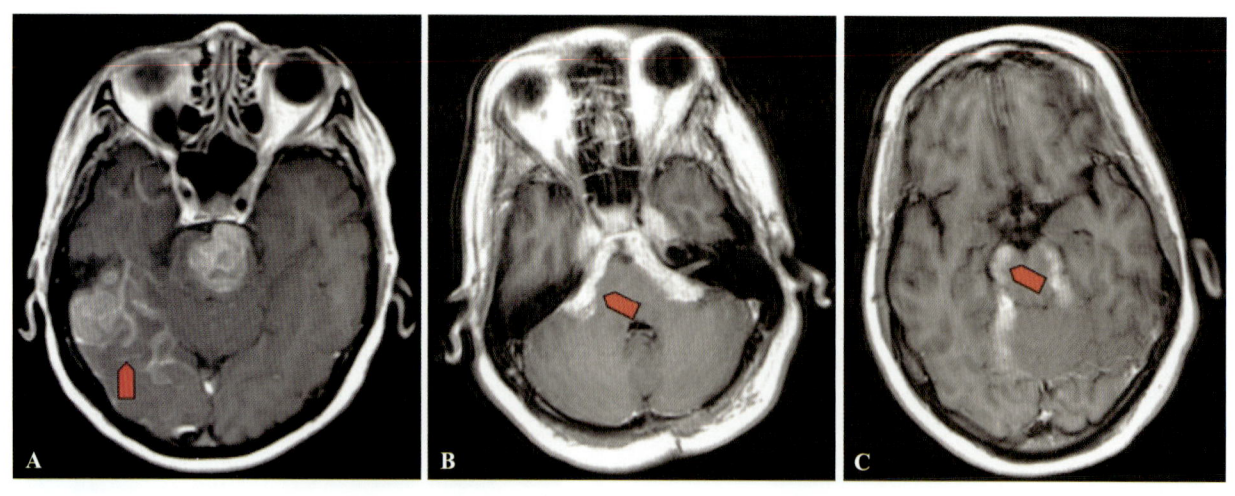

▲ 图 5-11 A. 轴位 T_1 加权增强 MR 图像显示右颞下软脑膜增强。注意特征性的脑沟强化信号；B 和 C. 轴位 T_1 加权增强 MR 图像显示硬脑膜增强，而不是软脑膜增强。注意脑膜表面的增强

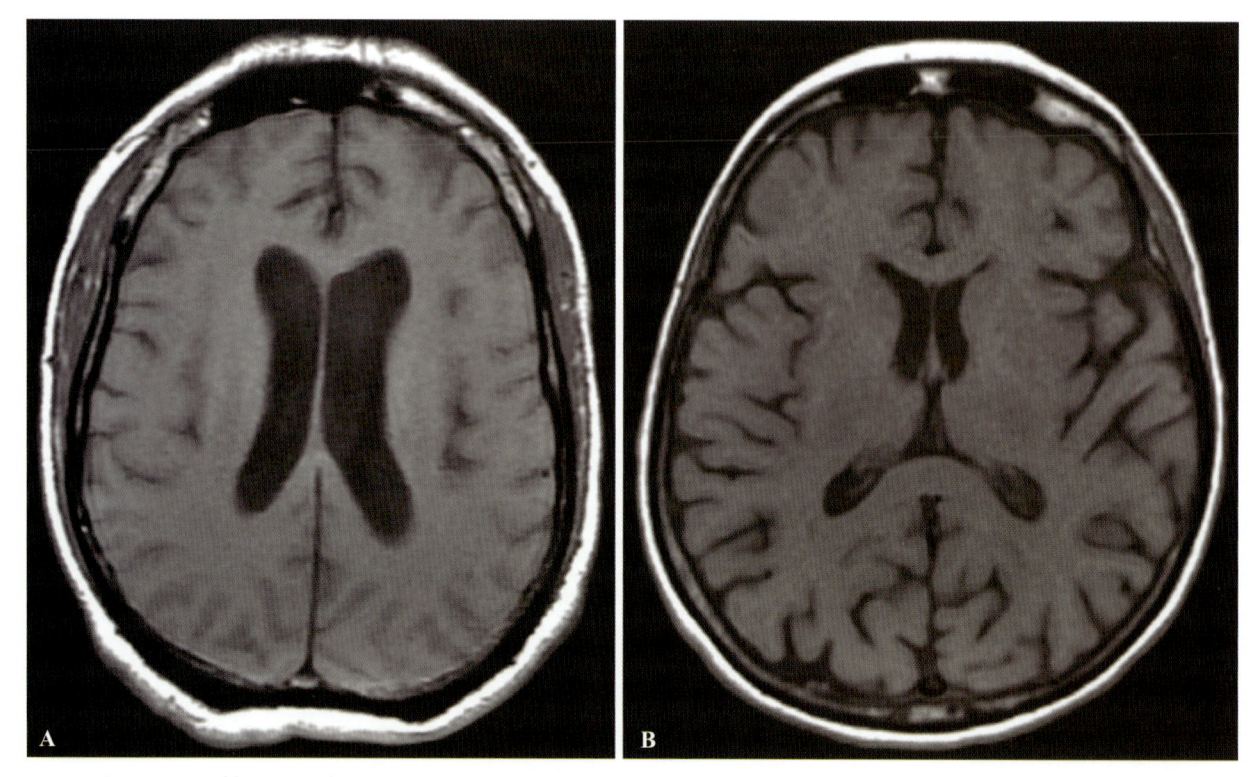

▲ 图 5-12 A. 轴位 T_1 加权图像显示侧脑室增大。患者出现急性脑积水，既往诊断为转移性滤泡性甲状腺癌，腰椎转移并伴有严重头痛和视盘水肿；B. 正常侧脑室无脑积水，用于比较

状，包括体位性头痛、恶心、呕吐和共济失调[16]（图 5-12）。患者也会因为颅内压升高而出现视盘水肿。在急性失代偿性脑积水的情况下，MR 影像显示脑室增大，脑室周围的 FLAIR 信号异常增高。

五、结论

静脉注射钆对比剂增强 MRI 检查是明确脑转移瘤的一个重要检查手段。临床症状通常与肿块对邻近神经结构的影响有关，特别是如果有明

显的血管源性水肿，患者可能表现为病理性神经功能缺陷或没有症状。全面评估（包含影像学和神经系统检查）将有助于诊断和管理。

> **要点**
> - 尽管不做 MRI 检查也可进行颅脑放射外科治疗和立体定向放射治疗，但是增强或平扫 MRI 提供了一种有效的检查方法，能实现 CT 成像无法达到的软组织清晰度。
> - 利用颅脑 MRI 成像的 3D 特性，并通过观察轴位、矢状位和冠状位的图像并相互交叉参考，可以帮助识别重要的解剖结构并确认勾画结构正确。
> - 扰相梯度回波序列（SPGR）T_1 加权图像对于识别转移瘤能提供重要帮助。
> - 其他特殊序列（如灌注成像）可能有助于区分坏死和有活性的转移灶。

参考文献

[1] Dolgushin M, Kornienko V, Pronin I. Magnetic resonance imaging (MRI). Brain metastases: advanced neuroimaging. New York: Springer International Publishing; 2018. p. 51–83.

[2] Erbil M, Onderoglu S, Yener N, Cumhur M, Cila A. Localization of the central sulcus and adjacent sulci in human: a study by MRI. Okajimas Folia Anat Jpn. 1998;75(2–3):155–62.

[3] Berger MS, Cohen WA, Ojemann GA. Correlation of motor cortex brain mapping data with magnetic resonance imaging. J Neurosurg. 1990;72(3):383–7.

[4] Kido DK, LeMay M, Levinson AW, Benson WE. Computed tomographic localization of the pre central gyrus. Radiology. 1980;135(2):373–7.

[5] Naidich TP, Daniels DL, Haughton VM, Williams A, Pojunas K, Palacios E. Hippocampal formation and related structures of the limbic lobe: anatomic-MR correlation. Part I. Surface features and coronal sec tions. Radiology. 1987;162(3):747–54.

[6] Lambiase LA, DiBella EM, Thompson BB. Neuroanatomy. In: White JL, Sheth KN, editors. Neurocritical care for the advanced practice clinician. New York: Springer International Publishing; 2018. p. 5–28.

[7] Pukenas B. Normal brain anatomy on magnetic resonance imaging. Magn Reson Imaging Clin N Am. 2011;19(3):429–37, vii.

[8] Choi CY, Han SR, Yee GT, Lee CH. Central core of the cerebrum. J Neurosurg. 2011;114(2):463–9.

[9] Wichmann W, Muller-Forell W. Anatomy of the visual system. Eur J Radiol. 2004;49(1):8–30.

[10] Angeles Fernandez-Gil M, Palacios-Bote R, Leo Barahona M, Mora-Encinas JP. Anatomy of the brain stem: a gaze into the stem of life. Semin Ultrasound CT MR. 2010;31(3):196–219.

[11] Rhoton AL. The middle cranial base and cavernous sinus. In: VVR D, Larry, editors. Cavernous sinus: developments and future perspectives. Austria: Springer-Verlag/Wien; 2009.

[12] Sabanci PA, Batay F, Civelek E, Al Mefty O, Husain M, Abdulrauf SI, et al. Meckel's cave. World Neurosurg. 2011;76(3–4):335–41. Discussion 266–7.

[13] Patchell RA, Tibbs PA, Walsh JW, Dempsey RJ, Maruyama Y, Kryscio RJ, et al. A randomized trial of surgery in the treatment of single metastases to the brain. N Engl J Med. 1990;322(8):494–500.

[14] Wang N, Bertalan MS, Brastianos PK. Leptomeningeal metastasis from systemic cancer: review and update on management. Cancer. 2018;124(1):21–35.

[15] Antony J, Hacking C, Jeffree RL. Pachymeningeal enhancement-a comprehensive review of literature. Neurosurg Rev. 2015;38(4):649–59.

[16] Ammar A. Hydrocephalus: what do we know? And what do we still not know? Cham: Springer; 2017.

第 6 章 手术和放射外科联合治疗的进展
The Evolution of Combination Therapies Involving Surgery and Radiosurgery

David Peters　Roshan Prabhu　Stuart Burri　Anthony Asher　著
刘铮铮　译
周　琴　校

一、病例介绍

（一）病例 1

37 岁女性，明显头痛、恶心和顽固性呕吐 1 周。头部影像学检查显示右侧额叶孤立性增强的肿块，约 3cm×3cm×3cm 大小，周围水肿面积约 7.6cm×6.8cm，中线向左移位 1.4cm（图 6-1）。

患者于 15 个月前确诊为三阴性乳腺癌（$T_2N_{3b}M_0$，ⅢC 期），BRCA 基因阳性，已行双侧乳房切除术和放化疗，治疗完成后无明显病灶残留，直到出现上述症状。

患者接受了神经外科的评估，使用了大剂量的地塞米松，并在重症监护室（ICU）接受治疗。胸腹盆平扫增强 CT 检查未发现颅外病变。尽管使用了大剂量类固醇激素，患者住院期间仍有持续性恶心和呕吐。鉴于患者的肿瘤体积大，广泛性周围水肿，严重的占位效应和中线偏移，且症状持续，颅外疾病控制良好，患者接受了开颅颅内肿块全切术（图 6-2）。术后病理证实为转移性乳腺癌。

患者出院后接受了术后辅助放射治疗。经过风险和利弊权衡，患者最终在立体定向放射外科（SRS）和全脑放射治疗（WBRT）中选择了 SRS。开颅术后 5 周，基于 1 周内新的 MRI 扫描，患者接受了 27Gy/3 次的 SRS。术腔外放 2mm，计划靶体积（planning target volume，PTV）为 21.5cm³。肿瘤内科医生不推荐患者进行全身治疗。

放射治疗后 6 周，患者再次行胸腹盆 CT 及头部 MRI 检查进行评估，结果均未发现异常。患者无任何症状，一般情况良好。又经过 6 周后，患者再次因头痛及呕吐就诊急诊科。轴位头部影像学检查显示右侧多发肿块伴软脑膜增强，以及术腔内部分增强囊肿。中线从右向左偏移 7mm（图 6-3）。

患者再次接受了神经外科和放射肿瘤科医生的评估，推荐进行姑息性 WBRT，30Gy/10 次。患者的症状在使用地塞米松和止吐药后得到了部分缓解。她很快就出院了，并开始在门诊接受 WBRT。

两周后，患者因难治性呕吐和神志不清再次就诊于急诊科。头部 CT 显示患者颅内病变进展，中线从右向左偏移 13mm。患者被送进 ICU 进行医治。在 ICU，患者的病情突然恶化，意识丧失，伴右侧瞳孔固定散大。给予 50g 甘露醇脱水后，患者的神经系统状况迅速改善，再次清醒。在和患者及患者丈夫充分沟通后，对患者进行了紧急的开颅手术，以防止高渗脱水疗法失效后因脑疝导致神经性死亡的发生。患者在手术室进行了右侧额叶囊肿引流术。由于广泛的右侧大脑半球及硬脑膜受侵，并且继发脑卒中或神经功能损伤的风险要明显高于软脑膜病变切除所带来的潜在收益，手术没有尝试切除病变的软脑膜。术

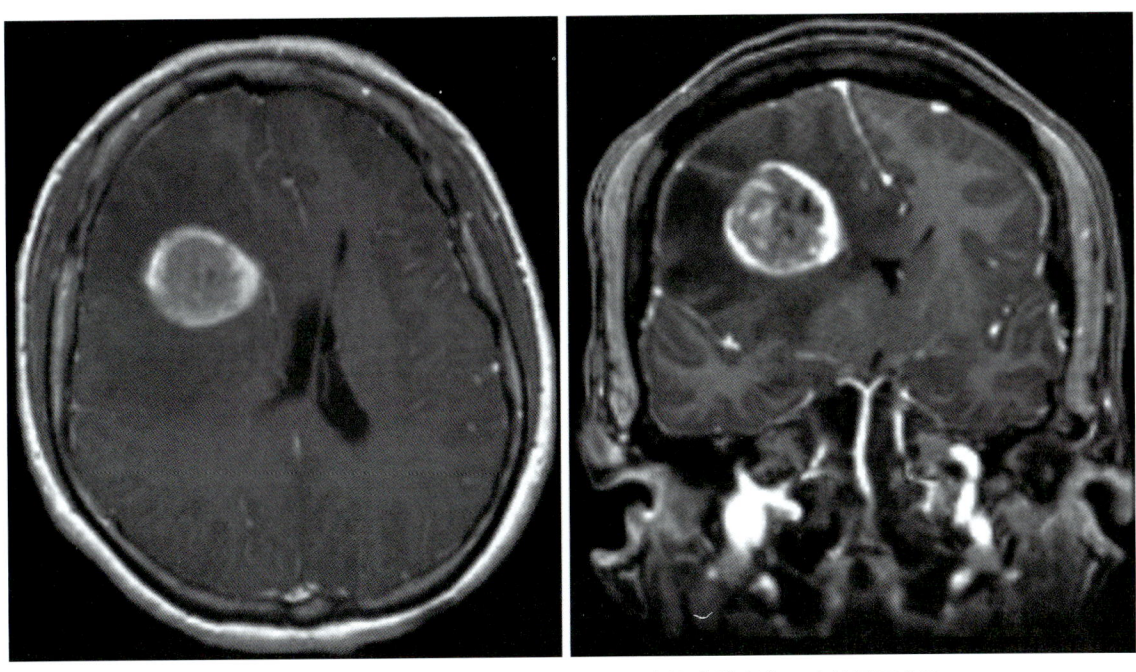

▲ 图 6-1 MRI T$_1$ 增强像显示右侧额叶孤立性病灶强化，病灶周围水肿

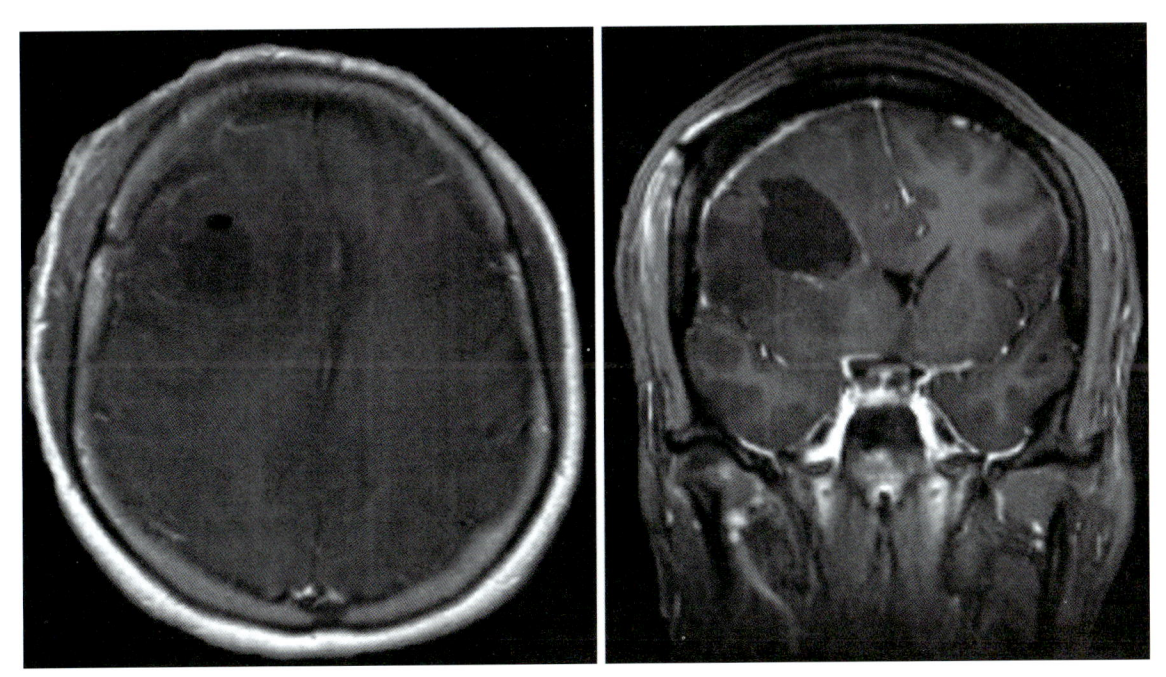

▲ 图 6-2 术后 MRI T$_1$ 增强显示大体肿瘤被完全切除

后，患者恢复了清醒，但仍然有持续恶心、呕吐和神志不清。患者和她的家人选择了寻求临终关怀护理，在临终关怀 1 个月后，患者死亡。

(二) 病例 2

74 岁男性患者，起病表现为隐匿性言语混乱和用词困难，并迅速恶化为严重的表达性失语症，入住了没有神经外科的农村医院。头部影像学检查显示左侧额叶孤立性增强肿块，约 3cm×3cm×4cm，周围中度水肿，中线向右移位 2mm (图 6-4)。

患者既往患有糖尿病，冠心病，50 包 / 年

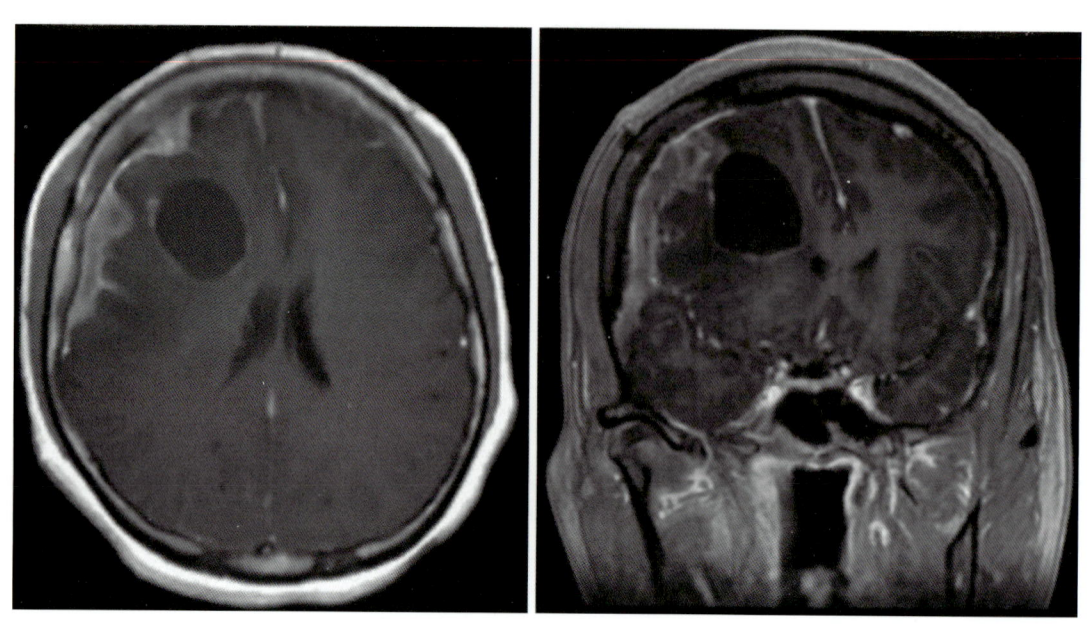

▲ 图 6-3 术后 4 个月 MRI T_1 增强像显示肿瘤复发，软脑膜转移性病变

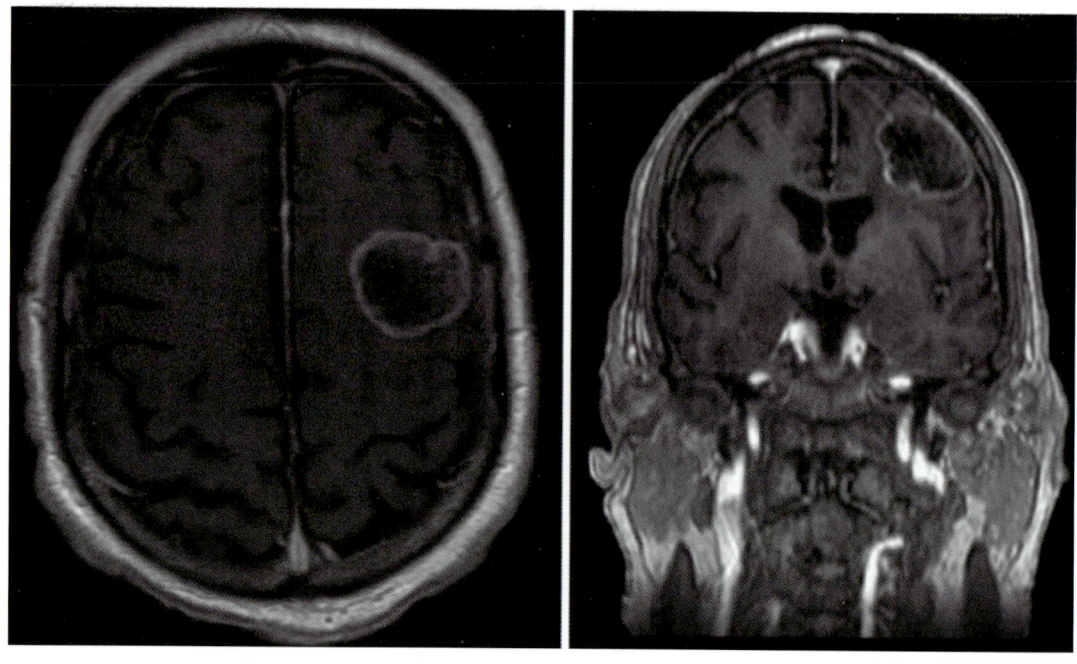

▲ 图 6-4 MRI T_1 增强显示左侧额叶灰白质交界处环形强化肿块

的吸烟史，慢性阻塞性肺疾病和心房颤动，房颤长期服用利伐沙班治疗。患者无恶性肿瘤病史。胸腹盆增强 CT 显示肺部肿块大小约为 3.2cm×1.2cm。因可疑局灶性癫痫发作，患者接受了大剂量的地塞米松和左乙拉西坦治疗。在使用这些药物治疗后患者的言语功能有了显著的改善。安排患者出院后 3 天来神经外科门诊随访。同时门诊进行肺穿刺活检，活检病理显示鳞状细胞癌。

鉴于患者颅内肿瘤单发，体积大且有症状，同时颅外病变局限，有手术治疗指针。在权衡风险与利弊后，决定对病灶进行术前 SRS。患者接受了 6MV 光子治疗，80% 的等剂量线治疗剂量为 14Gy。肿瘤病灶最大直径为 38.7mm，没有外放边界，因此，肿瘤大体体积（gross tumor volume，GTV）等于PTV，测得体积为22.4cm³。处方等剂量体积为29.46cm³。次日，患者接受了开颅左额叶病变切除术，术中肿块完全切除（图6-5）。

术后病理证实是肺部鳞状细胞癌转移。术后患者入住ICU，次日早晨出院回家，神经功能完整。出院后患者继续服用左乙拉西坦，地塞米松在2周内减量。他的家人发现他的言语混乱在术后到了显著改善。

随后，患者接受了胸外科、肿瘤内科、放射肿瘤科的评估。完善了PET检查，结果显示没有其他部位的转移。患者因为肺功能太差无法耐受肺部肿瘤的手术治疗。因此，肺部肿块采用了放射治疗，并且耐受性良好。肿瘤内科医师没有推荐进行全身化疗或免疫治疗。

随后患者每3个月进行头部磁共振检查。在肺部放疗后的6个月，PET检查发现了一个新的肝脏病变。随后对肝脏病变进行了放射治疗，患者耐受良好。目前，患者距离首次确诊1年，没有发现病灶残留或颅内复发病变，且颅外病变控制良好，卡诺夫斯基评分（KPS）为80分。

二、概述

放射治疗和手术切除是目前最有效、研究最深入的用于治疗脑转移瘤的两种方法。当这两种治疗手段使用恰当时能给患者带来明确的获益，而难点在于如何为患者制定最佳的个体化治疗方案。目前普遍接受的治疗方案组合包括单纯的WBRT，WBRT联合SRS，单纯SRS，手术切除后观察，手术切除后进行WBRT，手术切除后进行术后SRS，术前SRS后再进行手术。推荐采用保护海马的全脑放疗，并联合美金刚给药能尽可能地减少全脑放疗所带来的神经认知功能后遗症。同时，某些组织学类型的脑转移瘤对新的系统治疗反应良好，放射治疗通常可以考虑延后进行，在本书内其他地方讲述。

脑转移患者临床变化的多样性要求决策者全面了解所有的治疗方案。对于如何更好地将手术和放疗结合，指南一直在持续更新，目前一个非常有前景的研究得出的数据可能有助于为需要进行手术切除的脑转移瘤患者制定一个新的治疗标准。本章的目的是回顾现有治疗方法的选择，并为如何更好地将手术和放疗结合治疗脑转移瘤提

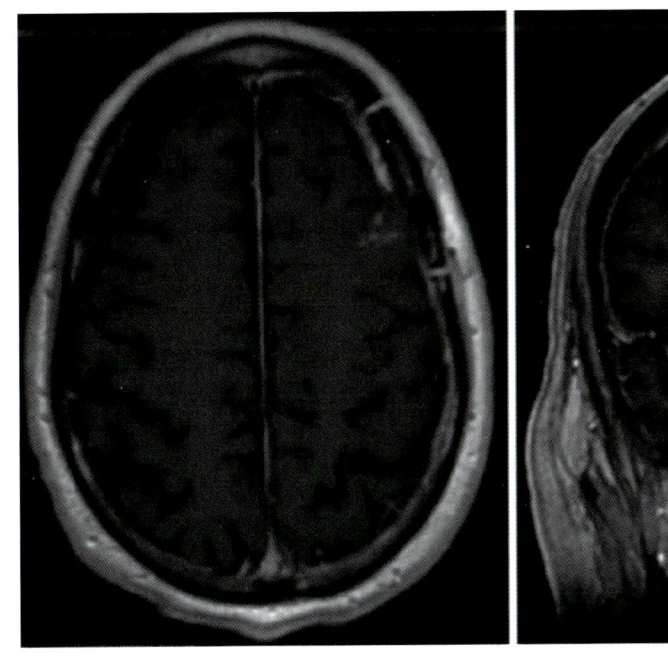

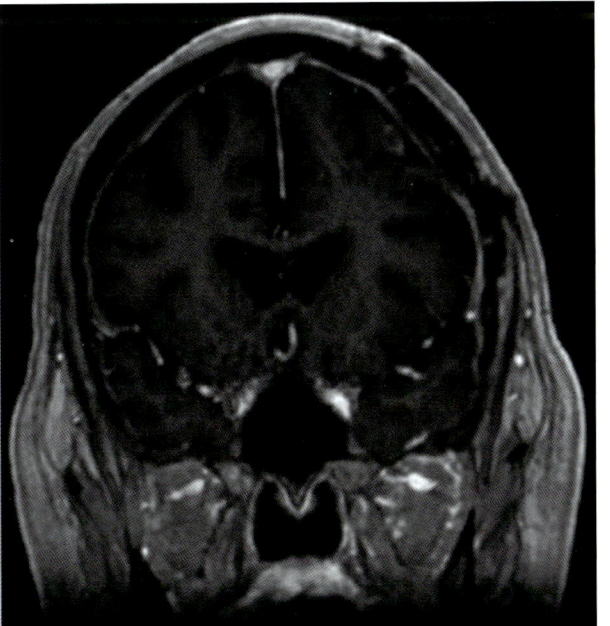

▲ 图 6-5 术后 MRI T₁ 增强显示肿瘤完全切除

供循证医学建议。

三、循证基础

放射治疗应用于脑转移瘤的治疗最早报道于20世纪50年代[1,2]，早期的放射治疗采用全脑放疗，不结合手术治疗，主要用于缓解症状，患者的总生存很差[1,3,4]。20世纪90年代Patchell等开展两项里程碑式的研究表明，单个脑转移瘤患者，采用手术联合WBRT的治疗方案对比单纯WBRT或者单纯手术，均有显著获益[5,6]。在第一项研究里纳入了单个脑转移瘤患者，随机分为手术联合WBRT组和单纯WBRT组。结果显示手术联合WBRT组的中位OS为40周，而单纯WBRT组的中位OS为15周（$P<0.01$）。随后开展的研究纳入了单个脑转移瘤患者，随机分为单纯手术组和手术联合WBRT组。这项研究结果显示手术联合WBRT组并没有带来生存获益（手术组和手术联合WBRT组中位OS分别为43周和48周，$P=0.39$），但它确实表明手术联合WBRT明显降低了颅内肿瘤的复发率和神经源性死亡。单纯手术组术腔的局部复发率为46%，而手术联合WBRT组的局部复发率为10%[5]。随后的研究证实了接受单纯手术治疗的患者局部复发率高（1~2年局部复发率为47%~59%）[7,8]。为了降低局部复发风险，脑转移瘤术后患者通常推荐进行辅助放疗。

多年来，WBRT一直是脑转移瘤患者手术切除后的标准放射治疗方案。然而，WBRT所导致的神经认知能力衰退和生活质量的下降引起了人们越来越多的关注[9-11]。从而开展了辅助SRS有效性的研究。多项研究比较了单纯SRS和SRS+WBRT治疗未手术的脑转移瘤患者（最多只有3~4个转移瘤）。这些研究结果一致显示与SRS+WBRT相比，单纯SRS的局部控制率更差，但两组间OS并无明显差异[9,10,12]。此外，单纯SRS组术后3~4个月神经认知功能下降的发生率显著降低[9,10]。多项研究还采用了生活质量评估量表对患者进行生活质量评估，结果发现与单纯SRS相比，WBRT联合SRS组明显降低了脑转移瘤患者的生活质量[9,11]。这些数据都支持SRS成为数量有限、一般状况良好的脑转移瘤患者的首选放射治疗方案[13]。

基于未经手术切除的脑转移瘤患者，放疗的数据可以应用于术后患者这个假设，同理推测放疗也适用于脑转移术后患者。推断术后辅助SRS可以降低单纯手术切除带来的局部复发高风险，同时也可以避免由WBRT所导致的神经认知功能障碍和生活质量的下降。正因为如此，对于数量有限的脑转移瘤患者，SRS逐渐成为临床实践中比WBRT更受青睐的术后辅助放疗方式。最初，只有少数回顾性研究和仅有的一项单臂前瞻性试验支持这种方法[14]。

最近，已有多项前瞻性临床研究提供了高级别的证据，对于脑转移瘤术后患者支持SRS优于WBRT进行辅助治疗。与单纯外科手术相比，术后辅助SRS提高了局控率；与WBRT相比，SRS降低了神经认知功能下降的风险[8,14,15]。此外，两项回顾性研究均显示与单纯SRS相比，手术联合术后SRS能显著降低局部复发率，提高患者的OS[16,17]。这两项研究纳入的患者都包括1~4个脑转移瘤，尽管大多数患者只有单个病变。在Prabhu等的研究中，所有患者至少有一个体积$\geqslant 4cm^3$的转移瘤。

回顾性研究显示术后行SRS的患者1年局部复发率（local recurrence，LR）为0%~39%，这些研究在治疗方案、患者人群、统计学方法和随访周期上有很大的差异[18]。表6-1列出了术后SRS的最佳研究数据。

这些回顾性研究也都存在偏倚，在所有接受了术后SRS的患者里，没有考虑到失访的患者，或者因为技术或其他因素不能接受术后SRS治疗的患者。一项前瞻性临床研究随机将患者分为两组，一组手术切除后观察，另一组手术切除后行SRS。术后SRS组1年的术腔局部复发率为28%，而术后观察组的复发率为57%（$P=0.015$）[8]。

两组间的 OS、其他颅内疾病控制率、神经系统死亡率、软脑膜疾病（leptomeningeal disease，LMD）转移率或后续接受 WBRT 的比率均无明显差异。这是术后 SRS 能有效降低术腔局部复发率的最有力的证据。

随着术后辅助 SRS 临床研究的增多和多项高质量前瞻性研究结果的公布，与此种治疗模式有关的重要原则和建议已经形成。首先，一个重要的技术要点是术后辅助 SRS 靶区需要在术腔周围外放 1~2mm。如果不外放 1~2mm，局部复发的风险会更高，这可能是因为精确勾画术腔边缘存在困难，以至于不能完全包括残留的肿瘤细胞[23, 24]。其次，术后接受 SRS 患者 LMD 可能比接受 WBRT 治疗的患者更高[19, 21, 25, 26]。LMD 定义为大脑周围脑膜的转移（图 6-6）。

一项回顾性研究比较了术后 SRS 和术后 WBRT，结果显示在 18 个月时，两组 LMD 的发生率分别为 31% 和 13%（P =0.045）[21]。另一项回顾性研究表明，单纯接受 SRS 的患者 1 年的 LMD 转移率为 5.2%，而手术联合 SRS 的患者 1 年的 LMD 转移率为 16.9%（$P < 0.01$）[25]。人们认为手术切除导致肿瘤扩散到软脑膜间隙，引起脑脊液播散。术后 WBRT 使整个颅内均受到照射，可限制或控制肿瘤通过脑脊液途径播散以及随后出现的软脑膜转移。单纯 SRS 比术后 SRS 软脑膜转移降低的原因是不存在术中医源性肿瘤细胞的播散。

术前行 SRS 是手术联合放疗治疗脑转移瘤的一种新的联合治疗方式。与术后 SRS 一样，术前 SRS 不仅能达到良好的局部控制，同时与 WBRT 相比，能明显降低神经认知功能的损伤。然而，这种治疗顺序也能避免术后 SRS 所观察到的一些不足。

从理论的角度来说术前 SRS 有几个优点。首先，与勾画术腔相比，术前 SRS 更容易勾画完整的转移瘤病灶。与术腔不同，完整脑转移瘤病灶的边界更好确定，因此，靶区不需要对病灶的边界进行外放。如前所述，术后 SRS 的最佳方式需要在不规则术腔边界周围外放 1~2mm，以确保靶区能完全包含所有残留的肿瘤细胞，但这也导致了更多的正常大脑组织受到照射[23, 24]（图 6-7 和图 6-8）。

众所周知，接受高剂量照射的正常脑组织体积的增加会增加放射性脑坏死率[27-29]，因此，从理论上来说，术前 SRS 能减少术后 SRS 所导致的放射性脑坏死的发生率。其次，已有数据证实，放射治疗在肿瘤有完整的血液供应和充分氧合的情况下能够更有效地杀灭肿瘤细胞。因此，

表 6-1 术后 SRS 数据总结 [8, 14, 15, 19–22]

研究机构	研究类型	患者数量	中位 SRS 边缘剂量（Gy）	总生存率	1 年复发率（%）	1 年放射性坏死	1 年软脑膜转移（%）
Atalar（Stanford）2013	回顾性研究	165	NR	1 年：66%	10	7（2+级，原发）	11
Iorio-Morin（Canada）2014	回顾性研究	110	16	中位：11 个月 1 年：56%	27	6	未报道
Patel（Emory）2014	回顾性研究	96	18	中位：22 个月	17	13	未报道
Ojerholm（UPenn）2014	回顾性研究	91	16	中位：12 个月	19	7（2+级，原发）	14（原发）
Brennan（MSKCC）2014	回顾性研究	39	18	中位：17 个月	22	18	未报道
Mahajan（MDACC）2017	回顾性研究	63（SRS 组）	16	中位：12 个月	28	0	28
Brown（N107C）2017	回顾性研究	98（SRS 组）	NR		39	4（2+级，原发）	7

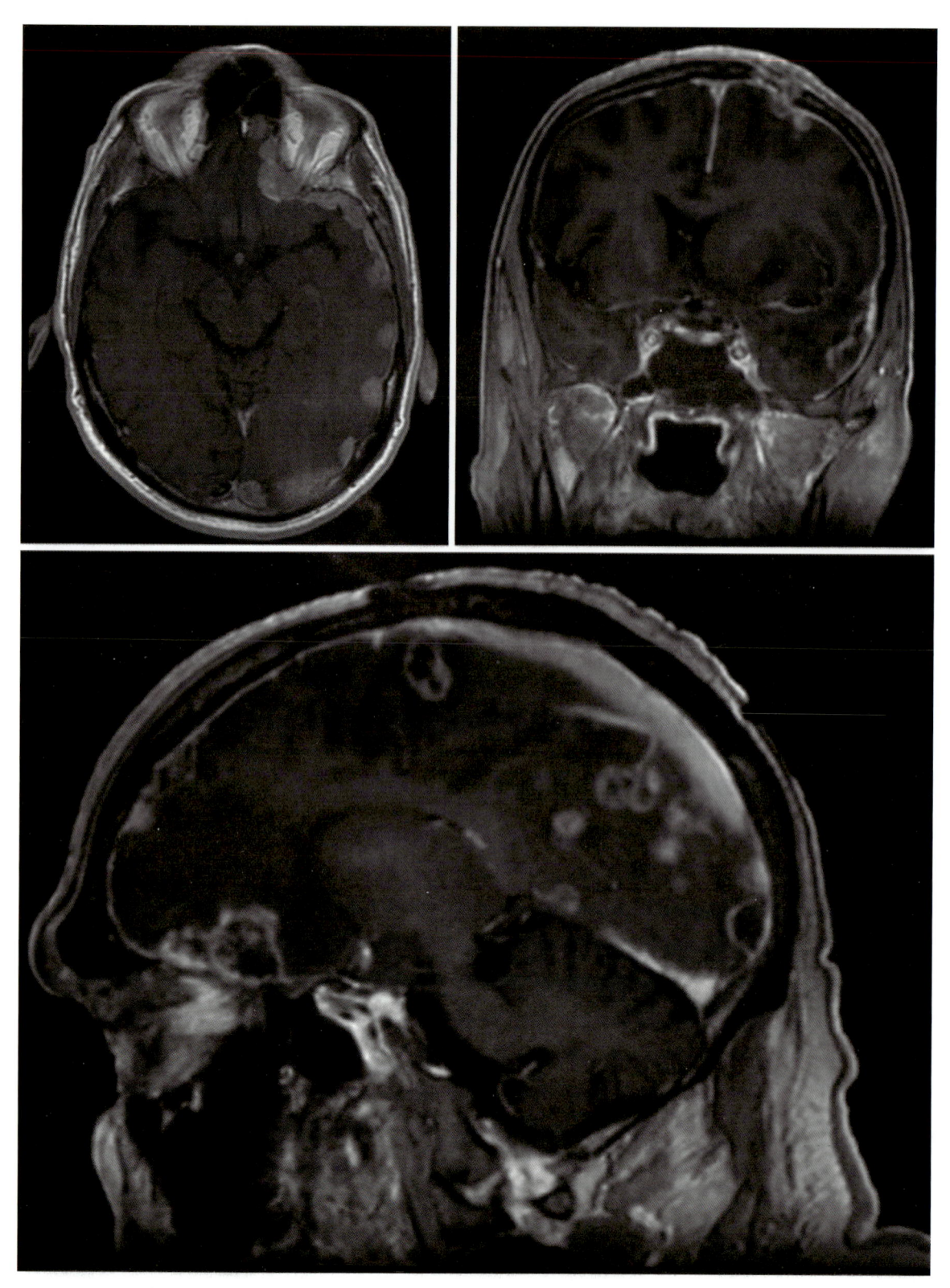

▲ 图 6-6　患者的 MRI T₁ 增强图像显示患者左侧额叶后部单发的转移病灶行手术及术后 SRS 改变，矢状位和冠状位上可见左侧额叶后部术腔局部复发。同时，此患者还出现额叶下、大脑镰后、左颞部和左侧顶叶凸出硬脑膜的转移

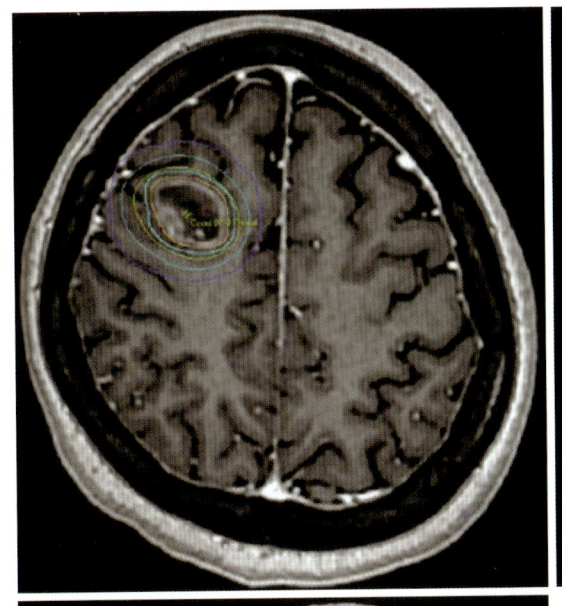

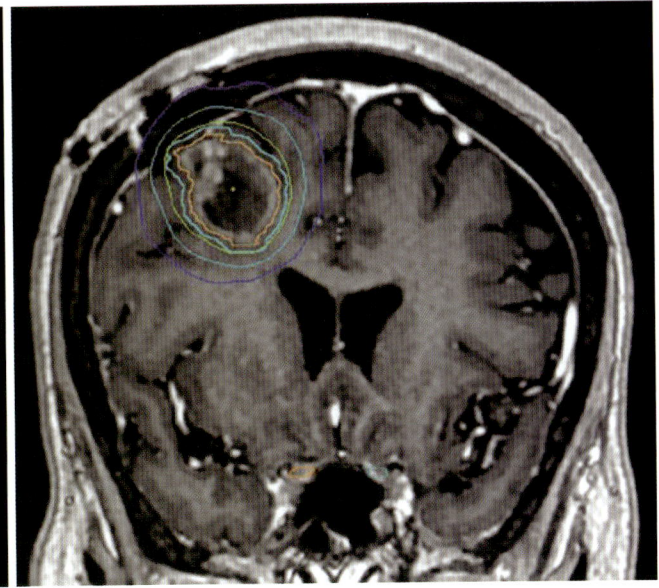

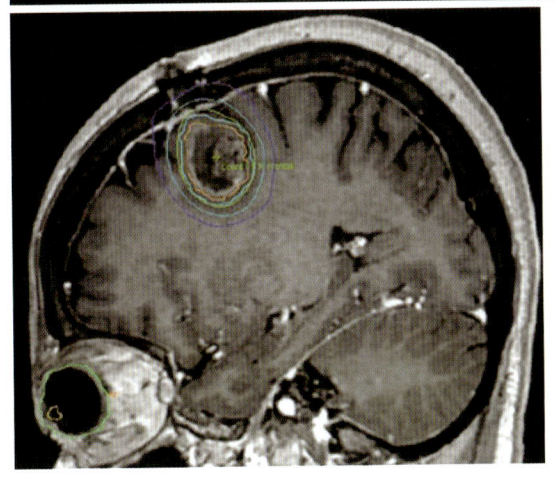

第 6 章 手术和放射外科联合治疗的进展
The Evolution of Combination Therapies Involving Surgery and Radiosurgery

▲ 图 6-7 54 岁女性患者，经手术切除颅内有症状的 5cm 单发肿块

病理证实为肺腺癌，术后立体定向外科治疗剂量为 15Gy/ 次。橙色 . 大体肿瘤体积（GTV）；蓝绿色 . 计划体积外放 1.5mm（PTV）；绿色 . 80% 等剂量线（处方剂量线）；浅蓝色 . 50% 等剂量线；深蓝色 . 30% 等剂量线

与术后乏氧、缺乏血供的瘤床相比，术前对完整的肿瘤进行放疗剂量更低。第三，术前 SRS 能减少存活肿瘤细胞的医源性脑脊液播散，因为这些肿瘤细胞在术前已经受到了辐射。因此，LMD 的发生率也会低很多。最后，术前 SRS 的可行性比术后 SRS 更高，手术通常在 SRS 后 48h 内进行或更早，而术后 SRS 通常要在手术后延迟数周才能进行。这种时间上的延迟使得 CNS 进展和全身进展出现更高和随访失败可能性更高。这在一个单臂前瞻性 Ⅱ 期临床研究中就有体现，纳入手术切除加术后 SRS 的患者中有 20% 未能接受按计划进行的术后 SRS [14]。

至今为止，尽管有一些研究正在开展，但还没有前瞻性的随机对照临床研究完成了术前 SRS 和术后 SRS 的比较。一项纳入了 180 例患者的回顾性临床研究显示，术前 SRS 与术后 SRS 在总生存率，局部复发率，脑转移发生率上无显著性差异。然而，2 年的随访数据显示术后 SRS 的 LMD（16.6% vs. 3.2%，$P=0.01$）和症状性放射性脑坏死（16.4% vs. 4.9%，$P=0.01$）的发生率明显高于术前 SRS [30]。表 6-2 列举了一些经典的术前 SRS 研究。

术前 SRS 与术后 SRS 相比，主要的缺点包括 CNS 病变缺乏病理学诊断，从理论上讲可能导致伤口愈合并发症，SRS 后无法全切肿瘤，以及可能因为患者存在神经功能不稳定或者需要急诊手术而无法进行术前 SRS [34]。缺乏 CNS 病变的病理诊断是客观的，但风险低，因为非转移性

063

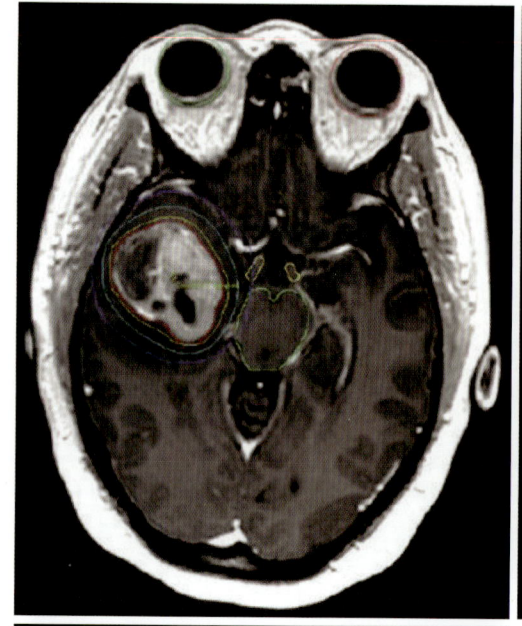

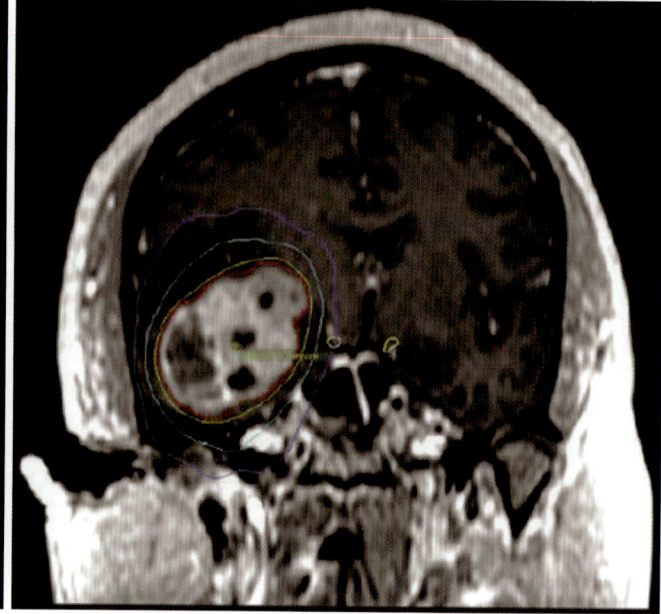

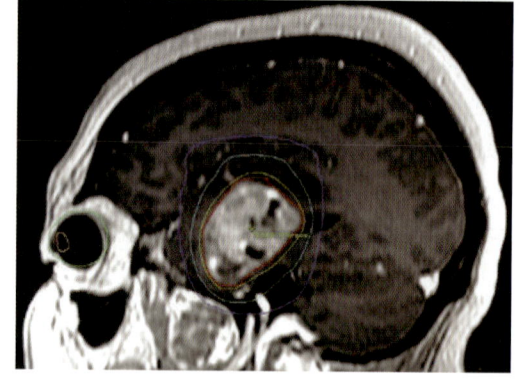

▲ 图 6-8 34 岁女性患者，既往有未分化多形性肉瘤病史，发现右侧颞叶前部单发的转移病灶

先行术前 SRS，第二天接受 SRS 后的手术切除术。术前立体定向外科治疗剂量为 13Gy/ 次。红色 . 大体肿瘤体积（GTV）；GTV. 计划靶区体积（PTV），没有外放边界；绿色 .80% 等剂量线（处方剂量线）；浅蓝色 .50% 等剂量线；深蓝色 .30% 等剂量线

病变的假阳性率为 2%~3%，并且绝大多数接受 SRS 或 WBRT 的患者在术前不需要对 CNS 病变进行病理证实。虽然很罕见，但仍有一些患者因为颅内占位性效应需要紧急手术治疗。这些患者手术前可能无法进行 SRS。影响伤口愈合问题大多是理论上的，因为与术后 SRS 或 WBRT 相比，术前 SRS 影响伤口愈合的风险并没有增加。SRS 后的次全切手术已经成为术前 SRS 的一个潜在的缺点。以前的报道显示术前 SRS 仅仅影响了患者全切术后的状态，但近来 Prabhu 等更新的报道显示，接受术前 SRS 的人群中只有 6 名（5%）患者因为 SRS 而导致了肿瘤的次全切。这 6 名患者中有 4 位患者出现局部复发。多变量分析表明，与全切术相比，次全切是影响术腔局部高复发率和高死亡率的一个显著的预测因素[31]。著者的结论是对患者进行选择非常重要，有可能导致次全切的患者不应接受术前 SRS。对接受了无法预期的次全切除术的患者应进行评估是否可以再次手术或进行放疗补量，以减少局部复发的风险。然而，对这一小部分患者寻求最佳的治疗仍然是目前研究的方向。

四、诊断和治疗

放射治疗是否联合手术治疗对于所有脑转移患者来说都是需要考虑的。因此，放射肿瘤科和神经外科需要对这些患者进行评估。制订最佳治疗方案时不同患者常常差异较大。因为治疗方案要考虑患者年龄、症状、肿瘤负荷、总体预后、肿瘤组织学、身体状态，以及脑转移瘤数量、大

表 6-2 术前 SRS 数据总结[30-33]

	研究方式	患者特点	术腔复发率	症状性放射性坏死	软脑膜转移
Asher 等（2014）	前瞻性和回顾性单臂研究相结合	47 个患者，51 个术腔	1 年：14%	未报道	1 年：0%
Patel 等（2016）	回顾性研究 术前 SRS vs. 术后 SRS	66 术前/114 术后 SRS	2 年：23% vs.16% （P=0.33）	2 年：5% vs.16% （P=0.02）	2 年：3% vs.17% （P=0.01）
Patel 等（2017）	回顾性研究 术前 SRS vs. 术后 WBRT	66 术前/36 后 WBRT	2 年：25% vs.25% （P=0.81）	原发：6% vs. 0% （P=0.29）	2 年：4% vs.9% （P=0.66）
Prabhu 等（2018）	前瞻性和回顾性单臂研究相结合	117 个患者，125 个术腔	2 年：25%	1 年：4.8%	1 年：4.3%

小和位置等问题。

首先应对患者进行详细全面的病史采集和体格检查。有 2%～14% 的脑转移患者没有确诊的肿瘤病史[35]。如果近期（<8 周内）未行检查，推荐进行胸腹盆增强 CT 或 PET-CT 扫描以评估肿瘤负荷和分期。对于没有确诊肿瘤病史的患者，这也有助于确定原发病灶，并对颅外病变部位进行活检。接下来需要根据病史进行进一步检查（如乳腺钼靶照片，结肠镜检查）以明确诊断或重新评估患者原发疾病的进展。如果没有明确的颅外病灶可以进行活检，那么需要进行开颅手术获得病理诊断。一般来说，颅外肿瘤组织活检比开颅活检更有效和安全。

一旦明确了病理诊断，应评估患者进行外科手术切除的潜在获益。67%～80% 的脑转移瘤患者原发肿瘤为非小细胞的肺癌、乳腺癌或黑色素瘤[13, 35]。有几种类型的肿瘤，尤其是小细胞肺癌、淋巴瘤和一些生殖细胞肿瘤对放射极为敏感，不能从手术中获益。这就显示出在开颅手术前明确病理诊断的重要性，如果可能，在开颅手术前要尽可能明确病理诊断。组织学诊断同样也可以明确靶向治疗的潜在获益，这个内容超越本章的范围。

对部分患者来说，外科手术是一种非常有效的治疗手段，但需要充分考虑风险效益比。手术适应证包括明确组织病理诊断需要、大转移灶（>2cm）、显著的占位效应或病灶周围水肿，以及神经系统症状无法用类固醇激素缓解而可以从手术减压中受益。手术的目的在于提高生存率，明确组织病理诊断和（或）缓解症状。手术禁忌证包括患者一般情况差、凝血功能障碍、软脑膜转移、肿瘤负荷大且预期生存期 <3 个月、多发性小病灶，以及对放疗、化疗或免疫治疗非常敏感的肿瘤组织学类型等（表 6-3）。图 6-9 至图 6-12 列举了可能从手术联合放疗中获益的患者。图 6-13 至图 6-15 列举了不能从手术切除中获益的患者。

对于接受手术的患者，目前的证据表明与部分切除相比，手术全切患者的 OS 更好，局部复发率更低[17, 22, 36-38]。Ⅲ类证据也显示对于孤立性肿瘤整块切除比分块切除 LMD 的发生率更低[36, 39-41]。对于已经接受了开颅手术的患者，肿瘤切除后出现术腔局部复发或非原位颅内复发不是再次手术的禁忌证。应该使用表 6-3 中列出的相同标准对这些患者进行再次评估，以确定他们是否适合再次接受外科手术，以及他们是否能从再次开颅手术中获益。Ⅲ类证据表明手术或 SRS 后对颅内复发转移灶进行再切除可以提高患者的总生存[36, 42, 43]。

最重要的是，手术的风险效益比最终需要由神经外科和放射肿瘤科医师团队，包括肿瘤内科医师以及护理小组，根据患者的具体情况进行评估。

著者所在的中心，多学科合作团队成员会对没有明显手术适应证的疑难病例是否接受手术进行评估，并给出治疗意见。对于前面所介绍的第一个病例患者，鉴于患者的年龄、巨大的孤立性病变、广泛的水肿、明显的颅内占位性效应、颅外病变控制良好、病变位置易于切除、难治性神经症状、PS 评分高以及需要获得组织学诊断，最初认为她非常适合手术治疗。患者的症状在术后立即获得了明显的改善。不幸的是，术后 4 个月左右患者出现了软脑膜转移。她的再次手术引起了争议。普遍认为软脑膜转移是手术的禁忌证，且预后极差，在这种情况下，预计她的生存期不超过 3 个月。然而，她的神经功能在接受高渗脱水治疗好转后又突然急剧下降。如果当时患者没有做手术，她肯定会在 24h 内因神经系统疾病的进展而导致死亡，因为脱水治疗只能暂时性地控制颅高压。在和患者家属进行充分沟通后急诊科医生对患者进行了紧急手术，只对额叶的囊肿进行了引流。如果一个具有软脑膜转移同时具有其他部位的转移的患者，考虑到其巨大的风险和最小的获益，接受手术治疗切除转移的软脑膜病灶很少尝试。最终，手术后患者有机会转到临终关怀中心，离开医院后超过 1 个月患者死亡。

第二个病例也是一个适合手术的患者，该患者具有症状性孤立性大肿瘤，肿瘤位置易于切除，且颅外病变局限。其与第一个患者不一样的是，肿瘤占位性效应和水肿不明显，且通过药物治疗后患者的症状得到明显改善。很快为他安排了放射治疗及肿瘤内科治疗计划。他在完成了术前 SRS 后 1 天，接受了手术治疗。术后 1 年患者仍状态良好，无局部复发及 LMD。该病例为术

表 6-3 外科手术决策制订

适合手术者	不适合手术者
• 肿瘤数目少（尤其是孤立性病灶）	• 肿瘤数目多（> 3）
• 肿瘤直径大（> 2cm）	• 肿瘤直径小（< 2cm）
• 肿瘤位置容易切除	• 肿瘤位置难以切除（功能区）
• 病灶周围广泛水肿或占位效应明显	• 软脑膜转移
• 症状难以用药物控制	• 凝血功能异常
• PS 评分高	• PS 评分低
• 颅外病变局限	• 颅外病变负荷重（生存期 < 3 月）
• 放疗后复发	• 肿瘤组织学类型对放疗、化疗、免疫治疗敏感
• 需要进行组织学诊断	

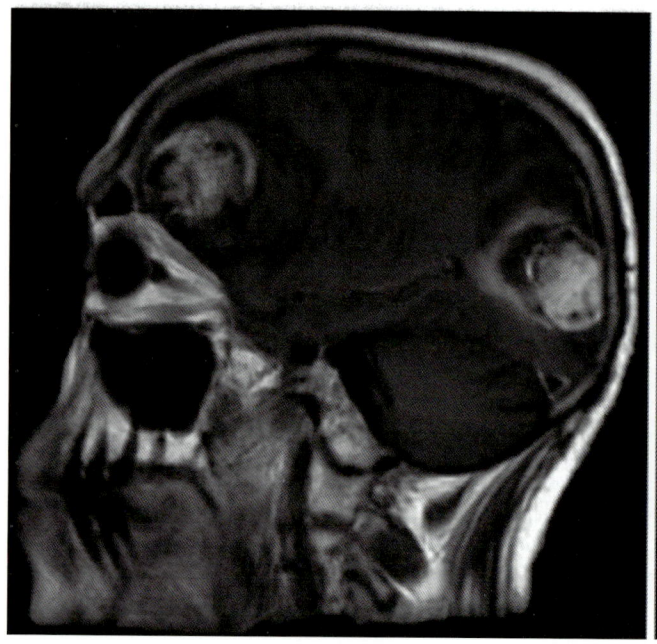

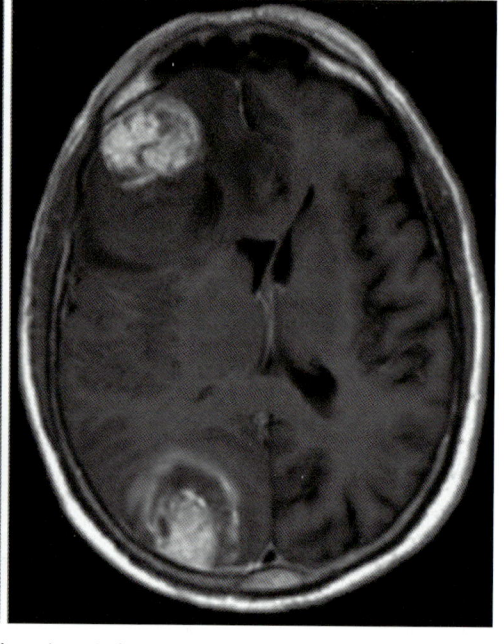

▲ 图 6-9 68 岁男性肝细胞癌患者头部有 2 个大转移瘤，在一次手术中采用 2 个不同的切口进行切除

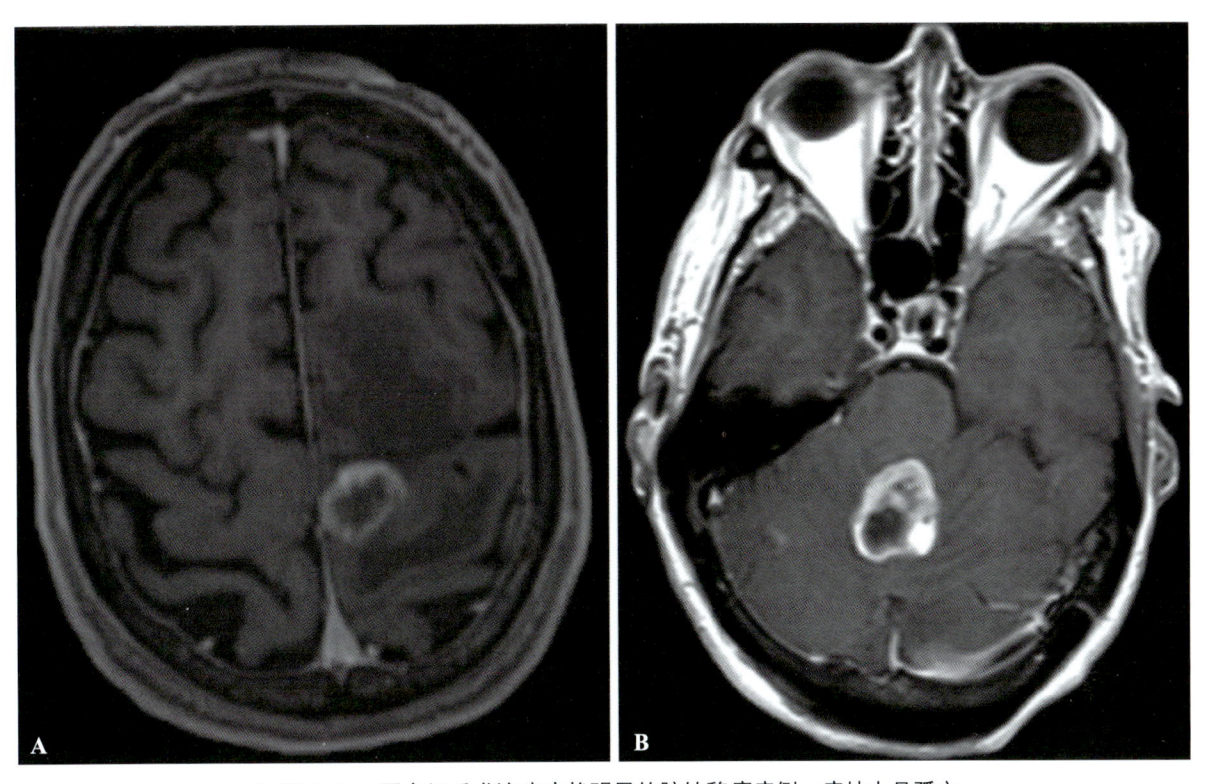

第 6 章　手术和放射外科联合治疗的进展
The Evolution of Combination Therapies Involving Surgery and Radiosurgery

▲ 图 6-10　两个经手术治疗症状明显的脑转移瘤病例，病灶小且孤立
A. 76 岁男性结直肠癌患者，其症状为右侧肢体无力和发音含糊；B. 72 岁女性乳腺癌患者，其症状为头晕、恶心、严重的共济失调

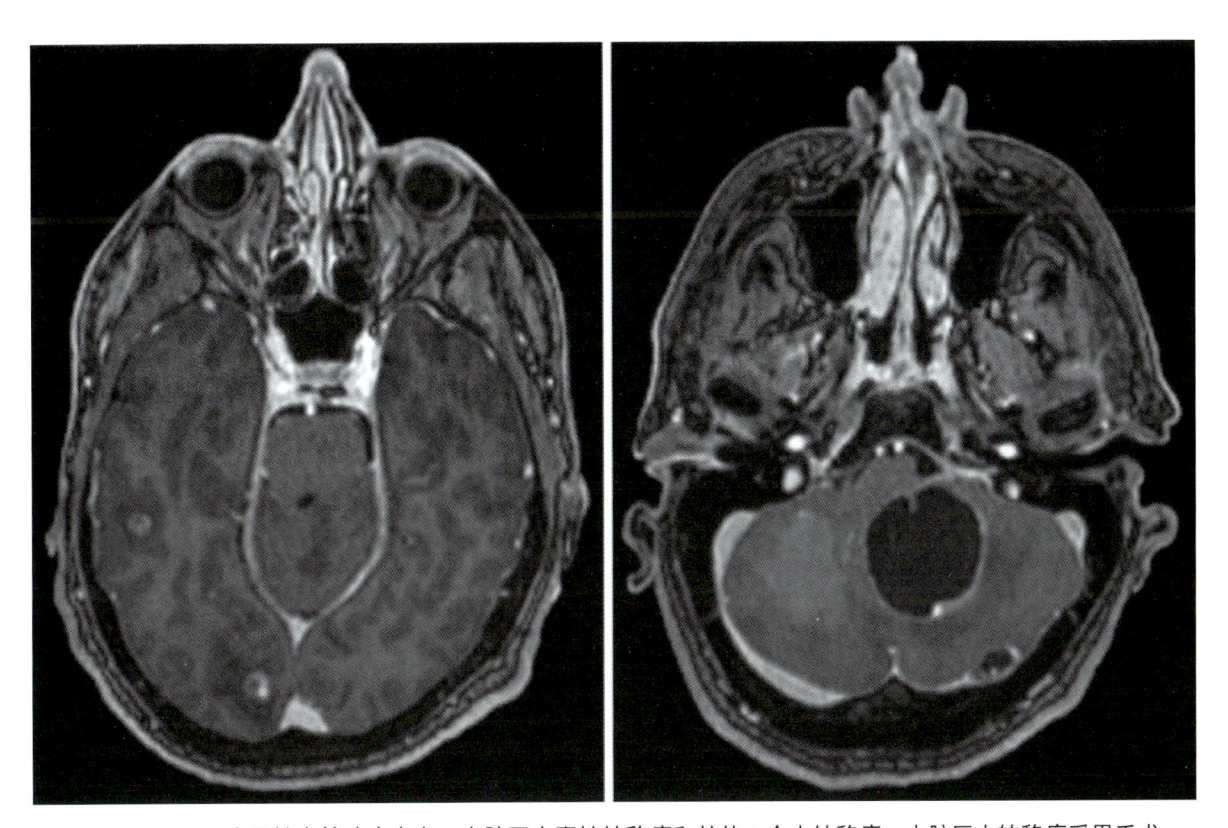

▲ 图 6-11　56 岁男性食管腺癌患者，小脑巨大囊性转移瘤和其他 3 个小转移瘤。小脑巨大转移瘤采用手术切除，其他三个病灶采用 SRS

067

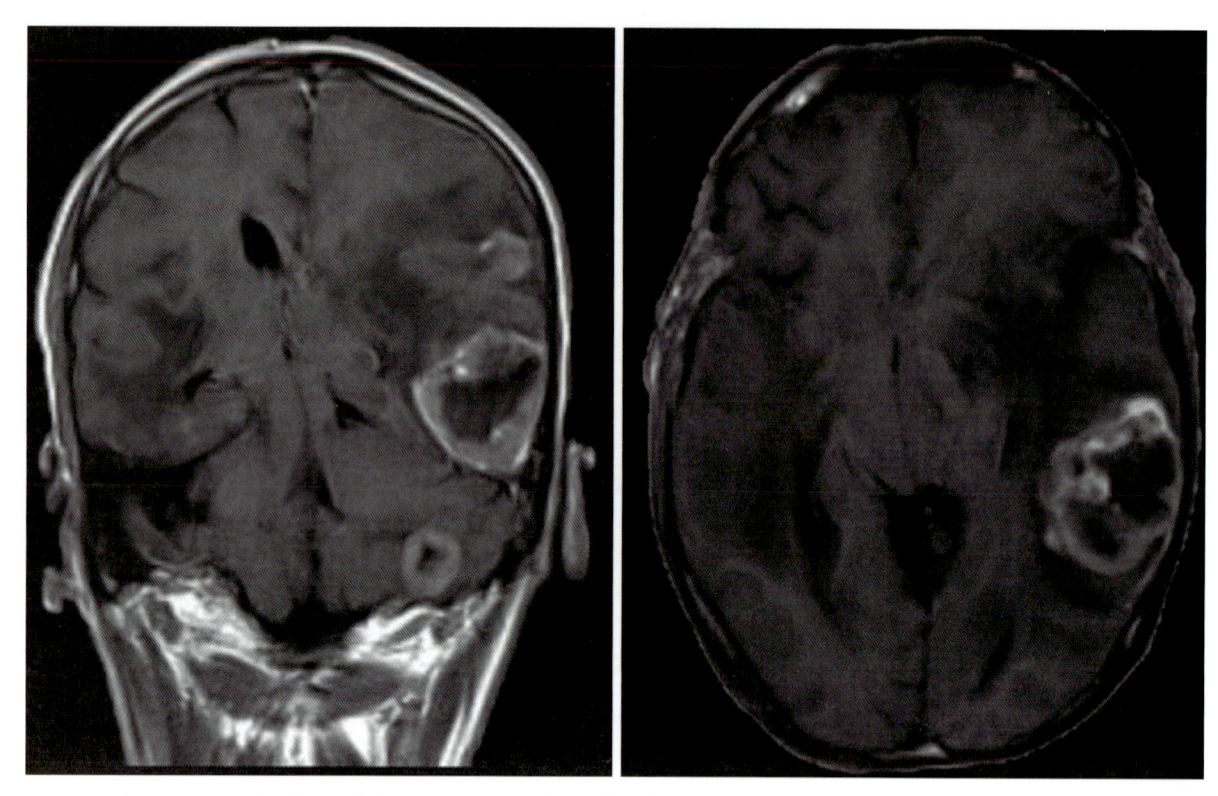

▲ 图 6-12 64 岁男性肺腺癌患者有 6 个脑转移病灶，主要的病灶位于左颞叶，也是唯一被切除的病灶
考虑到该病灶的显著占位效应是引起患者主要症状的原因，减轻症状是手术的目的。患者术后接受了 WBRT

前 SRS 相比术后 SRS 利弊提供了有效证据。

如果一个患者被认为是合适的手术对象，一定要做好如何进行辅助放疗的方案。每项治疗方案所带来的风险与获益都需要与患者进行充分讨论，并共同决定。一般来说，对于 1~4 个（或更多）脑转移瘤患者，SRS 在辅助治疗中优于 WBRT。较低的神经认知功能减退的发生率与复发的高风险相比是值得的，且两者的总生存率相似。对超过 4 个转移病灶的患者，WBRT 仍是首选辅助治疗方案，虽然 SRS 也经常用于治疗超过 4 个转移病灶的患者，但目前还没有权威的前瞻性随机对照临床试验，我们认为术前 SRS 优于术后 SRS。术前 SRS 通常在手术前 48 小时完成，也可以术前 1 周内完成。对于术前 SRS，我们更倾向于针对 GTV 进行 SRS，在靶区勾画时不需要外放边界。也就是说，PTV 就等于 GTV。基于 RTOG 90-05 的剂量标准，减少 10%~20% 进行单次给量。未被切除的脑转移瘤可以采用标准的 SRS 方案。虽然对大多数脑转移患者而言术前接受 SRS 更为安全，但对于具有严重水肿、肿瘤占位效应明显和（或）严重的难治性症状的患者，紧急手术后再进行 SRS 可能是更安全的治疗选择。

五、争议及未来发展方向

目前正在开展的前瞻性随机临床试验以证实早期有限的回顾性研究数据，表明术后 SRS 较术前 SRS 有更高的 LMD 和放射性坏死的风险。此外，需要更好地描述手术和 SRS 后 LMD 的复发特征，确定术后 LMD 最佳的治疗方案及可能的预后。最后，众所周知，放疗可以诱导肿瘤表面抗原表达的增加，从而提高免疫治疗药物的疗效。SRS 和手术时间对肿瘤表面抗原的表达影响在很大程度上仍然未知，正在开展相关研究以确定理想的 SRS 后手术的时间，从而使肿瘤表面抗原最大限度地表达以利于后续的免疫治疗。

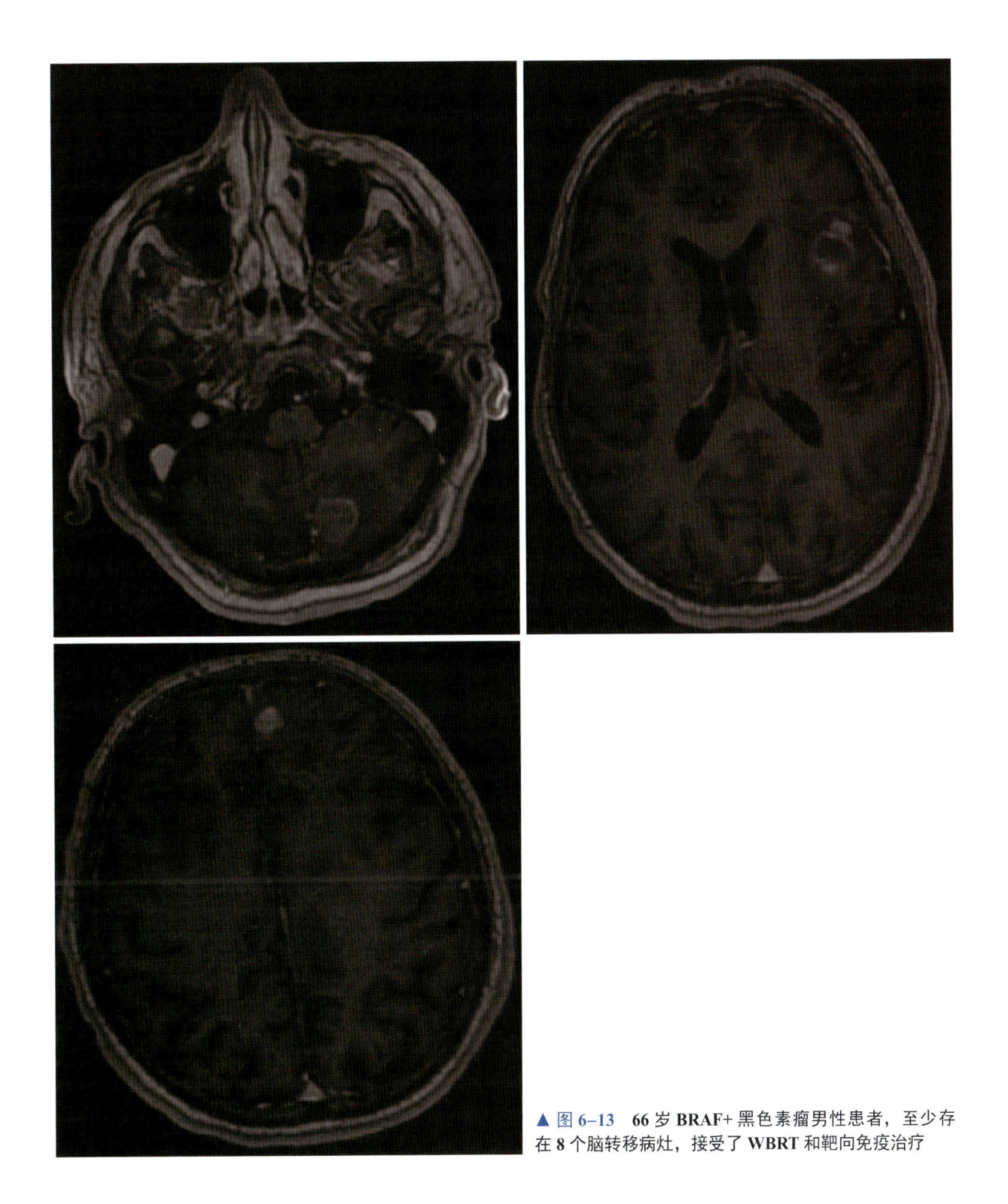

第 6 章 手术和放射外科联合治疗的进展
The Evolution of Combination Therapies Involving Surgery and Radiosurgery

▲ 图 6-13 66 岁 BRAF+ 黑色素瘤男性患者，至少存在 8 个脑转移病灶，接受了 WBRT 和靶向免疫治疗

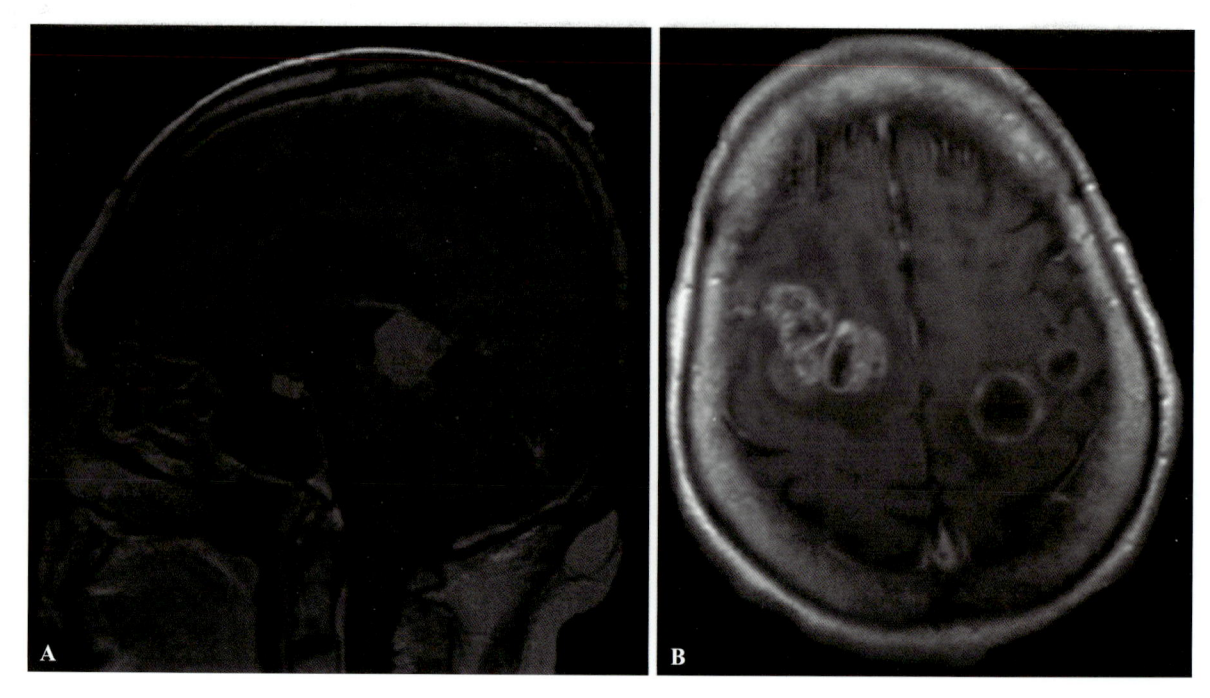

▲ 图 6-14 A. 84 岁男性患者松果体区孤立性占位，导致梗阻性脑积水。他首先接受了内镜下第三脑室引流术缓解梗阻性脑积水，同时行活检明确为黑色素瘤转移。考虑到患者高龄，肿瘤位于功能区难以切除，手术切除风险大，患者接受了 SRS 和免疫治疗。B. 63 岁女性患者双侧额顶叶非小细胞肺癌脑转移。患者颅外病变严重且有严重的并发症，接受了姑息性 WBRT，3 个月后死亡

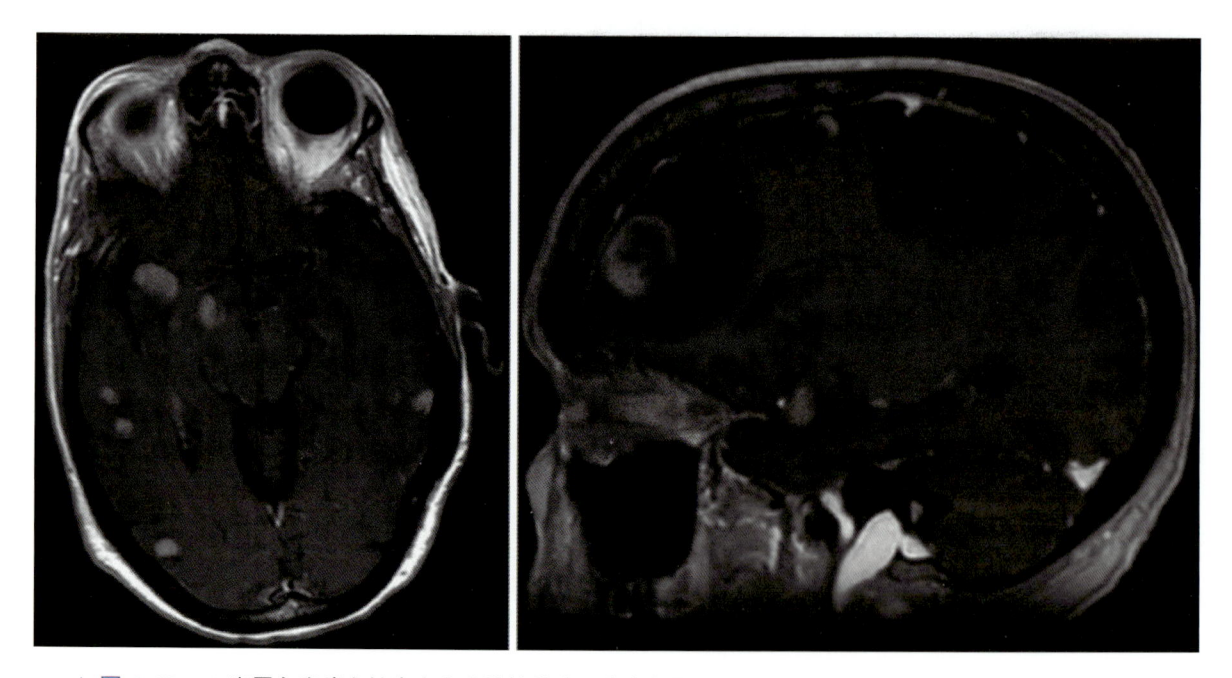

▲ 图 6-15 72 岁黑色素瘤女性患者多发脑转移瘤，病变主要位于右侧额叶和右侧额顶叶。考虑到肿瘤负荷重及不良预后，不适合接受手术

要 点

- 所有脑转移患者的治疗方案应该由放射肿瘤科、肿瘤内科、神经外科医生共同讨论决定。手术的适应证及禁忌证因素如表 6-3 所示。
- 对于接受手术切除的脑转移患者，建议进行辅助放疗以降低局部复发的风险。
- 最大限度地安全切除应是手术的目的。术后复发性病变可以从再次开颅手术中获益。
- 与辅助 SRS 相比，辅助 WBRT 更容易导致神经认知功能下降和生活质量下降，但颅内肿瘤控制率更高，而两者的总生存率相当。因此，对颅内转移数量有限的患者术后推荐进行 SRS 而非 WBRT。
- 术前 SRS 与术后 SRS 相比，肿瘤复发率相似，放射性脑坏死和软脑膜转移发生率更低。
- 接受了术前 SRS 的患者如果是次全切，强烈推荐再次手术或进行放疗补量。
- 尽管权威的研究仍在进行，我们仍然认为接受手术的患者术前 SRS 优于术后 SRS，除非因肿瘤占位危及生命需要紧急干预的患者。

参考文献

[1] Chao JH, Phillips R, Nickson JJ. Roentgen-ray therapy of cerebral metastases. Cancer. 1954;7:682–9.

[2] McTyre E, Scott J, Chinnaiyan P. Whole brain radiotherapy for brain metastasis. Surg Neurol Int. 2013;4(Suppl 4):S236–44.

[3] Borgelt B, Gelber R, Kramer S, et al. The palliation of brain metastases: final results of the first two studies by the Radiation Therapy Oncology Group. Int J Radiat Oncol Biol Phys. 1980;6(1):1–9.

[4] Gaspar L, Scott C, Rotman M, et al. Recursive partitioning analysis (RPA) of prognostic factors in three Radiation Therapy Oncology Group (RTOG) brain metastases trials. Int J Radiat Oncol Biol Phys. 1997;37(4):745–51.

[5] Patchell RA, Tibbs P, Regine WF, et al. Postoperative radiotherapy in the treatment of single metastases to the brain. JAMA. 1998;280(17):1485–9.

[6] Patchell RA, Tibbs P, Walsh JW, et al. A randomized trial of surgery in the treatment of single metastases to the brain. N Engl J Med. 1990;322(8):494–500.

[7] Kocher M, Soffietti R, Abacioglu U, et al. Adjuvant whole-brain radiotherapy versus observation after radiosurgery or surgical resection of one to three cerebral metastases: results of the EORTC 22952-26001 study. J Clin Oncol. 2011;29(2):134–41.

[8] Mahajan A, Ahmed S, McAleer MF, et al. Post-operative stereotactic radiosurgery versus observation for completely resected brain metastases, a single-centre randomised, controlled, phase 3 trial. Lancet Oncol. 2017;18(8):1040–8.

[9] Brown PD, Jaeckle K, Ballman KV, et al. Effect of radiosurgery alone vs radiosurgery with whole brain radiation therapy on cognitive function in patients with 1 to 3 brain metastases: a randomized clinical trial. JAMA. 2016;316(4):401–9.

[10] Chang EL, Wefel J, Hess KR, et al. Neurocognition in patients with brain metastases treated with radiosurgery or radiosurgery plus whole-brain irradiation: a randomised controlled trial. Lancet Oncol. 2009;10(11):1037–44.

[11] Soffietti R, Kocher M, Abacioglu UM, et al. A European Organisation for Research and Treatment of Cancer phase III trial of adjuvant whole-brain radiotherapy versus observation in patients with one to three brain metastases from solid tumors after surgical resection or radiosurgery: quality-of-life results. J Clin Oncol. 2013;31(1):65–72.

[12] Aoyama H, Shirato H, Tago M, et al. Stereotactic radiosurgery plus whole-brain radiation therapy vs stereotactic radiosurgery alone for treatment of brain metastases. JAMA. 2006;295(21):2483–91.

[13] Prabhu RS, Patel KR, Press RH, et al. Preoperative vs postoperative radiosurgery for resected brain metastases: a review. Neurosurgery. 2019;84(1):19–29.

[14] Brennan C, Yang TJ, Hilden P, et al. A phase 2 trial of stereotactic radiosurgery boost after surgical resection for brain metastases. Int J Radiat Oncol Biol Phys. 2014;88(1):130–6.

[15] Brown PD, Ballman K, Cerhan JH, et al. Postoperative stereotactic radiosurgery compared with whole brain radiotherapy for resected metastatic brain disease (NCCTG N107C/CEC3): a multicentre, randomised, controlled, phase 3 trial. Lancet Oncol. 2017;18(8):1049–60.

[16] Prabhu RS, Press R, Patel KR, et al. Single-fraction stereotactic

radiosurgery (SRS) alone versus surgical resection and SRS for large brain metastases: a multi-institutional analysis. Int J Radiat Oncol Biol Phys. 2017;99(2):459–67.

[17] Quigley MR, Bello N, Jho D, et al. Estimating the additive benefit of surgical excision to stereotactic radiosurgery in the management of metastatic brain disease. Neurosurgery. 2015;76(6):707–13.

[18] Roberge D, Parney I, Brown PD. Radiosurgery to the postoperative surgical cavity: who needs evidence? Int J Radiat Oncol Biol Phys. 2012;83(2):486–93.

[19] Atalar B, Modlin LA, Choi CY, et al. Risk of leptomeningeal disease in patients treated with stereotactic radiosurgery targeting the postoperative resection cavity for brain metastases. Int J Radiat Oncol Biol Phys. 2013;87(4):713–8.

[20] Iorio-Morin C, Masson-Cote L, Ezahr Y, Blanchard J, Ebacher A, Mathieu D. Early Gamma Knife stereotactic radiosurgery to the tumor bed of resected brain metastasis for improved local control. J Neurosurg. 2014;121(Suppl):69–74.

[21] Patel KR, Prabhu RS, Kandula S, et al. Intracranial control and radiographic changes with adjuvant radia- tion therapy for resected brain metastases: whole brain radiotherapy versus stereotactic radiosurgery alone. J Neuro-Oncol. 2014;120(3):657–63.

[22] Ojerholm E, Lee J, Thawani JP, et al. Stereotactic radiosurgery to the resection bed for intracranial metastases and risk of leptomeningeal carcinomatosis. J Neurosurg. 2014;121(2):75–83.

[23] Soltys SG, Adler J, Lipani JD, et al. Stereotactic radiosurgery of the postoperative resection cavity for brain metastases. Int J Radiat Oncol Biol Phys. 2008;70(1):187–93.

[24] Choi CY, Chang S, Gibbs IC, et al. Stereotactic radiosurgery of the postoperative resection cavity for brain metastases: prospective evaluation of target margin on tumor control. Int J Radiat Oncol Biol Phys. 2012;84(2):336–42.

[25] Johnson MD, Avkshtol V, Baschnagel AM, et al. Surgical resection of brain metastases and the risk of leptomeningeal recurrence in patients treated with stereotactic radiosurgery. Int J Radiat Oncol Biol Phys. 2016;94(3):537–43.

[26] Huang AJ, Huang KE, Page BR, et al. Risk factors for leptomeningeal carcinomatosis in patients with brain metastases who have previously undergone stereotactic radiosurgery. J Neuro-Oncol. 2014;120(1):163–9.

[27] Blonigen BJ, Steinmetz R, Levin L, et al. Irradiated volume as a predictor of brain radionecrosis after linear accelerator stereotactic radiosurgery. Int J Radiat Oncol Biol Phys. 2010;77(4):996–1001.

[28] Minniti G, Clarke E, Lanzetta G, et al. Stereotactic radiosurgery for brain metastases: analysis of outcome and risk of brain radionecrosis. Radiat Oncol. 2011;6(1):48.

[29] Sneed PK, Mendez J, Vemer-van den Hock JG, et al. Adverse radiation effect after stereotactic radiosurgery for brain metastases: incidence, time course, and risk factors. J Neurosurg. 2015;123(2):373–86.

[30] Patel KR, Burri S, Asher AL, et al. Comparing preoperative with postoperative stereotactic radiosurgery for resectable brain metastases. Neurosurgery. 2016;79(2):279–85.

[31] Prabhu RS, Miller KR, Asher AL, et al. Preoperative stereotactic radiosurgery before planned resection of brain metastases: updated analysis of efficacy and toxicity of a novel treatment paradigm. J Neurosurg. 2018:1–8.

[32] Patel KR, Burri SH, Boselli D, et al. Comparing pre-operative stereotactic radiosurgery (SRS) to post-operative whole brain radiation therapy (WBRT) for resectable brain metastases: a multi-institutional analysis. J Neuro-Oncol. 2017;131(3):611–8.

[33] Asher AL, Burri SH, Wiggins WF, et al. A new treatment paradigm: neoadjuvant radiosurgery before surgical resection of brain metastases with analysis of local tumor recurrence. Int J Radiat Oncol Biol Phys. 2014;88(4):899–906.

[34] Routman DM, Yan E, Vora S, et al. Preoperative stereotactic radiosurgery for brain metastases. Front Neurol. 2018;9:959.

[35] Nayak L, Lee EQ, Wen PY. Epidemiology of brain metastases. Curr Oncol Rep. 2012;14(1):48–54.

[36] Nahed BV, Alvarez-Breckenridge C, Brastianos PK, et al. Congress of neurological surgeons systematic review and evidence-based guidelines on the role of surgery in the management of adults with metastatic brain tumors. Neurosurgery. 2019;84(3):E152–5.

[37] Lee CH, Kim D, Kim JW, et al. The role of surgical resection in the management of brain metastasis: a 17-year longitudinal study. Acta Neurochir. 2013;155(3):389–97.

[38] Obermueller T, Schaeffner M, Gerhardt J, Meyer B, Ringel F, Krieg SM. Risks of postoperative paresis in motor eloquently and non-eloquently located brain metastases. BMC Cancer. 2014;14(1):21.

[39] Suki D, Hatiboglu M, Patel AJ, et al. Comparative risk of leptomeningeal dissemination of cancer after surgery or stereotactic radiosurgery for a single supratentorial solid tumor metastasis. Neurosurgery. 2009;64(4):664–76.

[40] Patel AJ, Suki D, Hatiboglu MA, Rao VY, Fox BD, Sawaya R. Impact of surgical methodology on the complication rate and functional outcome of patients with a single brain metastasis. J Neurosurg. 2015;122(5):1132–43.

[41] Patel AJ, Suki D, Hatiboglu MA, et al. Factors influencing the risk of local recurrence after resection of a single brainmetastasis. J Neurosurg. 2010;113(2):181–9.

[42] Stark AM, Stöhring C, Hedderich J, Held-Feindt J, Mehdorn HM. Surgical treatment for brain metastases: prognostic factors and survival in 309 patients with regard to patient age. J Clin Neurosci. 2011;18(1):34–8.

[43] Kano H, Kondziolka D, Zorro O, Lobato-Polo J, Flickinger JC, Lunsford LD. The results of resection after stereotactic radiosurgery for brain metastases. J Neurosurg. 2009;111(4):825–31.

第7章 激光间质热疗在脑转移瘤中的应用
Laser Interstitial Thermal Therapy for Brain Metastasis

Ahmet F.Atik　Krishna C.Joshi　Alireza Mohammad Mohammadi　Gene H.Barnett　著

井　笛　译

周　琴　校

一、病例介绍

（一）病例1

一名75岁的吸烟男性被诊断为肺鳞癌ⅢB期，患者接受了多西他赛联合卡铂的化疗。治疗结束6个月后，患者开始出现右手精细运动不协调的症状，后来出现右下肢乏力及行动不便。MRI检查结果显示患者颅内有两处病变，分别位于左额叶和左小脑。因为患者有原发肺癌病史，所以诊断为肺癌脑转移。颅内两处病灶均接受了伽马刀的治疗：左额叶病灶直径为16mm，68%的等剂量线为24Gy；左侧小脑病灶直径为25.3mm，首先接受18Gy伽马刀的治疗，然后接受了57%等剂量线为12Gy伽马刀的治疗。治疗后2年，复查左侧额叶和小脑病变均消失。第2年底，左侧小脑病变再次长大并且伴随辨距不良，左侧肢体运动障碍。磁共振灌注结果显示脑血容量增加（cerebral blood volume，CBV），治疗组讨论后决定采用激光间质热疗法（laser interstitial thermal therapy，LITT）治疗这种复发性病变。患者的LITT治疗路径见图7-1。随访2年多，影像学资料显示患者颅内病灶消失（图7-2）。患者神经系统的不适症状逐渐减轻。不幸的是由于原发病灶进展，患者在LITT治疗后3年去世。

（二）病例2

一名44岁的女性被诊断为三阴性乳腺癌伴区域淋巴结转移。患者接受了乳腺癌改良根治术，术后在其他医疗中心接受化疗。术后8个月，发现有两处颅内转移病灶，接受了分阶段的伽马刀治疗（第一阶段是50%的等剂量线为18Gy，第二阶段是50%的等剂量线为12Gy）。体积较小的病变对治疗敏感，而右侧丘脑较大的病灶对治疗不敏感且持续存在。伽马刀治疗4个月之后，位于丘脑的病灶开始长大，随后转诊至著者医疗中心。灌注MRI成像检查结果提示脑血容量增加，提示病变极有可能是颅内肿瘤复发而非放射性损伤。患者既往仅有乳腺癌病史，目前尚无神经系统功能障碍。

患者接受了立体定向活检确诊为肿瘤复发，随后行LITT治疗。从同一个穿刺孔沿着3条轨迹，进行LITT治疗（图7-3）。直径为41mm的颅内肿瘤被完整消融。患者术后病情平稳，手术后2天无任何并发症。随访发现肿瘤周围水肿带明显减少，在6个月时水肿带几乎完全消失（图7-4）。LITT后肿瘤体积缩小，6个月内肿瘤体积从18.9cm³缩小至14.7cm³（图7-5）。尽管水肿带明显减少，但是增强影像显示在肿瘤边界后缘出现增强，提示复发（图7-5D）。

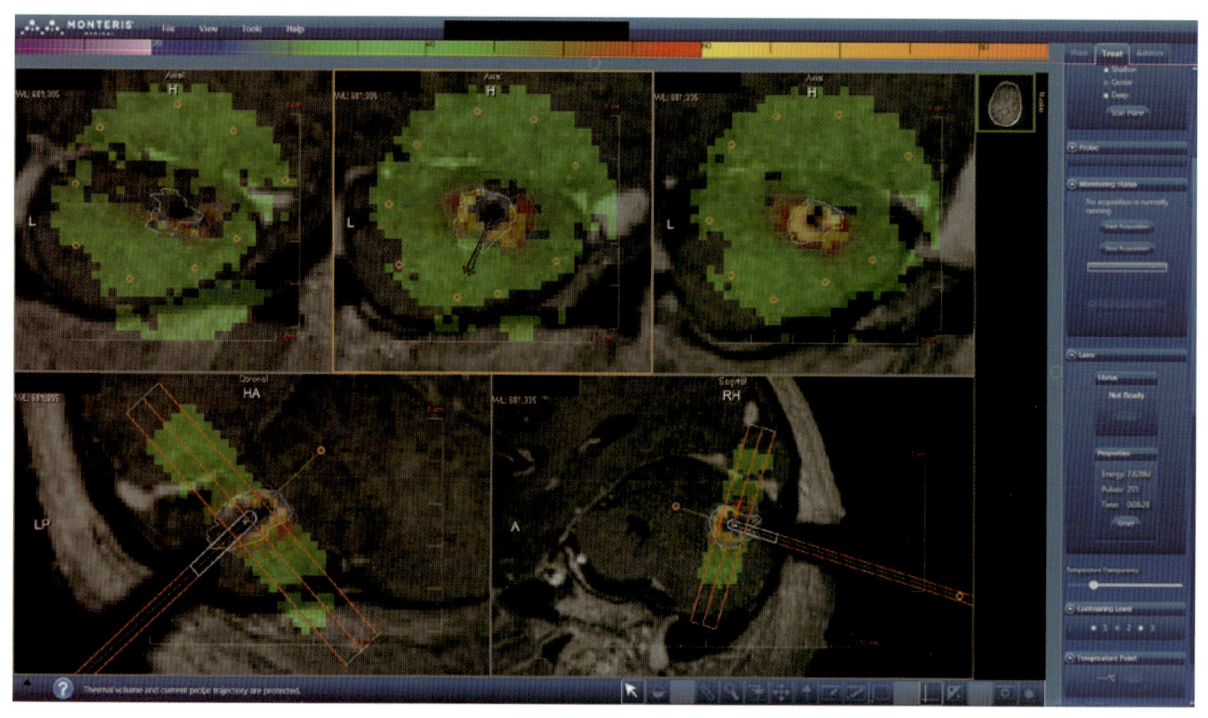

▲ 图 7-1 小脑转移病灶 LITT 手术期间的屏幕截图

蓝色线.凝固性坏死；蓝绿色线.肿瘤边界；绿色区域.MR 测温区域；绿色圆圈中的黄色圆圈.MR 测温的读数；蓝色箭头.计划方向；红色箭头.实际位置（红色将随后变为蓝色）；黄色直线.表示探测区域；黄色圆圈.探针可以达到的最大长度

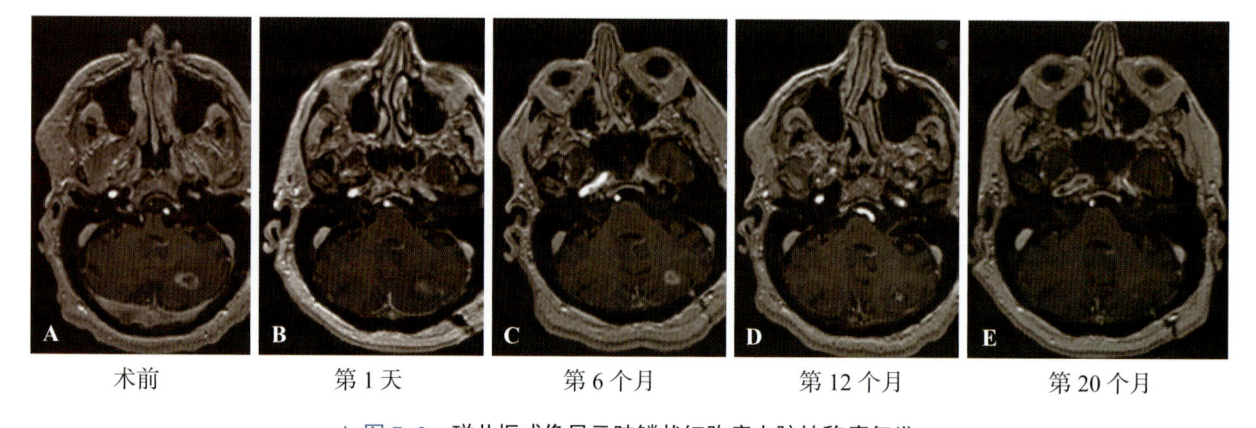

▲ 图 7-2 磁共振成像显示肺鳞状细胞癌小脑转移瘤复发

A.T_1 增强 MRI 显示术前病灶；B.手术后第 1 天；C.手术后第 6 个月；D.手术后第 12 个月；E.手术后第 20 个月

二、概述

肿瘤诊断能力的提升和新疗法的出现使得脑转移瘤的诊断率提高。在过去的 20 年里，脑转移病灶的治疗方式发生了转变。虽然以前脑转移的患者通常被认为是无法治愈，但是现在越来越多的患者经过治疗，脑部病灶明显缩小。这种现象在很大程度上可以归因于新型治疗方式的发展，而局部治疗也越来越受到重视。MRI 引导的 LITT 是神经外科最新的治疗方式之一，可用于各种颅内肿瘤的一种微创治疗方法。

激光（光的能量通过发射装置放大）探头直接对准需要热凝固的结构[1]。激光消融的机制依赖于将热能（生物热）传递到激光探针周围的组织[2]，产生凝固性坏死，以及通过光

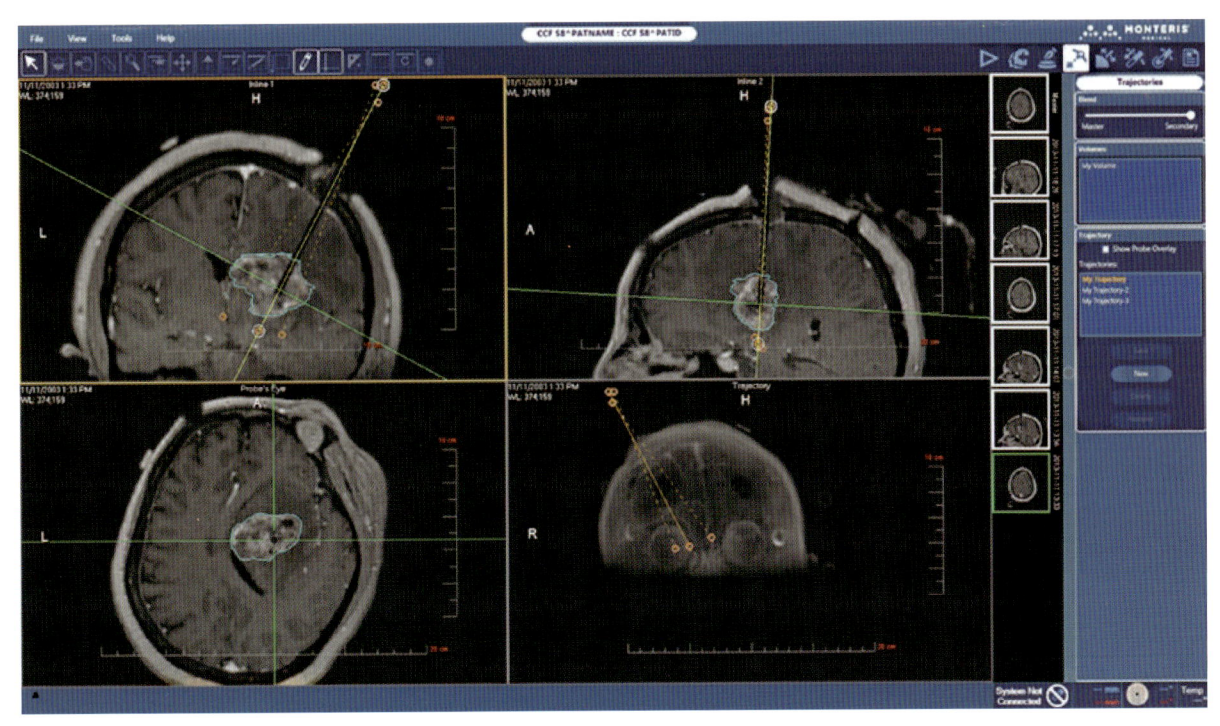

▲ 图 7-3　带有四个嵌入式窗口的 LITT 术中屏幕截图。三条直线显示 LITT 的每次治疗轨迹

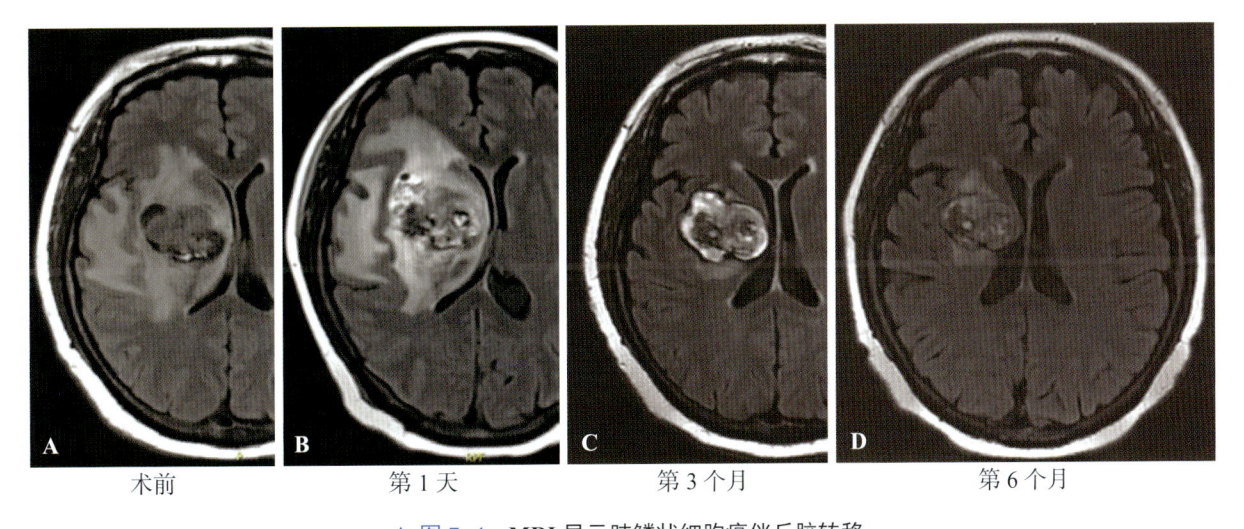

A 术前　　B 第 1 天　　C 第 3 个月　　D 第 6 个月

▲ 图 7-4　MRI 显示肺鳞状细胞癌伴丘脑转移
A. T$_2$ Flair MRI 显示术前复发病灶；B. 手术后第 1 天；C. 手术后第 3 个月；D. 手术后第 6 个月

凝固术使血管硬化[3]。同样的道理，微波或超声波都可以作为发热源靶向治疗区域[4]。目前这三种方法中的两种已经应用于神经外科。超声消融主要用于神经退行性病变的消融，如原发性震颤等[5]。LITT 首先由从事外科手术的 Bown 医师使用[6]，然后由神经外科医师 Kahn 等在 MRI 实时成像的辅助下应用于各种颅内肿瘤[7]，这种治疗方式经常用于不适合手术治疗的颅内肿瘤患者[8]。与传统外科手术模式相比，这种微创手术可以缩短住院时间并降低死亡率[9]。

LITT 的不良反应是碳化和汽化都会使组织

075

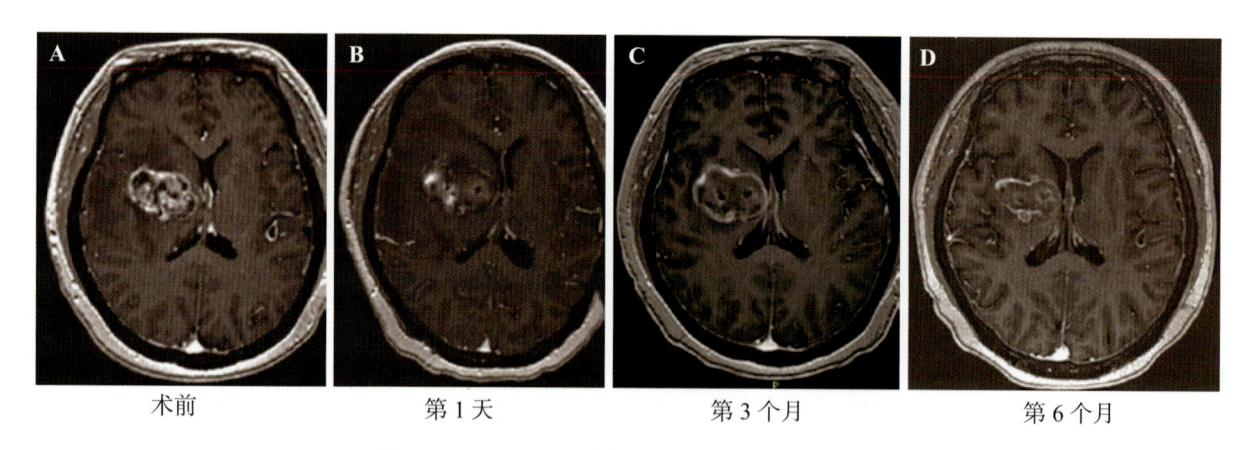

▲ 图 7-5 MRI 显示肺鳞状细胞癌患者的丘脑转移病灶
A. T₁ 加权 MRI 显示术前病变；B. 术后第 1 天；C. 术后第 6 个月；D. 术后 12 个月；E. 术后 20 个月

温度达到 100℃。通过 MR 实时测温监控病灶的内部温度是治疗过程中的关键步骤。

不同类型激光器的重要区别在于组织穿透深度的不一致。例如，掺钕的钇铝石榴石（Nd-YAG）激光器的穿透深度为 4mm，而氩气仅为 0.4mm。最常用的 CO_2 激光器其组织穿透力为 30μm。组织穿透力最好的是 Nd-YAG 激光器，因为它具有更长的波长。较短波长的激光产生的热量更多，组织穿透欠佳，导致颅内组织热坏死的风险更大。

在 20 世纪 60 年代，红宝石激光器在医疗领域最早用于去除文身[10]。红宝石激光器具有较短的波长（694nm），首次应用的领域是皮肤科。在 20 世纪 80 年代初期，Bown 等使用 CO_2 激光器治疗肿瘤，发现虽然长波长的激光可穿透更深的组织，适用于更大的病灶，但这种类型的激光可以瞬间（数秒内）达到最高温度，并且可以切割汽化组织而不产生凝固性坏死。所以，应用于深部组织并不实际[6]。

目前，处于近红外光波段（Nd-YAG 激光范围）的激光器可以用于 LITT。首先它们是长波，可以安全地治疗位置较深的肿瘤，其次其缓慢升温的特性可以在术中长时间停留在一个位置[6]。目前神经外科使用的两种技术分别是脑肿瘤激光消融系统 Neuroblate（美国明尼苏达州普利茅斯的蒙特里斯公司）和可视化酶技术

Visualase（美国明尼苏达州明尼阿波利斯的美敦力公司），它们在近红外范围内使用相同的固态激光器（1064nm，12W），但冷却系统却不一样。Neuroblate 系统使用的是 CO_2 气冷激光探头，而 Visualase 系统使用的是基于盐水循环系统围绕探针进行冷却[11]。

神经外科使用激光治疗可以追溯到 20 世纪 90 年代，Sugiyama 等证实了使用 Nd-YAG 激光器治疗颅内肿瘤的安全性[12]。这种长波激光器与 X 线断层扫描一起使用可成功切除病灶。尽管在 90 年代使用过这种长波和低功率的激光器，但是激光探头的不成熟设计和术中无法实时监测的缺点，给 LITT 在神经外科的临床应用带来了困难。然而，Nd-YAG 激光器非常适合用于灌注度良好的软组织，如脑白质[13]。

使 LITT 的利用实现突破的因素是 MRI 热成像技术的发展。在此技术之前，激光器在 20 世纪 80 年代引起了人们的兴趣，但是由于难以监测和预测热损伤程度，导致在十年内使用率下降。LITT 的相关文献向我们展示了在引入 MR 热成像技术（1994 年后），LITT 的文献数量呈指数增长（图 7-6）。MR 热成像技术能实时监测组织内部的热损伤，从而最大限度地消融病变，同时最大限度地减少对周围正常组织的损害[14]。提高激光的能量可以增加目标区域温度，破坏细胞内部氢键的同时增加自由水分子的数

量。MR 热像仪测量组织温度的方法称为质子共振频移（proton resonance frequency shift PRFS）[15]。MR 热像仪不仅仅限于 LITT，也可以用于颅内超声[16]，以及身体其他部位的射频消融[17]。

组织的光学特性取决于多个因素，如实质透明质酸的含量。研究已表明激光能量在灰质中的穿透能力远远高于白质[18]。此外，病变组织结构中激光能量的渗透/吸收率不同于健康组织。与高级别胶质瘤相比，低级别神经胶质瘤吸收的激光能量更少，但事实上低级别胶质瘤的灰质组织比正常的灰质吸收更多能量[18]。

病灶内部包含有三个热效应区域。第一个区域是探头周围可以吸收最大能量并产生真正的凝固性坏死，并伴随有碳化和（或）汽化，坏死程度取决于 LITT 达到的温度。当组织温度超过 50℃时，会发生凝固性坏死。当组织温度超过 100℃时会发生碳化和汽化。第二个区域也会发生凝固性坏死，第三区域可能会受到一定程度的热损伤，但该区域中的细胞可能会存活[19]。

本章中，我们讨论了 LITT 当前的适应证并回顾相关文献，阐明 LITT 在治疗脑转移瘤中的作用。

三、手术中的应用

在我们医疗中心，LITT 是联合脑肿瘤激光消融系统 Neuroblate 执行，该系统使用 Nd-YAG 范围内（1064nm，12W）的固态二极管激光器。激光能量通过 CO_2 气体冷却的定向激光探头传输到治疗区域。轨迹规划和激光探头插入肿瘤主要是通过使用外科手术导航设备和 NeuroBlate 系统特有的装置完成。激光探针在肿瘤内的位置通过术中 MRI 确定。在实时 MR 热成像技术辅助下，激光发射部分的控制主要是采用了 M° Vision™ 软件（Monteris 医疗公司，明尼苏达州，美国）的 NeuroBlate System。实时性热消融的控制主要通过公司 M° Vision 软件，该款软件基于热杀死细胞的算法（时间和温度之间的关系）和热损伤阈值线（thermal damage threshold TDT），分别包含了黄色、蓝色和白色三种热损伤阈值线。黄色的 TDT 线代表组织区域相当于加热到 43℃至少 2min；蓝色 TDT 线相当于加热到 43℃至

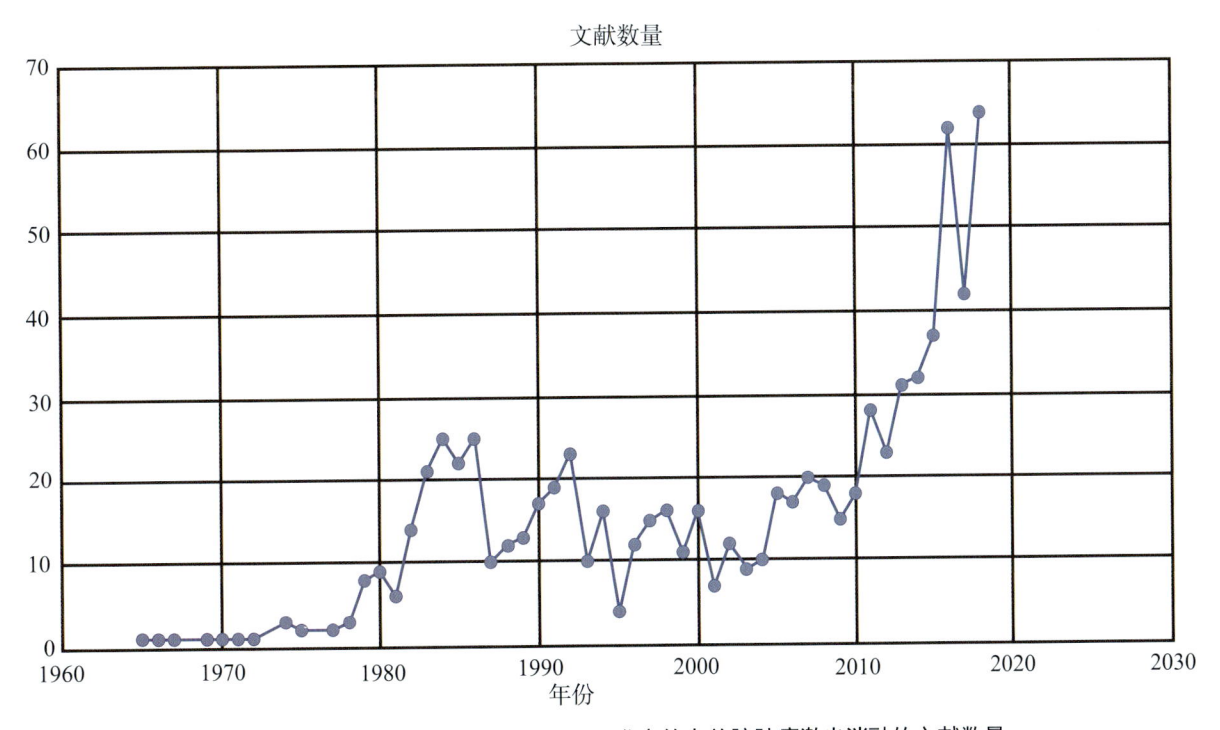

文献数量

▲ 图 7-6 自 1965 年以来在 PubMed 发表的有关脑肿瘤激光消融的文献数量

少 10min；白色的 TDT 线代表加热到 43℃达 60min，或较短时间间隔内加热到更高的温度。这些 TDT 线代表了肿瘤组织治疗效果的真实指标（图 7-4）[20]。

四、诊断与治疗

脑转移瘤源自多种不同的癌症，最常见的是肺癌，无性别差异；其次，女性常见的是乳腺癌和胃肠道恶性肿瘤，男性常见的是胃肠道恶性肿瘤和黑色素瘤[21]。如果原发肿瘤类型有扩散至大脑的可能而且有影像学支持，则颅内病变可以在无须进行活检的情况下诊断为转移。如果影像学特征不典型无法确诊，可以采用立体定向活检明确脑部病变性质的诊断。

最近的临床试验表明，对于脑转移瘤的治疗，立体定向放射外科（stereo tactic radiosurgery，SRS）的疗效相当于甚至优于全脑放疗（whole brain radiotherapy，WBRT）。SRS 可以用于多发脑转移病变，也可以与 WBRT 结合使用，或应用于手术残腔的照射。SRS 通常被认为是 1～3 处脑转移病灶患者的一线治疗方案[22]，放射性坏死是 SRS 常见的不良反应，而且难以明确诊断和治疗。随着成像技术的发展，如灌注 MRI 或脱氧葡萄糖正电子断层扫描（fluorodeoxyglucose positron emission tomography，FDG-PET）可以帮助医师区分放射性坏死与肿瘤复发或进展[23, 24]。

当存在诊断不明确或肿瘤迅速生长并引起神经系统症状时，应考虑进行手术切除脑转移病灶[25]。LITT 可以用于治疗顽固性转移性肿瘤，这些肿瘤通过其他治疗方式无法有效控制，LITT 被认为是治疗脑转移病灶的最后一招。Ahluwalia 等的研究表明颅内肿瘤进行完全消融 LITT，有 75% 达到完全缓解，但是当次全消融时有 62.5% 的肿瘤会出现进展[26]。Aliet 等的报道称 LITT 术后采用大分割立体定向放疗治疗复发性脑转移瘤的病灶局控率高达 100%，而仅采用 LITT 治疗病灶的局控率只有 57%[27]。

五、循证基础

激光在脑转移瘤中的首次应用可以追溯到 1986 年，Tobler 等报道了通过激光治疗脑转移病灶的成功病例[28]。当时，LITT 仍处于起步阶段，尚未与 MRI 热像仪联合使用。从那时起，出现了多种治疗脑转移瘤的新方法，尤其是 SRS。尽管 SRS 成功率很高，但仍有约 15% 的脑转移瘤对放疗抵抗[29]，LITT 可以作为这些病例的可选方案。脑转移瘤的原发病理类型是 SRS 治疗成败的重要预测因素。肾细胞癌[30]、大肠腺癌[31]、BRAF 野生型黑色素瘤[32] 及三阴性乳腺癌[33]，都被认为是 SRS 抵抗的组织病理学类型[34]。对于这些患者，LITT 可能是一个很好的选择，或者是 SRS 的补救性治疗措施。

使用 LITT 治疗脑转移瘤的成功病例报道较少。Carpentier 等早期有价值的研究包含了一些如化疗、放疗，以及免疫疗法治疗失败的病例，这些研究主要是复发转移的患者排除有放射性坏死的病例。Hawasli 等报道了可以使用 LITT 治疗的多种不同病理类型，其中有五种转移性肿瘤在无法手术切除的区域对激光消融反应敏感[35-37]。

六、LITT 治疗脑转移瘤的不确定领域

SRS 被广泛认为是许多颅内转移瘤患者的首选治疗方法[38]。然而，对于 SRS 治疗后的复发病灶的处理可能具有挑战性。这些病灶可能是复发转移灶，也可能是放射性坏死抑或两者均有。目前尚没有明确的影像学特征来区分，再程放疗可能会错将坏死病灶认为是疾病进展而加剧第一次放疗带来的损伤。放射性脑坏死目前有很多治疗选择，包括密切随访，高压氧、己酮可可碱、维生素 E、类固醇和贝伐珠单抗，但是这些治疗手段中没有哪一种治疗方式具有明显优势。手术切除诊断明确的病灶，减少病灶带来的占位效应。对于那些类固醇治疗无效的患者，VEGF 抑

制药如贝伐珠单抗有一定的效果[39]。但是，它尚未获得 FDA 批准治疗放射外科后影像学强化的病变。

有关 LITT 的近期研究主要是针对 SRS 治疗后影像学增强的病灶。它在诊断和治疗方面具有明显的优势，同时微小的创面有助于有全身合并症的患者避免大型的颅内手术[40, 41]。选择合适的患者是 LITT 治疗成功的关键，主要针对位置较深且难以进入的病变。然而，LITT 也可以用于浅表病变或由于先前的放疗或多次手术导致头皮变薄，不适宜开颅手术更倾向选择微创的患者。

另一个关注的问题是 LITT 治疗 SRS 治疗后的强化病灶，延缓了影像学强化病灶的复发。LITT 延缓复发的一种可能原因是病变确实是复发性肿瘤，而不是放射性坏死。以前发表的文献中没有清楚地描述他们的病理学诊断[42, 43]。在放射性坏死的情况下，脑水肿的短暂消退及细胞因子风暴的暂停引起的组织损伤不足以达到长期控制。相比之下，LITT 用于治疗复发性肿瘤可能需要加大消融范围以防止复发，特别在 LITT 治疗后还需要额外 SRS[44]。

七、LITT 的并发症

以前关于 LITT 的文献认为它是安全且耐受性良好，适用于各种颅内恶性肿瘤和转移性肿瘤的治疗。但是 LITT 导致的并发症以及技术局限性却很少被讨论。LITT 治疗的文献综述，包括 25 份临床报道和 243 名治疗患者，报道了并发症的发生率为 20%[45]，包括 4 例患者（1.6%）出现导管位置不正而产生的硬膜下血肿[46]、动脉损伤出血[47]及蛛网膜出血[48]，还有 1 例患者出现沿穿刺轨道肿瘤的种植[49]。然而，定位技术（尤其是颅骨锚定设备）的改进为放置导管提高了准确性。通过将 CT 血管造影与 MRI 融合，患者的出血风险将进一步降低，尤其是在较长轨迹的情况下。如之前文献所述，各种并发症与组织高温有关，其中包括新发或已有的神经功能损伤恶化（如语言障碍[36, 37]、同侧偏盲[50]、癫痫[51]）、感染（脑脓肿[52]）、恶性脑水肿[47]和脑脊液漏出[51]。在可能的情况下尽可能使用较小的扩散器尖端[45]，并通过使用纤维跟踪成像制定计划，用于治疗靠近语言功能区附近的肿瘤组织[53]。

> **要　点**
> - 目前没有足够的证据推荐 LITT 作为一线治疗用于脑转移瘤。
> - 它可能是 SRS 非常有效的辅助治疗手段，特别是对 SRS 疗效欠佳或在 SRS 之后发生放射坏死的转移性病灶。
> - LITT 可以考虑用于手术难以抵达的深部病灶，或者作为不适合 SRS 患者的替代治疗方式。
> - 需进一步前瞻性试验来探讨 SRS 与 LITT 两种治疗方式的安全性和有效性差异，特别是作为一线治疗应用。

参考文献

[1] Gologorsky Y, Ben-Haim S, Moshier EL, Godbold J, Tagliati M, Weisz D, et al. Transgressing the ventricular wall during subthalamic deep brain stimulation surgery for Parkinson disease increases the risk of adverse neurological sequelae. Neurosurgery. 2011;69(2):294–9; discussion 9–300.

[2] Fuentes D, Walker C, Elliott A, Shetty A, Hazle JD, Stafford RJ. Magnetic resonance temperature imaging validation of a bioheat transfer model for laser-induced thermal therapy. Int J Hyperth. 2011;27(5):453–64.

[3] Ryan RW, Spetzler RF, Preul MC. Aura of technology and the

[4] Skinner MG, Iizuka MN, Kolios MC, Sherar MD. A theoretical comparison of energy sources—microwave, ultrasound and laser—for interstitial thermal therapy. Phys Med Biol. 1998;43(12):3535–47.

[5] Quadri SA, Waqas M, Khan I, Khan MA, Suriya SS, Farooqui M, et al. High-intensity focused ultrasound: past, present, and future in neurosurgery. Neurosurg Focus. 2018;44(2):E16.

[6] Bown SG. Phototherapy in tumors. World J Surg. 1983;7(6):700–9.

[7] Kahn T, Bettag M, Ulrich F, Schwarzmaier HJ, Schober R, Furst G, et al. MRI-guided laser-induced interstitial thermotherapy of cerebral neoplasms. J Comput Assist Tomogr. 1994;18(4):519–32.

[8] Stafford RJ, Fuentes D, Elliott AA, Weinberg JS, Ahrar K. Laser-induced thermal therapy for tumor ablation. Crit Rev Biomed Eng. 2010;38(1):79–100.

[9] Leuthardt EC, Voigt J, Kim AH, Sylvester P. A single-center cost analysis of treating primary and metastatic brain cancers with either brain laser interstitial thermal therapy (LITT) or craniotomy. Pharmacoecon Open. 2017;1(1):53–63.

[10] Goldman L, Wilson RG, Hornby P, Meyer RG. Radiation from a Q-switched ruby laser. Effect of repeated impacts of power output of 10 megawatts on a tattoo of man. J Invest Dermatol. 1965;44:69–71.

[11] Mohammadi AM, Hawasli AH, Rodriguez A, Schroeder JL, Laxton AW, Elson P, et al. The role of laser interstitial thermal therapy in enhancing progression-free survival of difficult-to-access high-grade gliomas: a multicenter study. Cancer Med. 2014;3(4):971–9.

[12] Sugiyama K, Sakai T, Fujishima I, Ryu H, Uemura K, Yokoyama T. Stereotactic interstitial laser-hyperthermia using Nd-YAG laser. Stereotact Funct Neurosurg. 1990;54–55:501–5.

[13] Norred SE, Johnson JA. Magnetic resonance-guided laser induced thermal therapy for glioblastoma multiforme: a review. Biomed Res Int. 2014;2014:761312.

[14] Missios S, Bekelis K, Barnett GH. Renaissance of laser interstitial thermal ablation. Neurosurg Focus. 2015;38(3):E13.

[15] Chen Y, Ge M, Ali R, Jiang H, Huang X, Qiu B. Quantitative MR thermometry based on phase-drift correction PRF shift method at 0.35 T. Biomed Eng Online. 2018;17(1):39.

[16] Lewis MA, Staruch RM, Chopra R. Thermometry and ablation monitoring with ultrasound. Int J Hyperth. 2015;31(2):163–81.

[17] Kolandaivelu A, Zviman MM, Castro V, Lardo AC, Berger RD, Halperin HR. Noninvasive assessment of tissue heating during cardiac radiofrequency ablation using MRI thermography. Circ Arrhythm Electrophysiol. 2010;3(5):521–9.

[18] Eggert HR, Blazek V. Optical properties of human brain tissue, meninges, and brain tumors in the spectral range of 200 to 900 nm. Neurosurgery. 1987;21(4):459–64.

[19] Fuentes D, Feng Y, Elliott A, Shetty A, McNichols RJ, Oden JT, et al. Adaptive real-time bioheat transfer models for computer-driven MR-guided laser induced thermal therapy. IEEE Trans Biomed Eng. 2010;57(5):1024–30.

[20] Sloan AE, Ahluwalia MS, Valerio-Pascua J, Manjila S, Torchia MG, Jones SE, et al. Results of the NeuroBlate System first-in-humans Phase I clinical trial for recurrent glioblastoma: clinical article. J Neurosurg. 2013;118(6):1202–19.

[21] Louis DN, Perry A, Reifenberger G, von Deimling A, Figarella-Branger D, Cavenee WK, et al. The 2016 World Health Organization classification of tumors of the central nervous system: a summary. Acta Neuropathol. 2016;131(6):803–20.

[22] O'Beirn M, Benghiat H, Meade S, Heyes G, Sawlani V, Kong A, et al. The expanding role of radiosurgery for brain metastases. Medicines (Basel). 2018;5(3):pii: E90.

[23] Wadhwa EL, Franc BL, Aboian M, Kim JY, Pampaloni M, Nicolaides T. Delayed fluorodeoxyglucose positron emission tomography imaging in the differentiation of tumor recurrence and radiation necrosis in pediatric central nervous system tumors: case report and review of the literature. Cureus. 2018;10(9):e3364.

[24] Muto M, Frauenfelder G, Senese R, Zeccolini F, Schena E, Giurazza F, et al. Dynamic susceptibility contrast (DSC) perfusion MRI in differential diagnosis between radionecrosis and neoangiogenesis in cerebral metastases using rCBV, rCBF and K2. Radiol Med. 2018;123(7):545–52.

[25] Lamba N, Cagney DN, Brignell RH, Martin AM, Bessel LA, Catalano PR, et al. Neurosurgical resection and stereotactic radiation versus stereotactic radiation alone in patients with a single or solitary brain metastasis. World Neurosurgeon. 2019;122:e1557–61.

[26] Ahluwalia M, Barnett GH, Deng D, Tatter SB, Laxton AW, Mohammadi AM, et al. Laser ablation after stereotactic radiosurgery: a multicenter prospective study in patients with metastatic brain tumors and radiation necrosis. J Neurosurg. 2018;130(3):804–11.

[27] Ali MA, Carroll KT, Rennert RC, Hamelin T, Chang L, Lemkuil BP, et al. Stereotactic laser ablation as treatment for brain metastases that recur after stereotactic radiosurgery: a multiinstitutional experience. Neurosurg Focus. 2016;41(4):E11.

[28] Tobler WD, Sawaya R, Tew JM Jr. Successful laser-assisted excision of a metastatic midbrain tumor. Neurosurgery. 1986;18(6):795–7.

[29] Flickinger JC, Kondziolka D, Lunsford LD, Coffey RJ, Goodman ML, Shaw EG, et al. A multi-institutional experience with stereotactic radiosurgery for solitary brain metastasis. Int J Radiat Oncol Biol Phys. 1994;28(4):797–802.

[30] Kim YH, Kim JW, Chung HT, Paek SH, Kim DG, Jung HW. Brain metastasis from renal cell carcinoma. Prog Neurol Surg. 2012;25:163–75.

[31] Nozawa H, Ishihara S, Kawai K, Sasaki K, Murono K, Otani K, et al. Brain metastasis from colorectal cancer: predictors and treatment outcomes. Oncology. 2017;93(5):309–14.

[32] Gallaher IS, Watanabe Y, DeFor TE, Dusenbery KE, Lee CK, Hunt MA, et al. BRAF mutation is associated with improved

local control of melanoma brain metastases treated with gamma knife radiosurgery. Front Oncol. 2016;6:107.

[33] Rostami R, Mittal S, Rostami P, Tavassoli F, Jabbari B. Brain metastasis in breast cancer: a comprehensive literature review. J Neuro-Oncol. 2016;127(3):407–14.

[34] Eschrich SA, Pramana J, Zhang H, Zhao H, Boulware D, Lee JH, et al. A gene expression model of intrinsic tumor radiosensitivity: prediction of response and prognosis after chemoradiation. Int J Radiat Oncol Biol Phys. 2009;75(2): 489–96.

[35] Carpentier A, McNichols RJ, Stafford RJ, Itzcovitz J, Guichard JP, Reizine D, et al. Real-time magnetic resonance-guided laser thermal therapy for focal metastatic brain tumors. Neurosurgery. 2008;63(1 Suppl 1):ONS21–8; discussion ONS8–9.

[36] Carpentier A, McNichols RJ, Stafford RJ, Guichard JP, Reizine D, Delaloge S, et al. Laser thermal therapy: real-time MRI-guided and computer-controlled procedures for metastatic brain tumors. Lasers Surg Med. 2011;43(10):943–50.

[37] Hawasli AH, Bagade S, Shimony JS, Miller-Thomas M, Leuthardt EC. Magnetic resonance imaging-guided focused laser interstitial thermal therapy for intracranial lesions: single-institution series. Neurosurgery. 2013;73(6):1007–17.

[38] Ewend MG, Morris DE, Carey LA, Ladha AM, Brem S. Guidelines for the initial management of metastatic brain tumors: role of surgery, radiosurgery, and radiation therapy. J Natl Compr Cancer Netw. 2008;6(5):505–13; quiz 14.

[39] Levin VA, Bidaut L, Hou P, Kumar AJ, Wefel JS, Bekele BN, et al. Randomized double-blind placebo-controlled trial of bevacizumab therapy for radiation necrosis of the central nervous system. Int J Radiat Oncol Biol Phys. 2011;79(5):1487–95.

[40] Rahmathulla G, Recinos PF, Valerio JE, Chao S, Barnett GH. Laser interstitial thermal therapy for focal cerebral radiation necrosis: a case report and literature review. Stereotact Funct Neurosurg. 2012;90(3):192–200.

[41] Jolesz FA. Intraoperative imaging in neurosurgery: where will the future take us? Acta Neurochir Suppl. 2011;109:21–5.

[42] Fabiano AJ, Alberico RA. Laser-interstitial thermal therapy for refractory cerebral edema from post-radiosurgery metastasis. World Neurosurg. 2014;81(3–4):652.e1–4.

[43] Rao MS, Hargreaves EL, Khan AJ, Haffty BG, Danish SF. Magnetic resonance-guided laser ablation improves local control for postradiosurgery recurrence and/or radiation necrosis. Neurosurgery. 2014;74(6):658–67; discussion 67.

[44] Rammo R, Asmaro K, Schultz L, Scarpace L, Siddiqui S, Walbert T, et al. The safety of magnetic resonance imaging-guided laser interstitial thermal therapy for cerebral radiation necrosis. J Neuro-Oncol. 2018;138(3):609–17.

[45] Pruitt R, Gamble A, Black K, Schulder M, Mehta AD. Complication avoidance in laser interstitial thermal therapy: lessons learned. J Neurosurg. 2017;126(4):1238–45.

[46] Willie JT, Laxpati NG, Drane DL, Gowda A, Appin C, Hao C, et al. Real-time magnetic resonance-guided stereotactic laser amygdalohippocampotomy for mesial temporal lobe epilepsy. Neurosurgery. 2014;74(6):569–85.

[47] Jethwa PR, Barrese JC, Gowda A, Shetty A, Danish SF. Magnetic resonance thermometry-guided laser-induced thermal therapy for intracranial neoplasms: initial experience. Oper Neurosurg. 2012;71(suppl_1):ons133–ons45.

[48] Wilfong AA, Curry DJ. Hypothalamic hamartomas: optimal approach to clinical evaluation and diagnosis. Epilepsia. 2013;54:109–14.

[49] Sloan AE, Ahluwalia MS, Valerio-Pascua J, Manjila S, Torchia MG, Jones SE, et al. Results of the NeuroBlate System first-in-humans Phase I clinical trial for recurrent glioblastoma. J Neurosurg. 2013;118(6):1202–19.

[50] Esquenazi Y, Kalamangalam GP, Slater JD, Knowlton RC, Friedman E, Morris S-A, et al. Stereotactic laser ablation of epileptogenic periventricular nodular heterotopia. Epilepsy Res. 2014;108(3):547–54.

[51] Carpentier A, Chauvet D, Reina V, Beccaria K, Leclerq D, McNichols RJ, et al. MR-guided laser-induced thermal therapy (LITT) for recurrent glioblastomas. Lasers Surg Med. 2012;44(5):361–8.

[52] Leonardi M, Lumenta C. Stereotactic guided laser-induced interstitial thermotherapy (SLITT) in gliomas with intraoperative morphologic monitoring in an open MR: clinical expierence. Minim Invasive Neurosurg. 2002;45(4):201–7.

[53] Yin D, Thompson JA, Drees C, Ojemann SG, Nagae L, Pelak VS, et al. Optic radiation tractography and visual field deficits in laser interstitial thermal therapy for amygdalohippocampectomy in patients with mesial temporal lobe epilepsy. Stereotact Funct Neurosurg. 2017;95(2):107–13.

第 8 章 脑转移瘤的系统性治疗
Integrating Systemic Therapy into the Management of Brain Metastases

John B. Fiveash　Anatoly Nikolaev　Robert M. Conry　著
井　笛　译
周　琴　校

一、概述

美国食品药品管理局负责监管审批新药，以前没有批准用于人体的一类药物被称为"新分子实体"，美国食品药品管理局每年收到 35~45 种"新分子实体"的申请报告，其中约有 25 种申请获得批准。尽管每年获得批准的数目不尽相同，每年约有 10 种新的肿瘤药物在美国获得批准，其中不包括扩大适应证的药物。当这些新药与脑部放射治疗联合应用时，肿瘤学家将面临关于这些新药互相作用的安全性及疗效信息不完整的问题。新药联合脑部放疗的安全性可能与放疗体积、放疗剂量、药物作用机制、正常脑组织与脑肿瘤药物渗透率、半衰期、辐射时间、药物作用时间等因素相关。本章将对各类联合放疗应用于脑转移瘤的系统治疗药物的安全性进行综述。在某些情况下，安全地利用放疗结合系统性化疗，进一步产生协同效应的理论是可行的。在缺乏临床安全性数据的情况下，提出了利用新药治疗脑转移瘤的策略。

二、循证基础

部分因素将会影响脑部放疗和全身药物治疗如何更好地结合并应用到脑转移瘤患者的治疗中。放疗辐照体积（放射外科治疗 vs. 全脑放疗）和放疗剂量与放射性脑坏死和白质脑病的发生风险相关。在考虑新药如何影响放疗毒性时，药物的作用时间和药理学尤为重要。有些药物需要在放疗同步使用，而另一些药物发挥作用则可能需要在辐射作用的环境或引起炎症的环境中。许多类似于单克隆抗体的大分子药物可能不能穿透大脑的非增强区域，但可能到达对比剂强化的区域，主要因为强化区域的血脑屏障不完整。其他药物如贝伐珠单抗（Bevacizumab）等靶向血管生长的药物可能不需要穿过血脑屏障。

三、研究概述

从以往经验来看，脑转移瘤新药的研究通常都是在没有其他治疗的情况下开展的，与最后一次治疗（如放射治疗）之间通常有 3~4 周的洗脱期。临床研究的结果往往不能满足实际的临床需求，临床上系统性治疗后脑部放疗并不一定会延迟实施。实际上，被放射外科最常引用的 RTOG90-05 研究排除了计划在未来 3 个月内需要进行全身治疗的患者[1]。因此，活动性 CNS 疾病患者往往被排除在新药物的前瞻性研究之外。

两项大型回顾性研究旨在探讨脑部放疗联合系统性药物治疗的安全性。来自约翰斯·霍普金斯大学的研究人员报道了 193 名接受放射外科（SRS）联合系统性药物治疗的患者。在各种联合治疗中同步治疗被认为是安全的，没有明显增加骨髓抑制或神经毒性反应[2]。在克利夫兰医疗中心接受脑转移瘤放射治疗的 1650 名患者中，其中有 445 人接受了同步系统性治疗[3]。在该系列研究中，同步治疗被定义为在五个生物学半衰期内进行。总之，同步系统性治疗的患者没有增加放射性坏死的风险，但是部分患者可能产生中高风险的并发症，其中包括接受全脑放疗和 SRS 同步系统性治疗的患者及接受 VEGF 或 EGFR 抑制药治疗的患者。本研究的毒性反应包括有症状和无症状的放射性坏死。最近的一项综述试图评估系统性治疗联合放射外科的安全性，并认为吉西他滨、厄洛替尼和维莫非尼作为联合用药可能产生较高的神经毒性风险[4]。下文各小节将进一步探讨这些结论。

四、细胞毒性药物

一直以来，传统的化疗药物是非小细胞肺癌和乳腺癌等多种脑转移瘤的主要治疗手段。在常见的肿瘤里，当免疫治疗或靶向治疗效果欠佳时，化疗药物仍然是标准的挽救性治疗方案。其中许多化疗药物（如顺铂、紫杉烷类和吉西他滨）都是放疗增敏剂，在全脑放疗过程中可能影响非中枢神经系统的正常组织，如皮肤或黏膜。在实际应用中，化疗药物往往按照周期给药而非每周给药，而放射外科可以不在化疗同一周进行。全脑放疗比放射外科可能需要更长的时间，但在胶质母细胞瘤的 I 期临床试验结果中认为这种治疗模式可能是安全的。在本节中，我们将重点讨论几种药物联合放疗可能具有的毒性反应，这些毒性可能无法在序贯治疗中被观察到。

1. 铂类

在肿瘤治疗中，顺铂或卡铂联合放射治疗具有悠久的历史。针对脑转移瘤和脑胶质瘤的前瞻性和回顾性研究表明，这些药物在放射治疗期间使用通常比较安全，但尚未进行大规模随机临床研究。放疗同步顺铂可能导致耳毒性和骨髓抑制的发生率偏高，除此之外铂类药物联合脑部放疗被认为安全可行[5]。在接受中枢神经系统放射治疗的髓母细胞瘤患者中，联合使用卡铂可能会导致发生骨髓抑制的概率偏高[6]。奥沙利铂主要用于结直肠癌治疗，在脑转移瘤放疗患者中的研究较少。在实际应用中，将同步脑放疗延迟到化疗周期的非同周进行，尽量减少包括疲劳等因素在内的潜在叠加毒性。当考虑以顺铂为基础的化疗，推迟脑部放疗是否具有潜在风险，有一项随机临床试验试图探讨这个问题。Robinet 等入组了 176 名患者，随机分为早期全脑放疗组和延迟全脑放疗组，采用顺铂和长春瑞滨同步化疗[7]。具体方案如下，第 1 天用顺铂 100mg/m^2，第 1、8、15 和 22 天使用 30mg/m^2 的长春瑞滨，4 个星期为 1 个周期。患者被随机分为两组，第一组接受第 1 周期化疗的同时采用总剂量为 30Gy 的全脑放疗，分 10 次完成，另一组在 2 周期化疗后给予脑放射治疗（如果评估疗效有颅内进展），颅内病灶没有进展的患者可以继续单独化疗。早期放疗组和延迟放疗组在总生存率或毒性方面没有差异，研究结果提示放疗时间的选择并非重要因素。在一项伴有脑转移的非小细胞肺癌患者的前瞻性 II 期临床试验中，顺铂和培美曲塞联合全脑放疗被证明是安全的[8]。培美曲塞与叶酸有关，而叶酸是一类被称为叶酸抗代谢物的化疗药物，其作用机制是通过抑制二氢叶酸还原酶。培美曲塞与放射外科治疗患者的无症状放射性脑坏死（影像学改变）发生率较高有关，但与有症状的放射性脑坏死无关[9]。

2. 紫杉烷类药物

紫杉醇或多西紫杉醇是同步放疗常使用的细胞毒性药物，但是对正常脑组织的穿透能力有限[10]。脑胶质瘤的患者接受紫杉醇化疗同步大野放射治疗是可行的[11, 12]。但是，紫杉醇联合全脑放疗有可能导致皮肤和黏膜毒性的发生率较高。目前还没有完成的放射外科同步紫杉类药物的前瞻性临床试验，认为化疗后一周再接受放射外科治疗或者延长放射外科治疗与系统性治疗的间隔时间是可行的。

3. 抗代谢药物

抗代谢药物通常是干扰 DNA 合成的低分子量化合物。其中许多药物，包括吉西他滨和卡培他滨都具有放疗增敏作用。吉西他滨对正常脑的渗透有限，但剂量比每周 1000～1250mg/m² 低许多倍即可产生显著的放射性增敏，特别是在皮肤和黏膜上效果明显。临床前研究表明，在注射药物 48～72h 后放疗增敏的效果逐渐减弱，这表明每周两次的放疗增敏方案更具有可行性。研究显示，每周 2 次 50mg/m² 的小剂量吉西他滨具有放疗增敏作用，可用于全脑放疗增敏[13]。增加药物剂量会产生骨髓抑制，吉西他滨的周方案可应用于全脑放疗，但是超过 600mg/m² 的剂量患者难以耐受[14]。在治疗开始时护理不佳可能会加重皮肤和黏膜毒性反应，吉西他滨对于放疗的远期效应影响最明显的也是皮肤和黏膜，也有文献报道吉西他滨对和视神经的不良反应[15]。

卡培他滨及其代谢产物 5-氟尿嘧啶（5-FU）是治疗胃肠道肿瘤和乳腺癌的常用化疗药物。卡培他滨和拉帕替尼已被认为是 *HER2* 阳性乳腺癌脑转移患者的挽救性方案。卡培他滨比氟尿嘧啶具有一定的理论优势，包括口服给药，单一给药时颅内肿瘤的药物浓度较高，而且放射治疗可以提高抗肿瘤药物的浓度。卡培他滨通过胸苷磷酸化酶（thymidine phosphorylase，TP）调控最终转化为肿瘤细胞内 5-FU，电离辐射增加肿瘤细胞内的 TP 激活并持续数周。在这种情况下，细胞内的 5-FU 作为放疗增敏剂，而在放疗后数周仍可提高 5-FU 在瘤体内的浓度。卡培他滨同步全脑放疗治疗脑转移瘤是可行的，而且在胶质母细胞瘤患者接受 60Gy 局部照射中无额外的神经毒性[16-18]。卡培他滨联合颅脑放射治疗最有可能应用于复发的乳腺癌脑转移患者中，基于之前的治疗，这类患者的放射剂量可能受到限制。

甲氨蝶呤是一种用于治疗乳腺癌的化疗药物，在淋巴瘤和白血病的治疗中仍然是标准治疗方案。除了抗肿瘤的作用，低剂量口服还具有抗炎作用。较大的放疗体积联合高剂量的甲氨蝶呤可能增加脑白质病变的发病率[19]。虽然甲氨蝶呤本身也会引起这个问题，但先前的辐照可能会增加颅内药物穿透能力。老年中枢神经系统的淋巴瘤患者在全脑放疗后接受大剂量的甲氨蝶呤，发生高级别脑部病变更为常见。如果在大剂量甲氨蝶呤后进行全脑放疗，高级别脑部病变的发生风险较低。这一经验可能与甲氨蝶呤治疗软脑膜复发有关。虽然有些人提倡鞘内注射甲氨蝶呤联合颅脑放疗治疗软脑膜肿瘤，但一项前瞻性试验发现，44 例接受该方案治疗的患者有 30 例影像学提示出现脑部病变[20]。

4. 其他细胞毒性药物

替莫唑胺是脑胶质瘤中联合放疗最常使用的药物。临床上使用替莫唑胺增加了肿瘤假性进展和骨髓抑制的风险。由于它在颅内肿瘤中的渗透作用较好，在免疫治疗时代之前它通常被用于脑转移瘤的治疗。最近的一项 Meta 分析了 6 项全脑放疗伴或不伴化疗的随机试验，其中有 3 项使用替莫唑胺[21]。虽然这些治疗方案已经在临床上应用，但接受同步化疗的不良反应较多，总体生存率却没有提高。伯明翰阿拉巴马大学开展的 II 期临床试验发现，在没有接受其他药物全身治疗的患者中，放射外科治疗脑转移病灶后马上联合替莫唑胺治疗是有效的[22]。

五、分子靶向药物

分子靶向药物包括小分子酪氨酸激酶抑制药和大分子单克隆抗体。小分子抑制药通常是口服药物，半衰期较短，为了脑部放疗更安全也可以在治疗周期中停止或者迅速重启给药。单克隆抗体通常每 2 周或 3 周给药一次，停止几个半衰期的治疗在临床上是不建议的。尽管人们认为大分子药物不容易穿过血脑屏障，磁共振强化的肿瘤已经可以用 PET 标记的抗体成像，这表明该抗体可以突破血脑屏障聚焦于脑转移瘤[23]。此外，抗PD1 单克隆抗体纳武利尤单抗被认为主要通过激活耗竭的肿瘤浸润淋巴细胞发挥作用，在黑色素瘤脑转移的患者中有 20% 的颅内应答率[24]。

EGFR 靶向药物在 EGFR 阳性的非小细胞肺癌患者中尤为重要。厄洛替尼和吉非替尼是早期批准的该类药物，与放疗联合的研究最多。虽然几项回顾性或单臂研究已经证明厄洛替尼与放疗联合治疗具有较好的安全性，这里重点介绍一项随机研究。这些小分子药物具有 CNS 活性，并在不同的肿瘤部位中被作为放疗增敏剂来研究。RTOG0320 临床试验将患者随机分为三组，即全脑放疗/放射外科组（病情需要可予标准化疗）、加厄洛替尼组、加厄洛替尼联合替莫唑胺组，EGFR 突变的患者不纳入本临床试验。厄洛替尼组的生存率较差，且总体毒性明显，这可能与非 CNS 的不良反应有关，其中 1 例患者发生高级别脑坏死。尽管这项临床研究认为厄洛替尼具有更高级别的不良反应，但目前尚不清楚这类毒性反应是不是放疗的叠加作用，或者持续使用厄洛替尼同步放疗的患者是否应该进行相应的不同处理，必要时中断治疗。使用这些药物值得注意的第二个问题是，无症状的脑转移患者是否应该予以放射治疗。一项针对既往未接受过 EGFR-TKI 治疗的新诊断脑转移瘤患者的多中心回顾性研究发现，与接受全脑放疗或放射外科联合厄洛替尼的患者相比，仅接受厄洛替尼的患者总生存率较低[25]，类似的结论来自于回顾性研究的大样本 Meta 分析。奥西替尼和阿法替尼等新的一代靶向药物在 CNS 中的总反应率超过 80%～90%[25, 26]。因为没有前瞻性的临床研究，EGFR 药物和脑部放疗的最佳组合方案和介入时机仍然存在争议。

非小细胞肺癌患者中 ALK 融合的发生率为 3%～5%，还有 1%～2% 的患者有 ROS 突变。与 EGFR 阳性患者的疗效相似，ALK 或 ROS 阳性的患者对靶向药物也具有良好的反应。目前还没有前瞻性的研究来确定使用 ALK 靶向药物联合脑部放疗的安全性，因此在联合脑部放疗时可以考虑予以短暂的间隔。对于那些不适合放射外科的患者，如果需要全脑放疗可以考虑首先单用靶向治疗，因为靶向治疗具有很好的 CNS 反应率，患者也可能会获得较长的总生存。与克唑替尼相比，最新一代的 ALK 靶向药物阿来替尼，具有更好的 CNS 缓解率和更长的无进展生存时间[27]。

六、病例介绍

（一）病例 1

55 岁的女性被诊断为 BRAF 阳性的黑色素瘤，接受维莫非尼和曲美替尼联合治疗 4 个月后，疗效评价显示肺和肝脏病灶部分缓解。患者出现恶心和头痛，检查发现有 10 个脑转移病灶，其中最大转移灶的直径为 2.3cm。全身 CT 扫描显示除了中枢神经系统病灶外，全身其余病灶持续缓解。在考虑选择放疗时，主要是权衡联合系统治疗时改变照射体积大小的必要性。

BRAF 和 MEK 抑制药是一种小分子酪氨酸激酶抑制药，能渗透进入中枢神经系统，但渗透能力低于颅外部位[28]。这些药物主要用于治疗 BRAF 突变型黑色素瘤。BRAF 抑制药包括维莫非尼、达拉菲尼和康奈非尼，这些都可以作为潜在的放疗增敏剂。但是应尽量避免在包括全脑放疗在内的大范围体积放射治疗中使用，因为会导致皮肤和黏膜毒性发生率较高[29]，联合同步放疗有导致肺和肝脏出血的报道[30]。对于 BRAF 抑制药是否增加放射外科的毒性仍存在争议，但有较高概率的出现坏死和出血报道。ECOG 指南建议在全脑放疗前后至少休息 3 天，在放射外科前后至少休息 1 天[30]。联合 BRAF 和 MEK 抑制药在治疗晚期黑色素瘤的Ⅲ期临床试验中，报道了约在 2% 脑转移进展的患者中有 18% 出现致死性的颅内出血[31]。因此，在治疗出血性黑色素瘤脑转移患者时，急性期应考虑暂缓使用 BRAF 和 MEK 抑制药（如曲美替尼、卡比替尼、比美替尼）。

抗 HER2 治疗包括单克隆抗体（如曲妥珠单抗）和小分子抑制药（如拉帕替尼、奈拉替尼、图卡替尼）。服用曲妥珠单抗的患者经常出现孤立复发的 CNS 转移病灶，表明曲妥珠单抗穿透血脑屏障的能力较差。拉帕替尼作为小分子药物可以更好地穿透血脑屏障，并经常与卡培他滨联合治疗脑转移病灶。拉帕替尼联合全脑放疗的Ⅰ期临床试验结果报道了相关毒性的增加，但产生的原因尚不清楚[33]。NRG/RTOG 1119研究中有该药物与全脑放疗或放射外科联合使用。据报道，曲妥珠单抗与全脑放射治疗联合使用时毒性发生率较低[34]。曲妥珠单抗的一种新的衍生物是T-DM1或曲妥珠单抗美坦新耦联物。尽管这种药物是大分子，但它在CNS中可以发挥作用，有报道显示在接受放射外科和系统性治疗的过程中使用T-DM1的患者会发生严重的放射性坏死[35-38]。目前还不清楚如何降低这种潜在的风险，因为许多患者并没有同步治疗。

*VEGF*抑制药（血管内皮生长因子抑制药）

*VEGF*抑制药包括单克隆抗体（如贝伐珠单抗）和口服酪氨酸激酶抑制药（如舒尼替尼、索拉非尼）。贝伐珠单抗联合放射治疗在胶质瘤中已经进行了广泛的研究，联合头部放疗（包括全脑放疗）是安全的[39]。在贝伐珠单抗应用初期，临床上担心CNS出血的风险，但是包括脑转移患者在内的大量研究表现出CNS出血的风险较低[40,41]。贝伐珠单抗可以减少CNS的水肿，还可用于治疗脑部的放射性坏死[42]。所有的*VEGF*抑制药都有可能导致临床综合征，影像学发现是后部可逆性白质脑综合征（posterior reversible enceph alopathy syndrome, PRES）。PRES发生在包括先兆子痫在内的各种药物和血管介导的高血压疾病中，与MRI双侧对称的FLAIR异常相关，通常始于后循环并向前循环延伸[43]。

克利夫兰医疗中心的一项大型回顾性研究发现，口服*VEGF*抑制药与放射性坏死的风险增加有关（14.3% vs. 6.6%无*VEGF*抑制药）。研究一共分为四组，即放射外科治疗联合/不联合口服*VEGF*抑制药，放射外科+全脑放疗联合/不联合口服*VEGF*抑制药，但对于单独接受放射外科治疗没有全脑放疗的患者来说结果没有统计学意义。在克利夫兰医疗中心进行的另一项前瞻性Ⅱ期临床试验显示，舒尼替尼作为放射外科的辅助药物是安全可接受的方案[44]。在临床应用过程中，大多数口服酪氨酸激酶抑制药包括*VEGF*抑制药会根据药物半衰期短暂停药一段时间，以避免潜在毒性。

（二）病例2

45岁女性，有右下肢黑色素瘤（$T_{3b}N_0M_0$）切除的病史，肿瘤检测为BRAF野生型，患者未接受辅助治疗，头痛病史1个月，左侧肢体运动乏力逐渐加重。头部CT显示一直径约3cm的颅内单发结节，MRI如图8-1显示右侧丘脑病灶为2.4cm，胸部结节穿刺活检证实是转移性黑色素瘤。神经外科医生会诊后，根据肿瘤位置不建议采取手术切除。如果患者将接受免疫疗法，作为医生将如何制定放疗剂量和体积呢？

1. 免疫疗法

2018年，诺贝尔生理学或医学奖授予了James Allison和Tasuku Honjo，以表彰他们各自在CTLA-4和PD-1上的研究成果。他们从基础

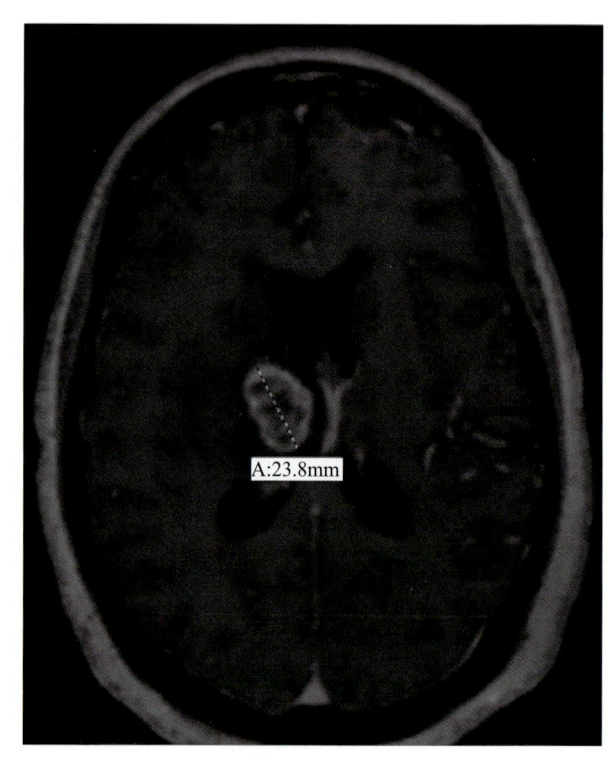

▲ 图8-1 病例2的头部T_1增强图像MRI显示右侧丘脑病变为2.4cm

科学研究到完全转化花了近二十年的时间，但免疫检查点抑制药现在是最常见的全身抗肿瘤疗法，应用于临床各类肿瘤，包括黑色素瘤、非小细胞肺癌、头颈部肿瘤、膀胱癌等。考虑到放疗对治疗肿瘤的潜在协同作用，用放射外科治疗已知的CNS肿瘤病灶可能增强其他部位对免疫治疗的反应。脑部放疗产生的远隔效应可能存在争议，但是在临床前模型和小样本的病案中有报道[45, 46]。其他免疫疗法如CAR-T细胞主要用于治疗血液恶性肿瘤和淋巴瘤，如何治疗实体肿瘤的脑转移病灶目前处在研究阶段。

易普利姆玛单克隆抗体（伊匹木单抗）是一种抗CTLA-4的单克隆抗体，2011年首次被批准用于治疗黑色素瘤。早期的回顾性研究发现，伊匹木单抗联合放射外科是安全的，可以提高CNS病灶的控制率，并延长生存时间[47, 48]。伊匹木单抗与全脑放疗或放射外科结合的安全性已经在一项Ⅰ期试验中进行了探讨[49]。目前，10mg/kg的伊匹木单抗在可耐受放射外科治疗的辅助治疗中被批准，在全脑放疗组，Ⅳ期黑色素瘤批准的治疗剂量不应超过3mg/kg。目前现有数据不支持伊匹木单抗与放射外科联合使用时中断免疫治疗。全脑放疗的潜在免疫抑制效应将在下一节中讨论，如果实施免疫治疗它将成为影响治疗决策的一个因素。

抗PD-1药物包括帕博利珠单抗和纳武利尤单抗，2014年首次被批准用于治疗转移性黑色素瘤。截至2019年，抗PD-1和抗PD-L1药物被批准用于治疗9种不同的癌症。与伊匹木单抗相似，使用抗PD-1药物与缓解率、CNS病灶控制率和总生存的改善密切相关，尤其是在与放射外科联合治疗时效果更好[50-52]。目前有多所机构都在开展前瞻性的临床研究探讨这些药物治疗脑转移的安全性和最佳时机。此外，大型随机试验（CheckMate 548和CheckMate 498）已经完成了60Gy的放射治疗联合抗PD-1药物治疗胶质母细胞瘤，但尚未报道相关毒性反应的数据。迄今为止，有许多回顾性研究表明其安全性，但因试验终点的设置不同而结果不一致[50, 51, 53-56]。表8-1总结了联合治疗方案中与抗PD-1相关的毒性反应研究数据。科罗拉多州和亚拉巴马州的单臂研究表明，放射外科3级毒性的发生率可能高于预期[52]。而来自MGH和John Hopkins的大型研究发现当放射外科联合抗PD-1药物时，多变量分析没有发现毒性反应有所增加[50, 57]。迄今为止最大的研究来自Dana Farber，该研究纳入接受了免疫治疗的115名患者[53]。在多变量分析中，接受抗PD-1免疫治疗的患者比未接受放射外科免疫治疗的患者发生有症状放射性坏死的风险高3倍以上。一项全脑放疗联合抗PD-1治疗的临床研究纳入了21名患者，其中报道1名患者出现3级神经认知功能减退，1名患者在肿瘤进展过程中出现严重水肿[55]。

与抗PD-1药物相比，双重免疫检查点抑制药联合放射外科是否具有更大的CNS毒性尚不清楚。在无脑转移的转移性黑色素瘤患者中，伊匹木单抗和纳武利尤单抗双重免疫检查点抑制药治疗肿瘤发生严重免疫相关不良事件（60%）比单独使用纳武利尤单抗要多3倍以上。在许多脑部放疗联合双重免疫检查点的回顾性报道中，缺乏联合治疗方案中关于时间和剂量的具体描述。对文献的进一步分析类固醇的使用及免疫治疗相关影像学变化的评估，这些问题将在后面的章节中讨论。

2. 放疗因素

当人们考虑系统治疗是否会增加脑部放疗的风险时，不应该忽视放射性脑损伤的固有风险。2009年以来发表的随机临床试验显示，全脑放疗后3~4个月后会出现神经认知功能障碍的高风险[58, 59]。随着许多恶性肿瘤系统治疗的发展，应尽最大努力降低放射性脑损伤的发生概率，确保具有较长生存时间的患者有良好的认知功能。例如，伊匹木单抗联合纳武利尤单抗治疗Ⅳ期黑色素瘤，获得了53%的4年总生存率[60]。对于放射外科，治疗体积仍然是放射毒性的主要决定因素。在RTOG90-05剂量递增研究中，治疗最大直

表 8-1　抗 PD-1 免疫疗法与脑部放疗的回顾性研究

	患者数目	肿瘤数目	毒 性
Moffitt	26	73	1 例（4%）2 级头疼
MSKCC	21		1 例（5%）3 级水肿
Colorado	38 SRS	—	2 级或 2 级以上（16%），3 级（8%）
UAB	43 SRS	126	11.6% 的患者出现毒性反应 4% 患者出现 3 级不可逆的毒性反应
Louisville	18 SRS	59	2 例（3.4%）坏死
Johns Hopkins	79 SRS	—	0%～3% 出现 3 级毒性反应
Brigham and Womens/Dana Faber	115 SRS		23/115（21%）有症状的坏死
Sydney	6 SRS 21 WBRT	—	约 1/6 出现 3 级坏死，2/21 出现 3 级神经认知功能和水肿的进展
MGH	50（各种放疗）	—	8%～10% 的出现 3 级毒性反应。与回顾性对照相比，3 级或 3 级以上的不良反应无区别

径为 3.1～4cm 的肿瘤产生的毒性风险比 2cm 或更小的肿瘤要高 16 倍。对于放疗剂量高达 24Gy 的小体积肿瘤，未发现剂量限制毒性。其他研究发现，给予不同体积 8～18Gy 的所有剂量梯度都可能产生放射性坏死[61]。实际上，无论系统治疗怎样调整，放射外科治疗体积较大的肿瘤将具有较高的毒性风险，而体积较小的肿瘤则风险较低。在临床治疗中，如果放射外科的靶体积处于临界状态或者新药物的安全性数据不足，降低风险的方法可能是大分割照射[62]。

七、不确定的领域和未来的方向

（一）病例

一名 57 岁男性，诊断为转移性黑色素瘤，出现头痛被诊断为单发脑转移。放射外科计划如图 8-2 所示，处方剂量中黄色代表的是 20Gy，绿色代表的是 10Gy。患者开始抗 PD-1 治疗，3 个月后随访，他状态良好且病灶缓解。你如何解读他的后续影像学图片？这是肿瘤还是治疗的结果？详情见下文关于 iRANO 标准的讨论。

（二）免疫治疗的影像改变

除脑转移本身外，免疫疗法也可以在脑实质、垂体和垂体柄中诱发炎症反应，这一过程称为"假性进展"。脑实质的炎症变化好发于受到高剂量辐射的部位。iRANO 的标准以胶质瘤在免疫治疗临床试验中的影像学反应而制定，但这些标准也与接受免疫治疗的脑转移患者的临床随访数据直接相关。从这些指南中得到的主要经验是 MRI T_1 增强开始会表现异常强化，然后会逐渐稳定下来。如果患者临床症状良好，并且在开始免疫治疗后早期出现，则强烈建议临床密切观察。上述病例 3 显示的是放射外科和抗 PD-1 治疗后 3 个月，转移灶的周围强化，对这名患者进行密切随访后判断该处肿瘤应属于完全缓解。

1. 单独的系统治疗

在精准筛选的患者中，由于靶向药物（ERFR、ALK、BRAF）或免疫治疗检查点药物的 CNS 反应率较高，因此有可能推迟在无症状脑转移患者中的脑部放疗。例如，在 76 名无症

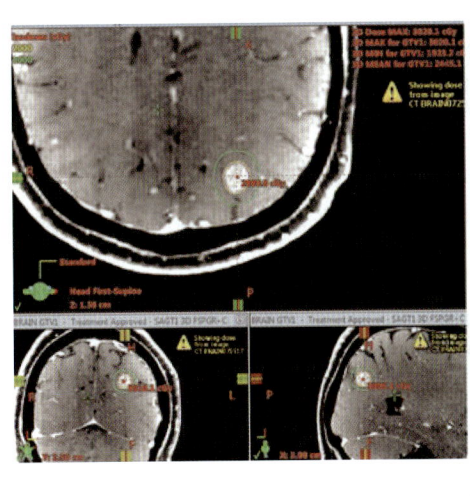

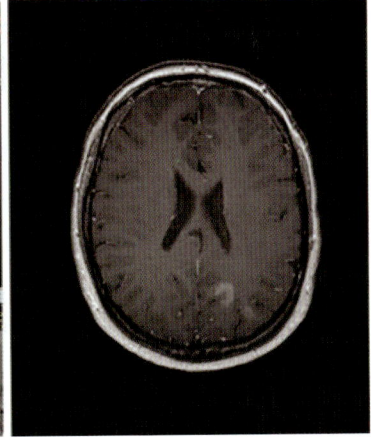

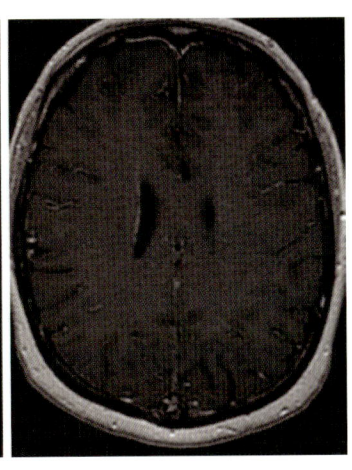

▲ 图 8-2 病例 3 的插图

放射外科计划（左图），处方剂量 20Gy 显示为黄色，10Gy 显示为绿色。患者开始抗 PD-1 治疗后 3 个月的随访（MRI 中间窗格）。治疗靶区周围有不规则强化的影像。虽然这可能被误认为是肿瘤进展，这例中患者的影像变化在 6 个月时恢复（右图）。这名患者随访 3 个月的影像显示为免疫治疗和放射外科引起的炎症改变

状黑色素瘤脑转移患者中，BRAF 联合 MEK 抑制药显示颅内病灶的有效率为 58%。与颅外结果一致，未放疗的持续有效中位缓解时间为 6.5 个月[63, 64]。对无症状黑色素瘤脑转移瘤的患者进行免疫治疗而不进行放射治疗的 II 期临床试验结果显示，只接受纳武利尤单抗治疗的患者中有 20% 出现颅内免疫应答反应，接受伊匹木单抗联合纳武利尤单抗双重检查点阻断的患者中有 56% 出现颅内免疫应答反应，其中 26% 的患者完全缓解和 67% 的患者无进展生存期为 6 个月，这是迄今为止对黑色素瘤脑转移瘤最有效的系统治疗[32, 65]。当需要使用类固醇药品时，检查点抑制药与放射外科联合使用时存在高毒性的风险，而且容易使系统治疗复杂化。迄今为止，还没有随机试验探究这些靶向药物或免疫治疗和放疗联用的最佳时机。系统治疗的大多数脑转移试验都招募无症状患者，因此关于较大的肿瘤、使用类固醇或软脑膜肿瘤的患者数据较少。NRG 一项试验计划选择患有 1～15 个黑色素瘤脑转移瘤的患者，单用双重免疫检查点抑制药与检查点抑制药加放射外科进行比较。在没有脑转移的情况下，大多数免疫检查点阻断药的临床试验允许最大类固醇剂量为泼尼松 10mg/d（约等于地塞米松 2mg/d）。伊匹木单抗治疗晚期黑色素瘤伴脑转移的一项临床试验，允许使用更高剂量的类固醇，即类固醇使用剂量约为限制量的 50%，且泼尼松 10mg/d 作为替代剂量有效。因此，当用免疫检查点抑制药治疗黑色素瘤脑转移瘤时，应尽一切努力将地塞米松限制在 2mg/d 或超出该剂量的时间尽量短，有一项前瞻性临床试验正在研究这个问题（如 NCT03563729）。

2. 淋巴细胞减少症—类固醇的作用和放疗体积

芝加哥大学的临床前研究表明，高剂量辐射需要完整的免疫系统功能才能达到最佳疗效[66]。这在接受免疫检查点抑制药和放射外科治疗的脑转移瘤患者中已得到了回顾性证明，其中低于 1000 个细胞 /μl 的淋巴细胞计数（ALC）与颅内病灶控制欠佳相关[48]。其他研究已经确定了放射外科联合免疫检查点抑制药的协同作用，部分依赖于淋巴计数超过 1000 个细胞 /μl[50]，不同肿瘤部位的大体积分割放疗与淋巴细胞减少有关[67]。此外，发现延长放疗时间（放疗次数 > 5）联合 PD-1 免疫检查点抑制药将增加抑制淋巴细胞的风险（ANC < 500）[68]。在接受抗 PD-1 治疗的转移性非小细胞肺癌患者中，使用泼尼松超过 10mg/d 与免疫反应、无进展生存期和总生存期密切相关[69]。综上所述，有充分的理由避免在脑转移患者中使用过量的类固醇，并对免疫检查

点抑制药治疗的患者中预防性使用类固醇提出质疑。

八、结论与建议

在全脑放射治疗应用减少的时代，包括放射外科在内的局部放射治疗具备更多的优势，最大限度地减少了系统治疗的延迟，降低骨髓抑制的风险。高剂量单次放疗联合免疫疗法在理论上具备一定的优势。由于大多数药物缺乏系统治疗和脑部放射治疗的临床数据，医生只能根据推断、临床前研究或药理学做出相应的临床决策，策略详见图 8-3。对于大多数药物来说，放射外科前后的停药时间仅限于数天或一周，而对于某些类别的药物则不建议停药，如免疫治疗检查点抑制药。

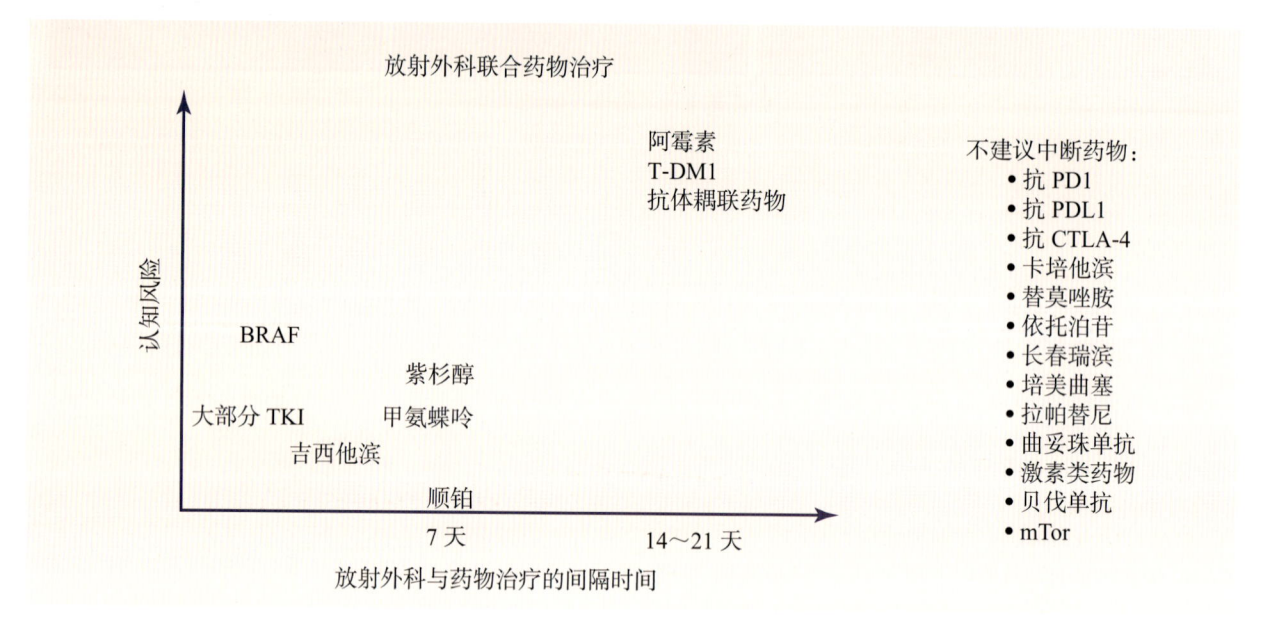

▲ 图 8-3 Alabama 大学伯明翰分校采用的管理 CNS 放射外科和全身药物结合风险的拟议方案
右侧列出了不建议中断的药物。其他药物标绘在图表上，x 轴标有建议的停药时间，如果没有规定中断，y 轴标有患者的感知风险。肿瘤体积的大小可能会促使治疗决策适度偏离该方案，并且该方案仅适用于放射外科患者，而不适用于接受全脑放射治疗的患者

> **要 点**
> - 照射体积是脑部放射外科不良反应的最强影响因素，体积小的肿瘤产生不良反应的风险很低。体积较大的肿瘤，尽管采取间隔较长时间分段治疗，但仍然具有较高的毒性风险。
> - 对于接受最常见细胞毒性药物的脑转移患者，放射外科可以在非化疗日安全地进行，但全脑放射治疗可能需要更长的间隔时间。
> - 对于接受大部分分子靶向药物治疗的患者来说，根据药物的半衰期，脑部放疗在较短的洗脱期内进行是安全的。
> - 对于接受最常见免疫治疗药物的患者来说，CNS 的病灶控制可能会得到改善，但关于毒性反应是否会更严重尚不清楚。使用类固醇来控制症状可能会降低免疫疗法的作用，而大体积的全脑放疗可能会进一步加重骨髓抑制。
> - 对于接受未知风险药物治疗且放射外科的靶体积处于临界状态时，大分割照射可能是降低毒副风险的有效措施。

参考文献

[1] Shaw E, Scott C, Souhami L, et al. Radiosurgery for the treatment of previously irradiated recurrent primary brain tumors and brain metastases: initial report of radiation therapy oncology group protocol (90-05). Int J Radiat Oncol Biol Phys. 1996;34(3): 647–54.

[2] Shen CJ, Kummerlowe MN, Redmond KJ, Rigamonti D, Lim MK, Kleinberg LR. Stereotactic radiosurgery: treatment of brain metastasis without interruption of systemic therapy. Int J Radiat Oncol Biol Phys. 2016;95(2):735–42.

[3] Kim JM, Miller JA, Kotecha R, et al. The risk of radiation necrosis following stereotactic radiosurgery with concurrent systemic therapies. J Neuro-Oncol. 2017;133(2):357–68.

[4] Verduin M, Zindler JD, Martinussen HM, et al. Use of systemic therapy concurrent with cranial radiotherapy for cerebral metastases of solid tumors. Oncologist. 2017;22(2):222–35.

[5] Quantin X, Bozonnat MC, Pujol JL. Recursive Partitioning Analysis Groups II–III brain metastases of non-small cell lung cancer: a phase II randomized study comparing two concurrent chemoradiotherapy regimens. J Thorac Oncol. 2010;5(6): 846–51.

[6] Jakacki RI, Burger PC, Zhou T, et al. Outcome of children with metastatic medulloblastoma treated with carboplatin during craniospinal radiotherapy: a Children's Oncology Group Phase I/II study. J Clin Oncol. 2012;30(21):2648–53.

[7] Robinet G, Thomas P, Breton JL, et al. Results of a phase III study of early versus delayed whole brain radiotherapy with concurrent cisplatin and vinorelbine combination in inoperable brain metastases of non-small-cell lung cancer: Groupe Francais de Pneumo-Cancerologie (GFPC) protocol 95-1. Ann Oncol. 2001;12(1):59–67.

[8] Dinglin XX, Huang Y, Liu H, Zeng YD, Hou X, Chen LK. Pemetrexed and cisplatin combination with concurrent whole brain radiotherapy in patients with brain metastases of lung adenocarcinoma: a single-arm phase II clinical trial. J Neuro-Oncol. 2013;112(3):461–6.

[9] Cagney DN, Martin AM, Catalano PJ, et al. Impact of pemetrexed on intracranial disease control and radiation necrosis in patients with brain metastases from non-small cell lung cancer receiving stereotactic radiation. Radiother Oncol. 2018;126(3):511–8.

[10] Glantz MJ, Choy H, Kearns CM, et al. Paclitaxel disposition in plasma and central nervous systems of humans and rats with brain tumors. J Natl Cancer Inst. 1995;87(14):1077–81.

[11] Glantz MJ, Chamberlain MC, Chang SM, Prados MD, Cole BF. The role of paclitaxel in the treatment of primary and metastatic brain tumors. Semin Radiat Oncol. 1999;9(2 Suppl 1):27–33.

[12] Lederman G, Wronski M, Arbit E, et al. Treatment of recurrent glioblastoma multiforme using fractionated stereotactic radiosurgery and concurrent paclitaxel. Am J Clin Oncol. 2000;23(2):155–9.

[13] Maraveyas A, Sgouros J, Upadhyay S, Abdel-Hamid AH, Holmes M, Lind M. Gemcitabine twice weekly as a radiosensitiser for the treatment of brain metastases in patients with carcinoma: a phase I study. Br J Cancer. 2005;92(5): 815–9.

[14] Huang YJ, Wu YL, Xie SX, Yang JJ, Huang YS, Liao RQ. Weekly gemcitabine as a radiosensitiser for the treatment of brain metastases in patients with non-small cell lung cancer: phase I trial. Chin Med J. 2007;120(6):458–62.

[15] Jeter MD, Janne PA, Brooks S, et al. Gemcitabine-induced radiation recall. Int J Radiat Oncol Biol Phys. 2002;53(2): 394–400.

[16] Grunda JM, Fiveash J, Palmer CA, et al. Rationally designed pharmacogenomic treatment using concurrent capecitabine and radiotherapy for glioblastoma; gene expression profiles associated with outcome. Clin Cancer Res. 2010;16(10): 2890–8.

[17] Niravath P, Tham YL, Wang T, et al. A phase II trial of capecitabine concomitantly with whole-brain radiotherapy followed by capecitabine and sunitinib for brain metastases from breast cancer. Oncologist. 2015;20(1):13.

[18] Chargari C, Kirova YM, Dieras V, et al. Concurrent capecitabine and whole-brain radiotherapy for treatment of brain metastases in breast cancer patients. J Neuro-Oncol. 2009;93(3):379–84.

[19] Low S, Han CH, Batchelor TT. Primary central nervous system lymphoma. Ther Adv Neurol Disord. 2018;11:1756286418793562.

[20] Pan Z, Yang G, He H, et al. Concurrent radiotherapy and intrathecal methotrexate for treating leptomeningeal metastasis from solid tumors with adverse prognostic factors: a prospective and single-arm study. Int J Cancer. 2016;139(8):1864–72.

[21] Qin H, Pan F, Li J, Zhang X, Liang H, Ruan Z. Whole brain radiotherapy plus concurrent chemotherapy in non-small cell lung cancer patients with brain metastases: a meta-analysis. PLoS One. 2014;9(10):e111475.

[22] Fiveash JB, Arafat WO, Naoum GE, et al. A phase 2 study of radiosurgery and temozolomide for patients with 1 to 4 brain metastases. Adv Radiat Oncol. 2016;1(2):83–8.

[23] Dijkers EC, Oude Munnink TH, Kosterink JG, et al. Biodistribution of 89Zr-trastuzumab and PET imaging of HER2-positive lesions in patients with metastatic breast cancer. Clin Pharmacol Ther. 2010;87(5):586–92.

[24] Long GV, Atkinson V, Lo S, et al. Combination nivolumab and ipilimumab or nivolumab alone in melanoma brain metastases: a multicentre randomised phase 2 study. Lancet Oncol. 2018;19(5): 672–81.

[25] Li SH, Liu CY, Hsu PC, et al. Response to afatinib in treatment-

naive patients with advanced mutant epidermal growth factor receptor lung adenocarcinoma with brain metastases. Expert Rev Anticancer Ther. 2018;18(1):81–9.

[26] Reungwetwattana T, Nakagawa K, Cho BC, et al. CNS response to osimertinib versus standard epidermal growth factor receptor tyrosine kinase inhibitors in patients with untreated EGFR-mutated advanced non-small-cell lung cancer. J Clin Oncol. 2018:JCO2018783118. https://doi.org/10.1200/JCO.2018.78.3118.

[27] Gadgeel S, Peters S, Mok T, et al. Alectinib versus crizotinib in treatment-naive anaplastic lymphoma kinase-positive (ALK+) non-small-cell lung cancer: CNS efficacy results from the ALEX study. Ann Oncol. 2018;29(11):2214–22.

[28] Mittapalli RK, Vaidhyanathan S, Dudek AZ, Elmquist WF. Mechanisms limiting distribution of the threonine-protein kinase B-RaF(V600E) inhibitor dabrafenib to the brain: implications for the treatment of melanoma brain metastases. J Pharmacol Exp Ther. 2013;344(3):655–64.

[29] Pulvirenti T, Hong A, Clements A, et al. Acute radiation skin toxicity associated with BRAF inhibitors. J Clin Oncol. 2016;34(3):e17–20.

[30] Anker CJ, Grossmann KF, Atkins MB, Suneja G, Tarhini AA, Kirkwood JM. Avoiding severe toxicity from combined BRAF inhibitor and radiation treatment: consensus guidelines from the Eastern Cooperative Oncology Group (ECOG). Int J Radiat Oncol Biol Phys. 2016;95(2):632–46.

[31] Dummer R, Ascierto PA, Gogas HJ, et al. Encorafenib plus binimetinib versus vemurafenib or encorafenib in patients with BRAF-mutant melanoma (COLUMBUS): a multicentre, open-label, randomised phase 3 trial. Lancet Oncol. 2018;19(5):603–15.

[32] Long GV, Stroyakovskiy D, Gogas H, et al. Combined BRAF and MEK inhibition versus BRAF inhibition alone in melanoma. N Engl J Med. 2014;371(20):1877–88.

[33] Lin NU, Freedman RA, Ramakrishna N, et al. A phase I study of lapatinib with whole brain radiotherapy in patients with Human Epidermal Growth Factor Receptor 2 (HER2)-positive breast cancer brain metastases. Breast Cancer Res Treat. 2013;142(2):405–14.

[34] Chargari C, Idrissi HR, Pierga JY, et al. Preliminary results of whole brain radiotherapy with concurrent trastuzumab for treatment of brain metastases in breast cancer patients. Int J Radiat Oncol Biol Phys. 2011;81(3):631–6.

[35] Carlson JA, Nooruddin Z, Rusthoven C, et al. Trastuzumab emtansine and stereotactic radiosurgery: an unexpected increase in clinically significant brain edema. Neuro-Oncology. 2014;16(7):1006–9.

[36] Geraud A, Xu HP, Beuzeboc P, Kirova YM. Preliminary experience of the concurrent use of radiosurgery and T-DM1 for brain metastases in HER2-positive metastatic breast cancer. J Neuro-Oncol. 2017;131(1):69–72.

[37] Vilela MD, Longstreth WT Jr, Pedrosa HAS, Gil GOB, Duarte JM, Filho MAD. Progressively enlarging cerebellar hematoma concurrent with T-DM1 treatment. World Neurosurg. 2018;111:109–14.

[38] Fabi A, Alesini D, Valle E, et al. T-DM1 and brain metastases: clinical outcome in HER2-positive metastatic breast cancer. Breast. 2018;41:137–43.

[39] Levy C, Allouache D, Lacroix J, et al. REBECA: a phase I study of bevacizumab and whole-brain radiation therapy for the treatment of brain metastasis from solid tumours. Ann Oncol. 2014;25(12):2351–6.

[40] Besse B, Lasserre SF, Compton P, Huang J, Augustus S, Rohr UP. Bevacizumab safety in patients with central nervous system metastases. Clin Cancer Res. 2010;16(1):269–78.

[41] Socinski MA, Langer CJ, Huang JE, et al. Safety of bevacizumab in patients with non-small-cell lung cancer and brain metastases. J Clin Oncol. 2009;27(31):5255–61.

[42] Levin VA, Bidaut L, Hou P, et al. Randomized double-blind placebo-controlled trial of bevacizumab therapy for radiation necrosis of the central nervous system. Int J Radiat Oncol Biol Phys. 2011;79(5):1487–95.

[43] Abbas O, Shamseddin A, Temraz S, Haydar A. Posterior reversible encephalopathy syndrome after bevacizumab therapy in a normotensive patient. BMJ Case Rep. 2013;2013:1–4.

[44] Ahluwalia MS, Chao ST, Parsons MW, et al. Phase II trial of sunitinib as adjuvant therapy after stereotactic radiosurgery in patients with 1–3 newly diagnosed brain metastases. J Neuro-Oncol. 2015;124(3):485–91.

[45] Pfannenstiel LW, McNeilly C, Xiang C, et al. Combination PD-1 blockade and irradiation of brain metastasis induces an effective abscopal effect in melanoma. Onco Targets Ther. 2019;8(1):e1507669.

[46] Grimaldi AM, Simeone E, Giannarelli D, et al. Abscopal effects of radiotherapy on advanced melanoma patients who progressed after ipilimumab immunotherapy. Onco Targets Ther. 2014;3:e28780.

[47] Kiess AP, Wolchok JD, Barker CA, et al. Stereotactic radiosurgery for melanoma brain metastases in patients receiving ipilimumab: safety profile and efficacy of combined treatment. Int J Radiat Oncol Biol Phys. 2015;92(2):368–75.

[48] An Y, Jiang W, Kim BYS, et al. Stereotactic radiosurgery of early melanoma brain metastases after initiation of anti-CTLA-4 treatment is associated with improved intracranial control. Radiother Oncol. 2017;125(1):80–8.

[49] Williams NL, Wuthrick EJ, Kim H, et al. Phase 1 study of ipilimumab combined with whole brain radiation therapy or radiosurgery for melanoma patients with brain metastases. Int J Radiat Oncol Biol Phys. 2017;99(1):22–30.

[50] Chen L, Douglass J, Kleinberg L, et al. Concurrent immune checkpoint inhibitors and stereotactic radiosurgery for brain metastases in non-small cell lung cancer, melanoma, and renal cell carcinoma. Int J Radiat Oncol Biol Phys. 2018;100(4):916–25.

[51] Anderson ES, Postow MA, Wolchok JD, et al. Melanoma brain metastases treated with stereotactic radiosurgery and concurrent

[52] Stokes WA, Binder DC, Jones BL, et al. Impact of immunotherapy among patients with melanoma brain metastases managed with radiotherapy. J Neuroimmunol. 2017;313:118–22.

[53] Martin AM, Cagney DN, Catalano PJ, et al. Immunotherapy and symptomatic radiation necrosis in patients with brain metastases treated with stereotactic radiation. JAMA Oncol. 2018;4(8):1123–4.

[54] Yusuf MB, Amsbaugh MJ, Burton E, Chesney J, Woo S. Peri-SRS administration of immune checkpoint therapy for melanoma metastatic to the brain: investigating efficacy and the effects of relative treatment timing on lesion response. World Neurosurg. 2017;100:632–40.. e634

[55] Liniker E, Menzies AM, Kong BY, et al. Activity and safety of radiotherapy with anti-PD-1 drug therapy in patients with metastatic melanoma. Onco Targets Ther. 2016;5(9):e1214788.

[56] Ahmed KA, Stallworth DG, Kim Y, et al. Clinical outcomes of melanoma brain metastases treated with stereotactic radiation and anti-PD-1 therapy. Ann Oncol. 2016;27(3):434–41.

[57] Hubbeling HG, Schapira EF, Horick NK, et al. Safety of combined PD-1 pathway inhibition and intracranial radiation therapy in non-small cell lung cancer. J Thorac Oncol. 2018;13(4):550–8.

[58] Chang EL, Wefel JS, Hess KR, et al. Neurocognition in patients with brain metastases treated with radiosurgery or radiosurgery plus whole-brain irradiation: a randomised controlled trial. Lancet Oncol. 2009;10(11):1037–44.

[59] Brown PD, Jaeckle K, Ballman KV, et al. Effect of radiosurgery alone vs radiosurgery with whole brain radiation therapy on cognitive function in patients with 1 to 3 brain metastases: a randomized clinical trial. JAMA. 2016;316(4):401–9.

[60] Wolchok JD, Chiarion-Sileni V, Gonzalez R, et al. Overall survival with combined nivolumab and ipilimumab in advanced melanoma. N Engl J Med. 2017;377(14):1345–56.

[61] Blonigen BJ, Steinmetz RD, Levin L, Lamba MA, Warnick RE, Breneman JC. Irradiated volume as a predictor of brain radionecrosis after linear accelerator stereotactic radiosurgery. Int J Radiat Oncol Biol Phys. 2010;77(4):996–1001.

[62] Minniti G, Scaringi C, Paolini S, et al. Single-fraction versus multifraction (9 Gy x 3) stereotactic radiosurgery for large (>2 cm) brain metastases: a comparative analysis of local control and risk of radiation-induced brain necrosis. Int J Radiat Oncol Biol Phys. 2016;95(4): 1142–8.

[63] Davies MA, Saiag P, Robert C, et al. Dabrafenib plus trametinib in patients with BRAF(V600)-mutant melanoma brain metastases (COMBI-MB): a multicentre, multicohort, open-label, phase 2 trial. Lancet Oncol. 2017;18(7):863–73.

[64] Drago JZ, Lawrence D, Livingstone E, et al. Clinical experience with combination BRAF/MEK inhibitors for melanoma with brain metastases: a real-life multicenter study. Melanoma Res. 2019;29(1):65–9.

[65] Tawbi HA, Forsyth PA, Algazi A, et al. Combined nivolumab and ipilimumab in melanoma metastatic to the brain. N Engl J Med. 2018;379(8):722–30.

[66] Lee Y, Auh SL, Wang Y, et al. Therapeutic effects of ablative radiation on local tumor require CD8+ T cells: changing strategies for cancer treatment. Blood. 2009;114(3):589–95.

[67] Ellsworth SG. Field size effects on the risk and severity of treatment-induced lymphopenia in patients undergoing radiation therapy for solid tumors. Adv Radiat Oncol. 2018;3(4):512–9.

[68] Pike LRG, Bang A, Mahal BA, et al. The impact of radiation therapy on lymphocyte count and survival in metastatic cancer patients receiving PD-1 immune checkpoint inhibitors. Int J Radiat Oncol Biol Phys. 2019;103(1):142–51.

[69] Arbour KC, Mezquita L, Long N, et al. Impact of baseline steroids on efficacy of programmed cell death-1 and programmed death-ligand 1 blockade in patients with non-small-cell lung cancer. J Clin Oncol. 2018;36(28):2872–8.

第 9 章 立体定向放射外科治疗多发脑转移瘤的指征
Indications for Stereotactic Radiosurgery: Multiple Brain Metastases

Anurag Saraf　Tony J. C. Wang　著
曾　瑜　译
周　琴　校

一、病例介绍

一位 63 岁的男性患者，2 年前诊断为肺腺癌ⅡA 期（$T_{2b}N_0M_0$），行立体定向体部放疗（stereotactic body radiotherapy，SBRT）（50Gy/5 次），既往有高血压、慢性阻塞性肺部疾病史。本次入院始发症状是他的妻子和旁人看到他在火车上抽搐发作，表现为强直性阵发性癫痫发作 2min，随后表现为癫痫发作后状态。患者被紧急带到急诊科，无发热，生命体征正常，血常规和心率正常。头部增强 CT 显示三处增强的幕上病灶。胸部/腹部/盆腔 CT 未见明显异常。头部增强磁共振显示四处幕上病灶（最大直径 0.3cm）以及两处幕下病灶（最大直径 0.5cm），总的肿瘤体积是 2.7cm³。

患者服用左乙拉西坦控制癫痫发作，偶感疲劳，无癫痫再次发作和其他不适。KPS 评分为 90 分。RPA 预后为Ⅰ类（KPS ≥ 70 分，年龄 < 65 岁，原发肿瘤已控制），分级预后评估（graded prognostic assessment，GPA）评分 2.0 且 Lung-mol GPA 评分 2.0。评估全脑放疗和立体定向放射外科（stereotactic radiosurgery，SRS）两种方案的优缺点后，患者选择接受 SRS 治疗所有 6 处病灶。

患者每 3 个月进行常规的脑部 MRI 随访。在第 3 个月和第 6 个月的随访中，患者有少许疲劳症状，但没有其他症状，头部 MRI 显示无新病变或原发病灶增大的迹象。

第 9 个月随访，患者身体状况良好。然而头部 MRI 显示两个新的幕上病灶，最大的转移灶直径为 0.3cm，体积总和为 1.2cm³。患者继续接受 SRS 治疗两个新发病灶，治疗过程中耐受良好，建议患者继续每 3 个月影像学复查随访。

第 12 个月随访，患者有短期的失忆以及疲劳不适。复查头部 MRI 显示 7 个新的颅内病灶，总体积为 5.1cm³。患者分 10 次接受总计 30Gy 的全脑放疗（whole brain radiation therapy，WBRT）。出院后开始每日服用美金刚缓释片。第 15 个月随访，患者表现出短期失忆进一步恶化和步态异常。此次预约后患者失访。

> **要　点**
> - 多发脑转移瘤中首先使用 SRS 治疗的适应证。
> - 重复 SRS 可作为有限数量脑转移复发的补救性治疗方式。
> - 多个复发的脑转移瘤，挽救性全脑放疗可能比重复 SRS 更可取。

二、概述

脑转移瘤（brain metastasis，BM）是最常见的颅内肿瘤，发生于10%～30%的癌症患者[1,2]。1/3～1/2的患者存在一个以上的脑转移瘤，并且出现超过3个脑转移瘤的患者比例在持续增加[3-5]。多发脑转移瘤的传统治疗方式为WBRT[6,7]。然而，大量研究发现，即使在多发脑转移的情况下，WBRT的认知毒性和生活质量（quality of life，QoL）受损也非常严重，而SRS已成为越来越多医生的选择[8-10]。

在本章中，多发脑转移瘤定义为任何多于一个脑转移瘤的情况。一些研究已经注意到局限性脑转移瘤（定义为2～4个）和广泛性脑转移瘤（定义为≥5个）两组患者在预后和治疗策略上的差异。

WBRT被推荐用于多发性脑转移瘤（特别是≥4个），主要基于以下几种观点：更好的治疗微转移病灶，正常脑组织所受总剂量比SRS更少，比多个等中心的SRS总治疗时间更少[1,11,12]。由于省略WBRT会增加复发的风险，因此SRS经常与WBRT一起使用，以最大限度地控制疾病[13]。在过去的几十年里，随机对照试验和前瞻性数据已经解决了这些问题，并开始将多发性脑转移瘤的治疗模式由WBRT转换为SRS。

SRS治疗多发性脑转移瘤相比WBRT的优点有：更好的局部控制，更好的保护正常组织，更少的资源消耗，更短的治疗天数以及更具成本效益。前瞻性研究表明，对于总生存期（overall survival，OS）相似的多发性脑转移瘤，单次高剂量放疗比常规放疗具有更持久的局部控制。即使是多发性或者弥漫性脑转移瘤，SRS也可以提供更多的局部治疗，能更好地保护正常脑组织，长期认知功能获益。随着现代治疗技术的发展，更容易通过单个等中心设置来治疗多发病灶，从而缩短治疗时间，减少治疗所需的资源。最后，数据表明，随着资源的减少和不良反应的减少，SRS可能比WBRT更具成本效益，即使在广泛转移的情况下也是如此[14,15]。

三、循证基础

（一）局限性转移

有限的脑转移瘤既往被定义为最多4个脑转移瘤，这是早期研究SRS治疗多发脑转移瘤安全性和有效性普遍的范畴。

SRS治疗脑转移瘤的循证始于几项比较WBRT和SRS的研究。首先，一些研究比较了WBRT和WBRT+SRS的优劣。RTOG 9508是第一个比较1～3个脑转移瘤患者行WBRT和WBRT+SRS的随机对照试验[6,7]。研究发现，与单纯WBRT相比，WBRT+SRS对预后良好（年龄小、工作状态好、原发肿瘤可控）的单发脑转移患者的生存期有优势（21.0个月 vs. 10.3个月），并发现随着时间的推移，KPS评分包括功能自主能力得到改善。本研究的一个不足是缺乏经证实的生活质量评估，因为与WBRT联合SRS推量组相比，单纯WBRT后接受挽救性SRS治疗对患者可能没有益处。

随后的几项随机研究进一步探讨了SRS与WBRT+SRS的差异[10,16-18]。这些研究发现，增加WBRT可以实现更广泛的颅内控制（从40%～70%提高到60%～90%）。然而，总生存期没有明显的获益，小于50岁的年轻患者单独使用SRS可能获得更好的总生存期。另一方面，增加WBRT后，患者的神经认知功能和生活质量显著下降。

最后，在WBRT和SRS两者相比较的问题上，一些研究已经注意到毒性和神经认知的差异。Brown等发布了一项涉及1～3个脑转移瘤患者对比使用SRS与SRS+WBRT治疗的研究，研究的主要指标为神经认知功能[10]。他们发现，单独使用SRS治疗3个月后患者的生活质量更高（$P=0.001$），增加WBRT后3个月认知功能降低更严重（91% vs. 63.5%，$P<0.001$），功能自主

性和中位总生存时间无差异。Chang 等报道了一项随机对照试验，将预后良好的 1~3 个脑转移瘤患者随机分为 SRS 组和 WBRT+SRS 组，发现 WBRT 的加入神经认知功能的下降率增加（23% vs. 49%，P =0.003），有趣的是，延迟 WBRT 对生存期有益处[16]。

除肿瘤直径较大（＞3cm）的情况外，有限脑转移瘤的患者应接受 SRS 治疗并定期监测。

（二）广泛转移

广泛性脑转移瘤传统定义上认为是 ≥ 5 个脑转移瘤。这类患者既往一般建议予以 WBRT 进行姑息性治疗而不宜采用 SRS。然而，最近的几项研究改变了这种观点。在采用 SRS 治疗脑转移瘤数量的问题，一些研究发现 SRS 处理有限脑转移瘤患者比起多发性脑转移瘤的患者，具有更好的生存结局和更少的长期不良反应。表 9-1 总结了一些研究的结果，这些研究纳入了至少 50 名广泛脑转移瘤患者予以 SRS 治疗的临床研究。在病例 1 中，患者最初显示为 6 个脑转移瘤。下面是先用 SRS 治疗广泛脑转移瘤患者获益的证据。

JLGK0901 是 Yamamoto 等在日本进行的一项研究，旨在观察 5~10 个脑转移瘤与 4 个以下脑转移瘤采用 SRS 治疗的生存期和预后的差异[8]。这是一项非劣效的前瞻性观察研究，共纳入 1194 例 1~10 个脑转移瘤患者，最大肿瘤体积 ＜ 10cm³，直径 ＜ 3cm，总累积体积 ＜ 15cm³。这是唯一采用 SRS 治疗 ＞ 5 个脑转移瘤的非回顾性研究，研究显示：更大的脑肿瘤负荷与更差的生存期或神经系统坏死无关。中位随访时间 20.9 个月，单发脑转移瘤组患者的总生存期为 13.9 个月，相比之下 2~4 个肿瘤组为 10.8 个月，5~10 个肿瘤组为 10.8 个月，两组多发性脑转移瘤的生存无明显差异（HR=0.97，95% CI 0.81~1.18，P=0.78）（图 9-1）。单发脑转移瘤组患者的神经系统坏死率为 10%，2~4 个脑转移瘤组患者的神经性死亡率为 6%，5~10 个脑转移瘤组患者的神经系统坏死率为 9%（P=0.27），这提示全身性疾

表 9-1 脑转移瘤的预后指标

预后指标	患者数目	年龄	评分标准	ECM	原发肿瘤控制情况	BM	脑转移瘤体积	对激素的反应	原发肿瘤分类	原发肿瘤特点	分子特征
RPA[19]	1200	X	KPS	X	X						
SIR[20]	65	X	KPS	X	X	X	X				
BSBM[21]	110		KPS	X	X						
Rotterdam[22]	1292		ECOG	X				X			
GGS[23]	479	X	KPS	X							
GPA[24]	1960	X	KPS	X		X					
DS-GPA[25]	4259	X	KPS	X		X			X		
Updated DS-GPA[26]	3940								X	X	
Modified Breast-GPA[27]	1552	X	KPS			X			X	X	X
Lung-molGPA[28]	1833	X	KPS	X		X			X	X	X

RPA. 递归分区分析；SIR. 放射外科评分指数；BSBM. 脑转移瘤基本评分；GGS. 黄金分级评分；GPA. 分级预后评估；DS-GPA. 诊断特异性分级预后评估；Lung-molGPA. 肺分子分级预后评估；KPS. Karnofsky 功能评分；ECM. 颅外转移；BM. 脑转移瘤

病进展是患者死亡的最大因素。更大的脑肿瘤负担并不影响颅内复发率，因为 1 个脑转移瘤患者的局部失败率为 16%，2~4 个脑转移瘤患者的局部失败率为 11%，5~10 个脑转移瘤患者的局部失败率为 10%，这表明三组的情况相似。三组患者 3~5 级毒性也相似，表明 SRS 治疗总体积大的脑转移瘤患者并不会增加治疗中产生不良反应的风险。

Yamamoto 报道显示，与单个脑转移瘤相比，SRS 治疗广泛脑转移瘤具有更高的颅内非照射区域的复发风险。然而，6 个月时统计，2~4 个脑转移瘤的失败率为 40.0%，5~10 个脑转移瘤的失败率为 45.9%（$P=0.067$），表明单纯 SRS 治疗多个脑转移瘤局部复发无统计学差异。随着转移负担的增加，软脑膜转移增加，5~10 个脑转移瘤在 24 个月后的失败率为 21.9%，而 2~4 个脑转移瘤为 13.2%（$P=0.035$）。然而，与特定分子亚型关联的相关研究数据有限，如 HER2 阳性乳腺癌或 ALK 阳性非小细胞肺癌（non-small-cell lung cancer，NSCLC）。

目前数据的一个限制因素是，多个研究纳入的 5 个脑转移瘤患者是否接受 WBRT 治疗以及 SRS 是挽救性还是初始治疗方面并不一致。目前还没有强有力的数据来比较挽救性 SRS 和初始 SRS 在总生存期、局部肿瘤控制或颅内非照射区域等方面的区别。

Hughes 等报道了对 2089 名最多达 15 个脑转移瘤的患者接受初始 SRS 治疗的多中心回顾性研究[29]。根据脑转移瘤个数对患者进行分组，其中 47%（989）为单发脑转移瘤，42%（882）为 2~4 个脑转移瘤，10%（212）为 5~15 个脑转移瘤。研究队列的中位总生存期为 14.6 个月（1 个脑转移瘤），9.5 个月（2~4 个脑转移瘤）和 7.5 个月（5~15 个脑转移瘤）；多变量分析显示 2~4 个脑转移瘤和 5~15 个脑转移瘤之间的总生存期没有差异。

一些研究报道的多发性脑转移患者需要频繁的挽救治疗。例如，Yamamoto 等开展的研究是目前最大的前瞻性试验之一，对 5~10 个脑转移瘤患者进行随访的结果显示总生存期没有差异，但据报道，50% 的患者出现了新的脑转移瘤，40% 的患者需要重复和多次 SRS 治疗[8]。多发性脑转移瘤患者需要通过频繁的连续 MRI 扫描进行密切监测。众所周知，非放疗区域出现新的脑转移随着时间的推移而增加，而磁共振监测可以发现患者出现症状或神经功能恶化前的新病变。

Chang 等报道了 323 例接受伽马刀立体定向放射外科（Gamma Knife stereotactic radiosurgery，GKRS）治疗的脑转移瘤患者，将 1~5 个、6~10 个、11~15 个和 > 15 个脑转移瘤患者分为 4 组[30]。虽然研究发现各组的总生存期或局部控制率没有差异，但报道显示脑转移瘤 > 15 个的患者颅内远处复发增加。

对超过 15 个脑转移瘤的患者开展的其他研究同样显示，脑转移瘤的数量不能预测 SRS 后患者的生存情况。Salvetti 等发表的一项单中心回顾性研究，96 例 5~15 个脑转移瘤的患者接受 SRS 治疗，平均总生存为 4.73 个月[31]。他们将转移个数为 5~15 作为连续变量并将 5~9 与 10~15 作为二分变量进行比较分析了他们的结果，在这两种情况下，他们发现脑转移瘤的数量与总生存无关。

（三）局部肿瘤控制

SRS 对脑转移瘤的局部肿瘤控制受多种因素的影响，包括肿瘤的直径、体积和处方剂量。局部肿瘤控制似乎不受转移瘤数量的影响。Yamamoto 等发现单发脑转移瘤患者 6 个月时的局部复发率为 6.5%（$P=0.45$），2~4 个脑转移瘤患者为 3.0%，5~10 个脑转移瘤患者为 4.3%（$P=0.70$），表明仅用 SRS 治疗时，脑转移肿瘤负荷不会影响局部控制[8]。

局部肿瘤控制的统计数据非常令人鼓舞。在多项研究中，6 个月的局部肿瘤控制率为 90%~95%，12 个月为 75%~90%，24 个月为 60%~75%[8, 16]。虽然患者可能经常治疗野外出现脑转移，但良好

组	中位总生存期（个月）(95% CI)	HR（95% CI）	P 值
1 个肿瘤	13.9（12.0~15.6）	0.76（0.66~0.88）	0.0004
2~4 个肿瘤	10.8（9.4~12.4）	参考	
5~10 个肿瘤	10.8（9.1~12.7）	0.97（0.81~1.18）	0.78

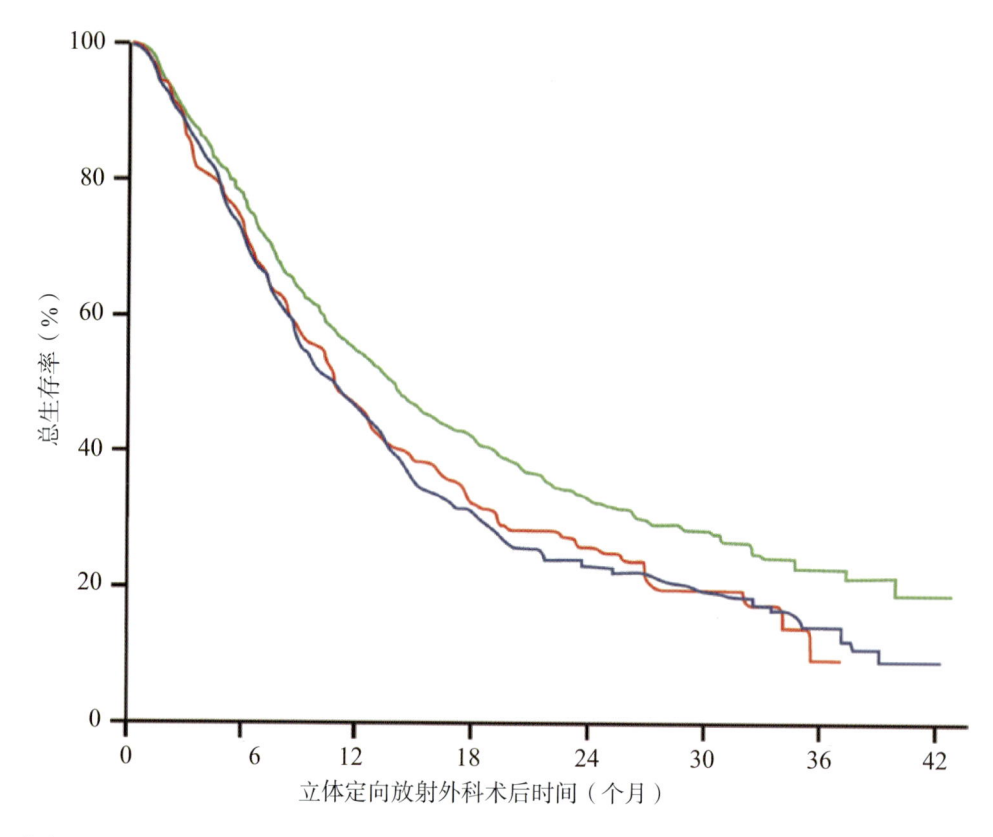

高危人群数量

1 个肿瘤	455	234	97	22
2~4 个肿瘤	531	215	61	16
5~10 个肿瘤	208	84	31	1

▲ 图 9-1　图示为单个脑转移瘤与 2~4 个脑转移瘤以及 5 个以上脑转移瘤的总生存期，按脑转移瘤的数量分级。一般来说，与多发性脑转移瘤患者相比，单发脑转移瘤患者的总生存期在统计学上显著增加；但是，与≥ 5 个脑转移瘤的患者相比，2~4 个脑转移瘤的患者没有明显的统计学差异（经 Elsevier 许可转载，引自 Yamamoto 等[8]）

的局部控制可以减少重复治疗的潜在不良反应，如神经认知功能下降和放射性坏死。

由于广泛性脑转移瘤的研究在肿瘤特征和治疗方案方面有很大差异，很难在不同的研究中进行比较。然而，单一研究机构比较了局限性脑转移和广泛性脑转移的局部肿瘤控制，结果没有发现显著差异。因此，大多数中心在同时治疗其他肿瘤时，将每个脑转移瘤视为一个独立的实体，不受考虑因素的影响。然而，剂量相互作用已经得到研究，并将在"剂量考虑因素"一节中详细介绍。

（四）颅内远处复发

颅内远处复发（distant brain failure，DBF）受多种因素的影响，包括脑转移瘤的数量、肿瘤的组织学和亚型及既往治疗。很多关于多发性脑转移瘤结果报道，包括既往予以 WBRT 治疗的患者，WBRT 是一种已知的降低治疗野外复发的因素。众所周知，DBF 会随着时间的推移而增加，40%~60% 的患者在接受 SRS 治疗后 1 年内很可能出现新的脑部病变[8, 32]。

单发脑转移瘤患者比 1 个以上脑转移瘤患者拥有更低的 DBF。然而，有限的脑转移瘤患者的 DBF 并不低于多发性脑转移瘤患者。Yamamoto 等的研究发现，单发脑转移瘤患者 6 个月时的 DBF 为 23.9%，而 2~4 个脑转移瘤患者的 DBF 为 40.0%，结果具有统计学意义（$P < 0.0001$）。然而，在 6 个月和 12 个月时，2~4 个脑转移瘤患者的 DBF 分别为 40.0% 和 54.5%，5~10 个脑转移瘤患者的 DBF 分别为 45.9% 和 63.8%（$P=0.067$），表明 > 1 个以上的多发性脑转移患者的 DBF 没有差异[8]。Hughes 等发现，单发脑转移瘤患者一年的 DBF 为 30%，2~4 个为 41%，5~15 个为 50%（$P < 0.01$）。与 2~4 个脑转移瘤相比，5~15 个脑转移瘤意味着更差的 DBF（HR 1.43，$P < 0.01$）；单发脑转移瘤的 DBF 比 2~4 个脑转移瘤更好（HR 0.70，$P < 0.01$）[29]。DBF 的预测因素包括年龄（≥ 65 岁）、边缘剂量、非肺、乳腺、肾细胞或原发性黑色素瘤（报告为"其他"）组织学来源。多发性脑转移瘤分组中，数据显示 5~10 个脑转移瘤患者 1 年时的 DBF 为 42%，11~15 个脑转移瘤为 73%。

很多报道显示有限个数和广泛脑转移瘤患者有着相似的 DBF。Chang 等按照 6~10 个、11~15 个和 > 15 个转移瘤将患者分为三组[30]。在这个队列中，仅 SRS 患者 1 年时的 DBF 为 73%，而 SRS+WBRT 患者为 45%（$P=0.02$）。因此，尽管数据有限，但数据显示脑转移瘤超过 10 个的患者的 DBF 更高。

（五）挽救性治疗

在病例 1 中，我们看到患者最初接受 SRS 治疗 6 个脑转移瘤，但在接受治疗 9 个月后因为治疗野外出现两个新的脑转移瘤。多发性脑转移瘤患者初始 SRS 后进展，根据临床情况有多种挽救治疗可供选择，如再次 SRS、挽救性 WBRT 或最佳支持治疗。

Hughes 等报道，随着脑转移瘤数量的增加，挽救性 SRS 的有效率降低，挽救性 WBRT 的有效率增加[29]。单发脑转移瘤的患者中，27% 的患者采用挽救性 SRS，13% 的患者采用 WBRT；在 2~4 个脑转移瘤的患者中，24% 的患者采用挽救性 SRS，15% 的患者采用 WBRT；在 5~15 个脑转移瘤的患者中，21% 的患者采用挽救性 SRS，18% 的患者采用 WBRT。与 2~4 个脑转移瘤患者相比，5~15 个脑转移瘤患者采用挽救性 SRS 治疗较低。2~4 个脑转移瘤组和 5~15 个脑转移瘤组患者到 WBRT 进行挽救性治疗的时间无统计学差异。作者认为这可能与 5~15 个脑转移瘤组在进展期采用非放射治疗方式进行挽救方式或予以最佳支持治疗的习惯性偏好有关。

（六）软脑膜病

软脑膜疾病（leptomeningeal disease，LMD）是 SRS 的一个关注点，与 WBRT 相比，局部治疗可减少对脑膜的伤害。肿瘤负荷增加与 LMD 的风险增加相关。Yamamoto 等发现，5~10 个脑转移瘤组的 LMD 发生率最高，2 年发生率为 21.9%，而 2~4 个脑转移瘤组和单发转移组的 LMD 发生率分别为 13.2% 和 11%[8]。值得注意的是，这些研究没有报道哪个亚组更有可能发生 LMD 的亚组差异，如 *EGFR* 阳性或 *ALK* 阳性的 NSCLC，或 *HER2* 阳性或三阴性乳腺癌。

（七）毒性

SRS 治疗多发脑转移瘤相关的毒性通常分为急性和迟发反应。急性反应往往发生在治疗开始的数周到数月内，通常是可逆的，包括疲劳、食欲不振、皮炎、脱发、恶心和呕吐、神经症状恶化。迟发反应发生在治疗数月后可能是不可逆的，最严重的可能包括放射性坏死和神经认知功能障碍。

现代NRG方案根据不良事件通用术语标准（common terminology criteria for adverse events，CTCAE）v5.0报告毒性。根据CTCAE，毒性可分为1~5级，3级毒性包括显著毒性但不立即危及生命、需要住院治疗或限制自我护理ADL；4级毒性包括危及生命的后果或指示紧急干预；5级毒性包括死亡。

多发性脑转移瘤患者的3~5级毒性并不比单发性转移患者严重。Yamamoto等报道，在他们纳入的1194名接受SRS治疗的患者队列中，8%的患者发生了与SRS相关的任何类型的不良事件，并且在脑转移瘤为1个、2~4个和5~10个的3组患者组中发生率没有差异。3~5级毒性每组均低于5%[8]。Brown等在他们的研究中发表了类似的结果，比较了SRS和SRS+WBRT对1~3个脑转移瘤的毒性，SRS组仅出现2.9%的3~5级毒性，而SRS+WBRT组的3~5级毒性为4.5%（P=0.72）[10]。对于多发性脑转移采用SRS治疗，患者的严重不良反应不会超过WBRT或SRS+WBRT联合治疗。

（八）神经认知

WBRT的主要关注点是对患者神经认知功能的影响及由此对生活质量的影响。放射治疗对海马神经有不良反应，主要影响记忆和回忆。虽然在早期的研究中，最小精神状态检查（miniMental status examination，MMSE）已经被用来测量神经认知功能，但该检查在检测和关联受放射治疗影响的更微妙的神经心理变化方面并不敏感。霍普金斯言语学习测验（Hopkins verbal learning test-revised，HVLT-R）是一种对测试者总回忆、延迟回忆和延迟再认的言语神经认知测验。随着时间的推移，它已经被证实并被纳入了几个随机试验中，更符合癌症患者在日常生活能力方面的需要。在多发性脑转移的问题中，颅内肿瘤总体积与基线的神经认知功能缺陷相关。几个随机对照试验直接解决了这个问题，这些试验观察了治疗后几个月患者的认知能力退化，包括学习和记忆能力。

Chang等将58例1~3个脑转移患者随机分为SRS+WBRT组和SRS组，治疗后4个月HVLT-R恶化为主要终点[16]。由于在4个月时有96%的置信度表明SRS+WBRT的总回忆能力低于单独SRS组，该试验提前终止。数据表明，神经认知能力的下降在治疗后持续了6个月。其他神经认知测试显示，与单纯SRS相比，SRS+WBRT组的执行功能（COWA测试，trail making test part B）下降更严重。SRS组具有更高的中位总生存期（15.2个月 vs. 5.7个月）和1年总生存期（63% vs. 21%，P= 0.003）。SRS组的1年局部控制率（67% vs. 100%，P= 0.012）和1年照射野外颅内肿瘤控制率（45% vs. 73%，P=0.02）较差。大多数单独SRS组的患者接受补救治疗，主要是手术或再次SRS。两组的3级和4级毒性相当。

Brown等将213名1~3个脑转移瘤患者随机分为SRS+WBRT组和SRS组，主要终点为治疗3个月后多项神经认知测试（包括HVLT-R）恶化，次要终点为生活质量[10]。Brown等发现，在接受SRS加WBRT治疗的患者治疗3个月后，在包括即时记忆、延迟记忆和语言流利性在内的多种不同认知测试中，神经认知能力显著下降。他们发现这些结果在超过6个月的患者中持续存在。他们观察了34名（16%）长期存活者（定义为12个月时评估的患者），发现3个月时SRS+WBRT组的神经认知能力下降更严重（94.1% vs. 45.5%，P=0.007），12个月时持续下降（94.4% vs. 60%，P=0.04），这表明WBRT的影响可能不是暂时的。SRS加WBRT组颅内肿瘤控制较好，但总生存期无显著差异（7.4个月 vs. 10.4个月，P =0.92）。这表明，虽然辅助性

WBRT 能更好地控制颅内肿瘤，但总生存期无明显差异，伴随神经认知功能恶化，但在 WBRT 急性反应后，生活质量持续良好。

两项试验都发现加入 WBRT 后患者的认知能力恶化率较高，颅内复发率较低，但对总生存期无影响。多个试验中的多个因素造成的 WBRT 的生存期缺乏改善，其中最突出的是常规随访发现颅内进展后挽救性治疗的有效性。

（九）生活质量

Brown 等利用癌症治疗功能评价量表来评估生活质量，以及日常生活活动的巴氏指数（activities of daily living，ADL 指数）来衡量治疗后患者的功能自主性[10]。与 SRS 加 WBRT 相比，单独使用 SRS 治疗的患者在 3 个月时的总体生活质量更好（与基线相比的平均变化为 –1.3 vs. –10.9，P =0.002），并且功能良好。Barthel-ADL 指数维持在较高水平，组间无显著性差异。研究发现，在长期存活 12 个月以上的患者中，单独 SRS 组 3 个月时的生活质量显著提高，有些入组区域持续超过 9 个月。其他研究表明，WBRT 后生活质量的下降持续超过 12 个月，而且这种现象部分不可逆转。

Kocher 等报道了纳入了 359 例 1～3 个脑转移瘤患者的 EORTC 22952–22601 研究，这些患者随机分为 SRS/ 手术 +WBRT 组、SRS/ 手术组和观察组[17]。主要终点是以世界卫生组织（World Health Organization，WHO）体力状态（performance status，PS）评分＞ 2（与自我护理能力有限、完全残疾或死亡相关）的功能自主时间的变化来衡量。WBRT 组和观察组之间没有差异（9.5 个月 vs. 10.0 个月，P=0.71）。随访第 2 年，22% 的患者存活，两组患者均功能良好。WBRT 组与观察组相比，颅内复发和颅内治疗野外复发较少。然而，WBRT 组与观察组之间的总生存期没有变化（10.9 个月 vs. 10.7 个月，P=0.89）。

对于＞ 5 个脑转移瘤的患者，单独 SRS 和其他治疗方式的神经认知功能或生活质量差异的高水平证据有限。北美伽马刀联盟（North American Gamma-knife Consortium，NAGKC）正在进行一项随机对照试验（NAGKC12–01），比较≥ 5 个脑转移瘤患者的放射外科治疗和 WBRT 治疗，主要终点是神经认知功能状态和肿瘤控制率。这些试验也可以阐明多发性脑转移瘤复发和患者生活质量的关系。与预先 WBRT 相比，连续 MRI 监测并挽救性治疗的患者可能具有更高的神经认知功能和生活质量，且对总生存期无影响。

（十）预后指数

在过去的几年里，已经制订、测试和验证了一些预后指标[19–28, 33, 34]。虽然较老的评分细则采用的临床风险因素往往更主观，但较新的评分细则发现脑转移的数量、同疾病亚型和分子 / 遗传因素一样与预后分级显著相关。表 9–2 显示了文献中的几个预后指标。

递归分区分析（recursive partitioning analysis，RPA）是脑转移患者最古老和最常用的预后指标。RPA 是一个简单但主观的指标，最初是在多个 RTOG 研究中对脑转移患者的结果进行分析描述，包括三个指标（年龄、KPS、原发肿瘤控制），将患者分为三类，即Ⅰ类、Ⅱ类和Ⅲ类。Ⅰ类患者的预后最好，包括 KPS 患者≥ 70 分，年龄＜ 65 岁，原发肿瘤控制良好且无颅外转移。Ⅲ类患者预后最差，KPS ＜ 70 分。Ⅱ类包括所有其他患者。一些分析 SRS 用于多发性脑转移瘤的研究发现，总生存期与较好的 RPA 分级有关，因此可用于进一步治疗。

表 9–3 总结了预后指数中不同分级的中位总生存期，其中包括脑转移瘤个数作为风险因素。分级预后评估（graded prognosis assessment，GPA）和诊断特异性分级预后评估（diagnosis-specific graded prognostic assessment，dsGPA）是两个较新的预后指标，试图利用更客观的指标对脑转移瘤患者进行分类。原始 GPA 利用年龄、KPS、颅外转移灶的存在、脑转移瘤的数量，得

分为 0~4 分，0 分为最差预后。虽然 GPA 评分在脑转移的一些研究中是有前景的，但在多发性脑转移瘤的 SRS 研究中，数据更为矛盾。新的 dsGPA 试图利用原发性癌症特异性因素来预测预后，如乳腺癌亚型和肺癌分子标志物。这一指标较新，可能在未来的研究中得到更多验证。

一些预后指标可用于评估前面所介绍的病例。根据 RPA 分级，患者 KPS > 70 分，年龄 < 65 岁，无颅外转移，分为 RPA Ⅰ级，中位总生存期为 7.1 个月。根据 GPA 分级，患者年龄 > 60 岁，KPS 90~100 分，脑转移瘤数 > 3 个，无颅外转移，GPA 评分为 2.0，中位总生存期为 6.5 个月。基于 Lung-mol GPA 分级，患者年龄 < 70 岁，KPS 90~100 分，无颅外转移，脑转移瘤 > 4 个，$EGFR/ALK$ 状态未知，Lung-molGPA 评分为 2.0，中位生存期为 13.7 个月。

表 9-2 根据预后指数分级的中位总生存期（包括脑转移瘤数量的指数）

预后指标	分级数量	中位生存（个月）	最差分级的中位 OS（个月）	中等分级的中位 OS（个月）	最佳分级的中位 OS（个月）
SIR [20]	3	6.8	2.9	7	31.4
GPA [24]	4	—	2.6	3.8~6.9	11
DS-GPA [25]	4	7.2	3.4	6.4~11.6	14.8
Updated ds-GPA [26]	4	7.2	3.1	5.4~8.7	16.7
Modified Breast-GPA [27]	4	8.5	2.6	9.2~19.9	28.8
Lung-molGPA（nonadenocarcinoma）[28]	3	9.2	5.3	9.8	12.8
Lung-molGPA（adenocarcinoma）[28]	4	15.2	6.9	13.7~26.5	46.8

SIR. 放射外科评分指数；GPA. 分级预后评估；DS-GPA. 诊断特异性分级预后评估；Lung-mol GPA. 肺分子分级预后评估

表 9-3 患者脑转移瘤 ≥ 5 个予以 SRS 治疗的研究综述

作者（年份）	转移瘤数目（患者例数）	中位随访时间（个月）	局部复发率	远处脑转移失败	总生存（个月）
Hughes 等（2019）[29]	5~15BM（212）	48.7	—	1 年 =50% 2 年 =54%	中位数 =7.5
Yamamoto 等（2014）[8]	5~10BM（208）	12	1yr=6.5% 2yr=9.8%	1 年 =63.8% 2 年 =72%	中位数 =10.8
Salvetti（2013）[31]	5~15BM（96）	4.1	1yr=15.2% 2yr=25.1%	总计 =41%	5~9BM=4.8 10~15BM=3.4
Mohammadi 等（2012）[35]	5~20BM（178）	6.2	3%	总计 =40% （中位数 =2.1 个月）	中位数 =6.7
Chang（2010）[30]	6~10BM（58） 11~15BM（17） > 15BM（33）	10.7 12.3 8.0	1 年 LC=83% 1 年 LC=92% 1 年 LC=89%	1 年 =47.2% 1 年 =53.1% 1 年 =80.3%	1 年 =83% 1 年 =92% 1 年 =88%
Bhatnagar（2006）[36]	4~18BM（205）	8	1 年 =29%	1 年 =43%	中位数 =8

—. 未报道；LC. 局部控制

（十一）治疗体积

最大脑转移瘤的大小可以决定治疗方案。>3cm 的大体积转移瘤应该首先考虑手术切除而不是 SRS，从而提高患者的总生存和功能独立生存期[37]。SRS 治疗大体积肿瘤会导致水肿，增加迟发性不良反应发生的风险。两项前瞻性对照试验将脑转移瘤患者随机分为 SRS 组和手术组，来探讨脑转移瘤的大小与治疗方式问题[38-40]。

一些研究表明，脑转移瘤总体积的大小比脑转移瘤的数量更能预测 SRS 治疗的临床结果。Bhatnagar 等发表了一个回顾性单中心临床研究结果，研究分析了接受 SRS 治疗的 205 名 ≥4 个脑转移瘤的患者，中位随访时间为 8 个月[36]。结果显示，总的治疗体积与总生存期和局部肿瘤控制有统计学关联；然而，脑转移的数量与临床结局没有统计学关联。

另一项小样本研究进一步证实了这一发现。Grandhi 等报道了 61 例仅接受 SRS 治疗的 ≥10 个脑转移瘤患者的单中心回顾性研究，显示中位生存期为 4 个月[41]。在这项研究中，多变量分析发现 ≥14 个脑转移瘤患者的总生存显著降低。然而，他们注意到，虽然其他亚组的脑转移瘤数量与局部控制或生存期无关，但治疗体积具有统计学意义，也许更能预测预后。

当一个有 2 个脑转移瘤且总治疗体积为 5cm³ 的患者与另一个有 5 个脑转移瘤且总治疗体积为 2cm³ 的患者比较时，后者的总生存期会更好，并且局部肿瘤控制是明显的。需要更多前瞻性和随机性的研究来进一步探讨这一结果。

我们可以将这些结果与病例 1 联系起来。患者最初有 6 个脑转移瘤，最大单个肿瘤大小为 0.5cm，肿瘤总体积为 2.7cm³，考虑先予以 SRS 治疗。患者在 9 个月时出现远处脑转移，最大单个肿瘤大小为 0.3cm，肿瘤总体积为 1.2cm³，行挽救性 SRS。患者在 12 个月时再次出现远处脑转移，肿瘤总体积为 5.1cm³，WBRT 被认为是更好的治疗选择。

（十二）治疗剂量

最近的研究发现，在 >3 个脑转移瘤的治疗方案中，正常脑组织受照射剂量可能会超量[42-45]。在多靶点治疗计划中，对第一个靶点的辐射必然会对随后的靶点产生背景剂量辐射，并被纳入后续靶点的治疗计划中。然而，随后靶区的辐射也会影响第一个靶点的剂量，从而产生一种相互作用的剂量效应[42, 43, 46]。被称为剂量相互作用效应，这是在多靶点计划中增加正常组织剂量限量的一个主要因素。这可能导致正常脑组织受到更高的剂量，如前所述，理论上可能导致包括认知功能下降和放射性坏死在内的毒性。

SRS 治疗设备不同也可能有不同的影响，这取决于射束的数量、辐射源和整体治疗方案。Ma 等研究了不同设备行 SRS 治疗多发性脑转移瘤的放疗计划，发现剂量适形度增加靶点数量时具有更大的可变性[43]。因此，医疗机构应意识到治疗所使用的特定设备的治疗差异，并根据靶区数目相应调整治疗计划。

Ma 等研究了在不同设备上开展 SRS 治疗不同数量脑转移瘤的放疗计划，发现增加 SRS 靶点的数量会导致适形度降低及等剂量体积变化[42]。作者建议减少 20%~30% 的处方剂量，以避免周围脑体积剂量适形度太差。另一项研究着眼于通过增加束数和正常组织最低剂量化来优化直线加速器容积调强弧形治疗（volumetric modulated arc therapy，VMAT）计划。作者建议，选择更多数量的优化射束（如调强射束的宽范围优化方法，简称 BROOMBA）能够通过多靶点治疗计划将正常脑组织的受照剂量降低高达 65%[45]。

四、诊断

既往未确诊为癌症而出现新的脑部病灶患者，应进行全面的癌症检查。病史和体格检查的联合应用有助于判断出 30% 的新诊断脑转移患者的原发癌。由于肺癌、乳腺癌和黑色素瘤是导致多发性脑转移瘤的最常见病种，因此应首先进行胸部 X 线检查，如果 CXR 不能诊断，则应进行胸部 CT 检查。并完善腹部/骨盆 CT 和骨扫描检查来明确是否有转移性病变。

诊断为多发性脑转移瘤的患者应完善病史和体格检查，并由包括神经外科、神经肿瘤学和放射肿瘤学的多学科团队完成。完整的脑转移瘤诊断检查包括影像学检查和组织活检。

（一）影像

疑似脑转移的患者应行脑部增强 MRI 来帮助诊断。增强 MRI 比未增强的 MRI 或 CT 更为敏感，尤其是在诊断那些无症状或未发现的颅内病变很重要。脑转移瘤的特征性表现是灰质和白质交界处的病变边缘强化信号，伴随周围水肿。

（二）组织活检

当对影像学诊断有疑问时可进行脑组织活检。颅内多发性病变的患者更具脑转移瘤特征，活检通常推迟进行。约 80% 的患者在原发肿瘤诊断后出现脑转移，称为异时性转移。然而，与原发肿瘤诊断同时出现的脑转移瘤（同时性转移瘤）和原发肿瘤诊断前出现的脑转移瘤（早期转移瘤）可进行脑部组织活检，以通过免疫组织化学帮助确认原发肿瘤部位，以及排除其他脑部病变的鉴别诊断，如原发性脑瘤、感染或炎症。

五、管理和指导方针

（一）初期管理

新诊断的脑转移瘤患者应首先处理症状（如果存在）。这可能包括用于颅内压升高的皮质类固醇、用于控制癫痫发作的抗癫痫药、血栓栓塞疾病的治疗和（或）用于减压的外科手术。患者应该有一个完整的分期检查，以确定转移性疾病的程度和预期寿命。

（二）预后指数

没有一个单一的预后指标优于其他任何指标被建议。常用的指标包括递归分区分析（recursive partitioning analysis，RPA）、分级预后评估（graded prognostic assessment，GPA）和较新的诊断特异性分级预后评估（diagnosis-specific graded prognostic assessment，dsGPA）。医生应利用工具更好地将患者进行预后分层，以便做出治疗决策、预测干预措施的结果和比较治疗结局。

（三）程序

患者可以选择具有立体定向放射外科功能的几种不同技术进行治疗，包括直线加速器、伽马刀放射外科（图 9-2）或射波刀放射外科。患者可以在一个疗程内接受治疗，包括在机器上定位、在计算机软件上绘制剂量曲线以及通过机器输送剂量。对于一个相对简单的病例，治疗时间通常为 45~90min，这取决于脑转移瘤的数量、机器的年份和放射性物质的使用年限。患者通常需要在诊所留观 12~24h。

（四）辐射剂量

一些试验研究了与治疗剂量和部位相关的不同疗效和不良反应。下面展示了两种不同的治疗方案。第一个是根据 RTOG90-05 的治疗指南，这是美国和世界各地临床医生经常使用的治疗策略。第二个是 JLGK0901（Yamamoto 等）的治疗方案，这是一项前瞻性观察试验。然而，该研究的局限性包括主要是日本人（具有更有利的特征）。医生制定治疗策略不仅取决于体积，还取决于 OAR 限制、之前的辐射剂量和其他临床因素。

根据 RTOG 90-05[47]，50%~90% 等剂量线（以最大直径测量）的治疗剂量。

- 肿瘤直径 < 2cm=20~24Gy
- 肿瘤直径 2~3cm=18Gy
- 肿瘤直径 3~4cm=15Gy

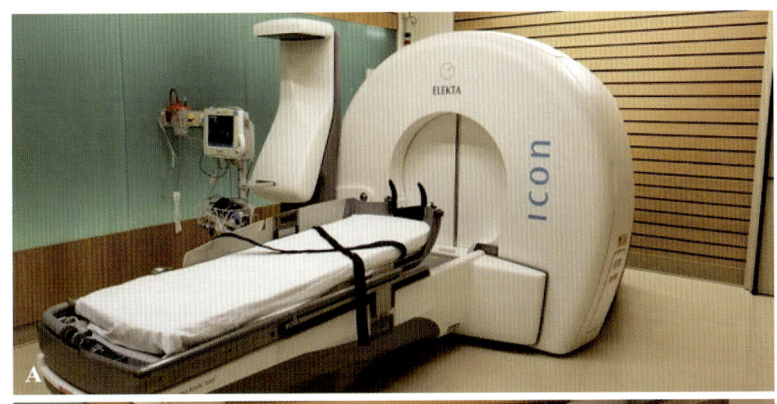

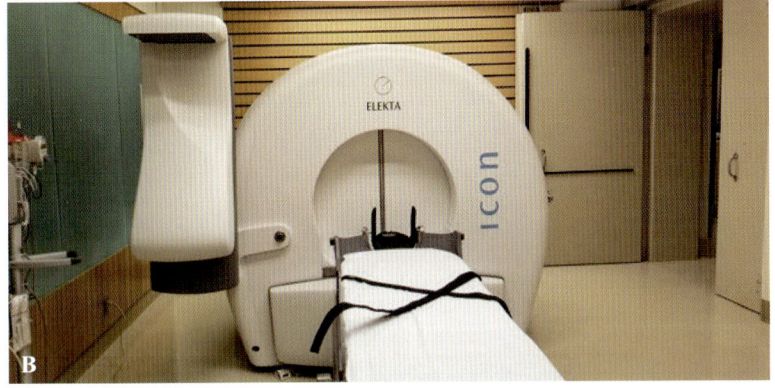

第 9 章 立体定向放射外科治疗多发脑转移瘤的指征
Indications for Stereotactic Radiosurgery: Multiple Brain Metastases

◀ 图 9-2 伽马刀 Icon 系统
（A）和（B）伽马刀 Icon 放射外科系统。该系统使用日常的锥形束 CT 对比计划 CT 共配准和立体定向成像来监测头部定位，内部探测器来确定精确的剂量沉积（图片由哥伦比亚大学肿瘤放疗科提供）

根据 JLGK0901[8]，病灶周围的治疗剂量随肿瘤部位不同而不同（根据临床判断 ±2Gy）。

- 肿瘤＜4cm³=22Gy
- 肿瘤 4～10cm³=20Gy
- 脑干肿瘤＜1cm³=20Gy
- 脑干肿瘤 1～4cm³=18Gy
- 脑干肿瘤 4～10cm³=16Gy

（五）WBRT 的角色

多发性脑转移瘤的患者除了 SRS 外，还可以进行 WBRT 治疗。众所周知，WBRT 虽然与肿瘤控制增加有关，但也与神经认知功能和生活质量降低有关，其生存期与 SRS 相似。保护海马的 WBRT 目前正在研究中（CC0001，见下文"未来方向"）。根据早期研究报道，可能是患者的一个合适选择。

（六）手术角色

直径＞3cm 的较大单发肿瘤应考虑手术或分次放射外科治疗。其他策略包括手术和辅助 SRS，新辅助 SRS 后再手术。

（七）姑息治疗的角色

对于预期寿命较短（＜3 个月）的患者，使用 WBRT 治疗可能不会明显改善 WBRT 治疗后的症状，舒适措施是患者的合理选择。QUARTZ 试验是一项Ⅲ期随机对照试验，共有 538 例非小细胞肺癌患者，其脑转移瘤不适合手术或 SRS，比较了最佳支持治疗 +WBRT 和单独最佳支持治疗[48]。两组患者的总生存期无统计学差异，经质量调整后的生存期差异为 4.7 天。在多发性脑转移的情况下，不良的机体状态和未积极控制的疾病是预期寿命短的危险因素。

（八）SRS 的时机

如果在放射外科当天的计划扫描中发现新的脑转移瘤，无论采用 SRS 治疗所有显示的病灶（即使超过 10 个病灶）或放弃 SRS 采用 WBRT 都是合理的；没有足够的高质量数据表明其中一个比另一个对患者更有利。

(九)随访

患者应在开始治疗6个月内每2~3个月进行一次脑部成像(最好是脑部MRI)的密切监视。如果患者出现新的病变,应该由多学科小组对患者进行重新评估,以便进行挽救性治疗或考虑临终关怀。在开始治疗6个月后没有出现新病灶的患者每3~4个月进行一次脑部成像随访。距初次治疗时间超过24个月的患者应继续随访,但筛查不需要那么频繁。

六、不确定领域及未来研究方向

大多数研究报道了5个以上脑转移患者的治疗数据,但都有一些局限性。患者的人种特征和肿瘤特征大不一致,包括脑转移数为2~37个,体积为3.2~10.9cm³。患者纳入标准差异很大,从KPS到不同治疗方式再到组织病理学。大多数研究包括在SRS之前接受过某些治疗的患者,包括WBRT。就局部控制率、头部非放疗区域控制率以及总生存期而言,首选SRS作为初始治疗还是挽救性治疗,目前仍无定论。

对于>5个的脑转移瘤,还没有直接比较WBRT和SRS的临床研究。北美伽马刀联盟开展的一项随机对照试验以≥5个脑转移瘤患者放疗后的神经认知状态和肿瘤控制情况作为主要终点(NAGKC 12-01;临床试验标识符:NCT01731704),探讨≥5个脑转移瘤患者进行放射外科治疗与WBRT治疗的比较。不幸的是,由于人手不足,实验在报名前就结束了。有一项丹麦研究比较全脑放射治疗(WBRT)和立体定向放射外科治疗(SRS)治疗4~10个脑转移瘤(WBRT对SRS)(临床试验标识符NCT02353000),具有类似的试验设计,目前正在进行中,还没有招募患者[49]。主要结果是生活质量,次要结果包括总生存期、KPS>70的时间、独立程度、类固醇使用和毒性。

在WBRT中和结束后应用美金刚,或在头部放射治疗后给予多奈哌齐等药理学药物已被用于预防认知功能障碍[50,51]。然而,尽管这些药物在降低WBRT后认知效应方面的作用是显著的,但是不能改善WBRT引起的生活质量下降和与WBRT相关的不良反应(如脱发、疲劳、放射性坏死)。

加拿大癌症试验小组(Canadian Cancer Trials Group,CCTG)/联盟小组合作开展了一项研究:立体定向放射外科与WBRT治疗5~15个脑转移瘤的比较,将5~15个脑转移瘤患者随机分为WBRT组每次30Gy/10次+每日美金刚对比SRS组为单次18~20或22Gy(CTI:NCT03550391)。主要目标是比较两组的总生存期和无神经认知功能下降进展生存期。次要终点包括局部/远处/软脑膜转移的时间、CNS衰竭模式的差异、挽救性治疗的数量、毒性和一些生活质量指标。

保护海马(hippocampal avoidance,HA)的WBRT是一种在治疗脑转移瘤的过程中避免对海马区的辐射剂量的计划技术,数据显示海马区很少出现脑转移。回顾性和小规模的前瞻性试验表明,延迟性神经认知功能下降没有恶化临床结果。盐酸美金刚和全脑放疗加或不加海马保护治疗减少脑转移患者神经认知功能下降(NRG CC001;CTI:NCT02360215)是一项Ⅱ期试验,评估保护海马的WBRT在延缓神经认知功能障碍的有效性。主要终点是在治疗后第2、4、6和12个月,利用HVLT-R、COWA和TMT测试评估神经认知功能。早期结果以摘要形式2018年的ASTRO展示,美金刚+HA WBRT降低了认知功能障碍的风险,并改善了患者症状。然而,应注意保护海马的WBRT的质量保障,与WBRT相比,治疗计划制定的复杂性更高、时间更长,以及治疗实施时间也会延长。

免疫治疗的迅速发展改变了一些患者的治疗方法,并显著改善了预后。近年来,SRS与免疫治疗相结合的治疗方法已被多次报道,其优点是增强了放疗后的抗肿瘤免疫应答。也被称为

abscopal 效应，对这些联合治疗方式的关注，未来将进行几项前瞻性随机试验。L19-IL2 联合 SABR 应用寡转移实体肿瘤（L19-IL2）患者的 I 期临床研究（临床试验标识符，NCT02086721），该研究将探讨寡转移灶行 SRS 后患者应用 L19-IL2（一种免疫细胞因子）剂量和毒性。虽然本试验将纳入多个疾病部位的寡转移灶，但脑转移瘤患者（尤其是肺和乳腺）的脑部病变多为寡转移病变，因此这项临床研究将为多发脑转移瘤行 SRS 联合免疫治疗提供相关数据。

七、结论与建议

- 多发性脑转移患者的治疗选择包括全脑放射治疗、外科手术、立体定向放射外科作为初始治疗和挽救性治疗的组合。多发性脑转移瘤的传统治疗方法是 WBRT。
- SRS 治疗脑转移的优势在于，避免了 WBRT 的很多急性反应和晚期毒性，包括脱发、神经认知能力下降，总疗程更短。
- SRS 治疗脑转移的缺点包括局部治疗增加了未照射脑组织转移的风险和治疗成本。
- 多发性脑转移的患者分为两组：局限性脑转移（1～4 个脑转移瘤）和多发性脑转移（≥5 个脑转移瘤）。
- 几项大型随机对照试验表明，有限脑转移的患者仅用 SRS 即可有效治疗，总生存期与单纯 WBRT 相似，神经认知功能和生活质量优于 WBRT。
- 尽管数据有限，但值得安慰的是，多发性脑转移瘤患者可以通过单纯的 SRS 得到有效治疗，与 WBRT 相比，总生存期相似，神经认知功能和生活质量得到改善。
- 仅仅接受 SRS 治疗的患者增加了未照射脑组织转移。然而，SRS 作为多次补救治疗耐受性良好，并且延迟了与神经认知毒性相关的 WBRT 的使用。
- 数据表明，与脑转移数量相比，肿瘤负荷总体积可能更能代表临床结果的风险。

八、未来发展方向

- WBRT 与 SRS：4～10 个脑转移瘤的 WBRT 与 SRS，主要终点：生活质量。
- CCTG 试验 / 联盟：WBRT/ 美金刚与 SRS 在 5～15 个脑转移瘤中的比较，主要终点：总生存期和神经认知功能。
- NRG CC001：WBRT/ 美金刚 ± 海马保护，主要终点：神经认知功能。

参考文献

[1] Wen PY, Loeffler JS. Management of brain metastases. Oncology (Williston Park). 1999;13(7):941–54, 957–61; discussion 961–2, 9.

[2] Johnson JD, Young B. Demographics of brain metastasis. Neurosurg Clin N Am. 1996;7(3):337–44.

[3] Villa S, et al. Validation of the new graded prognostic assessment scale for brain metastases: a multicenter prospective study. Radiat Oncol. 2011;6:23.

[4] Stelzer KJ. Epidemiology and prognosis of brain metastases. Surg Neurol Int. 2013;4(Suppl 4):S192–202.

[5] Tabouret E, et al. Recent trends in epidemiology of brain metastases: an overview. Anticancer Res. 2012;32(11):4655–62.

[6] Andrews DW, et al. Whole brain radiation therapy with or without stereotactic radiosurgery boost for patients with one to three brain metastases: phase III results of the RTOG 9508 randomised trial. Lancet. 2004;363(9422):1665–72.

[7] Sperduto PW, et al. Secondary analysis of RTOG 9508, a phase 3 randomized trial of whole-brain radiation therapy versus WBRT plus stereotactic radiosurgery in patients with 1-3 brain metastases; poststratified by the graded prognostic assessment (GPA). Int J Radiat Oncol Biol Phys. 2014;90(3):526–31.

[8] Yamamoto M, et al. Stereotactic radiosurgery for patients with multiple brain metastases (JLGK0901): a multi-institutional prospective observational study. Lancet Oncol. 2014;15(4):387–95.

[9] Chang EL, et al. A pilot study of neurocognitive function

in patients with one to three new brain metastases initially treated with stereotactic radiosurgery alone. Neurosurgery. 2007;60(2):277–83; discussion 283–4.

[10] Brown PD, et al. Effect of radiosurgery alone vs radiosurgery with whole brain radiation therapy on cognitive function in patients with 1 to 3 brain metastases: a randomized clinical trial. JAMA. 2016;316(4):401–9.

[11] Tsao MN, et al. Whole brain radiotherapy for the treatment of multiple brain metastases. Cochrane Database Syst Rev. 2006;(3):CD003869.

[12] Borgelt B, et al. The palliation of brain metastases: final results of the first two studies by the Radiation Therapy Oncology Group. Int J Radiat Oncol Biol Phys. 1980;6(1):1–9.

[13] Suzuki H, et al. Spontaneous haemorrhage into metastatic brain tumours after stereotactic radiosurgery using a linear accelerator. J Neurol Neurosurg Psychiatry. 2003;74(7):908–12.

[14] Muller-Riemenschneider F, et al. Medical and health economic assessment of radiosurgery for the treatment of brain metastasis. GMS Health Technol Assess. 2009;5:Doc03.

[15] Hall MD, et al. Cost-effectiveness of stereotactic radiosurgery with and without whole-brain radiotherapy for the treatment of newly diagnosed brain metastases. J Neurosurg. 2014;121(Suppl):84–90.

[16] Chang EL, et al. Neurocognition in patients with brain metastases treated with radiosurgery or radiosurgery plus whole-brain irradiation: a randomised controlled trial. Lancet Oncol. 2009;10(11):1037–44.

[17] Kocher M, et al. Adjuvant whole-brain radiotherapy versus observation after radiosurgery or surgical resection of one to three cerebral metastases: results of the EORTC 22952-26001 study. J Clin Oncol. 2011;29(2):134–41.

[18] Aoyama H, et al. Neurocognitive function of patients with brain metastasis who received either whole brain radiotherapy plus stereotactic radiosurgery or radiosurgery alone. Int J Radiat Oncol Biol Phys. 2007;68(5):1388–95.

[19] Gaspar L, et al. Recursive partitioning analysis (RPA) of prognostic factors in three Radiation Therapy Oncology Group (RTOG) brain metastases trials. Int J Radiat Oncol Biol Phys. 1997;37(4):745–51.

[20] Weltman E, et al. Radiosurgery for brain metastases: a score index for predicting prognosis. Int J Radiat Oncol Biol Phys. 2000;46(5):1155–61.

[21] Lorenzoni J, et al. Radiosurgery for treatment of brain metastases: estimation of patient eligibility using three stratification systems. Int J Radiat Oncol Biol Phys. 2004;60(1):218–24.

[22] Lagerwaard FJ, et al. Identification of prognostic factors in patients with brain metastases: a review of 1292 patients. Int J Radiat Oncol Biol Phys. 1999;43(4):795–803.

[23] Golden DW, et al. Prognostic factors and grading systems for overall survival in patients treated with radiosurgery for brain metastases: variation by primary site. J Neurosurg. 2008;109(Suppl):77–86.

[24] Sperduto PW, et al. A new prognostic index and comparison to three other indices for patients with brain metastases: an analysis of 1,960 patients in the RTOG database. Int J Radiat Oncol Biol Phys. 2008;70(2):510–4.

[25] Sperduto PW, et al. Diagnosis-specific prognostic factors, indexes, and treatment outcomes for patients with newly diagnosed brain metastases: a multi-institutional analysis of 4,259 patients. Int J Radiat Oncol Biol Phys. 2010;77(3):655–61.

[26] Sperduto PW, et al. Summary report on the graded prognostic assessment: an accurate and facile diagnosis-specific tool to estimate survival for patients with brain metastases. J Clin Oncol. 2012;30(4):419–25.

[27] Subbiah IM, et al. Validation and development of a modified breast graded prognostic assessment as a tool for survival in patients with breast Cancer and brain metastases. J Clin Oncol. 2015;33(20):2239–45.

[28] Sperduto PW, et al. Estimating survival in patients with lung cancer and brain metastases: an update of the graded prognostic assessment for lung cancer using molecular markers (lung-molGPA). JAMA Oncol. 2017;3(6):827–31.

[29] Hughes RT, et al. Initial SRS for patients with 5 to 15 brain metastases: results of a multi-institutional experience. Int J Radiat Oncol Biol Phys. 2019;104:1091–8.

[30] Chang WS, et al. Analysis of radiosurgical results in patients with brain metastases according to the number of brain lesions: is stereotactic radiosurgery effective for multiple brain metastases? J Neurosurg. 2010;113(Suppl):73–8.

[31] Salvetti DJ, et al. Gamma Knife surgery for the treatment of 5 to 15 metastases to the brain: clinical article. J Neurosurg. 2013;118(6):1250–7.

[32] Aoyama H, et al. Stereotactic radiosurgery with or without whole-brain radiotherapy for brain metastases: secondary analysis of the JROSG 99-1 randomized clinical trial. JAMA Oncol. 2015;1(4):457–64.

[33] Saraf A, et al. Breast cancer subtype and stage are prognostic of time from breast cancer diagnosis to brain metastasis development. J Neuro-Oncol. 2017;134(2):453–63.

[34] Tai CH, et al. Single institution validation of a modified graded prognostic assessment of patients with breast cancer brain metastases. CNS Oncol. 2018;7(1):25–34.

[35] Mohammadi AM, et al. Role of Gamma Knife surgery in patients with 5 or more brain metastases. J Neurosurg. 2012;117(Suppl):5–12.

[36] Bhatnagar AK, et al. Stereotactic radiosurgery for four or more intracranial metastases. Int J Radiat Oncol Biol Phys. 2006;64(3):898–903.

[37] Tsao MN, et al. Radiotherapeutic and surgical management for newly diagnosed brain metastasis(es): an American Society for Radiation Oncology evidence-based guideline. Pract Radiat Oncol. 2012;2(3):210–25.

[38] Lippitz B, et al. Stereotactic radiosurgery in the treatment of brain metastases: the current evidence. Cancer Treat Rev.

2014;40(1):48–59.

[39] Vecht CJ, et al. Treatment of single brain metastasis: radiotherapy alone or combined with neurosurgery? Ann Neurol. 1993;33(6):583–90.

[40] Patchell RA, et al. A randomized trial of surgery in the treatment of single metastases to the brain. N Engl J Med. 1990;322(8):494–500.

[41] Grandhi R, et al. Stereotactic radiosurgery using the Leksell Gamma Knife Perfexion unit in the management of patients with 10 or more brain metastases. J Neurosurg. 2012;117(2):237–45.

[42] Ma L, et al. Apparatus dependence of normal brain tissue dose in stereotactic radiosurgery for multiple brain metastases. J Neurosurg. 2011;114(6):1580–4.

[43] Ma L, et al. Variable dose interplay effects across radiosurgical apparatus in treating multiple brain metastases. Int J Comput Assist Radiol Surg. 2014;9(6):1079–86.

[44] McDonald D, et al. Comparison of radiation dose spillage from the Gamma Knife Perfexion with that from volumetric modulated arc radiosurgery during treatment of multiple brain metastases in a single fraction. J Neurosurg. 2014;121(Suppl):51–9.

[45] Dong P, et al. Minimizing normal tissue dose spillage via broad-range optimization of hundreds of intensity modulated beams for treating multiple brain targets. J Radiosurg SBRT. 2016;4(2):107–15.

[46] Sahgal A, et al. Prescription dose guideline based on physical criterion for multiple metastatic brain tumors treated with stereotactic radiosurgery. Int J Radiat Oncol Biol Phys. 2010;78(2):605–8.

[47] Shaw E, et al. Single dose radiosurgical treatment of recurrent previously irradiated primary brain tumors and brain metastases: final report of RTOG protocol 90-05. Int J Radiat Oncol Biol Phys. 2000;47(2):291–8.

[48] Mulvenna P, et al. Dexamethasone and supportive care with or without whole brain radiotherapy in treating patients with non-small cell lung cancer with brain metastases unsuitable for resection or stereotactic radiotherapy (QUARTZ): results from a phase 3, non-inferiority, randomised trial. Lancet. 2016;388(10055):2004–14.

[49] Zindler JD, et al. Whole brain radiotherapy versus stereotactic radiosurgery for 4-10 brain metastases: a phase III randomised multicentre trial. BMC Cancer. 2017;17(1):500.

[50] Brown PD, et al. Memantine for the prevention of cognitive dysfunction in patients receiving whole-brain radiotherapy: a randomized, doubleblind, placebo-controlled trial. Neuro-Oncology. 2013;15(10):1429–37.

[51] Rapp SR, et al. Donepezil for irradiated brain tumor survivors: a phase III randomized placebo-controlled clinical trial. J Clin Oncol. 2015;33(15):1653–9.

第 10 章 脑转移瘤的大分割立体定向放射外科治疗
Hypofractionated Stereotactic Radiosurgery for Intact and Resected Brain Metastases

Erqi L. Pollom   Siyu Shi   Scott G. Soltys   著
周 雪   周扬莹   译
周 琴   校

一、概述

根据神经外科和放射肿瘤学学会共识的定义[1]，立体定向放射外科治疗（stereotactic radiosurgery，SRS），是一种分成 1~5 次的立体定向放射治疗。单次 SRS 是未手术或已手术脑转移瘤患者一种有效的治疗方式。对于不适合手术的体积较大的脑转移瘤患者，既往研究认为，全脑放射治疗是标准治疗方案。考虑到全脑放射治疗的神经毒性及较差的局部控制，SRS 得到越来越多的应用。然而，单次 SRS 应用于体积较大、位于关键结构或语言功能区附近或内部（如脑干、视觉通路或运动皮质）的靶病灶可能会增加毒性。2~5 次的大分割 SRS 可能是一种替代治疗方法，它可以安全地将较高的累积剂量输送到由于大小或位置不适宜选用单次 SRS 的病灶。越来越多的临床证据表明，大分割 SRS 可以在保持较好局部控制率的同时将正常脑组织损伤的风险降至最低，尽管目前这种治疗方式的最佳剂量和分割方式尚未确定。其他综述也研究了 SRS 与大分割 SRS 对良、恶性脑肿瘤的治疗效果[2]。在此，我们会重点讨论大分割治疗脑转移瘤的作用和原理。

二、单次放射外科治疗的局限性

单次 SRS 的剂量受到 CNS 毒性的限制。不良辐射效应（adverse radiation effect，ARE），影像学上表现为相当于组织学上定义的脑放射性坏死，是 SRS 治疗颅内或邻近部位肿瘤后最常见的毒性反应，可能与神经功能缺损有关，需要激素、贝伐珠单抗治疗，甚至在某些情况下需要手术切除。

已发现与不良辐射效应发生相关的因素包括较高的辐射剂量、较大的肿瘤体积和正常脑组织照射的体积大小[3]。RTOG 90-05 发现，对于复发、不可切除、以及以前接受过放射治疗的原发脑瘤和脑转移瘤，采用递增剂量的单次 SRS 治疗后，肿瘤较大的患者容易出现 CNS 毒性。与最大直径 < 2cm 的肿瘤相比，最大直径为 2~3cm 和 3~4cm 的肿瘤发生不可逆转的 3 级或 4~5 级 CNS 毒性的风险分别高 7.3 倍和 16 倍[3]。除了与肿瘤大小有关外，增加放射剂量也与更高级别的脑组织毒性风险有关。有研究者发现 ARE 的风险与 10Gy 或 12Gy 等剂量线所覆盖的放射外科治疗体积相关[4]。包含 310 处脑转移病灶的 206 名患者接受单次 SRS 治疗后，接受 12Gy 照射剂量的体积超过 10.9cm³ 时，ARE 发生风险高达 51%[5]。Blonigen 等在分析 173 例脑转移瘤的 63

名患者的研究中同样发现，当接受 10Gy 和 12Gy 照射的瘤周正常脑组织体积分别大于 14.5cm^3 和 10.8cm^3 时，ARE 发生的风险高达 69%[6]。

对于已切除的脑转移瘤，放射性坏死的发生率与术前病灶的大小和接受 21Gy 照射的正常脑组织体积有关[7]。虽然增加术腔边缘照射改善了局部控制率[8]，但也增加了正常脑组织照射的体积，因此增加了发生毒性反应的风险[9,10]。

部分通过降低剂量来减少治疗毒性，一定程度上，较大的病灶在单次 SRS 后与较低的控制率相关。根据 RTOG 90-05 的结果，最大直径大于 2cm、2.1~3.0cm 和 3.1~4.0cm 的单次 SRS 的推荐剂量分别为 24Gy、18Gy 和 15Gy[3]。据报道，采用这些剂量，直径 2.1~3.0cm 和 3.1~4.0cm 的转移灶的一年局部控制率分别只有 49% 和 45%，而更小的病灶则为 85%[11]。Hasegawa 等也同样报道了使用单次 SRS 治疗体积大于 4cm^3 的肿瘤，1 年局部控制率为 49%[12]。Chang 等报道了 153 个脑转移瘤采用 20Gy 或更高剂量的单次 SRS 治疗后，直径 ≤1cm 的肿瘤 1 年局部控制率为 86%，>1cm 的肿瘤则仅为 56%[13]。最小的等剂量表面处方剂量 18Gy 或更高的处方剂量与局部控制率有关[14]。

三、大分割的放射生物学及理论基础

大分割 SRS 可以为较大的靶体积提供更高的累积剂量，同时将毒性风险降至最低。分次剂量照射是放射治疗的中心原则，它利用经典放射生物学的 4R 原则（修复、再增殖、再分布和再氧化）来扩大治疗窗口。单次 SRS 与传统的放射生物学原则相矛盾，但已证明对转移性和良性肿瘤均具有良好的局部控制和可接受的毒性反应。对小体积病灶给予高剂量辐射需要更高的精确度和准确度。以前，摆位固定是通过侵入性地将患者的头部固定并锁在治疗床上的框架上来实现。然而图像引导和基于自动控制系统技术的最新进展使得非侵入性、无框架放射外科治疗的发展成为可能，促使立体定向放射治疗可以精确地分次输送放射剂量[15-17]。此外，近年来有关单次大剂量 SRS 放射生物学的临床前和临床研究也揭示了其不同于常规分割放射治疗的放射机制，除了使 DNA 双链断裂外，单次高剂量 SRS 还可能通过鞘磷脂途径引起内皮细胞炎症和凋亡，从而导致微血管功能障碍和细胞死亡[18,19]。关于是否存在一种超越经典放射生物学分割模式的"新放射生物学"，或者仅采用更高的生物有效剂量（biological effective dose，BED）来解释单次 SRS 的疗效，目前仍存在争议[20]。

对于恶性肿瘤，人们会考虑单次 SRS 对肿瘤控制和远期疗效之间的次优选择。由于脑转移瘤由反应敏感的肿瘤细胞组成，周围被反应迟缓的正常脑组织包围，Hall 和 Brenner 认为，分次放射治疗能促进正常组织的修复，为探索肿瘤组织和正常组织对辐射的不同生物学反应和修复机制提供可能[21,22]。然而，单次照射后耐受辐射的乏氧细胞亚群可能存活[23]，导致肿瘤控制更差。分次照射遵循再氧化原理可能改善肿瘤的控制情况。对于使用立体定向技术治疗的小体积病灶，扩大治疗窗口不那么重要，因为在靶区范围内可达到足够的剂量。对于大体积的病灶，大分割 SRS 提供一种利用分次高剂量和分割方式的放射生物学优势的方法。模拟研究表明，对于增殖迅速的肿瘤，超过 5~10 次的分次治疗能最大限度地保留正常组织功能；改善率通常在分割次数较多（大于 10 次）时达到平衡[24]。最后，有新的证据表明，肿瘤的放射治疗可能通过免疫原性肿瘤细胞死亡和增强抗肿瘤 T 细胞的募集达到免疫刺激作用，并可与免疫治疗相结合来改善肿瘤治疗结果。不同的放射治疗方案可以与免疫治疗相结合，最近的数据表明，剂量分割方式可以决定联合治疗的疗效[25,26]。Dewan 等使用乳腺癌和结肠癌模型显示，虽然单次剂量 20Gy 在控制肿瘤生长方面与 8Gy/3 次和 6Gy/5 次的分割方式同样有效，但只有后两种分割方式能够与 CTLA-4 阻断药协同诱导抗肿瘤 T 细胞免疫，并抑制照射野外的第二个受影响的肿瘤（远隔效应）[27]。这可能是由于单次 SRS 损伤了血管结构，并损害抗原和免疫细胞的聚集和运输[28]。在体内外研究中也发现分次辐射细胞的分子反应与单次辐射不同，这可能是造成分次辐射和单次辐射效应不同的原因之一[29]。

四、大分割 SRS 的临床经验

（一）不可切除的脑转移瘤

表 10-1 总结了已发表的大分割 SRS 治疗不能手术切除脑转移瘤的研究，尽管许多研究中脑转移瘤的体积都较大，但总体体现了大分割治疗方案具有较好的局部控制率。此外，这些数据表明，与既往单次 SRS 相比，大分割 SRS 毒性反应更低。

Minniti 等纳入的 289 例患者的一项回顾性研究显示，与单次 SRS 相比，使用大分割 SRS（9Gy/3 次）治疗最大直径＞ 2cm 的脑转移瘤的局部控制率更高，1 年局部控制率分别为 77% 和 90%，同时大分割 SRS 发生 ARE 风险较低（9% vs. 18%）[45]。与此相反，Wiggenraad 等发现体积较大的脑转移瘤（体积＞ 13cm³），采用大分割 SRS（8Gy/3 次）和单次 SRS（15Gy）治疗的局部控制率及毒性无明显差异[52]。Fokas 等还发现，大分割 SRS（5Gy/7 次或 4Gy/10 次）与单次 SRS 的局部控制率相似；但单次 SRS 的 1 级～ 3 级毒性反应发生率（14%）明显高于大分割 SRS 的发生率（5Gy/7 次为 6%，4Gy/10 次为 2%）[34]。另一系列研究发现，30Gy/5 次的大分割 SRS 的局部控制率高于 24Gy/5 次照射（1 年局部控制率为 91% vs. 75%）[41]。另有研究报道了大分割 SRS 可能由于放射抵抗导致较差的局部控制率，这可能是因为分次照射的 BED 值较低[47]。这些数据表明大分割放疗具有安全性，为了达到最佳的局部控制率，临床医生应注意保证分次 SRS 的 BED 值，至少相当于单次 SRS 剂量的 BED。

虽然目前还缺乏比较大分割 SRS 与其他放疗技术的随机对照研究，但现有的临床经验表明对于较大的转移性脑瘤或靠近脑干或视交叉等功能区域的肿瘤，大分割 SRS 是一种更好的治疗选择。

（二）术腔

脑转移瘤仅做手术切除的局部控制率较低[53-55]。与术后全脑放射治疗相比，术后对术腔行 SRS 可以改善认知，而且不会影响总体生存率，现已成为标准治疗方案[56]。很多研究已经报道了单次 SRS 对小体积转移瘤术腔的结果，1 年局部控制率为 70%～ 90%[8, 55, 57, 58]。与接受 SRS 治疗的不可切除脑转移瘤一样，术前较大脑转移瘤（直径≥ 3cm）的术腔在 SRS 后局部复发可能性更大[59]。术腔体积的大小与毒性增加呈正相关[7, 60]。延迟进行 SRS 不能减少靶体积，因为手术到切除后 1 个月内的术腔缩小最不明显[61]，且延迟放疗可能影响肿瘤的局部控制[62]。针对术腔的大分割 SRS 已被证明有很好的局部控制率，即使对于较大的转移病灶也是如此。Minniti 等报道的 1 年和 2 年局部控制率分别为 93% 和 84%，接受 9Gy/3 次的术腔放疗后，有症状的放射性坏死发生率仅为 5%[60]。表 10-2 总结了已发表的关于已切除脑转移瘤的大分割 SRS 的研究。

五、最佳大分割 SRS 方案

大分割 SRS 的最佳剂量和分割方式尚未确定。虽然线性平方模型（L-Q 模型）的可靠性在 SRS 中受到了质疑[75]，但基于 L-Q 模型的 BED 值仍广泛应用于临床来比较各种分割方式的效果。局部控制率与 BED10 相关（肿瘤的

第 10 章 脑转移瘤的大分割立体定向放射外科治疗
Hypofractionated Stereotactic Radiosurgery for Intact and Resected Brain Metastases

表 10-1 大分割 SRS 治疗不可切除的脑转移瘤的系列研究

作　者	年　份	病灶数量	剂量（Gy/次）	病灶直径或体积（中位数，范围）	组织来源	边界（mm）	1 年局控率（%）	不良辐射反应率[a]（%）
Aoki 等[30]	2006	65	中位数 24（18～30）/（3～5）	>2cm（n=31）；≤2cm（n=34）	肺癌、其他	1	72	2
Aoyama 等[31]	2003	159	35/4	3.3cm³，0.006～48.3cm³	肺癌、其他	2	85	3
Ernst-stecken 等[32]	2006	72	（30～35）/5	2.27cm，0.85～5.22cm	肺、黑色素瘤、乳腺、结肠、肾细胞、其他	3	76	35
Fahrig 等[33]	2007	228	（30～35）/5；40/10；35/7	PTV：6.1cm³，0.02～95.97cm³	肺、黑色素瘤、乳腺、直肠、肾细胞癌、其他	3	72	1
Fokas 等[34]	2012	122	35/7；40/10	2.04cm³，0.02～27.5cm³（35/7）；5.93cm³，0.02～26.8cm³（40/10）	肺、乳腺、黑色素瘤、胃肠道、生殖性上皮、其他	3	75（35/7）；71（40/10）	6（35/7）；2（40/10）
Higuchi 等[35]	2009	46	30/3	17.6cm³（中位数；SD 6.3cm³）	肺、结肠、乳腺、其他	0	76	4
Kim 等[36]	2011	49	36/6	PTV：5.00cm³，0.14～37.80cm³	未说明	1	69	0
Kwon 等[37]	2009	52	25/5；20/5；30/5；36/6	1.16cm³，1.7～31.2cm	肺、黑色素瘤、其他	1～2	68	6
Lindvall 等[38]	2009	47	中位数 38（35～40）/5	6cm³，0.6～26cm³	肺、肾细胞癌、乳腺、黑色素瘤、其他	3	84（中位随访 3.7 个月）	0
Lockney 等[39]	2017	88	30/5	2.0cm³，0.4～4.6cm³	肺、乳腺、黑色素瘤、其他	2～5	81	4
Manning 等[40]	2000	57	中位数 27（12～36）/3	2.16cm³	肺、黑色素瘤、乳腺、胃肠道、甲状腺、其他	2	91（6 个月内）	6
Marcrom 等[41]	2017	182	2 或 30/5	1.68cm，0.31～5.50cm	肺、乳腺、黑色素瘤、胃肠道、生殖性上皮、其他	0～3	86	1
Märtens 等[42]	2012	108	30/6；30/5；35/5；（28～40）/（7～10）；25/5	1.0cm³，0.1～19.0cm³（前期 SRS）；2.0cm³，0.1～29.2cm³（挽救性 SRS）	肺、乳腺、黑色素瘤、肾细胞癌、其他	4	52	1
Matsuyama 等[43]	2013	573	外照射 BED10：中位数为 83.2（19.1～89.6）/ 平均 3（2～10）	1.4cm³，0.1～138.6cm³	肺	1	95	2

(续表)

作者	年份	病灶数量	剂量(Gy/次)	病灶直径或体积(中位数,范围)	组织来源	边界(mm)	1年局控率(%)	不良辐射反应率[a](%)
Minniti 等[44]	2014	171	27(≥2cm)或36(<2cm)/3	10.1cm³, 1.6~48.4cm³	肺、乳腺、胃肠道、肾细胞癌、其他	1~3	88	6
Minniti 等[45]	2016	138	27/3	17.9cm, 5.6~54cm	肺、乳腺、结肠、黑色素瘤、肾细胞癌、其他	1~2	91	3
Narayana 等[46]	2007	20	30/5	3.5cm, 2~5cm	肺、黑色素瘤、肾细胞癌、乳腺、胃肠道、卵巢、肉瘤	3	70	5
Oermann 等[47]	2013	74	20/2~5	2.5cm (IQR 0.8~2.2cm, 放疗抵抗的); 2.1cm (IQR 1.4~2.8cm, 放疗敏感)	黑色素瘤、肾细胞癌、肉瘤、乳腺、肺	未说明	中位数14.4个月(放疗抵抗); 中位数41.5个月(放疗敏感)	2
Ogura 等[48]	2012	27	20~25 或 35/5	1.8cm, 0.3~3.4cm	肺、乳腺、结肠、其他	2	87	5
Rajakesari 等[49]	2014	70	25/5(n=61); 30/10; 32/8; 33/11; 24/8	1.7cm, 0.4~6.4cm	肺、乳腺、黑色素瘤、胃肠道、肾细胞癌、其他	未说明	56	4
Saitoh 等[50]	2010	78	(39~42)/3	1.2cm, 0.4~3.8cm	肺	3	86	8
Tokuuye 等[51]	1998	95	42/7; 48/8; 52/13(>3cm或邻近关键部位)	未说明	肺、肾细胞癌、乳腺、其他	2~3	91	8
Wiggenraad 等[52]	2012	65	24/3	PTV>13cm³或病灶位于脑干附近(n=47)	肺、乳腺、黑色素瘤、其他	2	61	25%[b]

n.数目; cm³.立方厘米; PTV.计划治疗量; SD.标准差; IQR.四分位数范围; a.有临床意义, 需激素治疗; b.包括假性进展

表 10-2 大分割 SRS 治疗已切除脑转移瘤的系列研究

作者	年份	术腔数量	剂量（Gy/次）	术腔直径或体积（中位数，范围）	组织来源	边界（mm）	1年局控率（%）	不良辐射反应率（%）
Abuodeh 等[63]	2016	77	25/5	8.92cm³, 0.17~54.2cm³	肺黑色素瘤、肾细胞癌乳腺其他	1~2	89	3
Ahmed 等[64]	2014	65	（20~30）/5	8.06cm³, 0.13~54.25cm³	肺黑色素瘤肾细胞癌乳腺、其他	1~2	87	2
Ammirati 等[65]	2014	36	30/5	10.25cm³, 1.04~67.52cm³	肺、黑色素瘤、乳腺、其他	3	16%LF	8
Connolly 等[66]	2013	33	40.05/15	3.3cm, 1.7~5.7cm	肺、黑色素瘤、乳腺、其他	10	90	0
Do 等[67]	2009	33	（24~27.5）/（4~6）	>3cm（n=16）	肺、黑色素瘤、乳腺、其他	1~3	82	0
Dore 等[7]	2017	103	23.1/3	>3cm（n=48）	肺、肾细胞癌、乳腺、结肠、黑色素瘤其他	2	84	7
Keller 等[68]	2017	189	33/3	7.6cm³, 0.2~48.81cm³	肺乳腺胃肠道肾细胞癌黑色素瘤其他	2	88	19
Kumar 等[69]	2018	43	（28~30）/（3~5）	3.1cm（术前）	肺乳腺黑色素瘤其他	2	23% LF	0
Ling 等[70]	2015	100	中位数22（10~28）/平均3（1~5）	PTV: 12.9cm³, 0.6~51.1cm³	肺黑色素瘤肾细胞癌乳腺其他	0~1	72	6
Lockney 等[39]	2017	143	30/5	3.2cm, 0.7~6.3cm	肺乳腺黑色素瘤其他	2~5	84	4
Pessina 等[71]	2016	69	30/3	29cm³, 4.1~203.1cm³	肺黑色素瘤乳腺其他	3	100	9
Steinmann 等[72]	2012	33	40/10, 35/7, 30/5	9.7cm³, 0.95~52.6cm³	肺黑色素瘤肾细胞癌乳腺其他	4	71	0
Vogel 等[73]	2015	33	中位数30（16~35）/中位数5（1~5）	3.8cm, 2.8~6.7cm	肺乳腺黑色素瘤其他	2~3	69	10
Wang 等[74]	2011	37	24/3	>3cm	肺黑色素瘤乳腺、肾脏结肠	2~3	80	6

cm³. 立方厘米；cm. 厘米；mm. 毫米；LF. 局部复发；a. 有临床意义，需激素治疗的

α：β 为 10）：一个系列研究发现，BED10 大于 80Gy 的 1 年局部控制率为 97%，BED10 低于 80Gy 的 1 年局部控制率为 90%[43]。最近发表的一项关于脑转移瘤 SRS 治疗的综述比较了不同 SRS 治疗方案的 BED 值（α：β 为 12Gy），发现 BED12 ≥ 40Gy（相当于 25.5Gy 分 3 次照射或单次 20Gy 的剂量）是获得 1 年的局部控制率 > 70% 所必需的[52]。对术后脑转移瘤，术腔采

用 BED10 ≥ 48Gy 剂量的多次 SRS 可以改善局部控制率。接受 BED10 ≥ 48Gy（30Gy/5 次或 27Gy/3 次）治疗的术腔 1 年局部控制率为 100%，而使用较低 BED10 治疗的术腔 1 年局部控制率仅为 33%[69]。

在保证单次分割高剂量模式下，需要对总的治疗时间进行探索。在其他部位的研究表明，隔天放疗可提高疗效、降低毒性和改善生活质量[76-78]。放射生物学研究表明，脑坏死的修复半衰期相对较长，在 24 小时后仍有可能出现无法修复的损伤[79]。再氧合也同样需要更长的时间间隔，因为在对肺组织进行单次照射后 24~48h，仍在肺部肿瘤细胞中检测到缺氧状态[80]。通过增加放射治疗之间的时间间隔进行间断放疗，可以使剩余的肿瘤细胞再分布到细胞周期的 G2/M 期，并改善后续放疗的氧合情况和辐射敏感性，从而最大限度地提高放疗的疗效。治疗间隔为正常细胞的修复及再生提供了时间，从而将治疗风险降至最低。对于因肿瘤位置及大小不能接受单次 SRS 治疗的脑转移瘤患者，Narayana 等报道了 15% 对激素依赖的患者接受了每周 2 次，共 5 次 30Gy 的放射治疗，1 年的局部控制率为 70%[46]。然而也有其他研究发现，与每日治疗相比，隔日治疗并无获益[81]。

这概念进一步延伸为阶段性 SRS 治疗，在该治疗中，每次放疗间隔至少数周。阶段性 SRS 会随着时间的推移分配较高的累积剂量，并在随后的治疗过程中消除潜在的小病灶。Higuchi 等首次发表了阶段性 SRS 的结果，其中脑转移瘤体积 > 10cm³ 的患者接受了每次间隔 2 周，共 3 次总剂量 30Gy 的分阶段治疗[35]。其中肿瘤体积总体缩小了 91%，在第 2 次和第 3 次治疗时肿瘤体积分别缩小了 19% 和 40%。这种阶段性 SRS 的方法使得 1 年局部控制率为 76%，只有一名患者出现了需要手术的 3 级毒性反应。此后又有其他研究显示了类似的结果，采用总剂量 20~33Gy 的放疗，分两次的阶段性 SRS 治疗大的脑转移瘤同样有效，且与治疗相关的毒性反应发生率最低[82-84]。Angelov 等假设大脑中晚期辐射效应的修复半衰期为 76h，为了提供 10 个半衰期的时间进行修复，采用了 30 天的时间间隔[79]。据他们的研究报道，对于直径 > 2cm 的脑转移瘤采用中位剂量为 30Gy 分 2 次进行放疗，6 个月的局部控制率为 88%，有症状的放射性坏死发生率为 6%[83]。

六、大病灶的手术适应证（对比放射外科治疗）

大分割 SRS 已被证明是无法手术切除的大体积脑转移瘤的一种有效治疗方式。虽然较大的脑转移瘤（最大直径 > 2~3cm）通常先手术切除后辅以放射治疗，但有时由于患者的功能状态、并发症或疾病严重程度等因素，不宜采取手术切除。EORTC 22952-26001 的二次分析发现，在直径 ≤ 4cm 的一到两个脑转移瘤的患者中，与手术切除相比，SRS 的早期局部控制率更高[85]。但在以下情况下需要手术切除。

- 需要转移灶的病理诊断。
- 激素不能缓解的颅高压症状。
- 症状可用激素缓解，但患者会在肿瘤缩小前的数周到数月之间形成激素依赖者（即手术比单独 SRS 治疗更快消除颅高压症状）。

七、结论与展望

大分割放射外科治疗能最大限度提高脑转移瘤局部控制率的同时将毒性反应降至最低，特别是对于体积大或位于关键部位的病灶。虽然文献报道的可接受的分割方案范围很大，但维持较高的 BED 值（即 BED10 ≥ 48Gy，相当于 27Gy 分 3 次进行）才能达到最佳的局部控制[52, 69]。有待研究的问题包括大分割 SRS 与手术治疗在大体积脑转移瘤中的比较，以及大分割 SRS 与单次分割 SRS 在小体积脑转移瘤中的比较。关于 SRS 治疗的最佳间隔时间和新的放疗方案（如阶段性 SRS）也有待进一步研究。

第 10 章 脑转移瘤的大分割立体定向放射外科治疗
Hypofractionated Stereotactic Radiosurgery for Intact and Resected Brain Metastases

> **要　点**
> - 对于不可切除的转移瘤和直径＞2cm 的术腔，研究显示相较于单次 SRS，2~5 次的大分割 SRS 能更好控制肿瘤及降低治疗相关的毒性。
> - 大分割放疗要实现最佳局部控制（即 BED10 ≥ 48Gy，相当于 27Gy 分 3 次照射），需达到与单次剂量相当的等效生物剂量。不可切除脑转移瘤和术腔的推荐放射外科治疗剂量如表 10-3 所示。

表 10-3 本机构未行手术的转移瘤和术腔的推荐放射外科剂量

病灶最大直径（cm）	剂量（Gy/次）
＜2	（20~24）/1
2~3	（27~30）/3 或 18/1
3~4	27/3
4~5	24/3
＞5	25/5

八、病例介绍

（一）病例 1：较大术腔脑转移瘤的大分割 SRS，以及小体积不可切除脑转移瘤的单次 SRS

一位 59 岁的卵巢癌合并脑转移女性患者，表现为头痛、神志不清和视力障碍，检查发现左侧顶枕叶有 4.8cm×4.9cm 的出血性脑转移瘤，伴有边缘强化和周围血管源性水肿。在接受抗癫痫药物和激素治疗后症状完全消失。患者在开颅手术切除术后一周进行放射外科治疗。在制定放疗计划的磁共振上，左侧顶枕部病灶大小为 2.7cm×1.5cm。左侧中央前回和右侧额叶另有 2 个病灶，大小分别为 7mm×5mm 和 2mm。左侧顶枕部病灶未进行外扩，治疗剂量为 72% 的等剂量线达到 27Gy/3 次的处方剂量（图 10-1A），在另一个计划中，其余两个病灶一起接受放疗，72% 的等剂量线处方剂量为单次 24Gy（图 10-1B 和 C）。患者在接受放射外科治疗后 1 年内没有出现神经系统症状，局部控制良好。

（二）病例 2：巨大术腔的脑转移瘤予以超过 5 天的大分割 SRS

一位 64 岁性激素阳性的女性乳腺癌伴脑转移患者，表现为健忘和异常行为，发现右额叶有一个直径 5.5cm 巨大的囊性实性肿块，并伴有水肿、大脑镰下疝和中线移位。发现脑转移后，患者接受了脑转移瘤切除手术，在手术后两个月才接受辅助放疗。在制定放疗计划时，在术腔周围发现了较厚的边缘强化，怀疑肿瘤复发。该患者术腔及边缘 2mm 接受处方剂量为 25Gy/5 次的放射外科治疗。SRS 后 3 个月出现软脑膜结节，随后完成了全脑放疗（图 10-2）。

（三）病例 3：针对大体积及位于关键部位的脑转移瘤超过 3 天的大分割 SRS

一位 65 岁的女性卵巢癌伴脑转移患者，6 个月前曾因 4 处脑转移瘤接受 SRS 治疗，她表现为远侧凝视伴有轻度复视。MRI 显示脑桥有 2.7cm×2.7cm 的脑转移瘤。她接受了 72% 的等剂量线达到 24Gy/3 次（连续 3 天）的放疗。9 个月后随访，MRI 显示肿瘤持续缩小，无不良辐射效应（图 10-3）。

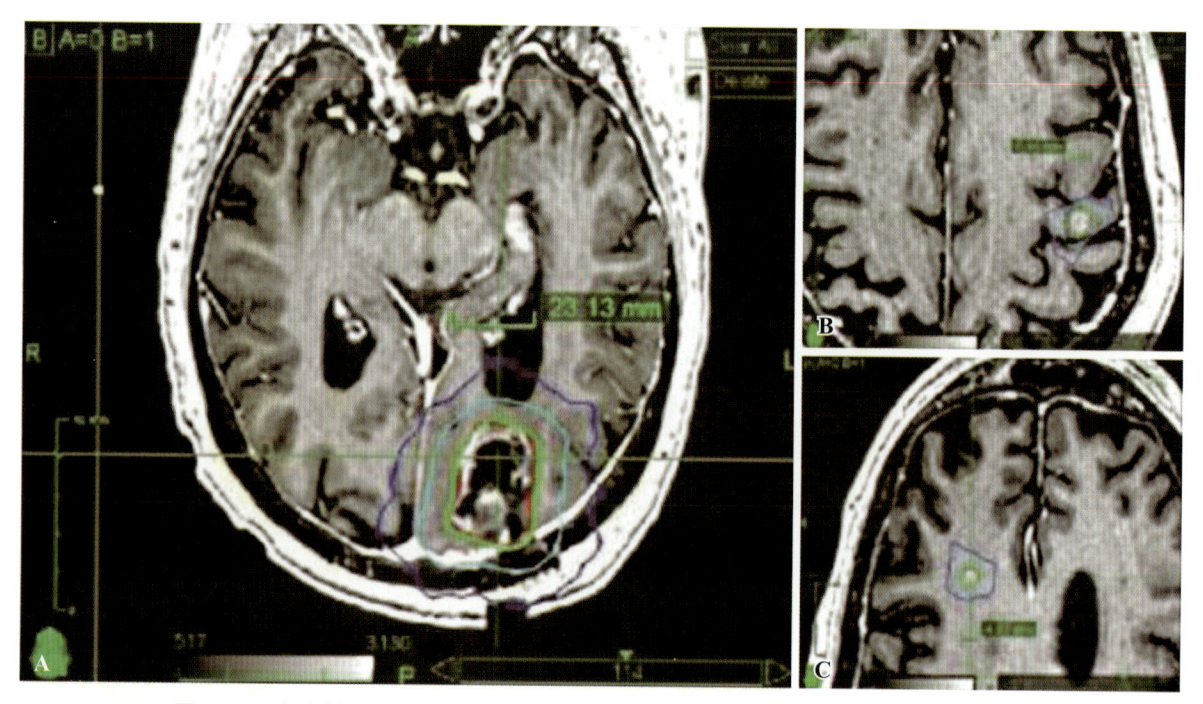

▲ 图 10-1 大分割 SRS 治疗大术腔脑转移瘤，以及单次 SRS 处理小体积未手术脑转移瘤

A. 左侧顶枕部病变（2.7cm×1.5cm），出血灶部分切除后放疗，72% 的等剂量线包含 27Gy/3 次（绿色线为 27Gy，浅蓝色线为 13.5Gy，深蓝色线为 6.75Gy）。B 和 C. 左侧中央前回病变（7mm×5mm）和右侧额叶病变（2mm），SRS 处方剂量为 72% 等剂量线包含单次 24Gy（绿色线 24Gy，浅蓝色线 12Gy，深蓝色线 6Gy）

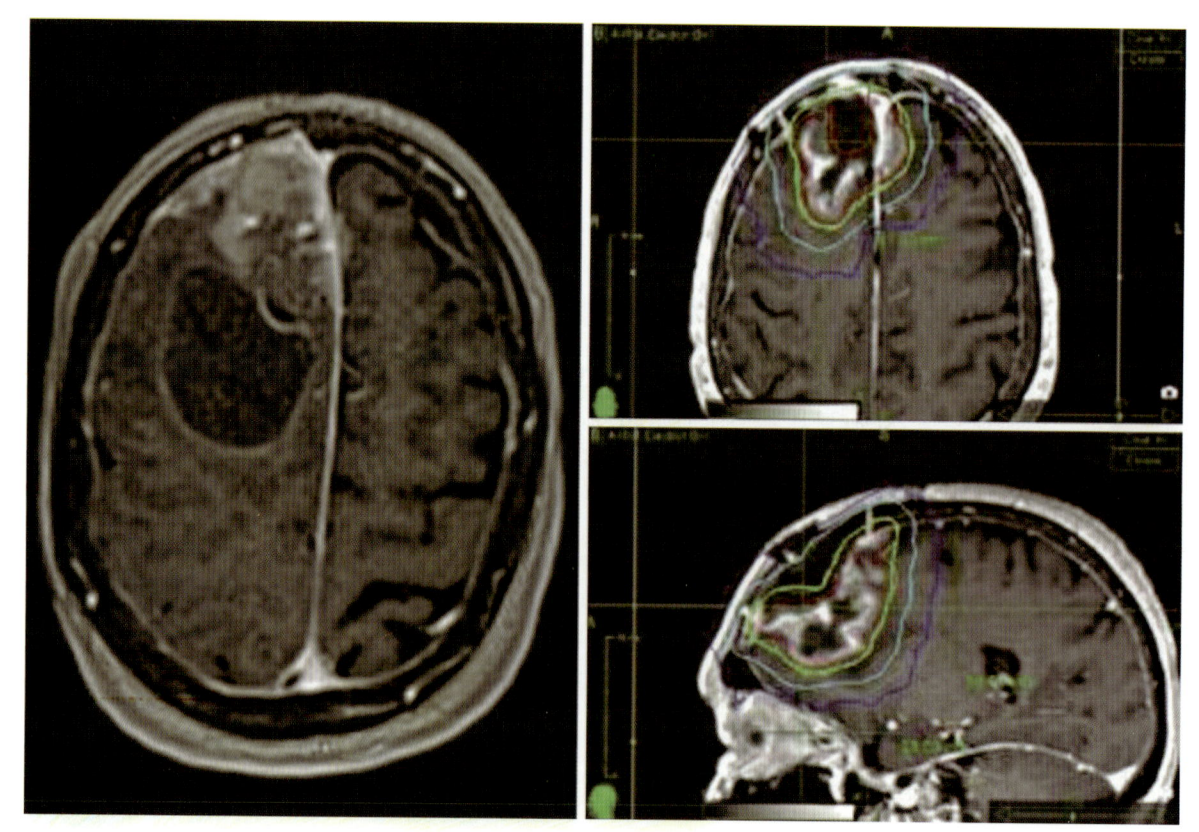

▲ 图 10-2 右额叶术腔及边缘 2mm 的轴位和矢状位图像，SRS 处方剂量为 72% 等剂量线包含 25Gy/5 次
勾画靶区时将术前术后 MRI 融合。靶区勾画按术前病灶范围而不是手术路径

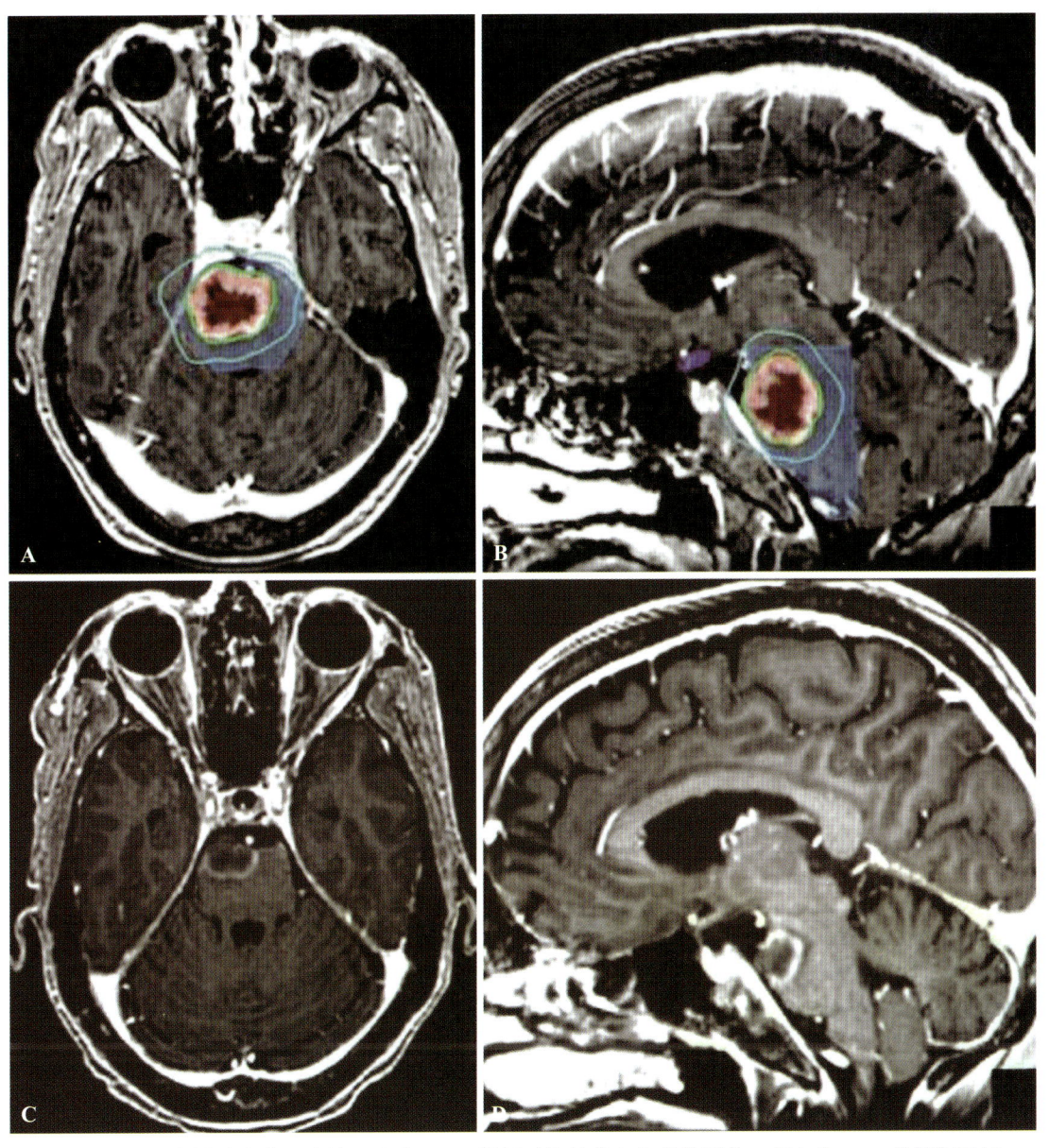

▲ 图 10-3 脑桥转移瘤经连续 3 次共 24Gy 照射后的轴位和矢状位图像，绿色为 72% 的等剂量线（A，B）。图中青色线为 50% 的剂量线（12Gy 等剂量线）。(C，D) 9 个月后随访的 MRI 显示肿瘤持续缩小，无不良辐射效应

参考文献

[1] Barnett GH, Linskey ME, Adler JR, Cozzens JW, Friedman WA, Heilbrun MP, et al. Stereotactic radiosurgery— an organized neurosurgery-sanctioned definition. J Neurosurg. 2007;106(1):1–5.

[2] Kirkpatrick JP, Soltys SG, Lo SS, Beal K, Shrieve DC, Brown PD. The radiosurgery fractionation quandary: single fraction or hypofractionation? Neuro Oncol. 2017;19(suppl_2):ii38–49.

[3] Shaw E, Scott C, Souhami L, Dinapoli R, Kline R, Loeffler J, et al. Single dose radiosurgical treatment of recurrent previously irradiated primary brain tumors and brain metastases: final report of RTOG protocol 90-05. Int J Radiat Oncol Biol Phys. 2000;47(2):291–8.

[4] Korytko T, Radivoyevitch T, Colussi V, Wessels BW, Pillai K, Maciunas RJ, et al. 12 Gy gamma knife radiosurgical volume is a predictor for radiation necrosis in non-AVM intracranial tumors. Int J Radiat Oncol Biol Phys. 2006;64(2):419–24.

[5] Minniti G, Clarke E, Lanzetta G, Osti MF, Trasimeni G, Bozzao

A, et al. Stereotactic radiosurgery for brain metastases: analysis of outcome and risk of brain radionecrosis. Radiat Oncol Lond Engl. 2011;6:48.

[6] Blonigen BJ, Steinmetz RD, Levin L, Lamba MA, Warnick RE, Breneman JC. Irradiated volume as a predictor of brain radionecrosis after linear accelerator stereotactic radiosurgery. Int J Radiat Oncol Biol Phys. 2010;77(4):996–1001.

[7] Doré M, Martin S, Delpon G, Clément K, Campion L, Thillays F. Stereotactic radiotherapy following surgery for brain metastasis: predictive factors for local control and radionecrosis. Cancer Radiother. 2017;21(1):4–9.

[8] Choi CYH, Chang SD, Gibbs IC, Adler JR, Harsh GR, Lieberson RE, et al. Stereotactic radiosurgery of the postoperative resection cavity for brain metastases: prospective evaluation of target margin on tumor control. Int J Radiat Oncol Biol Phys. 2012;84(2):336–42.

[9] Kirkpatrick JP, Wang Z, Sampson JH, McSherry F, Herndon JE, Allen KJ, et al. Defining the optimal planning target volume in image-guided stereotactic radiosurgery of brain metastases: results of a randomized trial. Int J Radiat Oncol Biol Phys. 2015;91(1):100–8.

[10] Nataf F, Schlienger M, Liu Z, Foulquier JN, Grès B, Orthuon A, et al. Radiosurgery with or without a 2-mm margin for 93 single brain metastases. Int J Radiat Oncol Biol Phys. 2008;70(3):766–72.

[11] Vogelbaum MA, Angelov L, Lee S-Y, Li L, Barnett GH, Suh JH. Local control of brain metastases by stereotactic radiosurgery in relation to dose to the tumor margin. J Neurosurg. 2006;104(6):907–12.

[12] Hasegawa T, Kondziolka D, Flickinger JC, Germanwala A, Lunsford LD. Brain metastases treated with radiosurgery alone: an alternative to whole brain radiotherapy? Neurosurgery. 2003;52(6): 1318–26.

[13] Chang EL, Hassenbusch SJ, Shiu AS, Lang FF, Allen PK, Sawaya R, et al. The role of tumor size in the radiosurgical management of patients with ambiguous brain metastases. Neurosurgery. 2003;53(2):272–81.

[14] Shiau C-Y, Sneed PK, Shu H-KG, Lamborn KR, McDermott MW, Chang S, et al. Radiosurgery for brain metastases: relationship of dose and pattern of enhancement to local control. Int J Radiat Oncol Biol Phys. 1997;37(2):375–83.

[15] Adler JR Jr, Chang SD, Murphy MJ, Doty J, Geis P, Hancock SL. The Cyberknife: a frameless robotic system for radiosurgery. Stereotact Funct Neurosurg. 1997;69(1–4):124–8.

[16] Fuss M, Salter BJ, Cheek D, Sadeghi A, Hevezi JM, Herman TS. Repositioning accuracy of a commercially available thermoplastic mask system. Radiother Oncol. 2004;71(3): 339–45.

[17] Li G, Ballangrud A, Chan M, Ma R, Beal K, Yamada Y, et al. Clinical experience with two frameless stereotactic radiosurgery (fSRS) systems using optical surface imaging for motion monitoring. J Appl Clin Med Phys. 2015;16(4):149–62.

[18] Paris F, Fuks Z, Kang A, Capodieci P, Juan G, Ehleiter D, et al. Endothelial apoptosis as the primary lesion initiating intestinal radiation damage in mice. Science. 2001;293(5528):293–7.

[19] Ch'ang H-J, Maj JG, Paris F, Xing HR, Zhang J, Truman J-P, et al. ATM regulates target switching to escalating doses of radiation in the intestines. Nat Med. 2005;11(5):484–90.

[20] Brown JM, Koong AC. High-dose single-fraction radiotherapy: exploiting a new biology? Int J Radiat Oncol Biol Phys. 2008;71(2):324–5.

[21] Brenner DJ, Martel MK, Hall EJ. Fractionated regimens for stereotactic radiotherapy of recurrent tumors in the brain. Int J Radiat Oncol Biol Phys. 1991;21(3):819–24.

[22] Hall EJ, Brenner DJ. The radiobiology of radiosurgery: rationale for different treatment regimes for AVMs and malignancies. Int J Radiat Oncol Biol Phys. 1993;25(2):381–5.

[23] Brown JM, Diehn M, Loo BW. Stereotactic ablative radiotherapy should be combined with a hypoxic cell radiosensitizer. Int J Radiat Oncol Biol Phys. 2010;78(2): 323–7.

[24] Ma L, Sahgal A, Descovich M, Cho Y-B, Chuang C, Huang K, et al. Equivalence in dose fall-off for isocentric and nonisocentric intracranial treatment modalities and its impact on dose fractionation schemes. Int J Radiat Oncol Biol Phys. 2010;76(3): 943–8.

[25] Demaria S, Golden EB, Formenti SC. Role of local radiation therapy in cancer immunotherapy. JAMA Oncol. 2015;1(9):1325.

[26] Demaria S, Bhardwaj N, McBride WH, Formenti SC. Combining radiotherapy and immunotherapy: a revived partnership. Int J Radiat Oncol Biol Phys. 2005;63(3):655–66.

[27] Dewan MZ, Galloway AE, Kawashima N, Dewyngaert JK, Babb JS, Formenti SC, et al. Fractionated but not single-dose radiotherapy induces an immune-mediated abscopal effect when combined with anti-CTLA-4 antibody. Clin Cancer Res. 2009;15(17):5379–88.

[28] Park HJ, Griffin RJ, Hui S, Levitt SH, Song CW. Radiation-induced vascular damage in tumors: implications of vascular damage in ablative hypofractionated radiotherapy (SBRT and SRS). Radiat Res. 2012;177(3):311–27.

[29] Tsai M-H, Cook JA, Chandramouli GVR, DeGraff W, Yan H, Zhao S, et al. Gene expression profiling of breast, prostate, and glioma cells following single versus fractionated doses of radiation. Cancer Res. 2007;67(8):3845–52.

[30] Aoki M, Abe Y, Hatayama Y, Kondo H, Basaki K. Clinical outcome of hypofractionated conventional conformation radiotherapy for patients with single and no more than three metastatic brain tumors, with noninvasive fixation of the skull without whole brain irradiation. Int J Radiat Oncol Biol Phys. 2006;64(2):414–8.

[31] Aoyama H, Shirato H, Onimaru R, Kagei K, Ikeda J, Ishii N, et al. Hypofractionated stereotactic radiotherapy alone without whole-brain irradiation for patients with solitary and oligo brain metastasis using noninvasive fixation of the skull. Int J Radiat Oncol Biol Phys. 2003;56(3):793–800.

[32] Ernst-Stecken A, Ganslandt O, Lambrecht U, Sauer R, Grabenbauer G. Phase II trial of hypofractionated stereotactic radiotherapy for brain metastases: results and toxicity. Radiother Oncol. 2006;81(1):18–24.

[33] Fahrig A, Ganslandt O, Lambrecht U, Grabenbauer G, Kleinert G, Sauer R, et al. Hypofractionated stereotactic radiotherapy for brain metastases: results from three different dose concepts. Strahlenther Onkol. 2007;183(11):625–30.

[34] Fokas E, Henzel M, Surber G, Kleinert G, Hamm K, Engenhart-Cabillic R. Stereotactic radiosurgery and fractionated stereotactic radiotherapy: comparison of efficacy and toxicity in 260 patients with brain metastases. J Neuro-Oncol. 2012;109(1):91–8.

[35] Higuchi Y, Serizawa T, Nagano O, Matsuda S, Ono J, Sato M, et al. Three-staged stereotactic radiotherapy without whole brain irradiation for large metastatic brain tumors. Int J Radiat Oncol Biol Phys. 2009;74(5):1543–8.

[36] Kim Y-J, Cho KH, Kim J-Y, Lim YK, Min HS, Lee SH, et al. Single-dose versus fractionated stereotactic radiotherapy for brain metastases. Int J Radiat Oncol Biol Phys. 2011;81(2):483–9.

[37] Kwon AK, DiBiase SJ, Wang B, Hughes SL, Milcarek B, Zhu Y. Hypofractionated stereotactic radiotherapy for the treatment of brain metastases. Cancer. 2009;115(4):890–8.

[38] Lindvall P, Bergström P, Löfroth P-O, Tommy Bergenheim A. A comparison between surgical resection in combination with WBRT or hypofractionated stereotactic irradiation in the treatment of solitary brain metastases. Acta Neurochir. 2009;151(9):1053–9.

[39] Lockney NA, Wang DG, Gutin PH, Brennan C, Tabar V, Ballangrud A, et al. Clinical outcomes of patients with limited brain metastases treated with hypofractionated (5 × 6 Gy) conformal radiotherapy. Radiother Oncol. 2017;123(2):203–8.

[40] Manning MA, Cardinale RM, Benedict SH, Kavanagh BD, Zwicker RD, Amir C, et al. Hypofractionated stereotactic radiotherapy as an alternative to radiosurgery for the treatment of patients with brain metastases. Int J Radiat Oncol Biol Phys. 2000;47(3):603–8.

[41] Marcrom SR, McDonald AM, Thompson JW, Popple RA, Riley KO, Markert JM, et al. Fractionated stereotactic radiation therapy for intact brain metastases. Adv Radiat Oncol. 2017;2(4):564–71.

[42] Märtens B, Janssen S, Werner M, Frühauf J, Christiansen H, Bremer M, et al. Hypofractionated stereotactic radiotherapy of limited brain metastases: a single-centre individualized treatment approach. BMC Cancer. 2012;12:497.

[43] Matsuyama T, Kogo K, Oya N. Clinical outcomes of biological effective dose-based fractionated stereotactic radiation therapy for metastatic brain tumors from non-small cell lung cancer. Int J Radiat Oncol Biol Phys. 2013;85(4):984–90.

[44] Minniti G, D'Angelillo RM, Scaringi C, Trodella LE, Clarke E, Matteucci P, et al. Fractionated stereotactic radiosurgery for patients with brain metastases. J Neuro-Oncol. 2014;117(2):295–301.

[45] Minniti G, Scaringi C, Paolini S, Lanzetta G, Romano A, Cicone F, et al. Single-fraction versus multifraction (3 × 9 Gy) stereotactic radiosurgery for large (>2 cm) brain metastases: a comparative analysis of local control and risk of radiation-induced brain necrosis. Int J Radiat Oncol Biol Phys. 2016;95(4):1142–8.

[46] Narayana A, Chang J, Yenice K, Chan K, Lymberis S, Brennan C, et al. Hypofractionated stereotactic radiotherapy using intensity-modulated radiotherapy in patients with one or two brain metastases. Stereotact Funct Neurosurg. 2007;85(2–3):82–7.

[47] Oermann EK, Kress M-AS, Todd JV, Collins BT, Hoffman R, Chaudhry H, et al. The impact of radiosurgery fractionation and tumor radiobiology on the local control of brain metastases: clinical article. J Neurosurg. 2013;119(5):1131–8.

[48] Ogura K, Mizowaki T, Ogura M, Sakanaka K, Arakawa Y, Miyamoto S, et al. Outcomes of hypofractionated stereotactic radiotherapy for metastatic brain tumors with high risk factors. J Neuro-Oncol. 2012;109(2):425–32.

[49] Rajakesari S, Arvold ND, Jimenez RB, Christianson LW, Horvath MC, Claus EB, et al. Local control after fractionated stereotactic radiation therapy for brain metastases. J Neuro-Oncol. 2014;120(2):339–46.

[50] Saitoh J, Saito Y, Kazumoto T, Kudo S, Ichikawa A, Hayase N, et al. Therapeutic effect of Linac-based stereotactic radiotherapy with a micro-multileaf collimator for the treatment of patients with brain metastases from lung cancer. Jpn J Clin Oncol. 2010;40(2):119–24.

[51] Tokuuye K, Akine Y, Sumi M, Kagami Y, Murayama S, Nakayama H, et al. Fractionated stereotactic radiotherapy of small intracranial malignancies. Int J Radiat Oncol Biol Phys. 1998;42(5):989–94.

[52] Wiggenraad R, Kanter AV, Kal HB, Taphoorn M, Vissers T, Struikmans H. Dose-effect relation in stereotactic radiotherapy for brain metastases. A systematic review. Radiother Oncol. 2011;98(3):292–7.

[53] Patchell RA, Tibbs PA, Regine WF, Dempsey RJ, Mohiuddin M, Kryscio RJ, et al. Postoperative radiotherapy in the treatment of single metastases to the brain: a randomized trial. JAMA. 1998;280(17):1485–9.

[54] Kocher M, Soffietti R, Abacioglu U, Villà S, Fauchon F, Baumert BG, et al. Adjuvant whole-brain radiotherapy versus observation after radiosurgery or surgical resection of one to three cerebral metastases: results of the EORTC 22952-26001 study. J Clin Oncol. 2011;29(2):134–41.

[55] Mahajan A, Ahmed S, McAleer MF, Weinberg JS, Li J, Brown P, et al. Post-operative stereotactic radiosurgery versus observation for completely resected brain metastases: a single-centre, randomised, controlled, phase 3 trial. Lancet Oncol. 2017;18(8):1040–8.

[56] Brown PD, Ballman KV, Cerhan JH, Anderson SK, Carrero XW, Whitton AC, et al. Postoperative stereotactic radiosurgery

compared with whole brain radiotherapy for resected metastatic brain disease (NCCTG N107C/CEC·3): a multicentre, randomised, controlled, phase 3 trial. Lancet Oncol. 2017;18(8):1049–60.

[57] Soltys SG, Adler JR, Lipani JD, Jackson PS, Choi CYH, Puataweepong P, et al. Stereotactic radiosurgery of the postoperative resection cavity for brain metastases. Int J Radiat Oncol Biol Phys. 2008;70(1):187–93.

[58] Brennan C, Yang TJ, Hilden P, Zhang Z, Chan K, Yamada Y, et al. A phase 2 trial of stereotactic radiosurgery boost after surgical resection for brain metastases. Int J Radiat Oncol Biol Phys. 2014;88(1):130–6.

[59] Ojerholm E, Miller D, Geiger GA, Lustig RA. Stereotactic radiosurgery to the resection bed for intracranial metastases and risk of leptomeningeal carcinomatosis. J Neurosurg. 2014;121:9.

[60] Minniti G, Esposito V, Clarke E, Scaringi C, Lanzetta G, Salvati M, et al. Multidose stereotactic radiosurgery (9 Gy × 3) of the postoperative resection cavity for treatment of large brain metastases. Int J Radiat Oncol Biol Phys. 2013;86(4):623–9.

[61] Atalar B, Choi CYH, Harsh GR, Chang SD, Gibbs IC, Adler JR, et al. Cavity volume dynamics after resection of brain metastases and timing of postresection cavity stereotactic radiosurgery. Neurosurgery. 2013;72(2):180 5.

[62] Iorio-Morin C, Ezahr Y. Early Gamma Knife stereotactic radiosurgery to the tumor bed of resected brain metastasis for improved local control. J Neurosurg. 2014;121:6.

[63] Abuodeh Y, Ahmed KA, Naghavi AO, Venkat PS, Sarangkasiri S, Johnstone PAS, et al. Postoperative stereotactic radiosurgery using 5-Gy × 5 sessions in the management of brain metastases. World Neurosurg. 2016;90:58–65.

[64] Ahmed KA, Freilich JM, Abuodeh Y, Figura N, Patel N, Sarangkasiri S, et al. Fractionated stereotactic radiotherapy to the post-operative cavity for radioresistant and radiosensitive brain metastases. J Neuro-Oncol. 2014;118(1):179–86.

[65] Ammirati M, Kshettry VR, Lamki T, Wei L, Grecula JC. A prospective phase II trial of fractionated stereotactic intensity modulated radiotherapy with or without surgery in the treatment of patients with 1 to 3 newly diagnosed symptomatic brain metastases. Neurosurgery. 2014;74(6):586–94.

[66] Connolly EP, Mathew M, Tam M, King JV, Kunnakkat SD, Parker EC, et al. Involved field radiation therapy after surgical resection of solitary brain metastases— mature results. Neuro Oncol. 2013;15(5):589–94.

[67] Do L, Pezner R, Radany E, Liu A, Staud C, Badie B. Resection followed by stereotactic radiosurgery to resection cavity for intracranial metastases. Int J Radiat Oncol Biol Phys. 2009;73(2):486–91.

[68] Keller A, Doré M, Cebula H, Thillays F, Proust F, Darié I, et al. Hypofractionated stereotactic radiation therapy to the resection bed for intracranial metastases. Int J Radiat Oncol Biol Phys. 2017;99(5):1179–89.

[69] Kumar AMS, Miller J, Hoffer SA, Mansur DB, Coffey M, Lo SS, et al. Postoperative hypofractionated stereotactic brain radiation (HSRT) for resected brain metastases: improved local control with higher BED10. J Neuro-Oncol. 2018;139(2):449–54.

[70] Ling DC, Vargo JA, Wegner RE, Flickinger JC, Burton SA, Engh J, et al. Postoperative stereotactic radiosurgery to the resection cavity for large brain metastases: clinical outcomes, predictors of intracranial failure, and implications for optimal patient selection. Neurosurgery. 2015;76(2):150–7.

[71] Pessina F, Navarria P, Cozzi L, Ascolese AM, Maggi G, Riva M, et al. Outcome evaluation of oligometastatic patients treated with surgical resection followed by hypofractionated stereotactic radiosurgery (HSRS) on the tumor bed, for single, large brain metastases. Sherman JH, editor. PLoS One. 2016;11(6): e0157869.

[72] Steinmann D, Maertens B, Janssen S, Werner M, Frühauf J, Nakamura M, et al. Hypofractionated stereotactic radiotherapy (hfSRT) after tumour resection of a single brain metastasis: report of a single-centre individualized treatment approach. J Cancer Res Clin Oncol. 2012;138(9):1523–9.

[73] Vogel J, Ojerholm E, Hollander A, Briola C, Mooij R, Bieda M, et al. Intracranial control after Cyberknife radiosurgery to the resection bed for large brain metastases. Radiat Oncol. 2015;10(1):221. Available from: http://www.ro-journal.com/content/10/1/221.

[74] Wang C-C, Floyd SR, Chang C-H, Warnke PC, Chio C-C, Kasper EM, et al. Cyberknife hypofractionated stereotactic radiosurgery (HSRS) of resection cavity after excision of large cerebral metastasis: efficacy and safety of an 800 cGy × 3 daily fractions regimen. J Neurooncol. 2012;106(3):601–10.

[75] Park C, Papiez L, Zhang S, Story M, Timmerman RD. Universal survival curve and single fraction equivalent dose: useful tools in understanding potency of ablative radiotherapy. Int J Radiat Oncol Biol Phys. 2008;70(3):847–52.

[76] Quon HC, Ong A, Cheung P, Chu W, Chung HT, Vesprini D, et al. Once-weekly versus every-other-day stereotactic body radiotherapy in patients with prostate cancer (PATRIOT): a phase 2 randomized trial. Radiother Oncol. 2018;127(2):206–12.

[77] Alite F, Stang K, Balasubramanian N, Adams W, Shaikh MP, Small C, et al. Local control dependence on consecutive vs. nonconsecutive fractionation in lung stereotactic body radiation therapy. Radiother Oncol. 2016;121(1):9–14.

[78] Jain S, Poon I, Soliman H, Keller B, Kim A, Lochray F, et al. Lung stereotactic body radiation therapy (SBRT) delivered over 4 or 11 days: a comparison of acute toxicity and quality of life. Radiother Oncol. 2013;108(2):320–5.

[79] Bender ET. Brain necrosis after fractionated radiation therapy: is the halftime for repair longer than we thought? Med Phys. 2012;39(11):7055–61.

[80] Kelada OJ, Decker RH, Nath SK, Johung KL, Zheng M-Q, Huang Y, et al. High single doses of radiation may induce elevated levels of hypoxia in early-stage non-small cell lung

[81] Samson P, Rehman S, Juloori A, DeWees T, Roach M, Bradley J, et al. Local control for clinical stage I non-small cell lung cancer treated with 5-fraction stereotactic body radiation therapy is not associated with treatment schedule. Pract Radiat Oncol. 2018;8(6):404–13.

[82] Yomo S, Hayashi M, Nicholson C. A prospective pilot study of two-session Gamma Knife surgery for large metastatic brain tumors. J Neuro-Oncol. 2012;109(1):159–65.

[83] Angelov L, Mohammadi AM, Bennett EE, Abbassy M, Elson P, Chao ST, et al. Impact of 2-staged stereotactic radiosurgery for treatment of brain metastases ≥ 2 cm. J Neurosurg. 2018;129:366–82.

[84] Yomo S, Hayashi M. A minimally invasive treatment option for large metastatic brain tumors: long-term results of two-session Gamma Knife stereotactic radiosurgery. Radiat Oncol Lond Engl. 2014;9:132.

[85] Churilla TM, Chowdhury IH, Handorf E, Collette L, Collette S, Dong Y, et al. Comparison of local control of brain metastases with stereotactic radiosurgery vs surgical resection: a secondary analysis of a randomized clinical trial. JAMA Oncol. 2019;5(2):243–7. Available from: https://jamanetwork.com/journals/jamaoncology/fullarticle/2713842.

第 11 章 脑转移放射外科治疗（含术后瘤腔）的靶区勾画

Target Delineation for Radiosurgery (Including Postoperative Cavity Radiosurgery) in Brain Metastases

Balamurugan A. Vellayappan　Mei Chin Lim　Clement Yong　Kejia Teo　Shawn Malone　Simon Lo　著
邓　俍　译
伍海军　校

一、病例介绍

（一）病例 1

一名 76 岁的老年女性患者，既往有转移性乳腺癌病史（*ER/PR* 阴性，*HER*2 阳性）。患者 2 年前出现额叶和左侧小脑转移病灶，行立体定向放射外科治疗（stereotactic radiosurgery，SRS）。目前临床表现为步态不稳。磁共振 T_1 对比增强显示小脑有两个病灶（小脑蚓体病灶大小为 1.9cm×1.6cm，右侧小脑半球病灶大小为 1.8cm×2.3cm），病灶具有肿块效应且引起第四脑室消失，从而导致早期脑积水，考虑转移瘤。位于右侧小脑半球较大的浅表病灶予以手术切除。全身评估显示颅外疾病控制良好。之后对患者的术后瘤床及残留转移灶实施超分割立体定向放疗（hypofractionated stereotactic radiotherapy，HSRT）（按 80% 等剂量线给予 25Gy，分 5 次完成）。患者病灶影像及靶区勾画如图 11-1 所示。

（二）病例 2

一名 70 岁的女性患者，因头痛、左侧偏瘫就诊。磁共振 T_1 对比增强显示右额叶有一囊性转移灶，大小约为 5cm×4cm，另有 5 个<1cm 的脑转移病灶。肺部病灶活检示非小细胞肺腺癌，分子亚型为 *EGFR* 外显子 20 突变（提示对酪氨酸激酶抑制药耐药），*ALK/ROS1* 阴性，PD-L$_1$ 评分为 11%。首先予以 Ommaya 储液囊植入术对大面积囊性转移灶进行引流后拟行 SRS。遗憾的是，囊性转移灶的液体再积聚速度相对快，因此患者不得不接受右侧额叶囊性脑转移瘤切除术，之后再对术腔行大分割立体定向放疗（hypofractionated stereotactic radiotherapy，HSRT）（按 80% 等剂量线给予 30Gy，分 5 次完成），其余病灶行 SRS。患者右侧额叶术腔的相关影像和靶区勾画见图 11-2。

二、概述

高达 60% 的癌症患者会出现脑转移（brain metastases，BM），进而导致发病和死亡[1]。因为有效的系统治疗能够控制颅外肿瘤，且灵敏度高的影像学检查能够发现小体积的脑转移瘤，脑转移瘤的发病率可能会增加。

约有 50% 的脑转移患者是单一的转移病灶[2]。由于大脑没有淋巴管，癌细胞只能通过血源性途径进入大脑[3]。一些癌症如原发性肺癌、黑色素瘤、乳腺癌和肾细胞癌较易发生颅内种植播散，占 BM 的 80%[4]。BM 通常位于大脑半球

第 11 章 脑转移放射外科治疗（含术后瘤腔）的 靶区勾画
Target Delineation for Radiosurgery (Including Postoperative Cavity Radiosurgery) in Brain Metastases

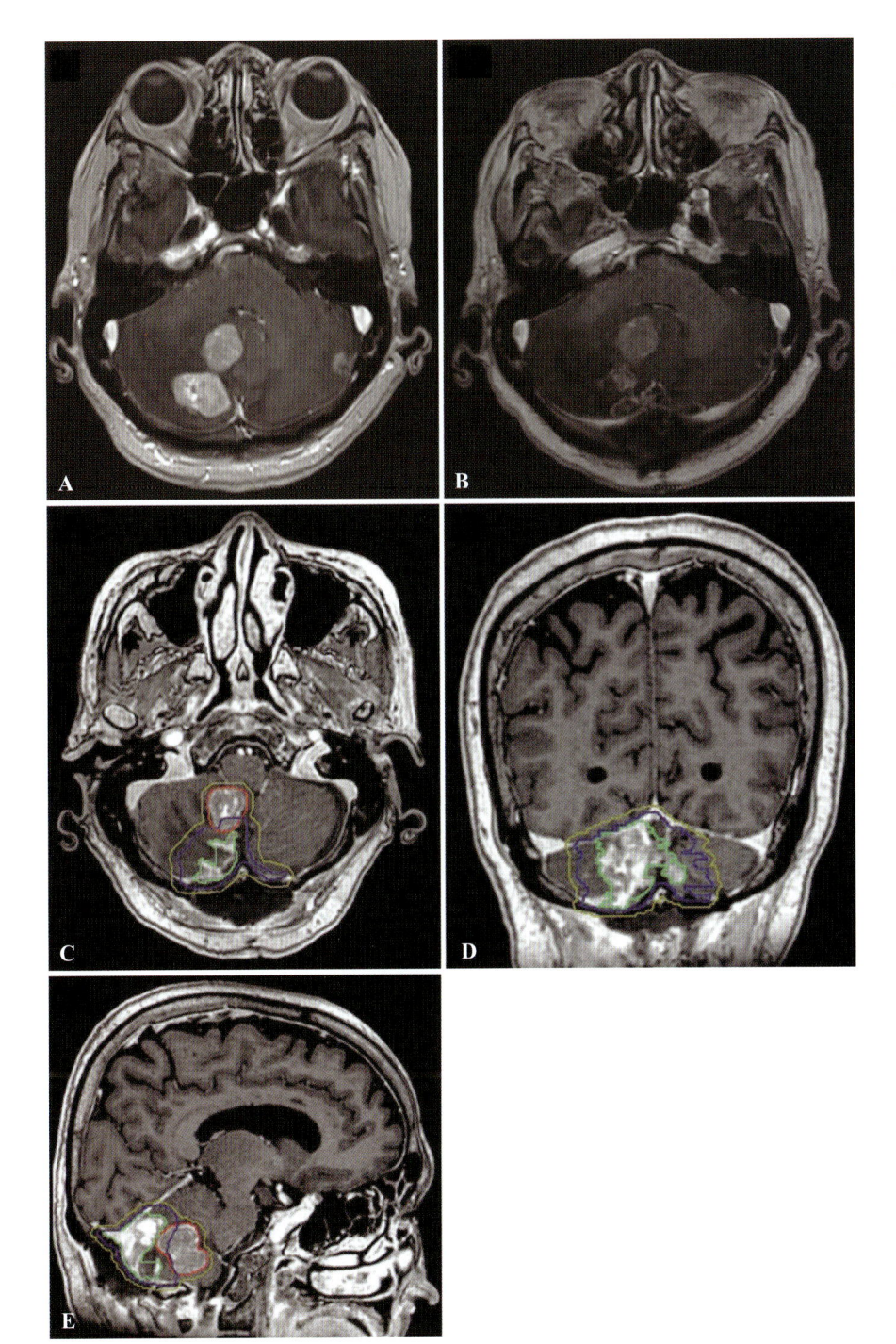

◀ 图 11-1 患者病灶影像及靶区体积

A. 术前轴位 T_1 对比成像显示两个小脑转移瘤导致第四脑室消失；B. 术后轴位 T_1 对比成像显示较大浅表病变的切除；C 至 E. 靶区体积勾画：术后瘤床（石灰绿色），瘤床临床靶区体积（蓝色），完整的转移大体肿瘤体积（红色）和计划靶区体积（橄榄绿）

的灰白质交界处（80%），肿瘤细胞聚集在毛细血管末端分支处[5]。小脑半球（15%）和基底节（3%）较少受累及[6]。

在本章中，我们将简要回顾 BM 的影像学特点和治疗方法。特别是我们将为脑转移的 SRS 应用提供一种实用的方法，包括术后治疗方案。

三、脑转移 CT 及 MRI 影像学特点

CT 常常是有症状患者的初步筛查工具，因为它能够早期识别一些危急情况，如颅内肿瘤占位效应、脑水肿及出血性事件[7]。当转移灶不够大，不足以引起肿块效应或导致明显的瘤周水肿

125

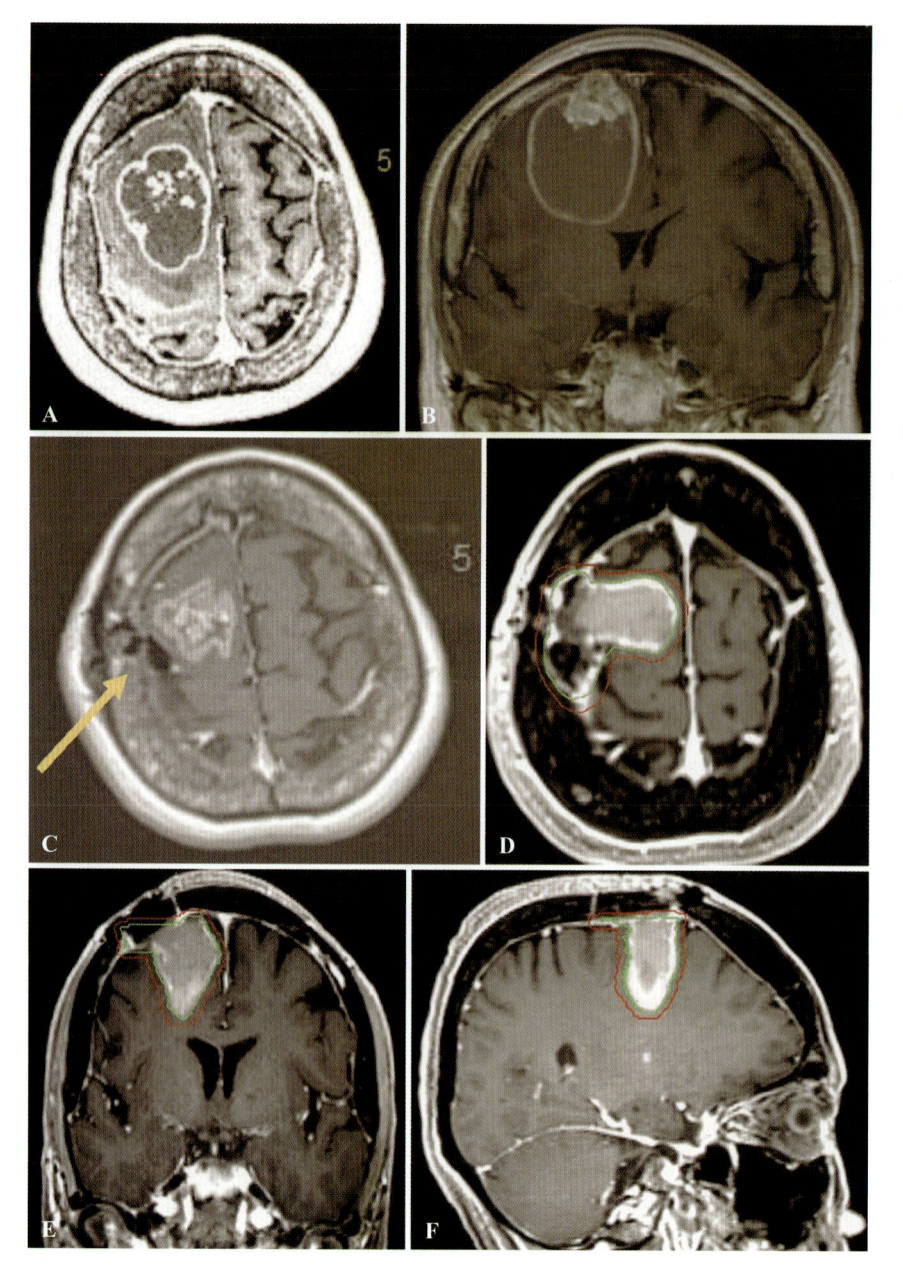

脑转移瘤放射治疗学：基于病例的研究
Radiotherapy in Managing Brain Metastases: A Case-Based Approach

◀ 图 11-2 患者右侧额叶术腔的相关影像和靶区体积

A 和 B. 轴位和冠状位 T₁ 增强 MRI 显示右侧额叶有一处大的囊性转移灶，边缘增强，且可见多个结节；（B）转移灶累及硬脑膜。C. 植入 Ommaya 储液囊后，囊性病变塌陷（黄箭）；D 至 F. 图像显示立体定向治疗的靶区体积。请注意，靶区体积包括了切除路径、病灶及其所累及的硬脑膜。CTV（绿色），PTV（红色）

时，静脉注射碘对比剂可以帮助诊断。但遗憾的是，单独增强 CT 的假阴性率可高达 19%，尤其是在低额颞区和后窝这些骨质含量大从而引起线束硬化的部位[8]。

MRI 无疑是评估和勾画 BM 的首选影像学检查方法。多项研究已证实其在检测 < 1cm 的病灶以及软脑膜癌变方面明显优于 CT[8-11]。在 T₁ 加权成像（T₁WI）中，BM 通常表现为等信号 / 低信号。出血性 BM 常见于肺癌和肾细胞癌，在 T₁WI 上呈高密度（图 11-3）。黑色素瘤在 T₁ 显示高信号，因此黑色素瘤的 BM 在 T₁WI 上也是高信号的。在 T₂ 加权成像（T₂WI）上，除非有潜在的出血，否则 BM 通常是高信号的。由于血脑屏障破坏所致的血管源性水肿的存在，T₂WI 能显示出 BM 周围白质的高信号变化，是最推荐的评估方法。通常情况下，BM 往往表现出弥散促进 [表观弥散系数（ADC）图上的数值升高，弥散加权成像（DWI）上高强度信号]，这和脑脓肿中所表现出的弥散限制（ADC 数值较低）相反[12]。

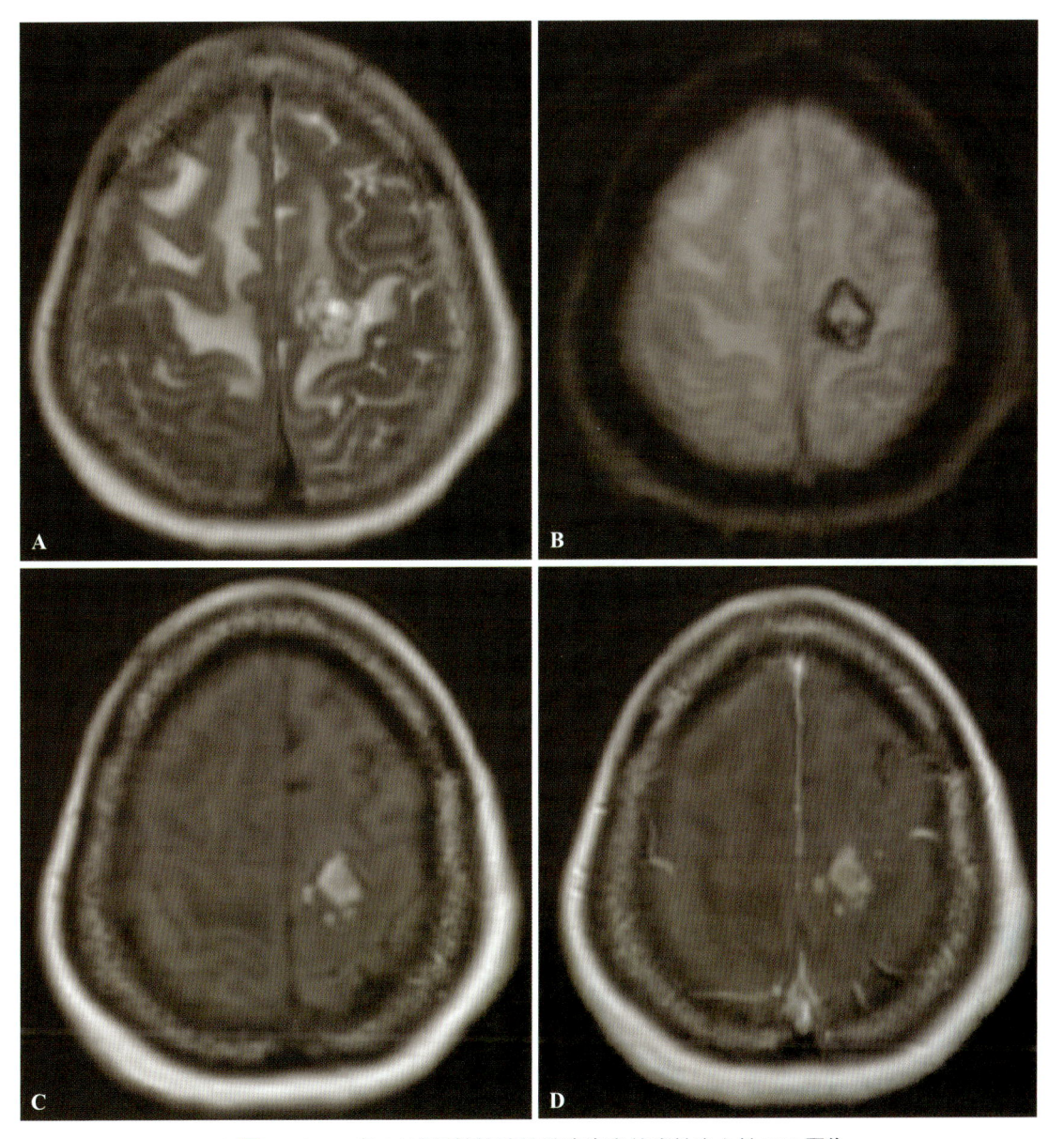

第 11 章 脑转移放射外科治疗（含术后瘤腔）的 靶区勾画
Target Delineation for Radiosurgery (Including Postoperative Cavity Radiosurgery) in Brain Metastases

▲ 图 11-3 一名 56 岁男性转移性肺癌患者的囊性出血性 BM 图像

A. 轴位 T_2WI 序列显示左额叶有一处分叶状 T_2WI 高信号肿块，周围有明显的血管源性水肿，且右额叶也存在血管源性水肿；B. 轴位 T_2 梯度回声序列显示，肿块周边存在慢性血液产物所致的含铁血黄素边缘；C. 增强前 T_1WI VIBE 序列显示，该肿块本身信号亮，提示存在亚急性血液产物中可见的高铁血红蛋白；D. 增强后 T_1WI VIBE 序列再次显示左额叶肿块 T_1WI 高信号在有出血的情况下，增强不能准确确定 BM 的真实情况

在图像采集过程中静脉输注钆，能提高脑转移的检出率。无论有无脂肪抑制，对比后的序列通常为 T_1WI。转移刺激生成的血管缺乏血脑屏障，有利于钆渗入间质组织，通过改变局部质子磁环境引起明显的实质增强（图 11-4）。在较大的，尤其是有出血或囊性改变的 BM 中，由于中心坏死，肿瘤增强往往是不均匀的。可能因为钆对比剂可以更易通过小转移灶新生血管中相对较小的表面积弥散出去，钆给药后延迟 10～15min 成像，能够提高小体积转移灶的显影和检测[13]。

四、BM 管理的进展

令人遗憾的是 BM 的患者死亡率很高，中

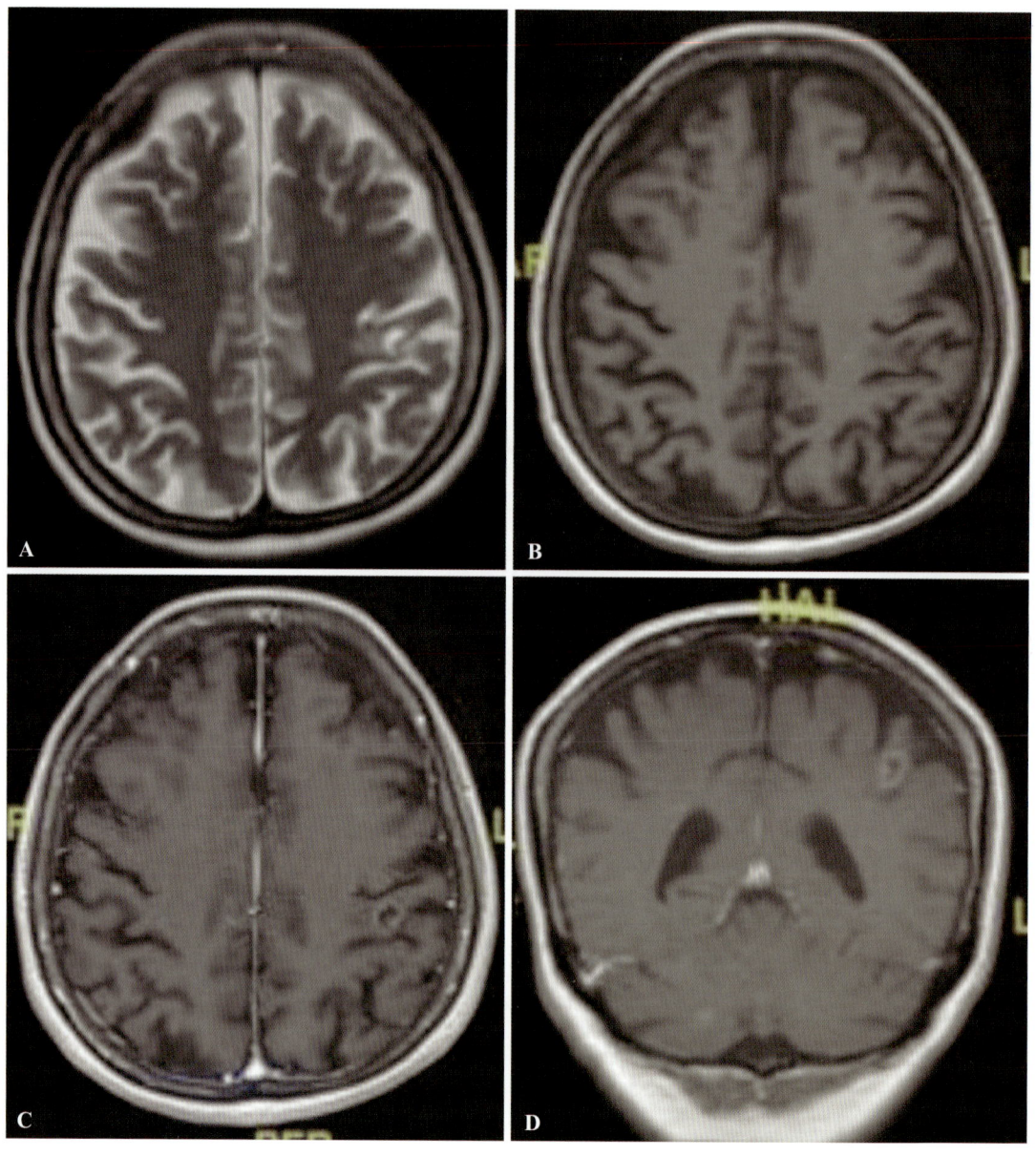

▲ 图 11-4 一名 73 岁男性转移性肺癌患者的环形增强 BM 图像

（A）轴位 T_2WI 序列显示左侧额叶有一个小的 T_2WI 高信号病灶，周围轻度水肿；（B）未增强的 T_1WI VIBE 序列显示稍低信号病变，在增强对比后的（C）轴位 T_1WI VIBE 序列和（D）冠状位 T_1WI 序列上显示环形增强；（D）另一个小的环状增强脑转移病灶见于右侧小脑半球

位生存期通常以月为单位计算，因此很多患者一旦确诊 BM 就不再进行积极的抗癌治疗。一项早期研究将全脑放疗（whole-brain radiotherapy，WBRT）与单纯使用皮质激素治疗历史的对照组进行比较，显示全脑放疗可以提高生存率，从而使其进入了人们的视野[14]。由于其广泛的可应用性、易于管理和相对较低的治疗成本，最近被认为是标准治疗方案。近年来，神经影像学、神经外科和全身治疗学的发展使患者的生存期延长，因此，WBRT 的长期疗效引起了高度关注[15]。此外，单用 WBRT 并不能有效持久的控制颅内病灶，人们开始期待更有效的治疗方式[16, 17]。

（一）立体定向放射外科（SRS）

SRS 是指在一次照射中，利用多束射线，以高度适形的方式将消融剂量汇集到肿瘤上（同时避免对周围脑组织的高剂量照射）。BM 表现为球形、边界清楚、肿瘤体积内无正常脑实质等固有特性，使得其适合 SRS 照射。

尽管没有发表过比较 SRS 和 WBRT 的随机对照试验（RCT）的文章，但许多前瞻性研究表明，单独应用 SRS 具有较好的局部控制率[18-22]。此外，WBRT 对生活质量（quality of life，QoL）和神经认知功能的损害也减少了辅助 WBRT 的常规使用[23]。现在有许多平台可用于实施颅内 SRS，这些平台包括 Gamma Knife、CyberKnife 或基于线性加速器的技术[24]。对这些技术的全面回顾超出了本章内容范围，鼓励读者通过查阅文献了解这些机器之间的复杂差异[25]。

（二）手术

随着 SRS 的兴起和其疗效的提高，手术切除的适应证通常为肿块占位效应明显的大体积肿瘤、导致神经功能障碍的术中可切除的病灶或疾病诊断不明确时用于明确诊断。手术目的是为了实现肿瘤的全切除。大多数转移性肿瘤都有一个假囊，便于进行整体切除。对于较大的肿瘤，只能进行病灶内切除（即减瘤）。如果分块切除，且不进行辅助治疗，局部复发的风险仍然非常高。例如，最近一项单中心 RCT 结果显示，切除术后 12 个月的局部复发风险高达 56%[26]。

20 年前，一项 RCT 就已证明辅助 WBRT 可以降低术后颅内复发的风险。然而，这种局部控制的提高是以 QoL 下降和神经认知障碍为代价的，并没有生存获益[27]。在 WBRT 的利弊权衡下，促使研究者尝试使用"有限"的脑部放疗，从而替代 WBRT。初步结果显示，其局部控制率与 WBRT 相当，优于单纯观察组[28]。令人意外的是，适形度最少的治疗组具有最佳的控制率，原因可能是欠理想的靶区勾画或局部肿瘤浸润引起靶区边界模糊。

一项后续研究表明，在不引起更大毒性的情况下，术腔边缘扩大 2mm 可降低局部失败率[29]。Brown 等最近报道了 NCCTG N107C/RTOG 12-70 试验，该试验对比了切除术腔的 SRS 与 WBRT[21]，虽然两组之间的总生存期没有差异，但单纯 SRS 组的无认知恶化生存期有所改善。此外，WBRT 组也改善了对颅内病灶的控制。对此可能的原因包括靶区勾画过于保守和（或）观察者靶区勾画的差异，以及对大的术腔放射外科处方剂量的不足。

五、SRS 的患者选择

一般情况下，应选择合适的患者予以 SRS。选择患者时需要考虑的因素包括年龄、全身状况、颅外肿瘤控制情况、脑转移的数量和体积。中位预期寿命可用预后算法如疾病特异性分级预后评估（disease-specific graded prognostic assessment，ds-GPA）[30]进行估算。关于最大病灶的大小，各种试验均允许最大病灶不超过直径 5cm 的患者入组[31]。由于并发症（尤其是症状性放射性坏死）发生的风险增加，大病灶可能不适合予以单次分割 SRS。本书在其他地方讨论了有关大体积脑 BM 的处理策略。

六、患者体位固定

患者体位固定是 SRS 的关键步骤，定位错误是导致治疗失败的主要原因[32, 33]。

SRS 传统采用的是基于框架的 SRS，通过使用销钉将与 MRI 兼容的立体定向金属框架牢固地固定到患者的颅骨外板上。基于框架的技术精度在亚毫米内。建立在金属框架系统的基准坐标在治疗过程中被用于定位等中心。基于框架的 SRS 有很好的耐受性，但在销钉的放置位置仍有小概率的感染和出血风险。

近年来，无框架 SRS 使用越来越多，在保持高水平精度的同时，提高了患者的舒适度并可重复设置。无框架 SRS 利用定制的接近刚性的热塑面罩、咬合器、真空缓冲的颈托或定制的热塑头枕来实施定位。采用图像引导系统如机载锥形束CT（cone-beam CT，CBCT）进行治疗前的图像验证或三维X线用于监测治疗过程中的头骨位置。为了提高患者的体位固定精准度，需要同时减少患者治疗时摆位误差和器官运动误差。利用在线成像，配合6度自由度的机器人监测平台，可以显著减少患者治疗时摆位误差。Guckenberger等报道，通过增加CBCT图像引导，摆位误差（在使用简单框架系统时）可从（3.9±1.7）mm减少到（0.9±0.6）mm [34]。然而，仍有0.9mm的残余误差（由器官内运动导致）。当使用特别配备额外的立体成像系统的直线加速器和CyberKnife平台时，可监测和纠正器官内运动。此外，咬合器的使用已经证明可以减少摆位所致的位置移动[35]。

在具有在线校正功能的单次分割SRS中，只需要考虑器官内运动所导致的位置移动。基于框架和无框架系统都已被证明具有低水平的器官内运动所导致的移动［平均移位（0.4±0.3）mm vs.（0.7±0.5）mm］[36]。然而同一研究中，分别有3%使用框架治疗的患者和22%使用无框治疗的患者出现了1mm或更多的器官内运动所致的移动。有文献报道，总体治疗时间延长会增加器官内运动所致的移动，因此我们应尽量将无框架SRS的治疗时间控制在20min以内[34]。

七、模拟及必要的预处理成像

除伽马刀以外的大多数治疗平台，CT模拟定位是必需的。CT成像对电子密度计算很有用，特别是在颅底位置，由于气腔可通过改变电子平衡造成剂量不均匀，CT模拟定位有利于获得精确图像。此外，与磁共振相比，CT具有优越的空间精度，不会失真变形。因此，如果在CT和MRI上都能识别出足够的位置标记，就可以验证MRI用于靶区勾画的空间精确性。

患者必须在整个模拟定位的过程中感到舒适和无痛。有幽闭恐惧症的患者可能不适合做SRS。过度使用镇静药或抗焦虑药会增加风险，因为在模拟定位和治疗过程中监测意识水平受损的患者非常具有挑战性。患者体位通常为仰卧位，身体摆直，双手置于身体两侧。垫膝盖枕使患者更舒适。如前所述，体位固定有多种选择，包括基于框架和无框架系统（热塑面罩有或无咬合器）。我们通常使用设置为120kV和350mA的CT对患者采用螺旋扫描方法从颅顶扫描到C_3椎体底部。可以把数据重建为任何断层厚度，我们建议水平断层厚度为1mm。在扫描前将一个CT定位盒放置于患者的头部上方，用于参考2D基准坐标，然后用于计算治疗等中心。黏性金属点标记用于建立模拟定位时的等中心（然后可用于建立治疗等中心）。CT模拟过程中可选择使用碘化对比剂进行增强，但对于采用MRI图像作为靶区勾画的患者，不常规推荐使用。

预处理成像

进行对比增强MRI检查对脑转移瘤予以SRS至关重要。每个治疗相关的部门都应为SRS计划匹配好MRI设置。推荐设置最小场强为1.5特斯拉（T），断层厚度为2mm或更小[37]。我们建议所有接受SRS的患者都要在治疗近期进行高分辨率容积MRI检查（邻近治疗时或至少在治疗前1~2周内）。Garcia等试验显示BM平均以0.02ml/d的速度生长，预计2周时间体积将增加到1.35倍[38]。同样，Salkeld等也提出，如果术腔SRS计划使用的MRI图像采集时间与实际SRS治疗的时间间隔超过1周，则需要重新进行MRI定位，及时调整治疗计划[39]。

目前NCIS使用的标准立体定向MR成像方案是在3T Siemens MAGNETOM Skyra MRI系统（Siemens Medical Solutions，埃尔兰根，德国）与西门子头/颈20通道线圈上进行的。SRS治疗方案用于诊断性MRI研究的补充，下面仅介绍SRS增强同位素T_1W梯度回波序列（gradient echo sequence，GRE）。使用的MRI对比剂是钆特酸葡胺（Dotarem®，Guerbet，Roissy CDG，法国），一种大环钆基对比剂。对比剂以 0.01mmol/kg 的标准剂量，$2cm^3/s$ 的速度从静脉注射，然后用 $10cm^3$ 的生理盐水冲洗。注射后约 10min 进行增强序列扫描[13]。所用的等容 T_1W GRE 成像为容积插值脑检查（volumetric interpolated brain examination，VIBE） T_1W 序列，该序列为射频破坏性 3D GRE 序列（TR/ TE=6.36/2.46ms，15°翻转角），层厚为 1.0mm 无间隙，矩阵为 256×256，视野（field of view，FOV）为 256mm。为了防止层面的混叠伪影，层面过采样为 15%。建议图像采集时不要有角度（以利于 CT-MR 配准）。

在检测小转移灶时，较高剂量的钆已被证明比标准剂量更有优势[40, 41]。一篇报道发现 3 倍剂量的对比增强 MRI 在检测转移方面优于标准剂量的延迟成像[42]，该报道是使用的 5～10mm 层厚，因此可能不适用于现代 SRS 应用。双倍剂量的钆被证明可以为放射外科提供更精确的肿瘤大体体积勾画[43]。尽管检测能力提高，但应用更高的对比剂量会增加假阳性的发生率（如将增强的小血管误认为是小的 BM）[44]。

需要特别强调的是，MRI 图像中存在固有空间和几何扭曲失真。虽然表现通常是细微的，但这种扭曲失真可以显著影响 SRS 的准确性。这些因素包括静电场不均匀、涡流和非线性梯度[45, 46]。磁场径向边缘（即大脑边缘）的病变失真更明显，据报道误差可达 2mm。Neumann 等的研究表明，与目前常用的 1.5T 和 3T 机器相比，高强度的梯度线圈的（如 7T 扫描仪）失真更为明显[47]。值得庆幸的是，大多数现代 MRI 扫描仪都带有失真校正算法，可以将这种误差降低 60%[47]。在不使用失真校正的情况下，Seibert 等报道了高达中位 4mm 的肿瘤大体体积（gross tumor volume，GTV）位移（MRI 与 CT 相比），其中 28% 的患者会出现几何错位[48]。

上述问题会导致配准错误（使用模拟 CT）。这些 MRI 扫描仪通常属于诊断放射学的范畴，虽然组织对比用于诊断是其主要目的，但仍应定期检查其毫米级空间分辨率。AAPM 已经成立了任务组 117 来提供指导，并推荐使用用于 SRS 成像数据的 MR 扫描仪来进行质量检查[49]。

自动配准工具通常与轮廓勾画软件一起提供，用于图像融合[50]。任何配准都应该在靶区勾画之前进行手动检查。在 CT 和 MRI 上容易看到的结构可以用来校验融合，包括硬脑膜表面（硬脑膜、脑室）、脑室系统（尤其是 CT 上常有的钙化的脉络丛）和骨性解剖结构（耳蜗、内耳道、视神经管、锁骨、鞍部）。病灶部位（即感兴趣的区域）的融合尤为重要。图 11-5 所示为一个图像配准验证的例子。通过比较肿瘤的轮廓，如前庭神经鞘瘤，其管腔内部分（在钆增强 MRI 上勾画）应完全贴合岩骨中内耳道（CT 上可见），评估整个图像采集、配准和靶区勾画过程的空间准确性。

八、有 MRI 禁忌证的情况

虽然靶区勾画首选高分辨率 MRI，但也存在 MRI 禁忌证的情形（如存在心脏起搏器或严重的肾功能不全的情况）。在这种情况下，我们建议用碘对比剂的高分辨率 CT（层厚 1mm）替代 MRI。在我们中心，采用 GE Healthcare Revolution 扫描仪进行 CT 成像（120kV、300mA、螺旋旋转、0.625mm 层厚的初级迭代重建），以 0.7ml/s 的速度注射 50 ml 碘对比剂（Omnipaque 350mg I/ml）。注射后 2min 进行扫描。之前的研究推荐使用注射 200ml 碘对比剂（Angiovist-370）的方案，延迟时间长达 1 小时，以提高检测效果[51, 52]。但随着时间的推移，增强的区域往往变大，其边缘变得不那么清晰[53]。这并不是常规方案，因为目前所用的螺旋 CT 层厚＜1mm，往往可以减少老式扫描仪中出现的部分容积效应的影响。肾透析的患者禁止使用钆对比剂用于行 MRI；但这类患者仍然可以接受用于 CT 的碘对比剂，因为碘对比剂会在透析过程中被清除。当禁止 MRI 检查时，建议 GTV 与临床靶区

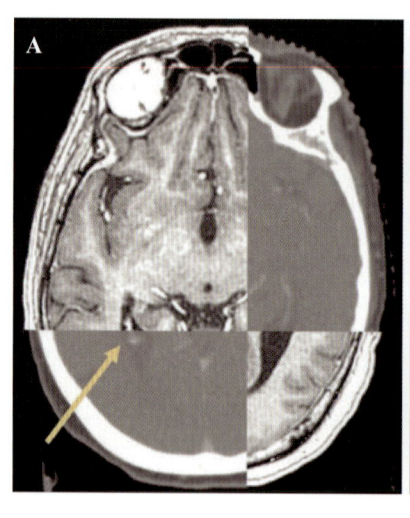

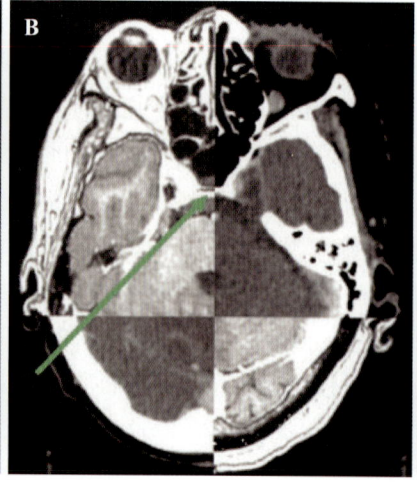

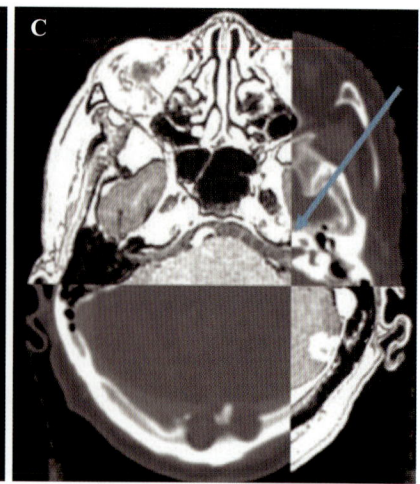

▲ 图 11-5 图像配准实例

A. CT/MR 使用校正框进行融合校验。侧脑室精确对准，MRI 和 CT 上均可见钙化的脉络丛（黄箭）；B. 斜坡在 CT 和 MRI 上对准（绿箭），用基底动脉验证左右融合；C. 内耳道和耳蜗对准（蓝箭）

体积（clinical target volume，CTV）的边缘相距 1～2mm。

九、BM 的靶区勾画（GTV、CTV）

图像融合完成校正后，就应开始进行靶区和危及器官的勾画。对于不确定的病例（如术后），我们建议让神经放射科医生和（或）神经外科医生参与靶区勾画。应调整 MRI 窗位以便清晰地识别病灶边界。与 CT 不同，MRI 的窗位没有预设。众所周知，MRI 的窗位受组织特异性参数和操作者特异性参数（如接收器带宽、翻转角度和矩阵大小）的影响，因此，我们建议使用视觉反馈手动调整窗位。

（一）分型

1. 新发 BM

新发 BM 的靶区勾画相对直观简单。大体肿瘤体积（gross tumor volume，GTV）在 T_1 对比增强 MRI 上应该很明显。对于小病灶，建议将影像放大。勾画的 GTV 应在矢状面和冠状面进行校验和调整。通常在边界清楚的 BM 旁可以看到扩大的分支血管。这些血管是否应包括在 GTV 中还存在争议。在 NCIS 和 UW 的实践中，我们并不常规将分支血管包括在 GTV 中。

通常，SRS 不要求临床靶区体积（以考虑显微镜下浸润）。Baumert 等通过尸检对 BM 的浸润进行了评估[54]。他们总共研究 76 份标本，63% 的标本显示肿瘤浸润超过了大体可见的边界。在不同的组织学亚型中，小细胞和黑色素瘤浸润深度＞1mm，其他亚型＜1mm。

Noel 等的研究表明，CTV 的边界扩大 1mm（在 1.5TMRI 上）可以增加 2 年的局部控制率[55]。然而，这项研究是在 2000 年前进行的，意味着有可能那个时代使用的 MRI 的分辨率不理想。Nataf 等对比了使用不外扩或与 2mm 的外扩（GTV-PTV），结果并没有改善局部控制，另外 2mm 边界组表现出更多的并发症[56]。同样来自杜克大学的随机对照试验（下文讨论）的结果也表明，PTV 边界越大，并发症的发生率越高[57]。

2. 侵袭硬脑膜的 BM 或硬脑膜 BM

临床工作中必须区分脑膜转移（leptomeningeal metastases，LM）和侵袭至脑膜中硬膜层（即硬脑膜）的 BM。LM 一般被认为是 SRS 的禁忌证，通常推荐 WBRT 或鞘内治疗。然而，对于侵袭硬脑膜的 BM，或硬脑膜受累的颅骨穹隆转移，可以安全进行 SRS。GTV 最好在 T_1 对比增强 MRI

序列上勾画。我们建议 CTV 边界沿硬脑膜扩大 5mm，以包括微小病灶。CTV 边界不需要包括脑实质。

根据之前一项观察者间对比研究（该研究仅以摘要形式呈现），最大的变异发生在脑膜受累和出血性病变这两种情况下[58]。因此，在这两种情况下可能需要更加慎重，建议征求神经放射科医生和神经外科医生的意见。

3. 有囊性或出血性成分的 BM

一些原发组织学亚型，特别是非小细胞肺癌，容易出现囊性 BM。囊性内容物在 T_2 序列上能更好地显示出来。然而囊壁可能是结节状且在 T_1 对比序列上常呈现增强。以往认为囊性 BM 整体预后较差，疗效不如实体 BM[59, 60]。有时大体积囊性 BM 不适合行单次分割 SRS。曾有治疗方案尝试过先将囊肿引流（使用 Ommaya 储液囊），之后再在同一天对病灶行 SRS（如病例 2）。目前尚不清楚这种方案与分割 SRT 相比效果如何。但在任何情况下，整个囊壁都应包括在 GTV 中。

出血性 BM 多见于黑色素瘤、RCC 和 NSCLC，但常见于绒毛膜癌或甲状腺乳头状癌转移。随着血块重吸收的发生，肿瘤内出血的程度有望减轻。但处于恢复期时，病变可能会进展或再出血。预计整个病灶都会被癌细胞污染，因此应全部纳入 GTV。

4. 术腔

BM 的切除通常是以分块切除的方式进行，多项研究显示局部复发率为 50%～85%，而且如果常规监测和挽救治疗不及时，有可能转变为较差的生存率[20, 26, 27, 61, 62]。有报道称，如果手术是通过整块切除技术完成，则局部复发率较低（1 年后为 14%）[63]，但这是文献数据中的一个特例。

切除路径是否应包括在术腔 SRS 的靶区勾画中存在争议[64]。例如，在 Kepka 等报道的随机试验及 N107C 试验中，CTV 不包括手术路径和术后水肿区[21, 65]。值得注意的是，早期报道显示腔镜 SRS 术后软脑膜播散的发生率较高，约为 10%[66]，乳腺癌被认为是软脑膜播散的一个危险因素。有人推测软脑膜播散可能是由于术腔 SRS 过程中的因病灶脱靶而非手术本身导致的[67]。因此，专家们对于术后 SRS 的应用制定了共识指南，这些指南总结在表 11-1 中，并在图 11-6 中展示了病例实例[68]。临床靶区体积显然应考虑到术后扫描所见的变化，且包括潜在邻近区域中所藏匿的微浸润病灶。

特别是在术腔 SRS 中，术后改变可能会使瘤床的边界不清楚，并可能类似残留肿瘤。推荐审阅手术操作记录以确定所做的手术类型，并在有疑问时征求外科医生和神经放射科医生的意见。根据共识指南，BM 位于幕下或靠近静脉窦和（或）硬脑膜的病例间的差异性最大。在所有病例中，CTV 的勾画应借助在切除术后 1～3 周做的 T_1 加权钆增强的 MRI 扫描来完成，并尽可能接近拟定的放射外科日期。

表 11-1 术后 CTV 勾画推荐

	推 荐
所有病例	融合术前 MRI（T_1 加权、钆增强）影像以帮助确定靶区体积 CTV 应包括整个手术通道（术后 CT 和轴向 T_1 加权钆增强 MRI 所见），且不包括术后水肿
分型	
术前累及硬脑膜	考虑到微浸润病灶，CTV 沿硬脑膜（骨瓣旁）外扩 5～10mm
无硬脑膜累及	CTV 沿骨瓣外扩 1～5mm
术前静脉窦累及	CTV 外扩 1～5mm 至邻近窦内

（二）PTV 边缘外扩

PTV 外扩距离高度依赖于治疗 BM 的平台。各个机构均不一致，应进行严格的内部质量保证以确定适当的 PTV。例如，当使用刚性固定时，0～1mm 的 PTV 边距通常就足够了[69, 70]。相反，使用热塑面罩时，可能需要 2～3mm 的边距。六自由度放射治疗床对于纠正旋转误差特别有效[71]。毫无疑问的是，PTV 外扩越大，病灶漏

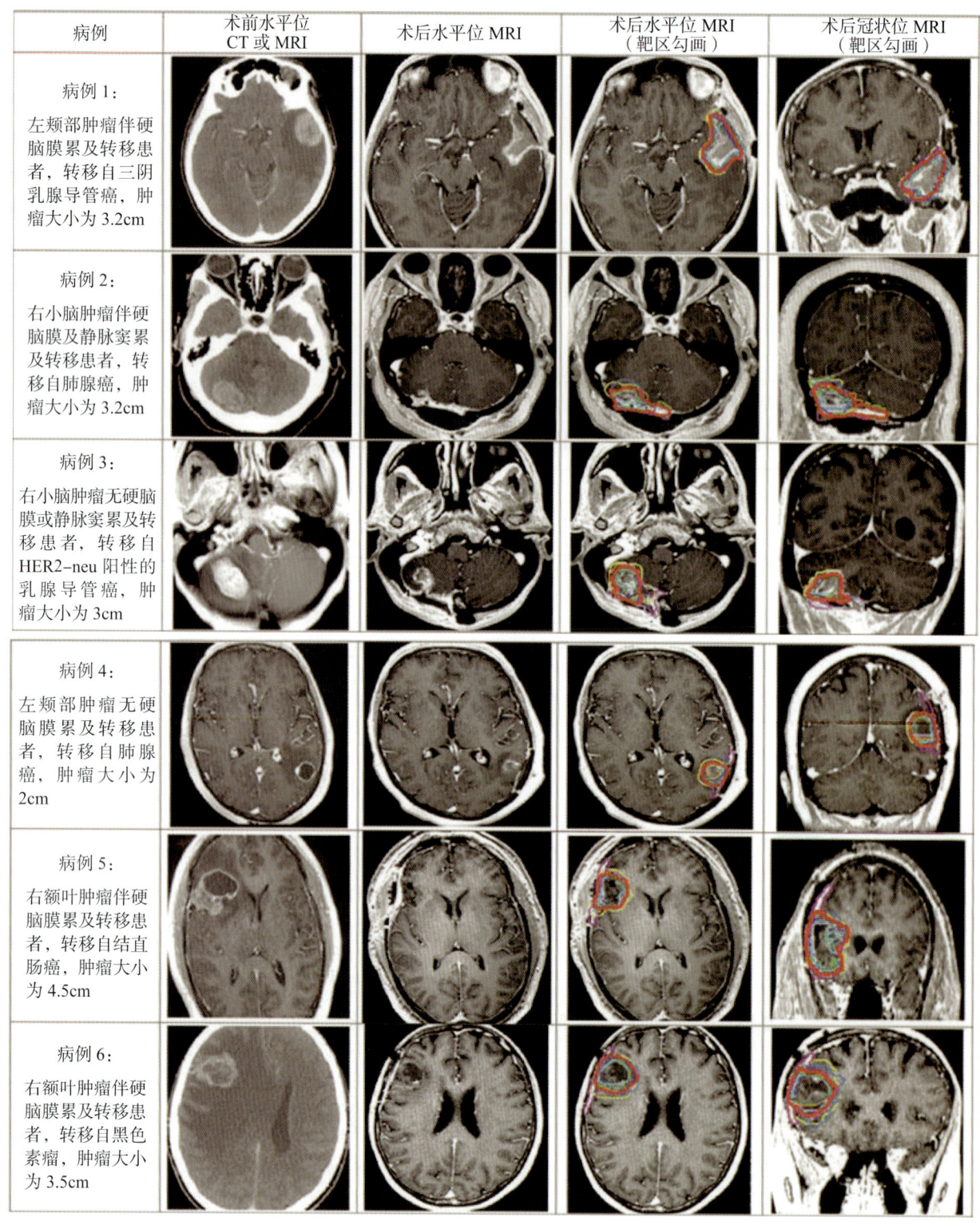

病例	术前水平位 CT 或 MRI	术后水平位 MRI	术后水平位 MRI（靶区勾画）	术后冠状位 MRI（靶区勾画）
病例 1：左颞部肿瘤伴硬脑膜累及转移患者，转移自三阴乳腺导管癌，肿瘤大小为 3.2cm				
病例 2：右小脑肿瘤伴硬脑膜及静脉窦累及转移患者，转移自肺腺癌，肿瘤大小为 3.2cm				
病例 3：右小脑肿瘤无硬脑膜或静脉窦累及转移患者，转移自 HER2-neu 阳性的乳腺导管癌，肿瘤大小为 3cm				
病例 4：左颞部肿瘤无硬脑膜累及转移患者，转移自肺腺癌，肿瘤大小为 2cm				
病例 5：右额叶肿瘤伴硬脑膜累及转移患者，转移自结直肠癌，肿瘤大小为 4.5cm				
病例 6：右额叶肿瘤伴硬脑膜累及转移患者，转移自黑色素瘤，肿瘤大小为 3.5cm				

▲ 图 11-6 切除脑转移瘤的个体化和共识靶区勾画

共识靶区勾画用深红色显示，个体化靶区勾画用其他颜色显示。CT. 计算机断层扫描；MRI. 磁共振成像。经 Elsevier 许可转载，引自 Soliman 等[68]

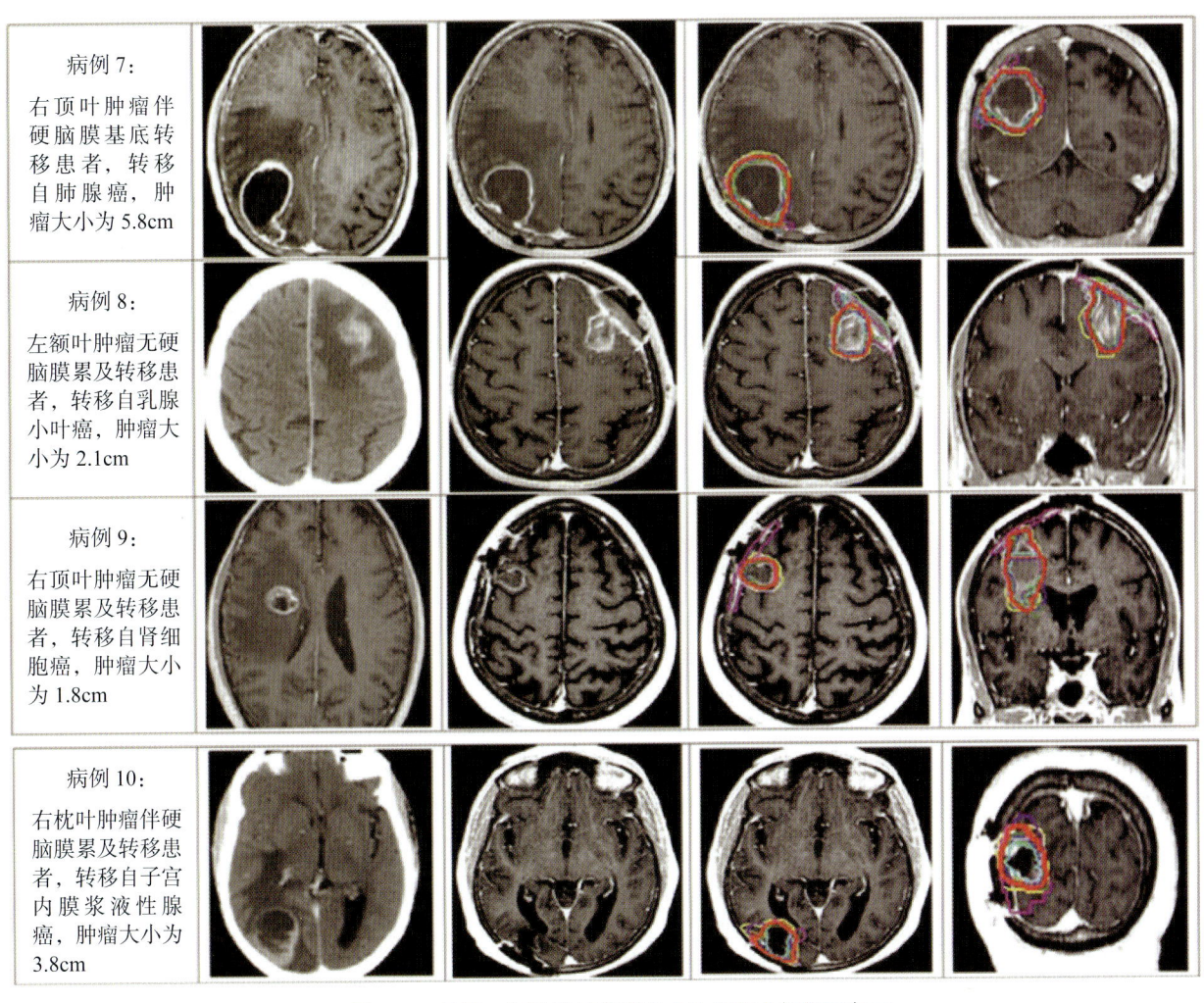

病例 7：右顶叶肿瘤伴硬脑膜基底转移患者，转移自肺腺癌，肿瘤大小为 5.8cm				
病例 8：左额叶肿瘤无硬脑膜累及转移患者，转移自乳腺小叶癌，肿瘤大小为 2.1cm				
病例 9：右顶叶肿瘤无硬脑膜累及转移患者，转移自肾细胞癌，肿瘤大小为 1.8cm				
病例 10：右枕叶肿瘤伴硬脑膜累及转移患者，转移自子宫内膜浆液性腺癌，肿瘤大小为 3.8cm				

▲ 图 11-6（续） 切除脑转移瘤的个体化和共识靶区勾画

诊的风险越小。然而这样的话，PTV 中接受到高剂量治疗的正常脑组织的体积越大。一项随机对照试验表明，当使用 3mm 的 PTV（vs. 1mm）外扩边距时，放射性坏死的风险会增加（12.5% vs. 2.5%）[57]。

（三）剂量选择

剂量的选择主要取决于 PTV 的体积或直径。为了减少治疗并发症的风险，体积大的 BM，其处方剂量反而会降低。这是基于 RTOG 90-05 I 期试验的数据[72]。≤ 20mm 的病灶采用 24Gy 治疗是安全的，而 21～30mm、31～40mm 大小的病灶用 18 Gy 和 15 Gy 治疗是安全的。然而，这些是基于复发的原发性及继发性脑肿瘤的混合数据所得出，所有患者之前都曾接受过放疗。

术后术腔往往呈不规则形状，通过病灶直径来选择剂量很难。N107C 试验（包括了切除的空腔）采用了基于体积的方法进行剂量选择[21]（表 11-2）。

在我们的临床实践中，对于直径 3cm 以上（14.1cm³）的病灶，我们更倾向于使用 3 或 5 次 HSRT 的方法[73]。无论分割次数多少，大体肿瘤体积的靶区勾画方法都是相似的。

十、OAR 的勾画

我们建议读者参考 Scoccianti 等在 2015 年发布的危及器官勾画指南[74]。

表 11-2 N107c 试验中使用的基于体积的单次 SRS 剂量选择建议[21]

N107c 试验中使用的基于体积的单次 SRS 剂量选择建议[21]		使用 5 次分割立体定向放疗的替代剂量
< 4.2cm³	20Gy	N/A
4.2~8cm³	18Gy	30~35Gy，5 次分割
8~14.4cm³	17Gy	25~30Gy，5 次分割
14.4~20cm³	15Gy	
20~30cm³	14Gy	25Gy，5 次分割
30cm³~5cm 的最大横向直径	12Gy	

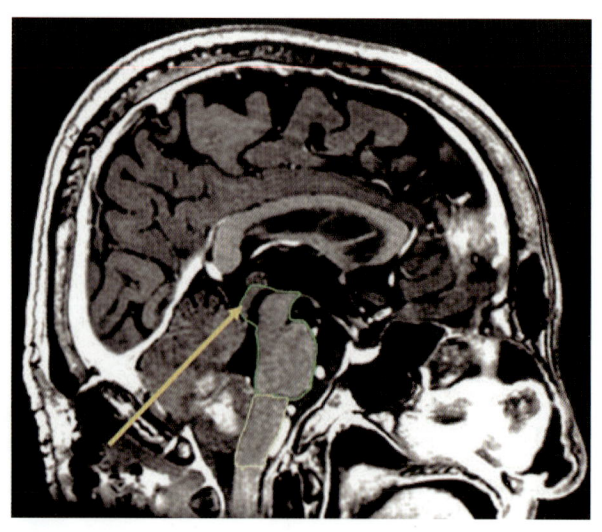

▲ 图 11-7 矢状位 T_1 MRI 显示中脑和脑桥（绿线）和延髓（黄线）

黄箭显示中脑后方的顶盖

1. 脑干

脑干是一个在 SRS 计划中被视为高度优先考虑的关键器官。超过脑干的剂量限制可能会导致放射性坏死以及随之而来的后果，如脑神经病变、运动无力，甚至最坏的情况会因呼吸抑制而死亡。脑干由三个子结构（中脑、脑桥和延髓）组成，位于后床突至枕骨大孔。

在勾画脑干的过程中，应注意到脑干被脑脊液包围。我们发现在矢状面上观察脑干对器官勾画很有帮助（图 11-7）。脑桥是脑干中最厚的部分，它的长度通常约为 3cm。脑干勾画中的错误比较常见，如没有包括位于中脑后部的四叠板（又称顶盖）。

据报道，脑干外围对放射的耐受性更强；但这并没有得到强有力的证据支持。延髓的剂量限制比中脑和脑桥低[75]。根据所使用的体位固定方式，我们推荐使用 1~2mm 的计划危及器官体积（planning organ-at-risk volume, PRV）。

2. 视觉器官

(1) 视觉器官由左、右视神经及视交叉组成。它们具有连续性且有相似的放射剂量限制，但仍应被分开勾画。这些结构的损伤表现为视力障碍（如视力模糊、色彩障碍或视野缺损）。

(2) 视神经在 CT 和 MRI 上都很容易识别。它们起源于球体后部，被眶内脂肪包围。视神经的管内部分位于视神经管内。视神经管最好在骨窗上使用冠状面进行识别。

(3) 视交叉位于鞍结节上方（脑垂体所在的位置）和颈内动脉的床突段之间。它被 CSF（交叉池）所包围。垂体柄是一个重要的标志，因为视交叉位于其前方。在高分辨率的 CT 和 MRI 图像上可以很容易地看到视交叉。需要注意的是，在矢状面上能最明显地看到视交叉通常是向上倾斜的（图 11-8）。

(4) 必须注意视神经和视交叉的勾画是连续的。如果勾画中留有空白，可能导致治疗计划系统无意中将高剂量放射至这些区域，但不会在剂量-体积直方图中被报道出来。

3. 耳蜗

耳蜗是一个小的螺旋形状充满液体的解剖结构，是听觉系统的组成部分。耳蜗位于颞骨的岩部，迷路的前方，内耳道的外侧。耳蜗功能受损可能会导致听力损失和（或）耳鸣。耳蜗最好在 T_2 序列或 CT 骨窗上识别（图 11-9）[76]。

十一、并发症及缓解策略

表 11-3 列出了危及器官的剂量限制。

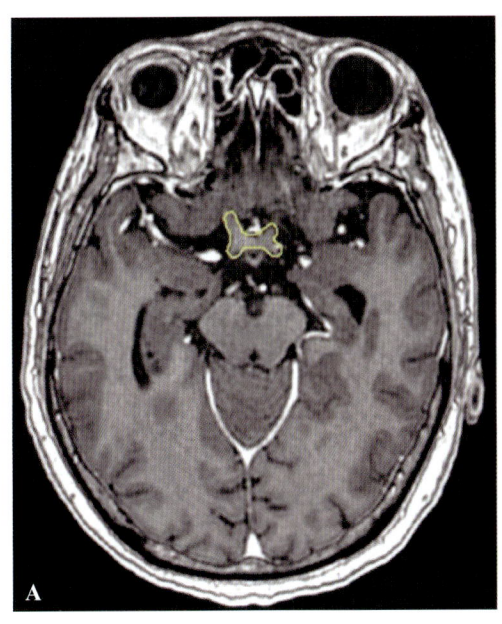

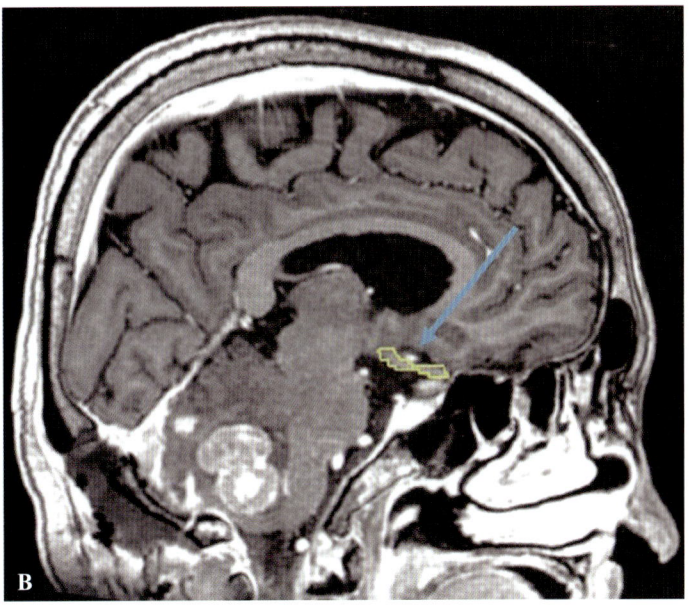

第 11 章 脑转移放射外科治疗（含术后瘤腔）的 靶区勾画
Target Delineation for Radiosurgery (Including Postoperative Cavity Radiosurgery) in Brain Metastases

▲ 图 11-8 视交叉在矢状面上明显向上倾斜
A. 轴位 T_1 MRI 显示视交叉；B. 轴位 T_1 MRI 显示视交叉向上倾斜（蓝箭）

（一）皮质类固醇的使用

SRS 期间常规使用皮质类固醇是有争议的。在 SRS 期间和之后短期使用类固醇可能会使有大量眼周水肿的患者受益。皮质类固醇的使用持续时间和剂量应根据症状决定，但通常持续 1~2 周[84]。

（二）抗惊厥药的使用

尽管有报道称 SRS 后会出现癫痫发作，但我们并不常规地预防性使用抗惊厥药。对于既往有癫痫发作史的患者，应继续使用抗惊厥药[84]。

（三）颅后窝位置

颅后窝的病变可能会压迫第四脑室从而导致阻塞性脑积水。SRS 引起的病灶周围水肿可能会导致这种效应的加重，患者在围术期应用地塞米松可能有用。但没有证据支持预防性脑室－腹膜引流术的使用。

（四）极后区位置

靠近极后区的 BM 行 SRS 可以诱发严重

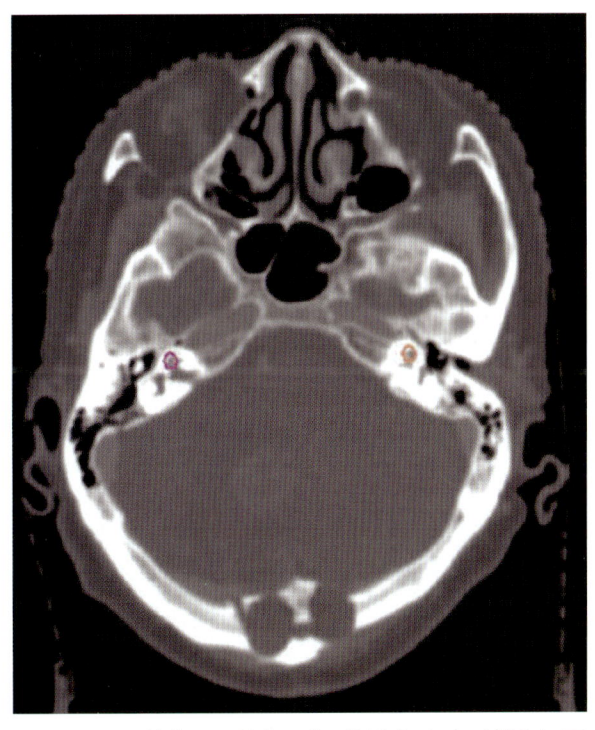

▲ 图 11-9 轴位 CT 骨窗，右（粉色）和左（橙色）耳蜗轮廓

的恶心呕吐。对于需要治疗这个区域的患者应预防性地使用药物，如 $5-HT_3$ 拮抗药，以防止恶心和呕吐，从而大大减少这种并发症的风险。

表 11-3 危及器官的建议剂量限值

器官	1分	3分	5分	参考文献	终点
脑干	D_{max}：15Gy	D_{max}：23.1Gy	D_{max}：31Gy	[77, 78]	G3+ 脑神经病变
	$D(0.5cm^3) < 10Gy$	$D(0.5cm^3) < 18Gy$	$D(0.5cm^3) < 23Gy$		
	D_{max}：12.5Gy	—	—	[78]	
视觉传导通路	D_{max}：10Gy	D_{max}：17.4Gy	D_{max}：25Gy	[79]	G3+ 视神经炎
	$D(0.2cm^3) < 8Gy$	$D(0.2cm^3) < 15.3Gy$	$D(0.2cm^3) < 23Gy$		
	D_{max}：12Gy	D_{max}：19.5Gy	D_{max}：25Gy	[80]	
耳蜗	D_{max}：12Gy	D_{max}：20Gy	D_{max}：27.5Gy	[77]	G3+ 听力损失
	D_{max}：4Gy			[81]	若 < 4Gy，则保存听力的可能性很大
脑（脑实质 -GTV）	$V_{10} < 10.5cm^3$，$V_{12} < 7.9cm^3$	N/A	$V_{20} < 20cm^3$	[82, 83]	症状性放射性坏死

十二、随访

使用单独 SRS 方案，1 年后仍有相对较高的远处脑转移风险（50%）。因此，需要定期影像监测。我们通常在 SRS 结束后 4～6 周行 MR 影像检查，此后每 2～3 个月检查 1 次。

十三、不确定性领域

（一）术后瘤床 SRS 的时机选择

在选择进行 SRS 的最佳时机时，必须考虑手术伤口愈合而不延迟局部和全身治疗之间的平衡。以往研究发现，如果从手术到实行 SRS 延期超过 3 周，局部复发的风险会增加[85]。Atalar 等的研究表明，大多数变化在术后即刻发生（0～3 天），之后术腔体积不会有明显缩小[86]。相反，Patel 等研究表明术后即刻的术腔与 3 周后的术腔大小相比中位数大小增加了 28%[87]。因此，大多数研究建议在术后 1～3 周进行 SRS。

（二）术前与术后 SRS 的比较

术前 SRS 是一个新的概念，即在切除前对肿瘤进行灭活。与切除腔 SRS 相比，术前 SRS 的个体间靶区勾画变化较小[88]。Atalar 等报道，术后靶区体积的平均尺寸要小一些，但他们的结果有很大的差异(-29%，范围为 -82%～1258%)[86]。此外，术后 SRS 的靶区可能需要包括手术通道以及加上 2mm 外扩的 PTV 边距，这使得术腔 SRS 的总体治疗体积较大。

北卡罗来纳州的研究者对此进行了前瞻性研究，手术平均在 SRS 之后 1 天(范围为 0～17 天) 进行，结果显示其有效安全，且没有出现发生放射性坏死的病例[89]。然而，目前还没有 1 级证据支持使用术前 SRS。术前 SRS 是否能使放射坏死和 LMD 的发生率降低还有待观察。这个话题在第 6 章中进一步详述。

十四、现行指南

已有一些临床学会指南可用于指导 BM 的整体管理[23, 90]。德国放射肿瘤学会已发表了关于 BM 的 SRS 实施指南[91]。关于完全切除的 BM 的靶区勾画共识指南也已发表[68]。

第 11 章 脑转移放射外科治疗（含术后瘤腔）的 靶区勾画
Target Delineation for Radiosurgery (Including Postoperative Cavity Radiosurgery) in Brain Metastases

> **要　点**
> - 每个实施 SRS 的机构都应商议好用于靶区勾画的 MRI 序列。
> - 应使用失真校正算法，并定期对 SRS 治疗计划中使用的 MRI 扫描仪运行质量保证程序。
> - 图像融合必须在靶区勾画之前由放射肿瘤学家进行手动校正。
> - MRI 采集和治疗实施之间的时间应尽量缩短。
> - 对于不确定的病例（如术后瘤床 SRS），建议采用多学科协作进行靶区勾画，包括神经放射科医生和（或）神经外科医生。
> - OAR 和靶区的勾画都应在 MRI 上进行，并在 CT 图像上进行交叉验证。
> - 当术腔贴于脑膜表面时，推荐在术后瘤床 SRS 中使用 CTV 边距，PTV 边距取决于体位固定和图像校正的类型。

参考文献

[1] Lassman AB, DeAngelis LM. Brain metastases. Neurol Clin. 2003;21(1):1–23. vii.

[2] Lohr F, Pirzkall A, Hof H, Fleckenstein K, Debus J. Adjuvant treatment of brain metastases. Semin Surg Oncol. 2001;20(1):50–6.

[3] Armulik A, Genove G, Mae M, Nisancioglu MH, Wallgard E, Niaudet C, et al. Pericytes regulate the blood-brain barrier. Nature. 2010;468(7323):557–61.

[4] Barnholtz-Sloan JS, Sloan AE, Davis FG, Vigneau FD, Lai P, Sawaya RE. Incidence proportions of brain metastases in patients diagnosed (1973–2001) in the Metropolitan Detroit Cancer Surveillance System. J Clin Oncol. 2004;22(14):2865–72.

[5] Hwang TL, Close TP, Grego JM, Brannon WL, Gonzales F. Predilection of brain metastasis in gray and white matter junction and vascular border zones. Cancer. 1996;77(8):1551–5.

[6] Fink KR, Fink JR. Imaging of brain metastases. Surg Neurol Int. 2013;4(Suppl 4):S209–19.

[7] Barajas RF Jr, Cha S. Imaging diagnosis of brain metastasis. Prog Neurol Surg. 2012;25:55–73.

[8] Schellinger PD, Meinck HM, Thron A. Diagnostic accuracy of MRI compared to CCT in patients with brain metastases. J Neuro-Oncol. 1999;44(3):275–81.

[9] Sze G, Milano E, Johnson C, Heier L. Detection of brain metastases: comparison of contrast-enhanced MR with unenhanced MR and enhanced CT. AJNR Am J Neuroradiol. 1990;11(4):785–91.

[10] Watanabe M, Tanaka R, Takeda N. Correlation of MRI and clinical features in meningeal carcinomatosis. Neuroradiology. 1993;35(7):512–5.

[11] Iaconetta G, Lamaida E, Rossi A, Signorelli F, Manto A, Giamundo A. Leptomeningeal carcinomatosis: review of the literature. Acta Neurol (Napoli). 1994;16(4):214–20.

[12] Al-Okaili RN, Krejza J, Wang S, Woo JH, Melhem ER. Advanced MR imaging techniques in the diagnosis of intraaxial brain tumors in adults. Radiographics. 2006;26(Suppl 1): S173–89.

[13] Kushnirsky M, Nguyen V, Katz JS, Steinklein J, Rosen L, Warshall C, et al. Time-delayed contrast-enhanced MRI improves detection of brain metastases and apparent treatment volumes. J Neurosurg. 2016;124(2):489–95.

[14] Chao JH, Phillips R, Nickson JJ. Roentgen-ray therapy of cerebral metastases. Cancer. 1954;7(4):682–9.

[15] Nieder C, Spanne O, Mehta MP, Grosu AL, Geinitz H. Presentation, patterns of care, and survival in patients with brain metastases: what has changed in the last 20 years? Cancer. 2011;117(11):2505–12.

[16] Patchell RA, Tibbs PA, Walsh JW, Dempsey RJ, Maruyama Y, Kryscio RJ, et al. A randomized trial of surgery in the treatment of single metastases to the brain. N Engl J Med. 1990;322(8):494–500.

[17] Kondziolka D, Patel A, Lunsford LD, Kassam A, Flickinger JC. Stereotactic radiosurgery plus whole brain radiotherapy versus radiotherapy alone for patients with multiple brain metastases. Int J Radiat Oncol Biol Phys. 1999;45(2):427–34.

[18] Aoyama H, Shirato H, Tago M, Nakagawa K, Toyoda T, Hatano K, et al. Stereotactic radiosurgery plus whole-brain radiation therapy vs stereotactic radiosurgery alone for treatment of brain metastases: a randomized controlled trial. JAMA. 2006;295(21):2483–91.

[19] Chang EL, Wefel JS, Hess KR, Allen PK, Lang FF, Kornguth DG, et al. Neurocognition in patients with brain metastases treated with radiosurgery or radiosurgery plus whole-brain irradiation: a randomised controlled trial. Lancet Oncol.

2009;10(11):1037–44.

[20] Kocher M, Soffietti R, Abacioglu U, Villa S, Fauchon F, Baumert BG, et al. Adjuvant whole-brain radiotherapy versus observation after radiosurgery or surgical resection of one to three cerebral metastases: results of the EORTC 22952-26001 study. J Clin Oncol. 2011;29(2):134–41.

[21] Brown PD, Ballman KV, Cerhan JH, Anderson SK, Carrero XW, Whitton AC, et al. Postoperative stereotactic radiosurgery compared with whole brain radiotherapy for resected metastatic brain disease (NCCTG N107C/CEC.3): a multicentre, randomised, controlled, phase 3 trial. Lancet Oncol. 2017;18(8):1049–60.

[22] Yamamoto M, Kawabe T, Sato Y, Higuchi Y, Nariai T, Watanabe S, et al. Stereotactic radiosurgery for patients with multiple brain metastases: a case-matched study comparing treatment results for patients with 2–9 versus 10 or more tumors. J Neurosurg. 2014;121(Suppl):16–25.

[23] Available from: https://www.astro.org/Patient-Care-and-Research/Clinical-Practice-Statements/ASTRO-39;s-guideline-on-brain-metasteses.

[24] Andrews DW, Bednarz G, Evans JJ, Downes B. A review of 3 current radiosurgery systems. Surg Neurol. 2006;66(6):559–64.

[25] Sahgal A, Ruschin M, Ma L, Verbakel W, Larson D, Brown PD. Stereotactic radiosurgery alone for multiple brain metastases? A review of clinical and technical issues. Neuro-Oncology. 2017;19(suppl_2):ii2–ii15.

[26] Mahajan A, Ahmed S, McAleer MF, Weinberg JS, Li J, Brown P, et al. Post-operative stereotactic radiosurgery versus observation for completely resected brain metastases: a single-centre, randomised, controlled, phase 3 trial. Lancet Oncol. 2017;18(8):1040–8.

[27] Patchell RA, Tibbs PA, Regine WF, Dempsey RJ, Mohiuddin M, Kryscio RJ, et al. Postoperative radiotherapy in the treatment of single metastases to the brain: a randomized trial. JAMA. 1998;280(17):1485–9.

[28] Soltys SG, Adler JR, Lipani JD, Jackson PS, Choi CY, Puataweepong P, et al. Stereotactic radiosurgery of the postoperative resection cavity for brain metastases. Int J Radiat Oncol Biol Phys. 2008;70(1):187–93.

[29] Choi CY, Chang SD, Gibbs IC, Adler JR, Harsh GR, Lieberson RE, et al. Stereotactic radiosurgery of the postoperative resection cavity for brain metastases: prospective evaluation of target margin on tumor control. Int J Radiat Oncol Biol Phys. 2012;84(2):336–42.

[30] Sperduto PW, Kased N, Roberge D, Xu Z, Shanley R, Luo X, et al. Summary report on the graded prognostic assessment: an accurate and facile diagnosis-specific tool to estimate survival for patients with brain metastases. J Clin Oncol. 2012;30(4):419–25.

[31] Andrews DW, Scott CB, Sperduto PW, Flanders AE, Gaspar LE, Schell MC, et al. Whole brain radiation therapy with or without stereotactic radiosurgery boost for patients with one to three brain metastases: phase III results of the RTOG 9508 randomised trial. Lancet. 2004;363(9422):1665–72.

[32] Lutz W, Winston KR, Maleki N. A system for stereotactic radiosurgery with a linear accelerator. Int J Radiat Oncol Biol Phys. 1988;14(2):373–81.

[33] Klein EE, Hanley J, Bayouth J, Yin FF, Simon W, Dresser S, et al. Task Group 142 report: quality assurance of medical accelerators. Med Phys. 2009;36(9):4197–212.

[34] Guckenberger M, Roesch J, Baier K, Sweeney RA, Flentje M. Dosimetric consequences of translational and rotational errors in frame-less image-guided radiosurgery. Radiat Oncol. 2012;7:63.

[35] Theelen A, Martens J, Bosmans G, Houben R, Jager JJ, Rutten I, et al. Relocatable fixation systems in intracranial stereotactic radiotherapy. Accuracy of serial CT scans and patient acceptance in a randomized design. Strahlenther Onkol. 2012;188(1):84–90.

[36] Ramakrishna N, Rosca F, Friesen S, Tezcanli E, Zygmanszki P, Hacker F. A clinical comparison of patient setup and intra-fraction motion using frame-based radiosurgery versus a frameless image-guided radiosurgery system for intracranial lesions. Radiother Oncol. 2010;95(1):109–15.

[37] Anzalone N, Essig M, Lee SK, Dorfler A, Ganslandt O, Combs SE, et al. Optimizing contrast-enhanced magnetic resonance imaging characterization of brain metastases: relevance to stereotactic radiosurgery. Neurosurgery. 2013;72(5):691–701.

[38] Garcia MA, Anwar M, Yu Y, Duriseti S, Merritt B, Nakamura J, et al. Brain metastasis growth on preradiosurgical magnetic resonance imaging. Pract Radiat Oncol. 2018;8(6):e369–e76.

[39] Salkeld AL, Hau EKC, Nahar N, Sykes JR, Wang W, Thwaites DI. Changes in brain metastasis during radiosurgical planning. Int J Radiat Oncol Biol Phys. 2018;102(4):727–33.

[40] Yuh WT, Engelken JD, Muhonen MG, Mayr NA, Fisher DJ, Ehrhardt JC. Experience with high-dose gadolinium MR imaging in the evaluation of brain metastases. AJNR Am J Neuroradiol. 1992;13(1):335–45.

[41] Sze G, Johnson C, Kawamura Y, Goldberg SN, Lange R, Friedland RJ, et al. Comparison of singleand triple-dose contrast material in the MR screening of brain metastases. AJNR Am J Neuroradiol. 1998;19(5):821–8.

[42] Yuh WT, Tali ET, Nguyen HD, Simonson TM, Mayr NA, Fisher DJ. The effect of contrast dose, imaging time, and lesion size in the MR detection of intracerebral metastasis. AJNR Am J Neuroradiol. 1995;16(2):373–80.

[43] Subedi KS, Takahashi T, Yamano T, Saitoh J, Nishimura K, Suzuki Y, et al. Usefulness of double dose contrast-enhanced magnetic resonance imaging for clear delineation of gross tumor volume in stereotactic radiotherapy treatment planning of metastatic brain tumors: a dose comparison study. J Radiat Res. 2013;54(1):135–9.

[44] Togao O, Hiwatashi A, Yamashita K, Kikuchi K, Yoshiura T, Honda H. Additional MR contrast dosage for radiologists' diagnostic performance in detecting brain metastases: a systematic observer study at 3 T. Jpn J Radiol. 2014;32(9):

[45] Sumanaweera TS, Glover GH, Binford TO, Adler JR. MR susceptibility misregistration correction. IEEE Trans Med Imaging. 1993;12(2):251–9.

[46] Baldwin LN, Wachowicz K, Fallone BG. A two-step scheme for distortion rectification of magnetic resonance images. Med Phys. 2009;36(9):3917–26.

[47] Neumann JO, Giese H, Biller A, Nagel AM, Kiening K. Spatial distortion in MRI-guided stereotactic procedures: evaluation in 1.5-, 3- and 7-Tesla MRI scanners. Stereotact Funct Neurosurg. 2015;93(6):380–6.

[48] Seibert TM, White NS, Kim GY, Moiseenko V, McDonald CR, Farid N, et al. Distortion inherent to magnetic resonance imaging can lead to geometric miss in radiosurgery planning. Pract Radiat Oncol. 2016;6(6):e319–e28.

[49] Available from: https://www.aapm.org/org/ structure/? committee_code=TG117.

[50] Knisely JP, Bond JE, Yue NJ, Studholme C, de Lotbinière AC. Image registration and calculation of a biologically effective dose for multisession radiosurgical treatments. Technical note. J Neurosurg. 2000 Dec;93 Suppl 3:208-18.

[51] Sighvatsson V, Ericson K, Tomasson H. Optimising contrast-enhanced cranial CT for detection of brain metastases. Acta Radiol. 1998;39(6):718–22.

[52] Davis PC, Hudgins PA, Peterman SB, Hoffman JC Jr. Diagnosis of cerebral metastases: double-dose delayed CT vs contrast-enhanced MR imaging. AJNR Am J Neuroradiol. 1991;12(2):293–300.

[53] Blatt DR, Friedman WA, Agee OF. Delayed computed tomography contrast enhancement patterns in biopsy proven cases. Neurosurgery. 1993;32(4):560–9.

[54] Baumert BG, Rutten I, Dehing-Oberije C, Twijnstra A, Dirx MJ, Debougnoux-Huppertz RM, et al. A pathology-based substrate for target definition in radiosurgery of brain metastases. Int J Radiat Oncol Biol Phys. 2006;66(1):187–94.

[55] Noel G, Simon JM, Valery CA, Cornu P, Boisserie G, Hasboun D, et al. Radiosurgery for brain metastasis: impact of CTV on local control. Radiother Oncol. 2003;68(1):15–21.

[56] Nataf F, Schlienger M, Liu Z, Foulquier JN, Gres B, Orthuon A, et al. Radiosurgery with or without A 2-mm margin for 93 single brain metastases. Int J Radiat Oncol Biol Phys. 2008;70(3):766–72.

[57] Kirkpatrick JP, Wang Z, Sampson JH, McSherry F, Herndon JE 2nd, Allen KJ, et al. Defining the optimal planning target volume in image-guided stereotactic radiosurgery of brain metastases: results of a randomized trial. Int J Radiat Oncol Biol Phys. 2015;91(1):100–8.

[58] Clavier J, Antoni D, Bauer N, Guillerme F, Truntzer P, Atlani D, et al. Delineation of brain metastases for stereotactic radiation therapy: an interobserver contour comparison. Int J Radiat Oncol Biol Phys. 2014;90(1):S311.

[59] Sun B, Huang Z, Wu S, Ding L, Shen G, Cha L, et al. Cystic brain metastasis is associated with poor prognosis in patients with advanced breast cancer. Oncotarget. 2016;7(45):74006–14.

[60] Goodman KA, Sneed PK, McDermott MW, Shiau CY, Lamborn KR, Chang S, et al. Relationship between pattern of enhancement and local control of brain metastases after radiosurgery. Int J Radiat Oncol Biol Phys. 2001;50:139-46.

[61] DeAngelis LM, Mandell LR, Thaler HT, Kimmel DW, Galicich JH, Fuks Z, et al. The role of postoperative radiotherapy after resection of single brain metastases. Neurosurgery. 1989;24(6):798–805.

[62] Smalley SR, Schray MF, Laws ER Jr, O'Fallon JR. Adjuvant radiation therapy after surgical resection of solitary brain metastasis: association with pattern of failure and survival. Int J Radiat Oncol Biol Phys. 1987;13(11):1611–6.

[63] Patel AJ, Suki D, Hatiboglu MA, Abouassi H, Shi W, Wildrick DM, et al. Factors influencing the risk of local recurrence after resection of a single brain metastasis. J Neurosurg. 2010;113(2):181–9.

[64] Brennan C, Yang TJ, Hilden P, Zhang Z, Chan K, Yamada Y, et al. A phase 2 trial of stereotactic radiosurgery boost after surgical resection for brain metastases. Int J Radiat Oncol Biol Phys. 2014;88(1):130–6.

[65] Kepka L, Tyc-Szczepaniak D, Bujko K, Olszyna-Serementa M, Michalski W, Sprawka A, et al. Stereotactic radiotherapy of the tumor bed compared to whole brain radiotherapy after surgery of single brain metastasis: results from a randomized trial. Radiother Oncol. 2016;121(2):217–24.

[66] Atalar B, Modlin LA, Choi CY, Adler JR, Gibbs IC, Chang SD, et al. Risk of leptomeningeal disease in patients treated with stereotactic radiosurgery targeting the postoperative resection cavity for brain metastases. Int J Radiat Oncol Biol Phys. 2013;87(4):713–8.

[67] Johnson MD, Avkshtol V, Baschnagel AM, Meyer K, Ye H, Grills IS, et al. Surgical resection of brain metastases and the risk of leptomeningeal recurrence in patients treated with stereotactic radiosurgery. Int J Radiat Oncol Biol Phys. 2016;94(3):537–43.

[68] Soliman H, Ruschin M, Angelov L, Brown PD, Chiang VLS, Kirkpatrick JP, et al. Consensus contouring guidelines for postoperative completely resected cavity stereotactic radiosurgery for brain metastases. Int J Radiat Oncol Biol Phys. 2018;100(2):436–42.

[69] Prabhu RS, Dhabaan A, Hall WA, Ogunleye T, Crocker I, Curran WJ, et al. Clinical outcomes for a novel 6 degrees of freedom image guided localization method for frameless radiosurgery for intracranial brain metastases. J Neuro-Oncol. 2013;113(1):93–9.

[70] Dhabaan A, Schreibmann E, Siddiqi A, Elder E, Fox T, Ogunleye T, et al. Six degrees of freedom CBCT-based positioning for intracranial targets treated with frameless stereotactic radiosurgery. J Appl Clin Med Phys. 2012;13(6):3916.

[71] Mancosu P, Reggiori G, Gaudino A, Lobefalo F, Paganini L,

[72] Palumbo V, et al. Are pitch and roll compensations required in all pathologies? A data analysis of 2945 fractions. Br J Radiol. 2015;88(1055):20150468.

[72] Shaw E, Scott C, Souhami L, Dinapoli R, Kline R, Loeffler J, et al. Single dose radiosurgical treatment of recurrent previously irradiated primary brain tumors and brain metastases: final report of RTOG protocol 90-05. Int J Radiat Oncol Biol Phys. 2000;47(2):291–8.

[73] Brenner DJ, Martel MK, Hall EJ. Fractionated regimens for stereotactic radiotherapy of recurrent tumors in the brain. Int J Radiat Oncol Biol Phys. 1991;21(3):819–24.

[74] Scoccianti S, Detti B, Gadda D, Greto D, Furfaro I, Meacci F, et al. Organs at risk in the brain and their dose-constraints in adults and in children: a radiation oncologist's guide for delineation in everyday practice. Radiother Oncol. 2015;114(2):230–8.

[75] Benedict SH, Yenice KM, Followill D, Galvin JM, Hinson W, Kavanagh B, et al. Stereotactic body radiation therapy: the report of AAPM Task Group 101. Med Phys. 2010;37(8): 4078–101.

[76] Pacholke HD, Amdur RJ, Schmalfuss IM, Louis D, Mendenhall WM. Contouring the middle and inner ear on radiotherapy planning scans. Am J Clin Oncol. 2005;28(2):143–7.

[77] Timmerman RD. An overview of hypofractionation and introduction to this issue of seminars in radiation oncology. Semin Radiat Oncol. 2008;18(4):215–22.

[78] Mayo C, Yorke E, Merchant TE. Radiation associated brainstem injury. Int J Radiat Oncol Biol Phys. 2010;76(3 Suppl):S36–41.

[79] Mayo C, Martel MK, Marks LB, Flickinger J, Nam J, Kirkpatrick J. Radiation dose-volume effects of optic nerves and chiasm. Int J Radiat Oncol Biol Phys. 2010;76(3 Suppl):S28–35.

[80] Grimm J, LaCouture T, Croce R, Yeo I, Zhu Y, Xue J. Dose tolerance limits and dose volume histogram evaluation for stereotactic body radiotherapy. J Appl Clin Med Phys. 2011;12(2):3368.

[81] Tamura M, Carron R, Yomo S, Arkha Y, Muraciolle X, Porcheron D, et al. Hearing preservation after Gamma Knife radiosurgery for vestibular schwannomas presenting with high-level hearing. Neurosurgery. 2009;64(2):289–96. Discussion 96.

[82] Ernst-Stecken A, Ganslandt O, Lambrecht U, Sauer R, Grabenbauer G. Phase II trial of hypofractionated stereotactic radiotherapy for brain metastases: results and toxicity. Radiother Oncol. 2006;81(1):18–24.

[83] Blonigen BJ, Steinmetz RD, Levin L, Lamba MA, Warnick RE, Breneman JC. Irradiated volume as a predictor of brain radionecrosis after linear accelerator stereotactic radiosurgery. Int J Radiat Oncol Biol Phys. 2010;77(4):996–1001.

[84] Soffietti R, Abacioglu U, Baumert B, Combs SE, Kinhult S, Kros JM, et al. Diagnosis and treatment of brain metastases from solid tumors: guidelines from the European Association of Neuro-Oncology (EANO). Neuro-Oncology. 2017;19(2): 162–74.

[85] Iorio-Morin C, Masson-Cote L, Ezahr Y, Blanchard J, Ebacher A, Mathieu D. Early Gamma Knife stereotactic radiosurgery to the tumor bed of resected brain metastasis for improved local control. J Neurosurg. 2014;121(Suppl):69–74.

[86] Atalar B, Choi CY, Harsh GR, Chang SD, Gibbs IC, Adler JR, et al. Cavity volume dynamics after resection of brain metastases and timing of postresection cavity stereotactic radiosurgery. Neurosurgery. 2013;72(2):180–5. Discussion 5.

[87] Patel RA, Lock D, Helenowski IB, Chandler JP, Sachdev S, Tate MC, et al. Postsurgical cavity evolution after brain metastasis resection: how soon should postoperative radiosurgery follow? World Neurosurg. 2018;110:e310–e4.

[88] Vellayappan BA, Doody J, Vandervoort E, Szanto J, Sinclair J, Caudrelier JM, et al. Pre-operative versus post-operative radiosurgery for brain metastasis: effects on treatment volume and inter-observer variability. J Radiosurg SBRT. 2018;5(2):89–97.

[89] Asher AL, Burri SH, Wiggins WF, Kelly RP, Boltes MO, Mehrlich M, et al. A new treatment paradigm: neoadjuvant radiosurgery before surgical resection of brain metastases with analysis of local tumor recurrence. Int J Radiat Oncol Biol Phys. 2014;88(4):899–906.

[90] Soffietti R, Cornu P, Delattre JY, Grant R, Graus F, Grisold W, et al. EFNS Guidelines on diagnosis and treatment of brain metastases: report of an EFNS Task Force. Eur J Neurol. 2006;13(7):674–81.

[91] Kocher M, Wittig A, Piroth MD, Treuer H, Seegenschmiedt H, Ruge M, et al. Stereotactic radiosurgery for treatment of brain metastases. A report of the DEGRO Working Group on Stereotactic Radiotherapy. Strahlenther Onkol. 2014;190(6):521–32.

第 12 章 全脑放疗的指征
Indications for Whole-Brain Radiation Therapy

Michael Huo　Fabio Ynoe de Moraes　Matthew Foote　Mark B. Pinkham　Gustavo N. Marta　John H. Suh　著

凡　丹　译

伍海军　校

一、病例介绍

一名 52 岁男性患者，白种人，因日益疲劳、咳嗽、体重减轻、头痛、恶心、共济失调、右上肢乏力就诊。患者合并慢性阻塞性肺疾病、高血压及高脂血症，吸烟史为 60 包 / 年，尚未戒烟。胸 / 腹 / 盆部 CT 显示左上肺叶有 5cm 大小的肿块，纵隔淋巴结肿大，左侧肾上腺 3cm 大小肿块。头部 CT 显示颅内共 16 处转移灶，大小 4mm～18mm，无脑积水，中线无明显移位，伴轻中度血管性水肿。除 CT 所示病灶外，头部 MRI（图 12-1）还显示出另外 9 个颅内病灶，最大者约为 4mm。

患者入院口服地塞米松（8mg/d）后症状好转。在 CT 引导下行肺肿块穿刺活检提示为肺腺癌，*TTF-1* 表达阳性，未检测到 *ALK* 或 *EGFR* 突变，PD-L$_1$ 表达< 1%。患者为进一步控制脑转移病灶，于肿瘤放疗科就诊。

鉴于脑转移病灶的数目及大小，患者不适合接受神经外科手术或放射外科治疗。患者的乏力、头痛及共济失调等症状在地塞米松治疗 24h 后明显好转，ECOG 功能状态评分也由入院时的 3 分改善至 1 分。放疗科医师评估患者后对其进行全脑放疗（30Gy/10 次）。放疗期间，患者出现乏力、恶心等不适，行昂丹司琼对症处理，总体上对放疗耐受良好。患者在 2 周内逐渐将地塞米松减量直至停药，并在之后的半年内进行了系统治疗。治疗后 3 个月复查头部 MRI 显示颅内所有病灶均维持稳定或部分缓解，且未见新发病灶。

二、概述

全脑放疗（whole-brain radiation therapy，WBRT）提高了许多脑转移患者的总生存期，是治疗脑转移的经典方法[1]。一项发表于 2005 年的系统性综述纳入了 8 项随机对照临床实验的研究结果，发现接受全脑放疗患者的总生存时间为 3.2～5.8 个月，而接受激素及最佳支持治疗患者的总生存时间仅为 2～3 个月[2]。此外，WBRT 的实施简单易行，如仅需适当保护晶体的前后野对穿照射（图 12-2），也使其成为全球广泛适用的治疗手段。WBRT 的典型剂量分布如图 12-3 所示。

然而，随着立体定向外科治疗（stereotactic radiosurgery，SRS）和对颅内病灶有效的系统治疗（如靶向治疗、免疫治疗等）等新型治疗手段的出现，脑转移瘤的治疗选择已发生巨大变化[3]。高级别循证医学数据指出，这些新型治疗手段在某些情况下与 WBRT 相比，是更安全的替代手段。近期的随机临床研究数据进一步指出，WBRT 对部分体能状态差的患者作用有限，这些研究均使 WBRT 在脑转移治疗中的作用被逐渐弱化[4]。

尽管如此，但手术或放射外科等局部治疗

143

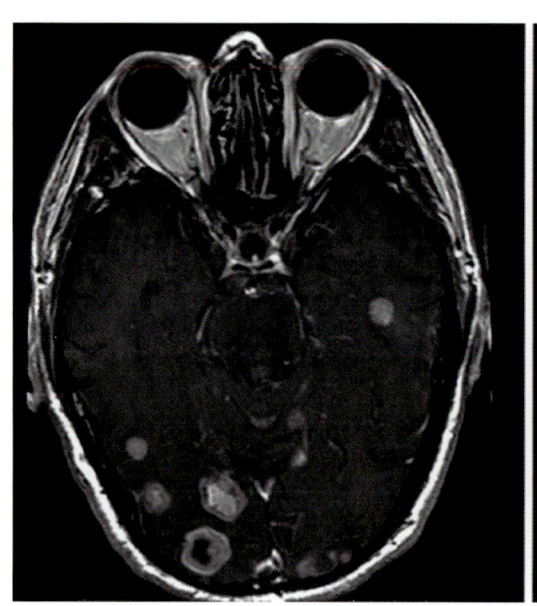

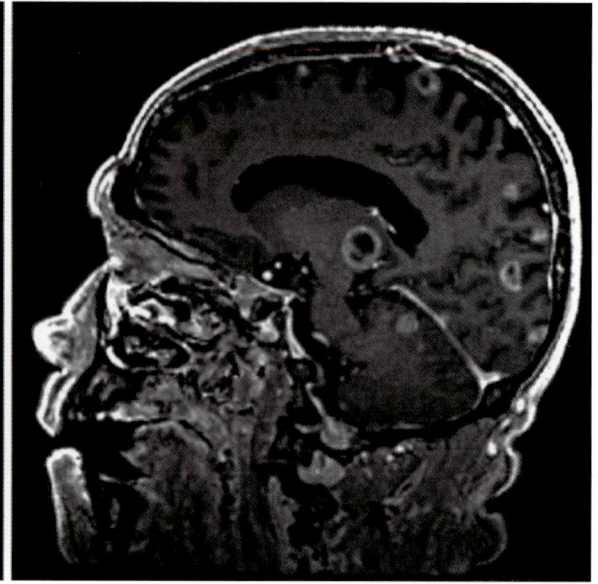

▲ 图 12-1　头部 MRI 显示非小细胞肺癌的广泛脑转移

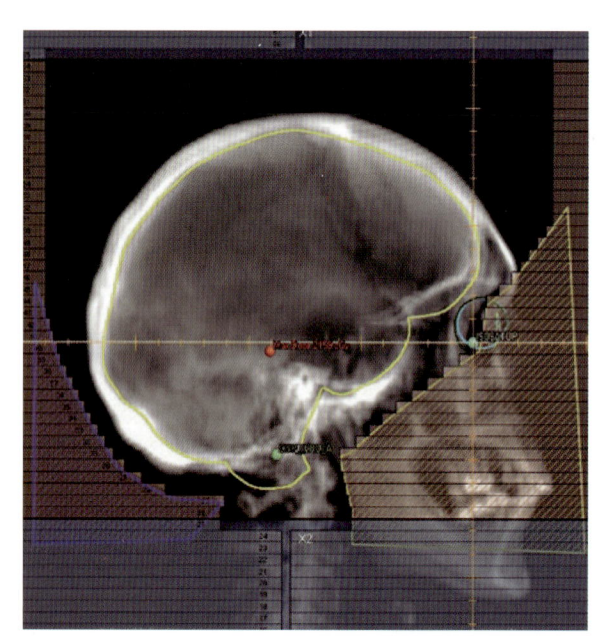

▲ 图 12-2　全脑放疗的照射野

手段对部分脑转移瘤患者并不适用，如患者颅内病灶体积大、高龄或体能状态差、全身肿瘤高负荷等。早期研究发现大部分脑转移为颅内多发转移灶，但局部治疗手段是否可用于 4 处以上的转移病灶仍需高质量的随机临床试验进行探索[5]。

WBRT 可同时治疗大体肿瘤及镜下病变，并有助于预防新转移灶和相关症状的发生。早期文献报道 WBRT 的反应持续时间为 1~8 个月[2]，症状缓解率较高，64%~83% 的患者可从早期研究中获益[6]。尽管缺乏确切的高质量数据支持，WBRT 还可用于软脑膜转移瘤的治疗以及既往已行 SRS 或 WBRT 的再程放疗。值得注意的是，以上随机试验的数据大多在靶向治疗、免疫治疗等有效的系统治疗问世之前发表，新的治疗手段的出现显著改善了大部分患者（如非小细胞肺癌）的预后，因此，WBRT 为患者带来更长生存的同时也可能增加患者晚期治疗毒性的风险。

尽管颅内病变通常是影响患者预后和生活质量的限制因素，但制定治疗决策时仍需综合考虑患者的生存期、生活质量及神经认知功能等方面。并非所有脑转移瘤都适合直接进行治疗，这取决于关于患者、肿瘤、治疗等多个因素，有时可能难以明确最佳的治疗方案。因此，脑转移的治疗在一定程度上需要进行个体化评估。

本章旨在回顾 WBRT 在脑转移治疗中的现状及其未来的研究方向。

三、患者选择

对于体能状态较差的患者，最佳支持治疗可

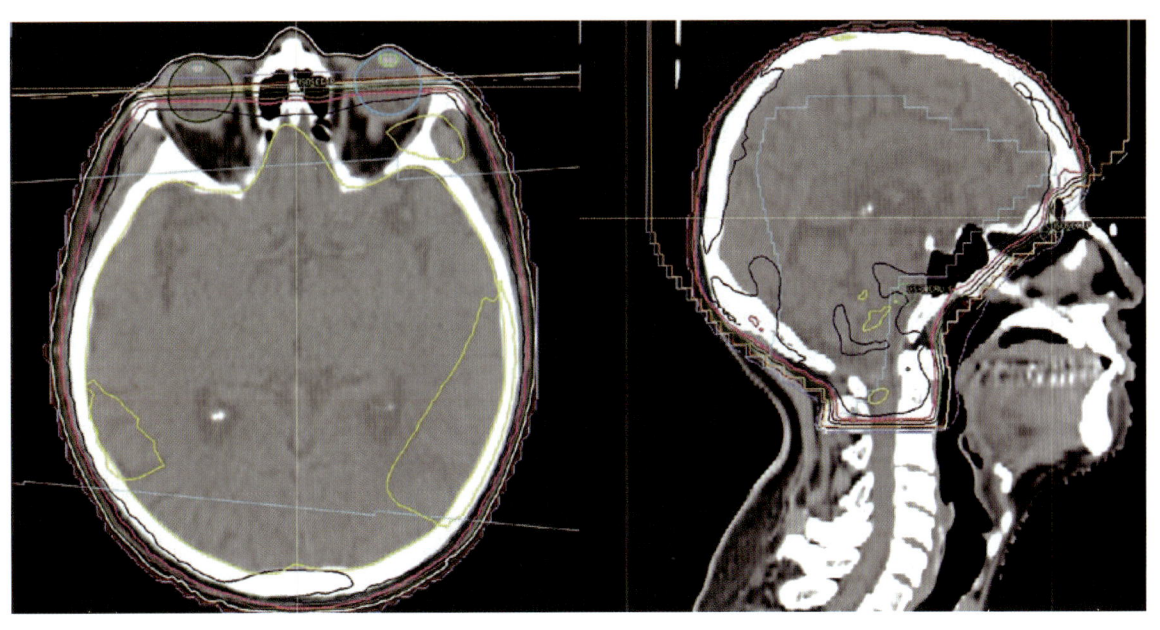

▲ 图 12-3　全脑放疗的常见剂量分布

作为代替 WBRT 的治疗手段。Pease 等在 2005 年发表的系统综述中指出：WBRT 的中位生存期与 Gaspar 等建立的 RPA 分类密切相关[2, 7]。具体来说，5 项观察性研究中报道的各类 RPA 的中位生存期分别为：RPA Ⅰ类为 8.3 个月，RPA Ⅱ类为 4.4 个月，RPA Ⅲ类为 2.4 个月[7]。一项英国和澳大利亚的 3 期非劣性研究，旨在非小细胞肺癌患者中比较 WBRT 和地塞米松支持治疗的效果，结果显示两组的生活质量无明显差异：两组的质量调整寿命时间分别为 46.4 天和 41.7 天，中位总生存期仅为 51 天和 49 天——这也符合该研究的纳入标准，如患者已不适合接受手术或 SRS 治疗[4]。值得注意的是，该研究结果比早期 WBRT 临床试验（并非均有断层影像）报道的平均生存期提高了 1 个月。然而，QUARTZ 临床试验发现部分患者仍可从 WBRT 中获益——WBRT 可提高 60 岁以下患者的生存率。此外，总生存期与 RPA 评分、GPA 评分、患者体能状态及可控的原发肿瘤之间有非统计学差异的相关性。

然而，将以上研究结果应用于所有体能状态差的患者时仍需谨慎。因为临床研究招募患者时可能存在选择偏倚，目前仍缺乏准确测量颅内病灶负荷的手段，且上述研究中并未提及其他抗肿瘤治疗，也并未报道神经系统相关死亡率，此外，暂无脑转移特异性的生活质量评分量表，其结果可能受到脑部病灶以外的多种因素影响。尽管 WBRT 的适应证仍需进行个体化的判定，上述研究仍提示最佳支持治疗可作为体能状态差的患者的合理治疗手段。

Gaspar 和 Sperduto 等发现通过递归分区分析（recursive partitioning analysis，RPA）和分级预后评估（graded prognostic assessment，GPA）可预测预后，并建立了相关的预后评分系统以帮助选择患者[7, 8]。2017 年，Sperduto 等进一步更新了肺癌和黑色素瘤分子标志物的 GPA 分组[9, 10]。在黑色素瘤中，*BRAF* 基因突变是一个阳性预后因子，其他预后因素还包括脑转移的数量、颅外病灶负荷、年龄及患者体能状态等；在肺腺癌中，*EGFR* 和 *ALK* 的突变状态是重要的预后指标。值得注意的是，结合患者年龄、体能状态、颅外病灶负荷、脑转移瘤的数量、基因突变状态等各个方面，最佳的中位生存期可长达 46.8 个月。尽管许多因素表明此类患者可行 SRS 或手术切除等局部治疗，但对于不适合局部治疗的患者，在评估 WBRT 的可行性时仍需考虑 *BRAF* 和 *EGFR/ALK* 的突变情况。

2018年美国国家癌症综合网络（National Cancer Comprehensive Network，NCCN）指南指出：对于初诊、局限的脑转移且全身病情稳定的患者，WBRT和SRS均可作为有效治疗手段——尽管SRS是首选[11]。值得注意的是，"局限的脑转移"（limited brain metastases）的定义在不断发展和变化，尽管临床具体情况各有不同，但通常指的是颅内病灶的体积相对较小和数量相对较少。对于全身广泛转移但脑转移病灶局限者，如果系统治疗的选择有限，可考虑予以WBRT或最佳支持治疗；颅内广泛转移的患者则不再受病灶数量和大小的限制，均可选择WBRT或SRS，但体能状态好的患者应首选SRS。尽管NCCN指南中未明确说明，免疫治疗或靶向治疗等系统治疗方法同样可用于广泛脑转移，尤其是病灶小、无症状的患者。此外，WBRT仍然是某些肿瘤（如小细胞肺癌）的标准治疗方法。

四、全脑放疗的分割方式

全脑放疗最常见的分割方式为30Gy/10次或20Gy/5次[2, 12]。基于多项临床试验的共识，放疗剂量、时间和分割方式并不会显著影响患者的生存预后[13]，2018年的Cochrane综述也进一步证实等效生物学剂量更高的分割方式并未带来任何获益[12]。然而，3项临床试验的数据显示，相比于30Gy/10次的分割方式，20Gy/5次、10Gy/1次、12Gy/2次等分割方式的总生存率似乎更差（HR=1.21，P=0.01）。另外两项随机临床试验则比较了20Gy/5次和30Gy/10次两种分割方案，结果显示两组的总生存期和神经功能状况相似，但低剂量WBRT组的神经功能改善较差（HR=1.74）。

五、术后全脑放疗

在SRS出现之前，术后WBRT一直是孤立性脑转移患者术后的首选治疗手段。

1990年，Patchell等的一项随机对照临床试验指出，相比于活检和WBRT，手术切除可为孤立性脑转移病灶的患者带来生存获益[14]。手术后WBRT组和活检后WBRT组的中位生存期分别为40周和15周，局部复发率分别为20%和50%。1998年，Patchell等的另一项随机对照临床试验则比较了手术联合WBRT和单纯手术的疗效[15]，尽管两组中位生存期均有限（43周 vs. 48周），但接受了WBRT组的局部复发率显著下降（10% vs. 46%），虽然手术联合WBRT组和单纯手术组的总生存率和功能独立维持时间无明显差异，但两组的总体颅内复发率分别为18%和70%，神经系统死亡率分别为14%和44%。

1994年Noordijk等的另一项随机临床试验进一步验证了以上结果。该研究指出，在孤立性脑转移病灶中，手术联合WBRT对比单纯WBRT可明显提高患者的总生存时间（10个月 vs. 6个月）[16]。此外，患者年龄和颅外病灶负荷是强有力的预后因子。

近期，EORTC22952-26001试验将359名出现1~3个脑转移病灶且已接受局部治疗（手术切除或放射外科）的患者随机分为WBRT组和观察组[17]，两组的总生存时间相近，分别为10.9个月和10.7个月，但手术联合WBRT的术后2年局部复发率从59%下降至27%，SRS联合WBRT的术后2年局部复发率从31%下降至19%。WBRT还可降低颅内远处进展率，外科术后WBRT使得颅内远处进展率从42%降至23%，SRS后WBRT使得颅内远处进展率从48%降至33%。挽救治疗在观察组中更为常见，两组挽救治疗率分别为16%和51%。然而，两组的主要研究终点——功能独立持续时间并无明显差异，这可能得益于适时监测及时发现并治疗了无症状的复发灶和可致残的颅外疾病进展。

多项回顾性研究及两项随机临床试验证实，SRS作为脑转移瘤术后的治疗手段同样可为患者带来局控率的改善。2017年，Mahajan等指出1~3个颅内转移灶经手术完全切除后，术腔行术后辅助 SRS（平均剂量 16Gy，剂量范围 12~18Gy）组的瘤床复发率显著低于单纯观察组[18]，SRS 组和观察组的 1 年瘤床控制率分别为 72% 和 43%。值得注意的是，局控率随着肿瘤体积的增大而降低，肿瘤最大径＜ 2.5cm 的局控率可超过 90%，最大径为 2.5~3.5cm 的局控率约为 46%，最大径＞ 3.5cm 的局控率仅为 43%，而术后辅助 SRS 为不同体积的肿瘤均带来局控率的改善。第二项随机临床试验中，Brown 等发现与术后 SRS 相比，术后 WBRT 除提高瘤床控制率、颅内控制率以外，还明显增加了患者 6 个月时认知功能下降的概率（85% vs. 52%），提示 WBRT 在神经认知功能方面的负面影响显著大于对疾病进展的影响[19]。同样，该研究中 WBRT 也并未带来总生存的获益。Kayama 等于 2018 年发表的临床试验将颅内转移灶不足 4 个的患者随机分为手术联合术后 WBRT 组（WBRT 组）、不可切除部分接受 SRS 组或不可切除部分接受 MRI 监测后行挽救性 SRS 组（SRS/ 观察组）[20]，尽管 SRS/ 观察组的颅内无进展生存时间显著短于 WBRT 组（WBRT 组 10.4 个月，SRS/ 观察组 4 个月），但其总生存期不劣于 WBRT 组（两组均为 15.6 个月）。值得注意的是，WBRT 组中有 16.4% 的患者在治疗后 3 个月内出现 2~4 度认知功能障碍，而 SRS/ 观察组的发生率仅为 7.7%。

Kepka 等的一项 3 期随机临床试验表明术后辅助 SRS 和术后辅助 WBRT 的瘤床控制率无显著差别（分别为 74% 和 75%），并且神经相关死亡率也无明显差别[21]。然而，该临床试验的统计效力过低，其结论有待进一步验证。

综上所述，目前已发表的研究表明，对于仅有 1~3 个脑转移病灶的患者，术后 WBRT 与术后 SRS 的总生存时间相近，但前者毒性更大，因此 WBRT 可能并不是最佳的术后治疗手段。基于目前已有的数据，针对瘤床行 SRS 应成为 1~3 个脑转移瘤患者术后的标准治疗。

六、全脑放疗后的再程放疗

脑转移瘤接受 WBRT 后进展在临床上十分常见。一般来说，对于体能状态好且病灶局限的患者，可再次选择手术切除或挽救性 SRS 且适应证和禁忌证与初治时类似。但对于不适合挽救性局部治疗的患者，再程 WBRT 尽管剂量低且控制时间相对较短，仍可能带来一定的获益。

1996 年发表的早期观察性研究数据显示再程 WBRT 可使 71% 的患者症状得到改善，中位生存期为 4 个月[22]。该回顾性研究中，86 例患者在初次 WBRT（中位剂量为 30Gy）后再次接受了 WBRT（中位剂量为 20Gy）。患者的中位年龄为 58 岁，大部分患者 ECOG 评分为 2 分或 3 分。值得注意的是，该研究中严重不良反应的发生率较低，这可能是因为患者的总生存时间较短，尚不足以发现严重的神经认知毒性。与之一致的是，中位反应持续时间仅为 2.75 个月。

Ammrati 等在 2010 年发表的文章中回顾了初次 WBRT 后再次接受 WBRT 的相关数据[23]，三项回顾性研究分别纳入 52 例、72 例、86 例患者，中位生存期为 4~5.6 个月[22, 24, 25]，再程放疗的平均剂量为 20~25Gy，神经功能改善率为 31%~70%。长期毒性方面，两项研究各报道了 1 例由于再程 WBRT 而出现痴呆症状的病例。

Son、Scharp、Oagen、Guo 等分别发表了纳入 10 例、134 例、28 例及 49 例患者的回顾性研究[26-29]，这些研究中再程放疗的中位生存期为 2.8~5.2 个月，未出现严重的不良反应。其中，3 项研究中 51%~83% 患者的症状部分缓解或维持稳定，一项研究显示 39% 的患者症状得到改善，但未报道症状稳定的病例数。其他近期的相关研究数据总结见表 12-1。

Logie 等回顾性分析了来自多中心的 205 例患者[30]，RPA Ⅰ类的患者接受再程 WBRT 后的中位生存期为 7.5 个月，RPA Ⅱ类和Ⅲ类患者分别为 5.2 个月和 2.9 个月。KPS 评分＜ 80、颅外

表 12-1　全脑放疗后再次接受全脑放疗的研究汇总

研究者	年份	病例数	中位年龄	初次放疗中位剂量（Gy）	再程放疗中位剂量（Gy）	疗效	中位 OS（月）
Wong 等	1996	86	58	30	20	临床症状缓解或改善 –70%	4
Cooper 等	1990	52	57.3	30	25	2～4 周维持稳定或临床症状改善 –94%	5
Sadikov 等	2007	72	56.5	20	25	维持稳定或临床症状改善 –73%	4.1
Son 等	2012	10	59（平均）	35	21.6	症状缓解或临床症状改善 –80%	5.2
Scharp 等	2014	134	57	30	20	维持稳定或临床症状改善 –83%	2.8
Ozgen 等	2013	28	52	30	25	症状缓解或临床症状改善 –39%	3
Guo 等	2016	49	56	30	20	神经功能症状稳定或缓解 –51%	3
Logie 等	2017	205	55	20	20	—	3.6

肿瘤负荷、两次放疗的间歇期 < 9 个月、小细胞组织学类型及无法控制的原发灶均与更短的中位生存期密切相关。

值得注意的是，可能由于患者的生存期有限，再程放疗的严重不良反应发生率相对较低[31]。而新的系统治疗手段在为患者带来更长生存获益的同时，也增加了发生晚期神经认知毒性的风险，再程放疗是否仍然具有低毒性仍待进一步证实。

七、立体定向外科治疗后的挽救性全脑放疗

脑转移瘤行 SRS 后进展、不能二次局部治疗的患者可考虑 WBRT。通常情况下，除在初治时已接近最高耐受剂量的脑干、视交叉等重要器官外，其他部位在 SRS 后行 WBRT 无须改变剂量及分割方式。

八、软脑膜病变

软脑膜转移（图 12-4）往往意味着不良预后，且大部分患者常合并有全身进展性疾病[32]，因此对于这部分患者，尤其当伴有严重的脑神经受损时，治疗的主要目的仅为缓解症状和维持生活质量。一般来说，单纯依赖激素治疗不足以控制软脑膜转移的并发症，而 WBRT 可通过缩小肿瘤体积、恢复脑脊液流量而起到一定的姑息性治疗目的[31]。

目前仍然缺乏 WBRT 有效缓解软脑膜转移瘤症状的确切数据。一项纳入 27 例乳腺癌和肺癌患者的回顾性研究显示，软脑膜转移行 WBRT 的中位总生存期仅为 8.1 周[33]。由于预后不佳，仅有 4 例患者有 MR 随访资料，其中 3 例的影像学表现有所改善，而生活质量的相关结果未见报道。

另一项纳入了 125 例非小细胞肺癌患者的研究则显示 WBRT 不能改善软脑膜转移患者的总生存[34]。值得注意的是，研究中有 34% 的患者有颅高压的症状，中位总生存时间为 3 个月，WBRT 的剂量范围为 30Gy/10 次至 37.5Gy/15 次。同样，该研究也未报道生活质量或症状缓解的相关数据。

总的来说，尽管缺乏生活质量相关的确切证据，WBRT 可能有助于缓解软脑膜转移患者的症状。

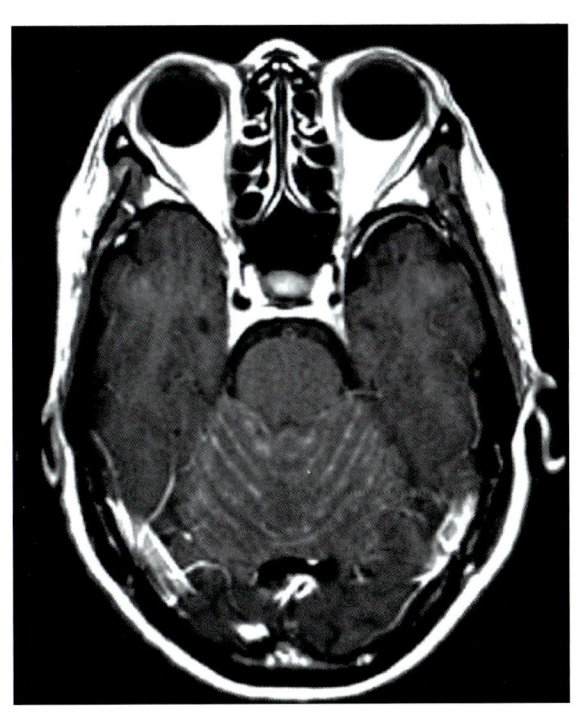

▲ 图 12-4 非小细胞肺癌患者颅后窝的软脑膜转移

表 12-2 预防性头部放疗研究汇总

分期	研究	生存预后	结果(%)
局限期	Meta 分析	PCI 后 3 年 OS	20
	Auperin 等	未接受 PCI 的 3 年 OS	15
		接受 PCI 的脑转移风险	33
		未接受 PCI 的脑转移风险	59
广泛期	随机临床试验	PCI 后 1 年 OS	27
		未接受 PCI 的 1 年 OS	13
	EORTC2007	接受 PCI 的 1 年有症状脑转移发生率	15
		未接受 PCI 的 1 年有症状脑转移发生率	40
	随机临床试验	PCI 后 1 年 OS	48
	Takahashi 等	未接受 PCI 的 1 年 OS	54
MRI 分期		有 MRI 分期的脑转移概率	48
		无 MRI 分期的脑转移概率	69

九、预防性头部放疗

预防性 WBRT 是小细胞肺癌的标准治疗手段之一，表 12-2 中归纳了相关的随机临床研究和系统性综述研究。

Auperin 等关于局限期小细胞肺癌的 Meta 分析发现，预防性头部放疗（prophylactic cranial irradiation，PCI）可将 3 年总生存率从 15.3% 提高至 20.7%，将脑转移风险从 59% 降低至 33%，同时还可提高患者的无病生存率[35]。值得注意的是，该研究中患者的肺部病灶在治疗后达到完全缓解，但研究中并未规范行 MRI 检查，治疗前也未常规进行 CT 扫描。

在广泛期小细胞肺癌方面，一项发表于 2007 年的 EORTC 临床研究指出 PCI 在提高总生存率的同时（1 年总生存率分别为 27% 和 13%）还有效地降低了有症状脑转移的发生率（1 年脑转移发生率分别为 15% 和 40%）[36]。因此，PCI 被认为是广泛期小细胞肺癌系统治疗有效后的标准治疗手段。然而，近期一项随机临床研究要求患者每 3 个月行头部 MRI 检查，其结果显示对于 MRI 无明显病灶的患者而言，PCI 与观察组的总生存率无明显差异（1 年总生存率分别为 48% 和 54%）[37]，但 PCI 仍可将脑转移的发生率从 69% 降至 48%。值得注意的是，58% 的患者接受观察后延迟了开始头部放疗的时间。该研究最主要局限性是在于参与试验的中心每年只招募约 1 例患者。因此，广泛期小细胞肺癌患者也可以将观察随访作为另一种选择，但目前尚未纳入实践标准。

为进一步指导放疗剂量及分割方式，一项随机临床试验比较分析了 25Gy/10 次的分割方式和高剂量的分割方式（36Gy/18 次和 36Gy/24 次每日两次的超分割方式），结果显示高剂量的放疗方式并未带来临床获益[38]。2012 年 RTOG0212 的一项研究指出，接受 36Gy 放疗患者发生慢性神经毒性的概率显著高于仅接受 25Gy 的患者[39]。因此，25Gy 的 PCI 仍然是目前的标准治疗模式。

PCI 在非小细胞肺癌中也有研究，但纳入了 356 例患者的 RTOG 临床研究显示其并未给总生存或无病生存带来获益[40]。因此，非小细胞肺癌并未常规推荐进行 PCI。值得注意的是，与小细胞肺癌的数据相比，非小细胞肺癌脑转移的概率相对较低，接受 PCI 或观察组的脑转移率分别为 7.7% 和 18%。

十、1~3 个脑转移瘤：WBRT±SRS

随着 SRS 的问世以及研究指出 WBRT 产生的迟发性神经认知毒性，WBRT 在脑转移治疗中的作用逐渐减弱，尤其在脑转移局限患者中更为显著。

RTOG9508 临床试验将初诊时 1~3 个脑转移瘤的患者随机分为两组：WBRT+SRS 组和 WBRT 组[41]。结果显示对于仅有 1 个不可切除的脑转移瘤的患者而言，WBRT+SRS 组的生存时间更长，KPS 评分得到明显改善，而两组的神经毒性无明显差别。2014 年发表的 RTOG9508 二次分析数据则指出，对于 GPA 评分 3.5 分~4 分的患者，WBRT+SRS 可使具有 1~3 个脑转移病灶的患者生存获益[42]，而对于 GPA 评分较低的患者则无此优势。

Patil 等发表的一项 Cochrane 系统综述比较了 WBRT 联合 SRS 与单纯 WBRT 的效果，其结果也证实了上述结论[43]。对于单个脑转移直径＜3cm 且原发病可控的患者，WBRT+SRS 不仅可显著提高患者的局控率、总生存率，还可改善患者的体能状态和对激素治疗的需求（6 个月时 KPS 保持不变的概率分别为 43% 和 28%）。值得注意的是，WBRT+SRS 在总的研究人群（包括脑转移病灶＞1 个的患者）中未发现明显生存获益。

十一、1~4 个脑转移瘤：SRS±WBRT

上述研究数据指出 WBRT 联合 SRS 可为 1~3 个脑转移病灶的患者带来明显获益。本节将基于非劣性生存和降低延迟神经认知功能毒性等方面评估未行 WBRT 的循证医学依据。

NCCTG N0574 临床研究（一项在 1~3 个脑转移病灶患者中比较 SRS 联合或不联合 WBRT 的 3 期随机对照临床试验）及 MD Anderson 癌症中心的研究数据均表明 SRS 后辅以 WBRT 会导致治疗后认知功能下降[44, 45]。尽管加用 WBRT 后颅内疾病控制有改善，但两组在总生存期方面并无明显差别。单独 SRS 组的 1 年 CNS 进展率更高，分别为（73% vs. 27%，35% vs. 12%）。此外，N0574 研究提示 SRS+WBRT 可导致瞬时回忆、记忆力及语言流利度等方面的缺陷（92% vs. 64%），MD Aderson 的研究也指出 SRS+WBRT 引起学习和记忆功能的下降。因此，SRS 后避免接受 WBRT 可能有助于减少神经认知毒性，缩短患者的恢复时间，并有利于尽快重启系统治疗。

Churilla 等对 NCCTG N0574 研究中预后较好的非小细胞肺癌患者进行了亚组分析，结果指出尽管 WBRT+SRS 可提高颅内病灶控制率，但 WBRT+SRS 组与 SRS 组的总生存时间并无明显差异[46]。这一结果与 JROSG-99 临床试验的结果不符，后者表明在预后较好的非小细胞肺癌患者中，WBRT+SRS 可以带来明显的总生存获益[47]。然而，考虑到日本人群中 EGFR 突变阳性率高而预后更好，综合两项研究结果可得出结论：WBRT+SRS 在西方人群中不能带来总生存的获益，即使单纯 SRS 的颅内复发率较高，但仍有挽救治疗可供选择。

日本另一项临床试验纳入了 132 例有 1~4 个脑转移病灶的患者，比较单纯 SRS 和 WBRT 联合 SRS 的疗效。结果显示 WBRT+SRS 组较 SRS 组局控率更高，分别为 89% 和 73%[48]，颅内远处转移率更低，分别为 42% 和 64%。与其他临床试验结果相一致的是，两组的总生存率无明显区别，神经系统死亡率也无明显差异。另一项常用于评价两组间差别的指标为功能独立性，EORTC 22952-26001 研究针对性地评估了 WBRT+SRS 组和 SRS 组功能独立性的持续时间，结果显示两组并无明显差别[17]，总生存期也相近。

一项纳入 3 项随机对照临床试验的 Meta 分析（共纳入 364 例患者）比较了 SRS 联合或不联合 WBRT 在 1~4 个脑转移患者中的疗效，结果显示孤立脑转移的总生存期更长且远处脑转移率更低[49]，年龄与疗效有相关性——尤其对于 50 岁以下的患者来说，尽管 SRS 联合 WBRT 的颅内控制率更高，总生存率却更差。这可能是由于 SRS 治疗后挽救性治疗的有效性，以及 WBRT 导致系统治疗的延迟。值得注意的是，相比于病灶进展后再行 WBRT，SRS 后行辅助 WBRT 可降低神经相关性死亡的风险，尽管无明显的统计学差异，但这一结果在 50 岁以下的人群中表现最为明显，神经系统相关死亡风险从 39% 降至 22%。这也提示尽管辅助 WBRT 的作用尚不明确，但在某些高风险人群中仍可能起到一定的作用。

SRS 联合 WBRT 所涉及的时间因素也可能对患者的疗效产生影响。Chang 等发现与接受 SRS+WBRT 的患者相比，仅接受 SRS 的患者可提前至少 1 个月接受系统治疗[45]，即平均多接受至少 2 周期的系统治疗。

EORTC 22952-26001 研究的数据指出，在有 1~3 个脑转移瘤的患者中，单纯局部治疗（手术或放射外科）的生活质量明显高于局部治疗联合 WBRT[50]，尤其表现在以下几方面：9 个月时的整体健康状况、2 个月时的身体功能及疲劳、12 个月时的认知功能等——提示 WBRT 不仅单纯影响早期或晚期的某个时间点。WBRT 的不良反应主要包括脱发、食欲减退、纳差、嗜睡及社交功能障碍等。

基于以上研究结果，体能状态尚可且有限的脑转移患者的标准治疗为单纯 SRS。额外的 WBRT 不仅没有改善患者的总生存率，反而因不良反应的增加而降低了患者的生活质量。即使仅行 SRS，也可在治疗后通过 MRI 监测而发现早期无症状的脑转移病灶，并且在患者病情恶化前进行有效的挽救性治疗。

十二、未来研究方向：4 个以上的脑转移瘤

由于早期观察性数据指出 SRS 也可应用于 4 个以上的脑转移病灶，WBRT 在脑转移瘤中的作用在未来仍会继续发生变化，相关随机临床研究仍在进行中。

2014 年，Yamamoto 等发表了一项多中心前瞻性观察性研究（JLGK0901），旨在探讨单纯 SRS 在 1~10 个脑转移病灶中的作用[51, 52]。研究发现若颅内病灶体积局限，患者的脑转移数目与其预后不相关，当患者 KPS ≥ 80 分且肿瘤总体积 ≤ 15cm³ 时，SRS 是一种合适的治疗手段。仅有 9% 的患者接受了挽救性 WBRT，5~10 个脑转移瘤与 2~4 个脑转移瘤的总生存期相近（均为 10.8 个月），神经性死亡率相近（分别为 4.3% 和 1.7%），颅内远处进展率相近（分别为 63.8% 和 54.5%）。值得注意的是，12 个月时超过 90% 的患者和 48 个月时超过 86% 的患者的简易智力状况检查（mini-mental state examination，MMSE）评分与基线相似。此外，无论是孤立转移病灶、2~4 个转移灶还是 5~10 个转移灶，不良反应发生率均无明显差别（约 12% 的患者出现不同程度的不良反应；2%~3% 的患者出现 3 度或以上的不良反应）。

目前尚无发表的随机对照研究比较 SRS+/- WBRT 在 4 个以上脑转移瘤中的作用。MD Anderson 的一项研究旨在探索 SRS 或 WBRT 在 4~15 个脑转移病灶中的作用（NCT01592968），荷兰的一项临床试验也试图比较 WBRT 和 SRS 在 4~10 个脑转移瘤中的疗效，主要研究终点是治疗 3 个月时的生活质量（NCT02353000）[53]。如果这些临床研究能取得阳性结果，WBRT 在多发脑转移中的作用将被进一步削弱。

十三、具有中枢神经系统活性的系统治疗在脑转移中的作用

靶向治疗和免疫治疗能增加血脑屏障的渗透性，在部分患者中可影响 WBRT 的作用[54]。这些治疗在大部分常见脑转移（如非小细胞肺癌、黑色素瘤等）中的作用越来越重要[5, 55]。总的来说，体积小、无症状的脑转移患者更适合接受系统治疗，如图 12-5 所示。

以黑色素瘤为代表，免疫治疗、靶向治疗已改变多种恶性肿瘤（包括脑转移瘤）的原有治疗模式。研究证实达拉菲尼、维莫菲尼和曲美替尼对 BRAF 突变的脑转移瘤具有一定的治疗效果。早期研究指出，尽管达拉菲尼、维莫菲尼单药治疗脑转移的无进展生存期未超过 4 个月，但肿瘤反应率为 6.7%～39%[56, 57]。而达拉菲尼与口服 MEK 抑制药曲美替尼相结合的疗效更加显著[58]，颅内反应率为 44%～60%，颅内无进展生存期为 5～7 个月。

伊匹木单抗是一种抗 CTLA-4 的单克隆抗体，在无症状黑色素瘤脑转移中的反应率为 24%[59]。但临床上常用于控制患者症状的激素可显著降低其效力，使用激素后有效率仅为 10%。此外，中位颅内无进展生存时间仅为 6 周。迄今为止，最有前景的免疫治疗可能是以帕博利珠单抗为代表的抗 PD-L1 抗体。2016 年，Goldberg 等发现帕博利珠单抗在黑色素瘤患者中的颅内反应率为 22%，而在病灶大小不足 1.9cm 的非小细胞肺癌中反应率为 33%[60]。近期，一项随机 II 期临床研究指出纳武利尤单抗联合伊匹木单抗的反应率可达到 46%，而纳武利尤单抗和伊匹木单抗单药治疗时的反应率分别为 20% 和 6%[61]。54% 接受双药联合治疗的患者出现 3 度或以上的不良反应。在靶向治疗后进展的 BRAF 突变患者中，联合免疫治疗的反应率仅为 16%，提示这部分患者不良的生物学行为。而对于软脑膜转移或正在接受激素治疗的患者，其反应率不足 10%。一项单臂 II 期临床试验进一步证实了上述结果，94 例无症状患者接受上述系统治疗后，58% 的患者病灶有效，其中 2% 的患者维持稳定、30% 获得部分缓

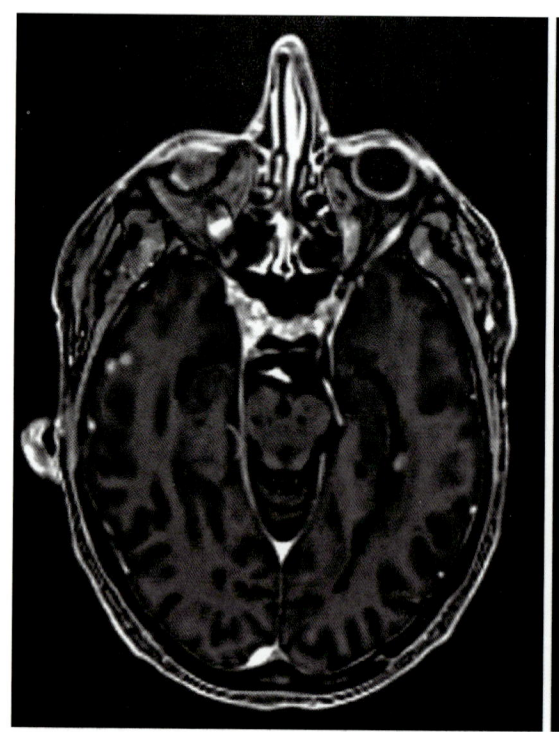

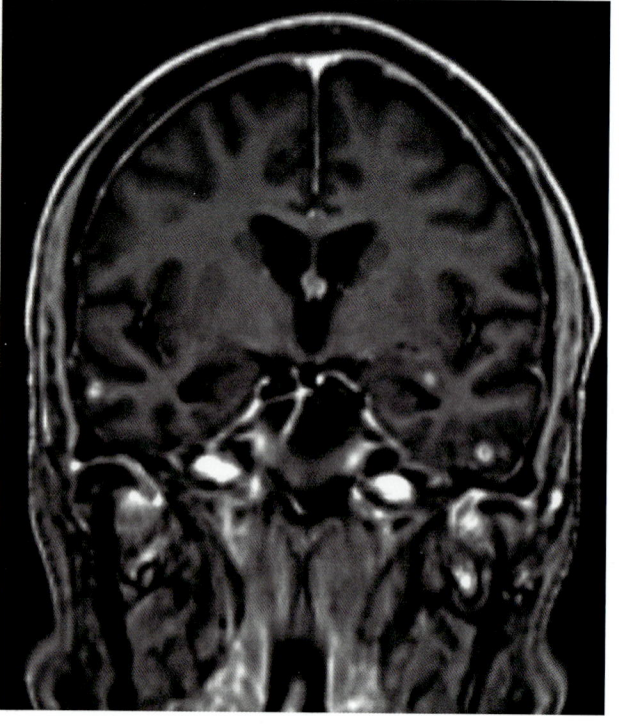

▲ 图 12-5　脑转移病灶较小、适合靶向治疗的患者头部 MRI

解、26%达到完全缓解[62]，76%的患者仅有1～2个脑转移瘤，最大者直径约为3cm，55%的患者出现3度或3度以上的不良反应，该结论与其他研究结果相一致。

因此，免疫治疗和靶向治疗适用于无症状且病灶位于非语言中枢的转移性黑色素瘤，即使病灶进展也不会立即出现严重症状。此外，鉴于目前研究报道的PFS有限，需要重视MRI随访监测的重要性，若病灶进展或复发，SRS或WBRT也可作为挽救治疗手段。

常规化疗方案难以透过肺癌患者的血脑屏障[63]。Sperduto等在一项Ⅲ期RTOG临床试验中探索替莫唑胺或厄洛替尼联合WBRT和SRS在非小细胞肺癌中的作用[64]。由于纳入病例数有限，研究并未发现总生存获益，且不良反应增加，结果显示出无统计学差异的不良反应（13.4个月 vs. 6.3个月和6.1个月）。

靶向治疗对EGFR突变和ALK基因重排非小细胞肺癌的脑转移同样有效，这使体积小、无症状脑转移的治疗模式发生了巨大变化[54, 65, 66]，然而，这仅仅是小部分非小细胞肺癌患者，尤其西方人群中EGFR和ALK的突变更为罕见。对于EGFR突变的NSCLC，厄洛替尼、吉非替尼和奥希替尼的颅内反应率相对较高，约为50%～80%，PFS为6～12个月。对于ALK重排的NSCLC，克唑替尼的颅内反应率约为20%，而阿来替尼、布加替尼、色瑞替尼等新药可将反应率提高至50%～70%[67-70]，其中布加替尼可使颅内PFS高达18个月。因此，对于EGFR突变和ALK重排的NSCLC，若患者无明显症状且肿瘤体积较小，可通过系统治疗及密切随访取得较好疗效时，WBRT或SRS可适当延迟。挽救性SRS或WBRT的疗效目前仍不确切。免疫治疗在无驱动基因突变的NSCLC脑转移治疗中的作用仍需进一步探讨，有待更确切的数据予以支持。

另一方面，尽管有上述研究，但在考虑放弃脑部放疗时仍需谨慎。2016年发表的回顾性研究数据指出EGFR突变的NSCLC中推迟放疗与较短的总生存期相关[71]。尽管该研究中纳入的大部分临床试验仅为Ⅱ期的单臂研究，但大部分药物的反应持续时间相对较短。2017年研究团队更新数据指出接受SRS、WBRT以及EGFR-TKI的初治患者的中位OS分别为46个月、30个月和25个月[72]。这一研究结果更加突出了前瞻性随机研究数据指导最佳治疗顺序的重要性，而最佳的治疗时机和治疗顺序同样有待明确。临床上制定治疗决策时，需要全面考虑各项临床指标，包括病灶大小、部位、颅内及颅外肿瘤负荷、系统性治疗的预期疗效、疾病进展速度等。

靶向治疗在HER2阳性乳腺癌的脑转移中同样有效。Ⅱ期临床试验LANDSCAPE研究指出，在45例HER2阳性转移性乳腺癌患者中，拉帕替尼和卡培他滨治疗脑转移病灶的反应率达65.9%[73]，尽管有49%的患者出现3或4度不良反应，中位颅内无进展生存率可达5.5个月。而在这之前的研究结果则令人沮丧，Freedman等的一项前瞻性临床试验表明，40例HER2阳性转移性乳腺癌患者接受来那替尼后CNS的客观缓解率仅为8%，中位PFS为1.9个月（每2个月规律复查影像学资料），3度不良反应发生率超过20%[74]。

系统治疗与放疗的最佳治疗顺序仍有待进一步探讨。2016年Kroeze等发表的一项综述研究指出靶向治疗或免疫治疗联合立体定向放疗的耐受性好，且增加的不良反应发生率较低，仅联合BRAF抑制药的严重不良反应发生率较高[75]。然而，帕博利珠单抗、纳武利尤单抗等免疫治疗的数据仍然有限。因此，临床医生在治疗前后仍需保持谨慎并与肿瘤内科医生保持密切联系。

十四、神经毒性和避免照射海马的全脑放疗（HA-WBRT）

WBRT主要的不良反应之一就是迟发的神经认知功能毒性。然而，颅内病灶进展同样可对认知功能造成影响，有时甚至超过治疗所带来的不良反应。早期评估 WBRT 后神经认知功能的研究中大部分脑转移患者生存期不超过 6 个月[76]，尽管如此，与 WBRT 相关的痴呆非常罕见，但在单次高剂量照射（＞3.5Gy）或总剂量高时症状较为突出[77]。这一点在问询患者时值得引起重视。

研究指出放疗对神经干细胞造成的损伤，尤其是对海马区的损伤，可导致放疗后认知功能的下降[78, 79]。IMRT 的出现使放疗可适形地避开海马神经干细胞区域，即避免照射海马的 WBRT（hippocampal-avoidance WBRT HA-WBRT）[80, 81]。表 12-3[82, 83] 中列出了 HA-WBRT 的技术要求，图 12-6 和图 12-7 分别显示出 HA-WBRT 的靶区勾画和剂量分布。

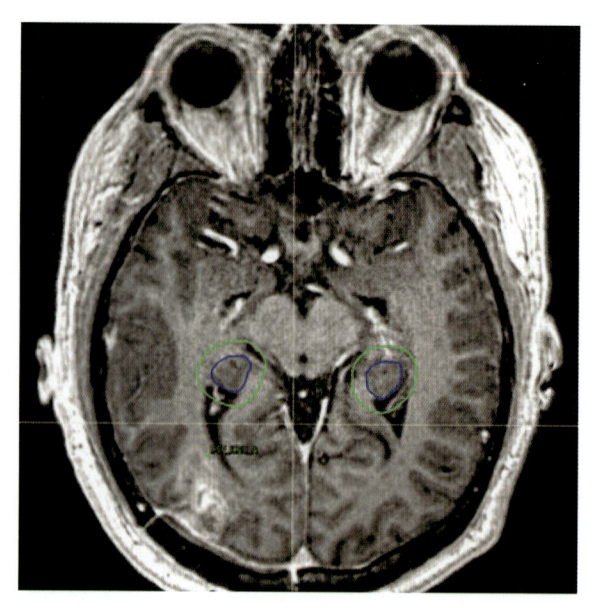

▲ 图 12-6 MRI 海马区的靶区勾画

表 12-3 HA-WBRT 的要求和剂量限制

	要 求
影像学	3D 轴向薄层 MRI（＜1.5mm）
定位	与放疗计划 CT 融合（≤2.5mm）
技术	调强适形放疗（IMRT），旋转容积调强放疗（VMAT），螺旋断层放疗
靶区勾画	勾画海马
	避免照射海马的靶区（海马区外扩 5mm）
剂量限制	海马：最大剂量 16Gy
	海马：＜9Gy 100%
	避免照射海马的靶区：最大剂量 30Gy

为了证明 HA-WBRT 的有效性，Ⅱ 期单臂的 RTOG0933 临床试验发现接受 HA-WBRT 后霍普金斯语言学习测试修订版（hopkins verbal learning test-Revised，HVLT-R）的延迟回忆相对于基线下降 7%，远低于传统 WBRT 的 30%[82]。此外，生活质量评分并无明显下降。基于该研究结果，海马区的平均推荐剂量为＜9Gy，最大剂量＜16Gy。具体剂量限制见表 12-3。

Gondi 等的前瞻性研究进一步指导了海马区

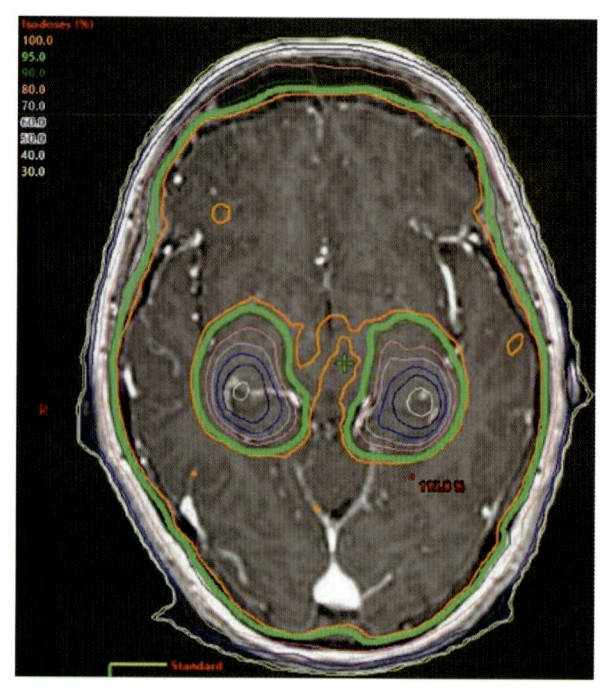

▲ 图 12-7 HA-WBRT 的剂量分布

的剂量限制，该研究在接受立体定向放疗的良性或低级别脑肿瘤患者中评估了海马剂量和长期神经认知功能之间的关系[84]，指出双侧海马区达到 7.3Gy（2Gy 分割的等效剂量）的体积≥40% 与 18 个月时延迟回忆的受损相关。

RTOG 0614 等研究报道了美金刚（Memantine）等放射保护剂的应用。这项多中心的随机对照研究发现在进行 WBRT 时应用 N- 甲基 –D- 天冬氨酸（NMDA）受体拮抗药美金刚并未显著降低 24 周时延迟回忆的下降率[85]，但美金刚组认知功能下降的时间明显长于对照组（24 周时分别为 54% 和 65%），并且具有更高的执行功能、处理速度和延迟识别，不良反应较小。但鉴于大部分患者在 24 周时出现进展或死亡导致仅 149 例患者可供分析，该研究结果仍存在一定的不确定性。

NCT02360215 的初步结果近期发表[86]。这是一项比较美金刚联合 WBRT 和美金刚联合 HA-WBRT 的 III 期临床试验，主要研究终点是神经认知衰竭的时间。截至 2018 年 10 月，结果指出美金刚联合常规 WBRT 和联合 HA-WBRT 具有相近的颅内控制率和总生存率，但后者的神经认知功能衰竭率有所下降：6 个月时的神经认知功能衰竭率由 69.1% 下降至 58%。该结果也有待更全面的数据予以证实。

NCT02635009 研究将探索 HA-WBRT 在小细胞肺癌预防性颅内放疗中的应用，主要研究终点之一是情景记忆的受损时间。

综上所述，尽管研究仍在进行，早期数据已提示海马保护、美金刚等对神经认知功能可起到一定的保护作用，但其对 WBRT 的作用仍然未知，而对 SRS 在 4~15 个脑转移病灶中的作用也仍在研究中。

> **要 点**
>
> - 随着放射外科和系统治疗的发展以及其良好的疗效和毒性管理，WBRT 在脑转移中的作用已逐渐弱化。SRS 已取代 WBRT 成为有限数目的脑转移瘤患者的标准治疗。
> - 对于不适合 SRS 且体能状态良好的患者，WBRT 仍具有一定作用——尤其对于软脑膜转移和小细胞肺癌的颅内预防性照射。此外，WBRT 还可用于 SRS 或 WBRT 后的再程放疗，但这些患者的预后通常很差。
> - 体能状态差的患者需根据自身各项因素综合评估是否行最佳支持治疗代替 WBRT。靶向治疗和免疫治疗可作为小体积、无症状的脑转移瘤患者有效治疗手段，部分患者可在病灶进展后再行 SRS 和 WBRT。但暂缓放疗的决策仍需谨慎，需遵循个体化治疗的原则，并积极开展与肿瘤内科医生、神经外科医生的多学科合作。
> - 研究指出 HA-WBRT 不仅可以避免照射海马有助于改善 WBRT 所致的延迟神经毒性，而且能带来明显获益。SRS 和 WBRT 在 4~15 个脑转移瘤中的研究仍在进行，可能会进一步影响脑转移的治疗模式，尤其是 WBRT 的地位，其结果值得期待。

参考文献

[1] Borgelt B, Gelber R, Kramer S, Brady LW, Chang CH, Davis LW, Perez CA, Hendrickson FR. The palliation of brain metastases: final results of the first two studies by the Radiation Therapy Oncology Group. Int J Radiat Oncol Biol Phys. 1980;6(1):1–9.

[2] Pease NJ, Edwards A, Moss LJ. Effectiveness of whole brain radiotherapy in the treatment of brain metastases: a systematic review. Palliat Med. 2005;19(4):288–99.

[3] Moraes FY, Taunk NK, Marta GN, Suh JH, Yamada Y. The rationale for targeted therapies and stereotactic radiosurgery in the treatment of brain metastases. Oncologist. 2016;21(2):244–51.

[4] Mulvenna P, Nankivell M, Barton R, Faivre-Finn C, Wilson P, McColl E, Moore B, Brisbane I, Ardron D, Holt T, Morgan S, Lee C, Waite K, Bayman N, Pugh C, Sydes B, Stephens R, Parmar MK, Langley RE. Dexamethasone and supportive care with or without whole brain radiotherapy in treating patients with non-small cell lung cancer with brain metastases unsuitable for resection or stereotactic radiotherapy (QUARTZ): results from a phase 3, non-inferiority, randomised trial. Lancet. 2016;388(10055):2004–14.

[5] Delattre JY, Krol G, Thaler HT, Posner JB. Distribution of brain

[6] McTyre E, Scott J, Chinnaiyan P. Whole brain radiotherapy for brain metastasis. Surg Neurol Int. 2013;4(Suppl 4):S236–44.

[7] Gaspar L, Scott C, Rotman M, Asbell S, Phillips T, Wasserman T, McKenna WG, Byhardt R. Recursive partitioning analysis (RPA) of prognostic factors in three Radiation Therapy Oncology Group (RTOG) brain metastases trials. Int J Radiat Oncol Biol Phys. 1997;37(4):745–51.

[8] Sperduto PW, Kased N, Roberge D, Xu Z, Shanley R, Luo X, Sneed PK, Chao ST, Weil RJ, Suh J, Bhatt A, Jensen AW, Brown PD, Shih HA, Kirkpatrick J, Gaspar LE, Fiveash JB, Chiang V, Knisely JP, Sperduto CM, Lin N, Mehta M. Summary report on the graded prognostic assessment: an accurate and facile diagnosis-specific tool to estimate survival for patients with brain metastases. J Clin Oncol. 2012;30(4):419–25.

[9] Sperduto PW, Jiang W, Brown PD, Braunstein S, Sneed P, Wattson DA, Shih HA, Bangdiwala A, Shanley R, Lockney NA, Beal K, Lou E, Amatruda T, Sperduto WA, Kirkpatrick JP, Yeh N, Gaspar LE, Molitoris JK, Masucci L, Roberge D, Yu J, Chiang V, Mehta M. Estimating survival in melanoma patients with brain metastases: an update of the graded prognostic assessment for melanoma using molecular markers (melanoma-molGPA). Int J Radiat Oncol Biol Phys. 2017;99(4):812–6.

[10] Sperduto PW, Yang TJ, Beal K, Pan H, Brown PD, Bangdiwala A, Shanley R, Yeh N, Gaspar LE, Braunstein S, Sneed P, Boyle J, Kirkpatrick JP, Mak KS, Shih HA, Engelman A, Roberge D, Arvold ND, Alexander B, Awad MM, Contessa J, Chiang V, Hardie J, Ma D, Lou E, Sperduto W, Mehta MP. Estimating survival in patients with lung cancer and brain metastases: an update of the graded prognostic assessment for lung cancer using molecular markers (lung-molGPA). JAMA Oncol. 2017;3(6):827–31.

[11] National Comprehensive Cancer Network. Central nervous system cancers (version 1. 2018). https://www.nccn.org/professionals/physician_gls/pdf/cns.pdf. Accessed 22 Oct 2018.

[12] Tsao MN, Xu W, Wong RK, Lloyd N, Laperriere N, Sahgal A, Rakovitch E, Chow E. Whole brain radiotherapy for the treatment of newly diagnosed multiple brain metastases. Cochrane Database Syst Rev. 2018;1:CD003869.

[13] Khuntia D, Brown P, Li J, Mehta MP. Whole-brain radiotherapy in the management of brain metastasis. J Clin Oncol. 2006;24(8):1295–304.

[14] Patchell RA, Tibbs PA, Walsh JW, Dempsey RJ, Maruyama Y, Kryscio RJ, Markesbery WR, Macdonald JS, Young B. A randomized trial of surgery in the treatment of single metastases to the brain. N Engl J Med. 1990;322(8):494–500.

[15] Patchell RA, Tibbs PA, Regine WF, Dempsey RJ, Mohiuddin M, Kryscio RJ, Markesbery WR, Foon KA, Young B. Postoperative radiotherapy in the treatment of single metastases to the brain: a randomized trial. JAMA. 1998;280(17):1485–9.

[16] Noordijk EM, Vecht CJ, Haaxma-Reiche H, Padberg GW, Voormolen JH, Hoekstra FH, Tans JT, Lambooij N, Metsaars JA, Wattendorff AR, et al. The choice of treatment of single brain metastasis should be based on extracranial tumor activity and age. Int J Radiat Oncol Biol Phys. 1994;29(4):711–7.

[17] Kocher M, Soffietti R, Abacioglu U, Villà S, Fauchon F, Baumert BG, Fariselli L, Tzuk-Shina T, Kortmann RD, Carrie C, Ben Hassel M, Kouri M, Valeinis E, van den Berge D, Collette S, Collette L, Mueller RP. Adjuvant whole-brain radiotherapy versus observation after radiosurgery or surgical resection of one to three cerebral metastases: results of the EORTC 22 952–26 001 study. J Clin Oncol. 2011;29(2):134–41.

[18] Mahajan A, Ahmed S, McAleer MF, Weinberg JS, Li J, Brown P, Settle S, Prabhu SS, Lang FF, Levine N, McGovern S, Sulman E, McCutcheon IE, Azeem S, Cahill D, Tatsui C, Heimberger AB, Ferguson S, Ghia A, Demonte F, Raza S, Guha-Thakurta N, Yang J, Sawaya R, Hess KR, Rao G. Post-operative stereotactic radiosurgery versus observation for completely resected brain metastases: a single-centre, randomised, controlled, phase 3 trial. Lancet Oncol. 2017;18(8):1040–8.

[19] Brown PD, Ballman KV, Cerhan JH, Anderson SK, Carrero XW, Whitton AC, Greenspoon J, Parney IF, Laack NNI, Ashman JB, Bahary JP, Hadjipanayis CG, Urbanic JJ, Barker FG 2nd, Farace E, Khuntia D, Giannini C, Buckner JC, Galanis E, Roberge D. Postoperative stereotactic radiosurgery compared with whole brain radiotherapy for resected metastatic brain disease (NCCTG N107C/CEC·3): a multicentre, randomised, controlled, phase 3 trial. Lancet Oncol. 2017;18(8):1049–60.

[20] Kayama T, Sato S, Sakurada K, Mizusawa J, Nishikawa R, Narita Y, Sumi M, Miyakita Y, Kumabe T, Sonoda Y, Arakawa Y, Miyamoto S, Beppu T, Sugiyama K, Nakamura H, Nagane M, Nakasu Y, Hashimoto N, Terasaki M, Matsumura A, Ishikawa E, Wakabayashi T, Iwadate Y, Ohue S, Kobayashi H, Kinoshita M, Asano K, Mukasa A, Tanaka K, Asai A, Nakamura H, Abe T, Muragaki Y, Iwasaki K, Aoki T, Watanabe T, Sasaki H, Izumoto S, Mizoguchi M, Matsuo T, Takeshima H, Hayashi M, Jokura H, Mizowaki T, Shimizu E, Shirato H, Tago M, Katayama H, Fukuda H, Shibui S, Japan Clinical Oncology Group. Effects of surgery with salvage stereotactic radiosurgery versus surgery with whole-brain radiation therapy in patients with one to four brain metastases (JCOG0504): a phase III, noninferiority, randomized controlled trial. J Clin Oncol. 2018:JCO2018786186.

[21] Kępka L, Tyc-Szczepaniak D, Bujko K, Olszyna-Serementa M, Michalski W, Sprawka A, Trąbska-Kluch B, Komosińska K, Wasilewska-Teśluk E, Czeremszyńska B. Stereotactic radiotherapy of the tumor bed compared to whole brain radiotherapy after surgery of single brain metastasis: results from a randomized trial. Radiother Oncol. 2016;121(2):217–24.

[22] Wong WW, Schild SE, Sawyer TE, Shaw EG. Analysis of outcome in patients reirradiated for brain metastases. Int J Radiat Oncol Biol Phys. 1996;34(3):585–90.

[23] Ammirati M, Cobbs CS, Linskey ME, Paleologos NA, Ryken TC, Burri SH, Asher AL, Loeffler JS, Robinson PD, Andrews

[23]... DW, Gaspar LE, Kondziolka D, McDermott M, Mehta MP, Mikkelsen T, Olson JJ, Patchell RA, Kalkanis SN. The role of retreatment in the management of recurrent/progressive brain metastases: a systematic review and evidence-based clinical practice guideline. J Neuro-Oncol. 2010;96(1):85–96.

[24] Cooper JS, Steinfeld AD, Lerch IA. Cerebral metastases: value of reirradiation in selected patients. Radiology. 1990; 174(3 Pt 1):883–5.

[25] Sadikov E, Bezjak A, Yi QL, Wells W, Dawson L, Millar BA, Laperriere N. Value of whole brain reirradiation for brain metastases–single centre experience. Clin Oncol (R Coll Radiol). 2007;19(7):532–8.

[26] Son CH, Jimenez R, Niemierko A, Loeffler JS, Oh KS, Shih HA. Outcomes after whole brain reirradiation in patients with brain metastases. Int J Radiat Oncol Biol Phys. 2012;82(2):e167–72.

[27] Scharp M, Hauswald H, Bischof M, Debus J, Combs SE. Re-irradiation in the treatment of patients with cerebral metastases of solid tumors: retrospective analysis. Radiat Oncol. 2014;9:4.

[28] Ozgen Z, Atasoy BM, Kefeli AU, Seker A, Dane F, Abacioglu U. The benefit of whole brain reirradiation in patients with multiple brain metastases. Radiat Oncol. 2013;8:186.

[29] Guo S, Balagamwala EH, Reddy C, Elson P, Suh JH, Chao ST. Clinical and radiographic outcomes from repeat whole-brain radiation therapy for brain metastases in the age of stereotactic radiosurgery. Am J Clin Oncol. 2016;39(3):288–93.

[30] Logie N, Jimenez RB, Pulenzas N, Linden K, Ciafone D, Ghosh S, Xu Y, Lefresne S, Wong E, Son CH, Shih HA, Wong WW, Tyldesley S, Dennis K, Chow E, Fairchild AM. Estimating prognosis at the time of repeat whole brain radiation therapy for multiple brain metastases: the reirradiation score. Adv Radiat Oncol. 2017;2(3):381–90.

[31] Nguyen TD, DeAngelis LM. Brain metastases. Neurol Clin. 2007;25(4):1173–92.

[32] Wang N, Bertalan MS, Brastianos PK. Leptomeningeal metastasis from systemic cancer: review and update on management. Cancer. 2018;124(1):21–35.

[33] Gani C, Müller AC, Eckert F, Schroeder C, Bender B, Pantazis G, Bamberg M, Berger B. Outcome after whole brain radiotherapy alone in intracranial leptomeningeal carcinomatosis from solid tumors. Strahlenther Onkol. 2012;188(2):148–53.

[34] Morris PG, Reiner AS, Szenberg OR, Clarke JL, Panageas KS, Perez HR, Kris MG, Chan TA, DeAngelis LM, Omuro AM. Leptomeningeal metastasis from non-small cell lung cancer: survival and the impact of whole brain radiotherapy. J Thorac Oncol. 2012;7(2):382–5.

[35] Aupérin A, Arriagada R, Pignon JP, Le Péchoux C, Gregor A, Stephens RJ, Kristjansen PE, Johnson BE, Ueoka H, Wagner H, Aisner J. Prophylactic cranial irradiation for patients with small-cell lung cancer in complete remission. Prophylactic Cranial Irradiation Overview Collaborative Group. N Engl J Med. 1999;341(7):476–84.

[36] Slotman B, Faivre-Finn C, Kramer G, Rankin E, Snee M, Hatton M, Postmus P, Collette L, Musat E, Senan S, EORTC Radiation Oncology Group and Lung Cancer Group. Prophylactic cranial irradiation in extensive small-cell lung cancer. N Engl J Med. 2007;357(7):664–72.

[37] Takahashi T, Yamanaka T, Seto T, Harada H, Nokihara H, Saka H, Nishio M, Kaneda H, Takayama K, Ishimoto O, Takeda K, Yoshioka H, Tachihara M, Sakai H, Goto K, Yamamoto N. Prophylactic cranial irradiation versus observation in patients with extensive-disease small-cell lung cancer: a multicentre, randomised, open-label, phase 3 trial. Lancet Oncol. 2017;18(5):663–71.

[38] Le Péchoux C, Dunant A, Senan S, Wolfson A, Quoix E, Faivre-Finn C, Ciuleanu T, Arriagada R, Jones R, Wanders R, Lerouge D, Laplanche A, Prophylactic Cranial Irradiation (PCI) Collaborative Group. Standard-dose versus higher-dose prophylactic cranial irradiation (PCI) in patients with limited-stage small-cell lung cancer in complete remission after chemotherapy and thoracic radiotherapy (PCI 99–01, EORTC 22003–08004, RTOG 0212, and IFCT 99–01): a randomised clinical trial. Lancet Oncol. 2009;10(5):467–74.

[39] Wolfson AH, Bae K, Komaki R, Meyers C, Movsas B, Le Pechoux C, Werner-Wasik M, Videtic GM, Garces YI, Choy H. Primary analysis of a phase II randomized trial Radiation Therapy Oncology Group (RTOG) 0212: impact of different total doses and schedules of prophylactic cranial irradiation on chronic neurotoxicity and quality of life for patients with limited-disease small-cell lung cancer. Int J Radiat Oncol Biol Phys. 2011;81(1):77–84.

[40] Gore EM, Bae K, Wong SJ, Sun A, Bonner JA, Schild SE, Gaspar LE, Bogart JA, Werner-Wasik M, Choy H. Phase III comparison of prophylactic cranial irradiation versus observation in patients with locally advanced non-small-cell lung cancer: primary analysis of radiation therapy oncology group study RTOG 0214. J Clin Oncol. 2011;29(3):272–8.

[41] Andrews DW, Scott CB, Sperduto PW, Flanders AE, Gaspar LE, Schell MC, Werner-Wasik M, Demas W, Ryu J, Bahary JP, Souhami L, Rotman M, Mehta MP, Curran WJ Jr. Whole brain radiation therapy with or without stereotactic radiosurgery boost for patients with one to three brain metastases: phase III results of the RTOG 9508 randomised trial. Lancet. 2004;363(9422):1665–72.

[42] Sperduto PW, Shanley R, Luo X, Andrews D, Werner-Wasik M, Valicenti R, Bahary JP, Souhami L, Won M, Mehta M. Secondary analysis of RTOG 9508, a phase 3 randomized trial of whole-brain radiation therapy versus WBRT plus stereotactic radiosurgery in patients with 1–3 brain metastases; poststratified by the graded prognostic assessment (GPA). Int J Radiat Oncol Biol Phys. 2014;90(3):526–31.

[43] Patil CG, Pricola K, Sarmiento JM, Garg SK, Bryant A, Black KL. Whole brain radiation therapy (WBRT) alone versus WBRT and radiosurgery for the treatment of brain metastases. Cochrane Database Syst Rev. 2017;9:CD006121.

[44] Brown PD, Jaeckle K, Ballman KV, Farace E, Cerhan JH, Anderson SK, Carrero XW, Barker FG 2nd, Deming R, Burri SH, Ménard C, Chung C, Stieber VW, Pollock BE, Galanis E, Buckner JC, Asher AL. Effect of radiosurgery alone vs radiosurgery with whole brain radiation therapy on cognitive function in patients with 1 to 3 brain metastases: a randomized clinical trial. JAMA. 2016;316(4):401–9.

[45] Chang EL, Wefel JS, Hess KR, Allen PK, Lang FF, Kornguth DG, Arbuckle RB, Swint JM, Shiu AS, Maor MH, Meyers CA. Neurocognition in patients with brain metastases treated with radiosurgery or radiosurgery plus whole-brain irradiation: a randomised controlled trial. Lancet Oncol. 2009;10(11):1037–44.

[46] Churilla TM, Ballman KV, Brown PD, Twohy EL, Jaeckle K, Farace E, Cerhan JH, Anderson SK, Carrero XW, Garces YI, Barker FG 2nd, Deming R, Dixon JG, Burri SH, Chung C, Ménard C, Stieber VW, Pollock BE, Galanis E, Buckner JC, Asher AL. Stereotactic radiosurgery with or without whole-brain radiation therapy for limited brain metastases: a secondary analysis of the North Central Cancer Treatment Group N0574 (Alliance) randomized controlled trial. Int J Radiat Oncol Biol Phys. 2017;99(5):1173–8.

[47] Aoyama H, Tago M, Shirato H, Japanese Radiation Oncology Study Group 99–1 (JROSG 99–1) Investigators. Stereotactic radiosurgery with or without whole-brain radiotherapy for brain metastases: secondary analysis of the JROSG 99–1 randomized clinical trial. JAMA Oncol. 2015 Jul;1(4):457–64.

[48] Aoyama H, Shirato H, Tago M, Nakagawa K, Toyoda T, Hatano K, Kenjyo M, Oya N, Hirota S, Shioura H, Kunieda E, Inomata T, Hayakawa K, Katoh N, Kobashi G. Stereotactic radiosurgery plus whole-brain radiation therapy vs stereotactic radiosurgery alone for treatment of brain metastases: a randomized controlled trial. JAMA. 2006;295(21):2483–91.

[49] Sahgal A, Aoyama H, Kocher M, Neupane B, Collette S, Tago M, Shaw P, Beyene J, Chang EL. Phase 3 trials of stereotactic radiosurgery with or without wholebrain radiation therapy for 1 to 4 brain metastases: individual patient data meta-analysis. Int J Radiat Oncol Biol Phys. 2015;91(4):710–7.

[50] Soffietti R, Kocher M, Abacioglu UM, Villa S, Fauchon F, Baumert BG, Fariselli L, Tzuk-Shina T, Kortmann RD, Carrie C, Ben Hassel M, Kouri M, Valeinis E, van den Berge D, Mueller RP, Tridello G, Collette L, Bottomley A. A European Organisation for Research and Treatment of Cancer phase III trial of adjuvant whole-brain radiotherapy versus observation in patients with one to three brain metastases from solid tumors after surgical resection or radiosurgery: quality-of-life results. J Clin Oncol. 2013;31(1):65–72.

[51] Yamamoto M, Serizawa T, Shuto T, Akabane A, Higuchi Y, Kawagishi J, Yamanaka K, Sato Y, Jokura H, Yomo S, Nagano O, Kenai H, Moriki A, Suzuki S, Kida Y, Iwai Y, Hayashi M, Onishi H, Gondo M, Sato M, Akimitsu T, Kubo K, Kikuchi Y, Shibasaki T, Goto T, Takanashi M, Mori Y, Takakura K, Saeki N, Kunieda E, Aoyama H, Momoshima S, Tsuchiya K. Stereotactic radiosurgery for patients with multiple brain metastases (JLGK0901): a multi-institutional prospective observational study. Lancet Oncol. 2014;15(4):387–95.

[52] Yamamoto M, Serizawa T, Higuchi Y, Sato Y, Kawagishi J, Yamanaka K, Shuto T, Akabane A, Jokura H, Yomo S, Nagano O, Aoyama H. A multiinstitutional prospective observational study of stereotactic radiosurgery for patients with multiple brain metastases (JLGK0901 study update): irradiation-related complications and long-term maintenance of mini-mental state examination scores. Int J Radiat Oncol Biol Phys. 2017;99(1):31–40.

[53] Zindler JD, Bruynzeel AME, Eekers DBP, Hurkmans CW, Swinnen A, Lambin P. Whole brain radiotherapy versus stereotactic radiosurgery for 4–10 brain metastases: a phase III randomised multicentre trial. BMC Cancer. 2017;17(1):500.

[54] Venur VA, Ahluwalia MS. Targeted therapy in brain metastases: ready for primetime? Am Soc Clin Oncol Educ Book. 2016;35:e123–30.

[55] Yawn BP, Wollan PC, Schroeder C, Gazzuola L, Mehta M. Temporal and gender-related trends in brain metastases from lung and breast cancer. Minn Med. 2003;86(12):32–7.

[56] Long GV, Trefzer U, Davies MA, Kefford RF, Ascierto PA, Chapman PB, Puzanov I, Hauschild A, Robert C, Algazi A, Mortier L, Tawbi H, Wilhelm T, Zimmer L, Switzky J, Swann S, Martin AM, Guckert M, Goodman V, Streit M, Kirkwood JM, Schadendorf D. Dabrafenib in patients with Val600Glu or Val600Lys BRAF-mutant melanoma metastatic to the brain (BREAK-MB): a multicentre, open-label, phase 2 trial. Lancet Oncol. 2012;13(11):1087–95.

[57] McArthur GA, Maio M, Arance A, Nathan P, Blank C, Avril MF, Garbe C, Hauschild A, Schadendorf D, Hamid O, Fluck M, Thebeau M, Schachter J, Kefford R, Chamberlain M, Makrutzki M, Robson S, Gonzalez R, Margolin K. Vemurafenib in metastatic melanoma patients with brain metastases: an open-label, single-arm, phase 2, multicentre study. Ann Oncol. 2017;28(3):634–41.

[58] Davies MA, Saiag P, Robert C, Grob JJ, Flaherty KT, Arance A, Chiarion-Sileni V, Thomas L, Lesimple T, Mortier L, Moschos SJ, Hogg D, Márquez-Rodas I, Del Vecchio M, Lebbé C, Meyer N, Zhang Y, Huang Y, Mookerjee B, Long GV. Dabrafenib plus trametinib in patients with BRAF(V600)-mutant melanoma brain metastases (COMBI-MB): a multicentre, multicohort, open-label, phase 2 trial. Lancet Oncol. 2017;18(7):863–73.

[59] Margolin K, Ernstoff MS, Hamid O, Lawrence D, McDermott D, Puzanov I, Wolchok JD, Clark JI, Sznol M, Logan TF, Richards J, Michener T, Balogh A, Heller KN, Hodi FS. Ipilimumab in patients with melanoma and brain metastases: an open-label, phase 2 trial. Lancet Oncol. 2012;13(5):459–65.

[60] Goldberg SB, Gettinger SN, Mahajan A, Chiang AC, Herbst RS, Sznol M, Tsiouris AJ, Cohen J, Vortmeyer A, Jilaveanu L, Yu J, Hegde U, Speaker S, Madura M, Ralabate A, Rivera A, Rowen E, Gerrish H, Yao X, Chiang V, Kluger HM. Pembrolizumab for patients with melanoma or non-small-cell

lung cancer and untreated brain metastases: early analysis of a non-randomised, open-label, phase 2 trial. Lancet Oncol. 2016;17(7):976–83.

[61] Long GV, Atkinson V, Lo S, Sandhu S, Guminski AD, Brown MP, Wilmott JS, Edwards J, Gonzalez M, Scolyer RA, Menzies AM, McArthur GA. Combination nivolumab and ipilimumab or nivolumab alone in melanoma brain metastases: a multicenter randomised phase 2 study. Lancet Oncol. 2018;19(5):672–81.

[62] Tawbi HA, Forsyth PA, Algazi A, Hamid O, Hodi FS, Moschos SJ, Khushalani NI, Lewis K, Lao CD, Postow MA, Atkins MB, Ernstoff MS, Reardon DA, Puzanov I, Kudchadkar RR, Thomas RP, Tarhini A, Pavlick AC, Jiang J, Avila A, Demelo S, Margolin K. Combined nivolumab and ipilimumab in melanoma metastatic to the brain. N Engl J Med. 2018;379(8):722–30.

[63] Postmus PE, Smit EF. Chemotherapy for brain metastases of lung cancer: a review. Ann Oncol. 1999;10(7):753–9.

[64] Sperduto PW, Wang M, Robins HI, Schell MC, Werner-Wasik M, Komaki R, Souhami L, Buyyounouski MK, Khuntia D, Demas W, Shah SA, Nedzi LA, Perry G, Suh JH, Mehta MP. A phase 3 trial of whole brain radiation therapy and stereotactic radiosurgery alone versus WBRT and SRS with temozolomide or erlotinib for non-small cell lung cancer and 1 to 3 brain metastases: Radiation Therapy Oncology Group 0320. Int J Radiat Oncol Biol Phys. 2013;85(5):1312–8.

[65] Welsh JW, Komaki R, Amini A, Munsell MF, Unger W, Allen PK, Chang JY, Wefel JS, McGovern SL, Garland LL, Chen SS, Holt J, Liao Z, Brown P, Sulman E, Heymach JV, Kim ES, Stea B. Phase II trial of erlotinib plus concurrent whole-brain radiation therapy for patients with brain metastases from non-small-cell lung cancer. J Clin Oncol. 2013;31(7):895–902.

[66] Mok TS, Wu Y-L, Ahn M-J, Garassino MC, Kim HR, Ramalingam SS, Shepherd FA, He Y, Akamatsu H, Theelen WS, Lee CK, Sebastian M, Templeton A, Mann H, Marotti M, Ghiorghiu S, Papadimitrakopoulou VA, AURA3 Investigators. Osimertinib or platinum-pemetrexed in EGFR T790M-positive lung cancer. N Engl J Med. 2017;376(7):629–40.

[67] Costa DB, Shaw AT, Ou SH, Solomon BJ, Riely GJ, Ahn MJ, Zhou C, Shreeve SM, Selaru P, Polli A, Schnell P, Wilner KD, Wiltshire R, Camidge DR, Crinò L. Clinical experience with crizotinib in patients with advanced ALK-rearranged non-small-cell lung cancer and brain metastases. J Clin Oncol. 2015;33(17):1881–8.

[68] Gadgeel SM, Gandhi L, Riely GJ, Chiappori AA, West HL, Azada MC, Morcos PN, Lee RM, Garcia L, Yu L, Boisserie F, Di Laurenzio L, Golding S, Sato J, Yokoyama S, Tanaka T, Ou SH. Safety and activity of alectinib against systemic disease and brain metastases in patients with crizotinib-resistant ALK-rearranged non-small-cell lung cancer (AF-002JG): results from the dose-finding portion of a phase 1/2 study. Lancet Oncol. 2014;15(10):1119–28.

[69] Crinò L, Ahn MJ, De Marinis F, Groen HJ, Wakelee H, Hida T, Mok T, Spigel D, Felip E, Nishio M, Scagliotti G, Branle F, Emeremni C, Quadrigli M, Zhang J, Shaw AT. Multicenter phase II study of whole-body and intracranial activity with ceritinib in patients with ALK-rearranged non-small-cell lung cancer previously treated with chemotherapy and crizotinib: results from ASCEND-2. J Clin Oncol. 2016;34(24):2866–73.

[70] Kim DW, Tiseo M, Ahn MJ, Reckamp KL, Hansen KH, Kim SW, Huber RM, West HL, Groen HJM, Hochmair MJ, Leighl NB, Gettinger SN, Langer CJ, Paz-Ares Rodríguez LG, Smit EF, Kim ES, Reichmann W, Haluska FG, Kerstein D, Camidge DR. Brigatinib in patients with crizotinib-refractory anaplastic lymphoma kinase-positive non-small-cell lung cancer: a randomized, multicenter phase II trial. J Clin Oncol. 2017;35(22):2490–8.

[71] Magnuson WJ, Yeung JT, Guillod PD, Gettinger SN, Yu JB, Chiang VL. Impact of deferring radiation therapy in patients with epidermal growth factor receptor-mutant non-small cell lung cancer who develop brain metastases. Int J Radiat Oncol Biol Phys. 2016;95(2):673–9.

[72] Magnuson WJ, Lester-Coll NH, Wu AJ, Yang TJ, Lockney NA, Gerber NK, Beal K, Amini A, Patil T, Kavanagh BD, Camidge DR, Braunstein SE, Boreta LC, Balasubramanian SK, Ahluwalia MS, Rana NG, Attia A, Gettinger SN, Contessa JN, Yu JB, Chiang VL. Management of brain metastases in tyrosine kinase inhibitor-naïve epidermal growth factor receptor-mutant non-small-cell lung cancer: a retrospective multi-institutional analysis. J Clin Oncol. 2017;35(10):1070–7.

[73] Bachelot T, Romieu G, Campone M, Diéras V, Cropet C, Dalenc F, Jimenez M, Le Rhun E, Pierga JY, Gonçalves A, Leheurteur M, Domont J, Gutierrez M, Curé H, Ferrero JM, Labbe-Devilliers C. Lapatinib plus capecitabine in patients with previously untreated brain metastases from HER2-positive metastatic breast cancer (LANDSCAPE): a single-group phase 2 study. Lancet Oncol. 2013;14(1):64–71.

[74] Freedman RA, Gelman RS, Wefel JS, Melisko ME, Hess KR, Connolly RM, Van Poznak CH, Niravath PA, Puhalla SL, Ibrahim N, Blackwell KL, Moy B, Herold C, Liu MC, Lowe A, Agar NY, Ryabin N, Farooq S, Lawler E, Rimawi MF, Krop IE, Wolff AC, Winer EP, Lin NU. Translational breast cancer research consortium (TBCRC) 022: a phase II trial of neratinib for patients with human epidermal growth factor receptor 2-positive breast cancer and brain metastases. J Clin Oncol. 2016;34(9):945–52.

[75] Kroeze SG, Fritz C, Hoyer M, Lo SS, Ricardi U, Sahgal A, Stahel R, Stupp R, Guckenberger M. Toxicity of concurrent stereotactic radiotherapy and targeted therapy or immunotherapy: a systematic review. Cancer Treat Rev. 2017;53:25–37.

[76] Brown PD, Ahluwalia MS, Khan OH, Asher AL, Wefel JS, Gondi V. Whole-brain radiotherapy for brain metastases: evolution or revolution? J Clin Oncol. 2018;36(5):483–91.

[77] DeAngelis LM, Delattre JY, Posner JB. Radiation-induced dementia in patients cured of brain metastases. Neurology. 1989;39(6):789–96.

[78] Monje ML, Mizumatsu S, Fike JR, Palmer TD. Irradiation induces neural precursor-cell dysfunction. Nat Med. 2002;8(9):955–62.

[79] Monje ML, Vogel H, Masek M, Ligon KL, Fisher PG, Palmer TD. Impaired human hippocampal neurogenesis after treatment for central nervous system malignancies. Ann Neurol. 2007;62(5):515–20.

[80] Gondi V, Tomé WA, Mehta MP. Why avoid the hippocampus? A comprehensive review. Radiother Oncol. 2010;97(3):370–6.

[81] Kazda T, Jancalek R, Pospisil P, Sevela O, Prochazka T, Vrzal M, Burkon P, Slavik M, Hynkova L, Slampa P, Laack NN. Why and how to spare the hippocampus during brain radiotherapy: the developing role of hippocampal avoidance in cranial radiotherapy. Radiat Oncol. 2014;9:139.

[82] Gondi V, Pugh SL, Tome WA, Caine C, Corn B, Kanner A, Rowley H, Kundapur V, DeNittis A, Greenspoon JN, Konski AA, Bauman GS, Shah S, Shi W, Wendland M, Kachnic L, Mehta MP. Preservation of memory with conformal avoidance of the hippocampal neural stem-cell compartment during whole-brain radiotherapy for brain metastases (RTOG 0933): a phase II multi-institutional trial. J Clin Oncol. 2014;32(34):3810–6.

[83] Gondi V, Tolakanahalli R, Mehta MP, Tewatia D, Rowley H, Kuo JS, Khuntia D, Tomé WA. Hippocampal-sparing whole-brain radiotherapy: a "how-to" technique using helical tomotherapy and linear accelerator-based intensity-modulated radiotherapy. Int J Radiat Oncol Biol Phys. 2010;78(4):1244–52.

[84] Gondi V, Hermann BP, Mehta MP, Tomé WA. Hippocampal dosimetry predicts neurocognitive function impairment after fractionated stereotactic radiotherapy for benign or low-grade adult brain tumors. Int J Radiat Oncol Biol Phys. 2013;85(2):348–54.

[85] Brown PD, Pugh S, Laack NN, Wefel JS, Khuntia D, Meyers C, Choucair A, Fox S, Suh JH, Roberge D, Kavadi V, Bentzen SM, Mehta MP, Watkins-Bruner D, Radiation Therapy Oncology Group (RTOG). Memantine for the prevention of cognitive dysfunction in patients receiving whole-brain radiotherapy: a randomized, double-blind, placebo-controlled trial. Neuro-Oncology. 2013;15(10):1429–37.

[86] Gondi V, Deshmukh S, Brown P, Wefel J, Tome W, Brune D, Bovi J, Robinson C, Khuntia D, Grosshans DR, Konski AA, Roberge D, Kundapur V, Devisetty K, Shah SA, Usuki KY, Anderson BM, Mehta MP, Kachnic LA. Preservation of neurocognitive function (NCF) with conformal avoidance of the hippocampus during whole brain radiotherapy (HA-WBRT) for brain metastases: preliminary results of phase III trial NRG oncology CC001. Int J Radiat Oncol Biol Phys. 2018;102(3):s5.

第13章 粒子治疗在脑转移瘤治疗中的应用
Particle Therapy for the Treatment of Brain Metastases

Jeremy Brownstein　Hooney D. Min　Marc Bussiere　Helen A. Shih　**著**
周　雪　周扬莹　**译**
伍海军　**校**

缩略语

ASL	Acute Severe Lymphopenia	急性重型淋巴细胞减少
CIT	Carbon Ion Therapy	碳离子治疗
IMPT	Intensity Modulated Proton Therapy	调强质子治疗
IMRT	Intensity Modulated Radiation Therapy	调强放射治疗
LET	Linear Energy Transfer	线性能量传递
MGH	Massachusetts General Hospital	马萨诸塞州总医院
PBS	Pencil Beam Scanning	笔形束扫描
PBT	Proton Beam Therapy	质子治疗
PSP	Passively Scattered Protons	被动散射质子
RBE	Relative Biological Effectiveness	相对生物效应
SOBP	Spread-Out Bragg Peak	扩展布拉格峰
SRS	Stereotactic Radiosurgery	立体定向放射外科
VMAT	Volumetric Modulated Arc Therapy	容积弧形调强放疗

一、病例介绍

（一）病例1

一名55岁的转移性非小细胞肺癌患者，男性，无吸烟史，3年前首发表现为持续性咳嗽3个月，予以抗哮喘药物和激素治疗均无效。检查发现右上肺肿块合并纵隔淋巴结肿大，活检为中分化腺癌，分期检查显示多发骨转移和多发脑转移。患者在接受全身系统治疗的同时予以了全脑放射治疗，剂量30Gy/10次，3年内颅内病变无进展。在常规复查时发现左额叶两个无症状的新发转移瘤，患者再次接受了质子SRS治疗，每个病灶的相对生物效应（relative biological effectiveness，RBE）为18Gy。质子SRS不仅耐受性好、一致性高，而且能最大限度地减少正常脑组织的二次照射（图13-1A和B）。

（二）病例2

一名46岁女性，4年前在切除瘙痒性色素沉着性头皮病变后确诊为*BRAF*突变型转移性黑色素瘤。进一步扩大切除发现，病变深度为5mm，

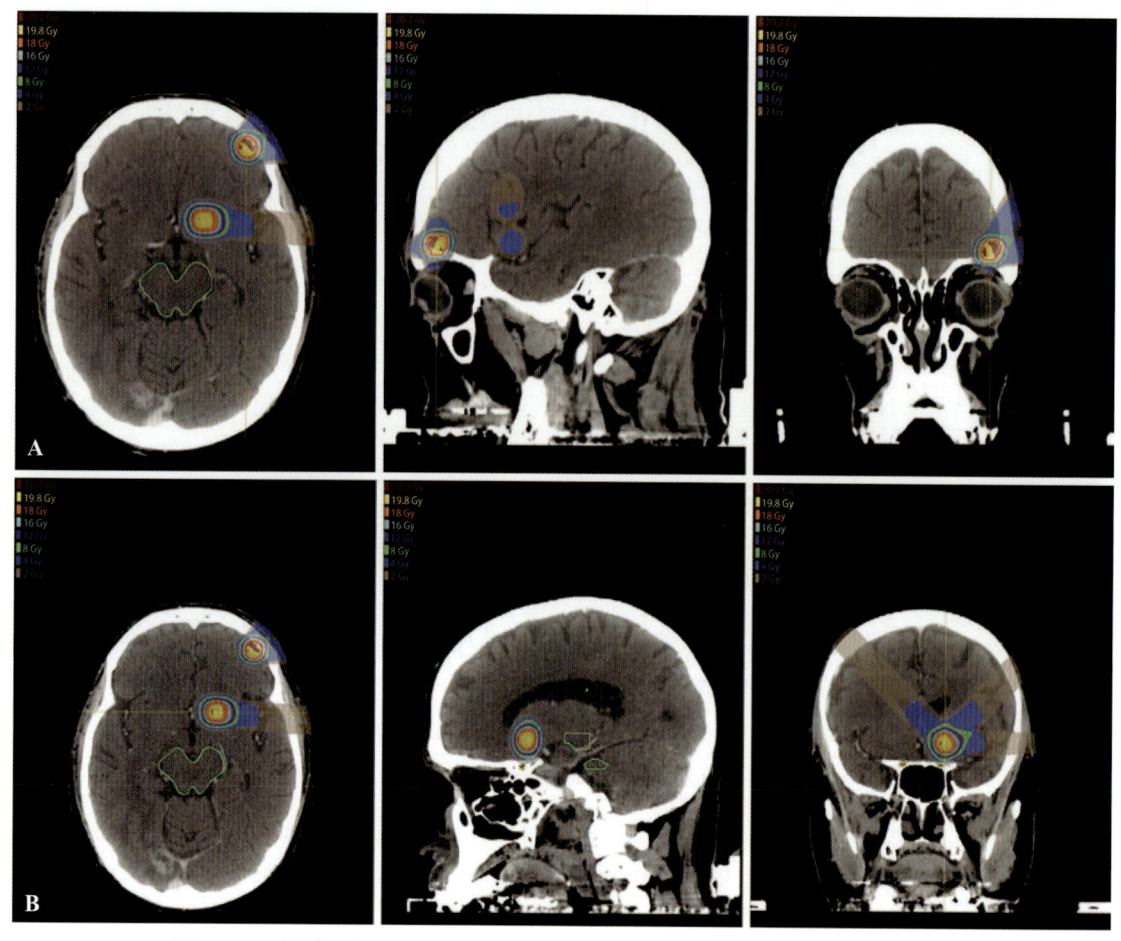

▲ 图 13-1 非小细胞肺癌左额叶及前颅底脑转移瘤同时接受质子治疗的 SRS 计划

A. 病灶位于左侧眼眶上方；B. 病灶位于左侧视神经上方、视交叉前方。质子治疗可最大限度地保护周围正常组织

前哨阳性淋巴结 2/5，尽管后续更广泛的局部和淋巴结切除未发现其他病变，但患者在首次诊断后 14 个月出现肺转移，并接受了 5 个月的 BRAF 靶向治疗，在病情进展后接受了免疫治疗。4 个月后，首次发现右枕叶和左丘脑的颅内转移瘤，并接受放疗；1 年后，再次出现无症状的右颞叶和左前额叶脑转移瘤，考虑到左前额叶病变为中等大小，为减少周边正常结构的照射，患者接受了质子 SRS 治疗（图 13-2A 和 B）。

二、质子的基本特点

（一）剂量分布

质子治疗（proton beam therapy，PBT），是一束质子被回旋加速器或同步加速器加速到高能状态，然后通过调强、聚焦和塑形以达到所需的治疗体积。由于质子治疗主要通过质子-电子反应与物质发生相互作用，因此沉积剂量不同于外照射放射治疗中使用的光子（如兆伏 X 线和高能 γ 射线），后者主要通过康普顿散射与物质相互作用[1]。光子具有很强的穿透性，在初始剂量积累之后，光子的沉积剂量在整个光束路径中逐渐减少[2]。而质子在穿过组织时会减慢速度，最终停止运动；与光子均匀减少的剂量分布相反，质子沉积的剂量随着质子束的减速而急剧增加，在较小的范围内爆发达到顶峰（称为布拉格峰），然后随着质子运动的突然停止而骤降至 0（图 13-3）。由于质子在布拉格峰外组织的剂量沉积很少，因此用于治疗与危及器官邻近的靶区是其相较于光子的潜在优势。

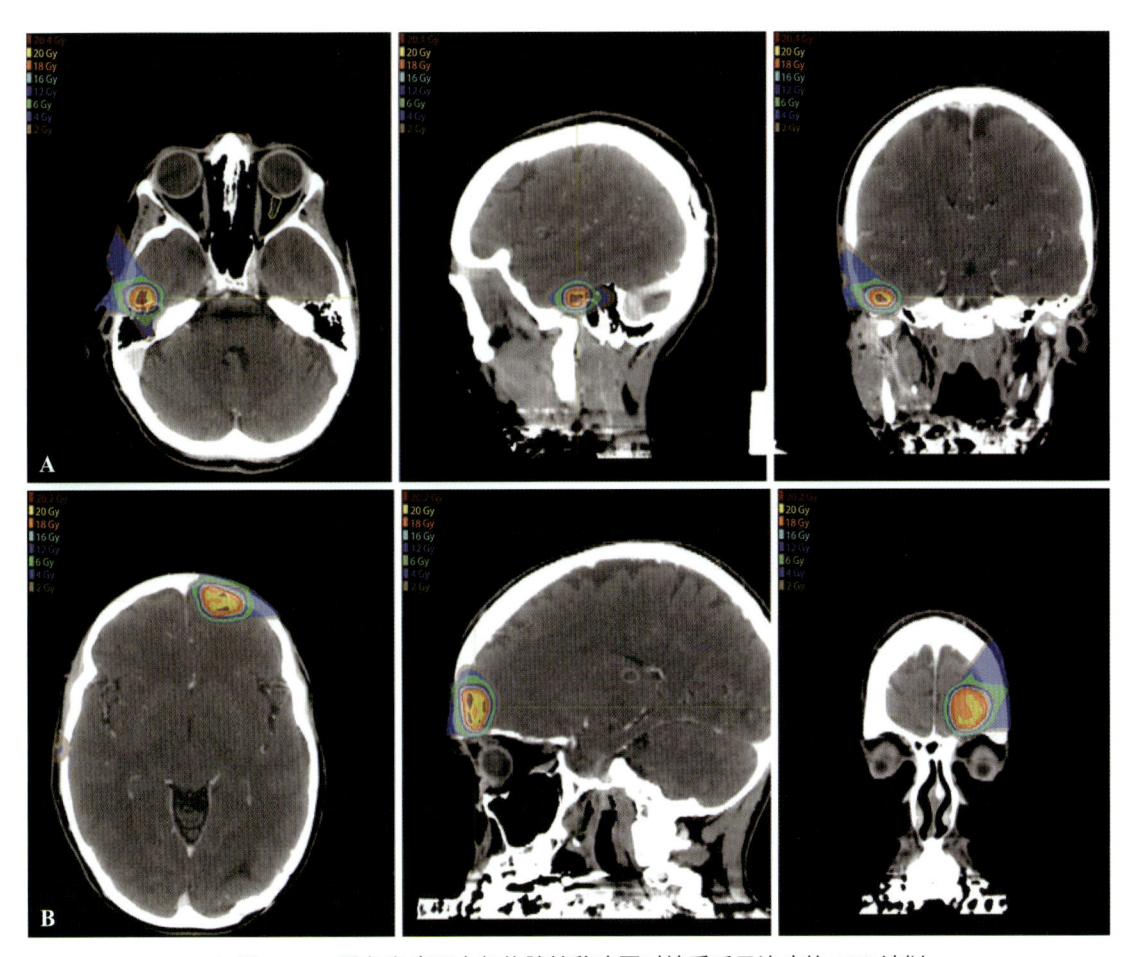

▲ 图 13-2 黑色素瘤两个部位脑转移瘤同时接受质子治疗的 SRS 计划

A. 病灶位于右侧颞骨颅底和耳蜗前方；B. 病灶（中等大小）沿左前额叶外凸。每个计划都能最大限度地保护周围脑组织

（二）散射与调强

布拉格峰的水当量深度与能量有关，大致与初始能量的平方成正比 $[D_{WET}{}^{[3]}=0.0022 \times E (MeV)^{1.77}]^{[4]}$。单能质子以保持直径几毫米，类似"笔形束"的形式离开加速器，通过沉积剂量只需几毫米深度的布拉格峰效应在组织中形成非常小的照射野。由于大多数临床病灶跨度为 1~20cm，单能质子笔形束不足以用于大部分的治疗。因此，必须使用多能质子束，通过散射和扫描技术让能量在靶区的深度范围内产生重叠的布拉格峰，并且改变光束方向以覆盖整个治疗靶区。

散射，又称被动散射，是最初几十年中临床应用的主流治疗技术。通过调强设备可以叠加不同能量的单能光束，在一定深度上产生均匀的剂量分布。一种常见的方法是让笔形质子束通过含有不同厚度辐条的旋转补偿器轮，当笔形质子束遇到逐渐加厚的辐条时，所得质子的能量将逐渐降低，并产生越来越浅的布拉格峰。每根辐条的弧长反映了相应峰值的相对权重。或者，笔形质子束可以通过脊形滤过器——一种表面有许多参差交错的，呈细脊状尖凸的静态块状物，遇到尖端的质子比遇到低谷的质子的能量低。上述两种方法均能产生多个布拉格峰，这些峰结合在一起形成所谓的"扩展布拉格峰"（spread-out Bragg peak，SOBP）。经过特别设计的调强设备，可以使 SOBP 在整个靶区产生均匀的物理剂量（图 13-4）。有关被动散射技术的详细说明，见参考文献 [5-7]。通过被动散射，窄的多能光束通过

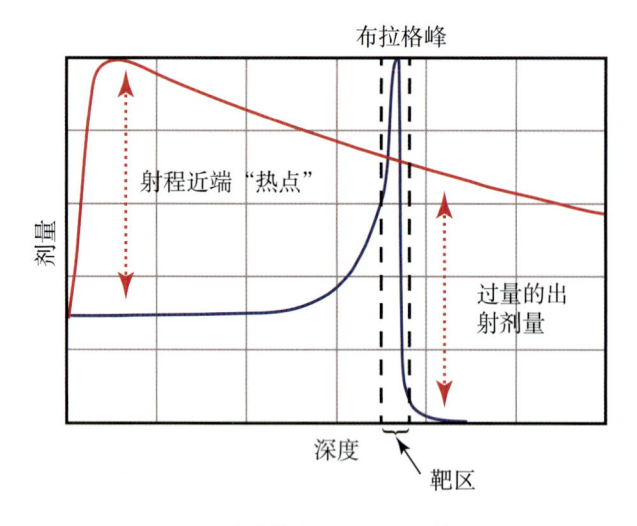

▲ 图 13-3　治疗性光子和质子束的剂量分布

光子（红色）和质子（蓝色）的剂量随深度而变化。光子的最大剂量出现在靶点附近。在光束路径内，"热点"将接受比靶点更高的剂量。光子还会在靶点的远端继续沉积剂量，从而产生过量的射出剂量。在质子束内，剂量随深度增加而增加，在布拉格峰处达到最大值，只需让质子束能量的布拉格峰值落在靶区范围内。在布拉格峰的远端，剂量急剧下降，仅沉积少量的射出剂量

一个或多个散射装置进行拓宽，这有助于横向剂量分布（即双散射）。由黄铜、合金或用多叶准直器制成的患者和靶区特异性的孔径使质子束与靶区和周围重要结构的形状一致。由塑料或蜡制成的患者和靶区特异性的距离补偿器也被用来进一步使扩展布拉格峰与靶区的远端边缘形状达到一致[7]。

相反，扫描系统（即笔形束扫描，PBS）利用弯曲磁铁将单能笔形质子束横向扫过治疗野（就像老式阴极射线电视中的电子束扫过磷光屏幕一样），从而使剂量在特定深度像"绘图"一样均匀分布到组织上。靶区的内层首先用最高能量的质子处理，然后主光束能量递减，较浅层面依次类似地接受剂量。由于笔形质子束在穿过治疗靶区时的强度和（或）停留在特定位点的时间均能被调控，因此该技术通常被称为调强质子治疗（intensity modulated proton therapy，IMPT）。与基于X线的调强放射治疗（intensity modulated radiation therapy，IMRT）一样，IMPT也采用逆向计划和优化；质子具有布拉格峰效应，IMPT

消除出口剂量所需的范围更小，所以与调强放射治疗相比，IMPT显著降低了累积剂量[8]。虽然被动散射和扫描系统各有优缺点，但大多数新系统采用扫描技术（即IMPT），因为这项技术使靶区的远端和近端边缘的适形度更好。大多数被动散射质子束的调强距离基本一致（即SOBP的"厚度"近似恒定），使用距离补偿器使靶区远端SOBP适应近端轮廓，也必然会影响近端SOBP，潜在地导致靶区表面出现热点。相比之下，扫描技术为笔形质子束的剂量分割提供了更大的自由度，从而具有更大的调控范围。此外，IMPT还能够在某一特定的治疗方案中给予靶区不同的剂量强度（即同步集成补量）[9]，允许进行额外的优化以解决范围不确定性[10]和（或）纳入生物学因素[11]（见下文）。

（三）生物因素

电离辐射有多种形式，从无质量的光子到以相对论速度运动的重原子核。辐射的生物学效应不仅取决于辐射的剂量，还取决于辐射与物质相互作用的方式。光子沉积的能量比较稀疏，导致的DNA损伤通常能被修复（单链断裂）。重离子比光子更有效，因为重离子在其布拉格峰内将辐射沉积在致密的电离轨道中，从而造成高度聚集的、不可修复的DNA损伤（双链断裂、双着丝粒环等）。例如，碳和重离子造成的损害可以等同于3倍的X线剂量造成的损害[12]，与低线性能量传递（linear energy transfer，LET）辐射的光子相比，大量能量在较短的距离内沉积，因此，重离子被称为高LET辐射[13]。为比较两种不同线性能量传递模式的剂量，引入了RBE，即引起相同生物效应所需的X线与目标粒子的剂量比（在上面的例子中，碳离子的RBE是3，因为需要高出3倍的X线剂量才能引起相同的损伤）[14]。

质子被认为是"低LET"辐射，但仍然比X线强。在大多数临床应用中，质子通常被假定具有1.1的恒定RBE，意味着质子治疗在生物学上

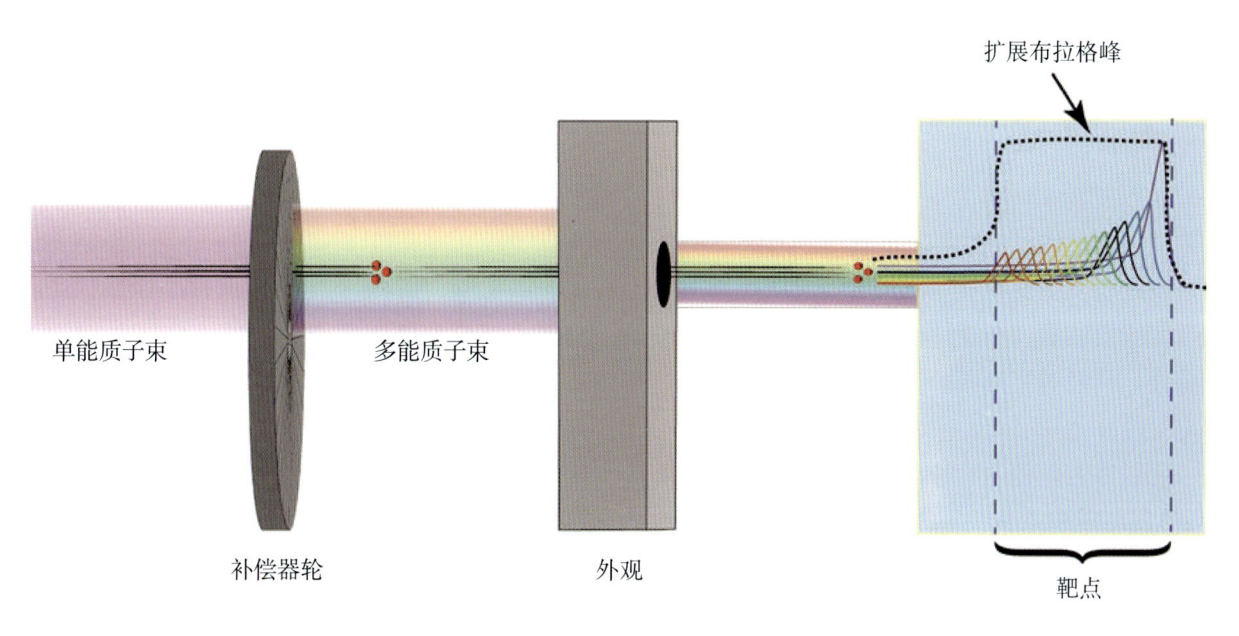

▲ 图 13-4　质子束被动调强示意图

离开回旋加速器或同步加速器的单能质子束与旋转的调强轮相互作用（未显示调强轮的可变深度），产生的多能质子束在到达靶点之前会通过一个光圈校准。调整调强轮的配置，以产生在整个靶区范围内沉积布拉格峰的能量谱，称为 SOBP。经 Brownstein 等许可修改

等同于增加 10% 剂量的 X 线[15]。因此，质子剂量通常以 Gy（RBE）表示，以确定 X 线的等效剂量[14]。然而，越来越多的文献表明，假设将质子的 RBE 统一为 1.1，可能会忽略临床上的细微差别。与碳离子类似，当质子沿着其路径减速时，它会随着强度和密度的增加而沉积能量。因此，移动缓慢的质子接近其射程末端时，具有更高的 LET，其 RBE > 1.1。由于靶区的远端边缘比近端边缘含有更多的慢速质子，假设整个靶区范围的物理剂量一致，则 RBE 随着深度的增加而增加。Paganetti 等（2014）描述了在剂量一致的扩展布拉格峰中质子 RBE 的递增情况：入口的 RBE 约为 1.1，中心约为 1.15，远端边缘约为 1.35，远端脱落处约为 1.7[16]。因此，如果假设 RBE 均为 1.1，在放射敏感器官中靶区远端边缘的有效生物剂量可能会超量 20%。Peeler 等回顾性研究了一系列接受质子治疗室管膜瘤的儿童患者，并使用蒙特卡罗模拟回顾性计算了 LET。研究显示，在单变量分析中，T_2 加权 MRI 上与治疗相关的改变与 CTV 内较高的 LET_{max} 显著相关[17]。

RBE 的计算是复杂的，依赖于许多变量。除了 LET 和分次剂量外，RBE 还受到生物学因素的影响，如组织学、组织固有的放射敏感性 / 修复能力及肿瘤的氧合情况[18]。最近一些研究团队发现细胞遗传学也可能影响 RBE 值，如 DNA 同源修复的突变和 Fanconi 贫血途径会增加质子杀伤细胞的敏感性，从而产生更高的 RBE[3, 19]。虽然目前正在研究包括物理和生物因素在内的许多 RBE 建模技术，但如何将可变 RBE 纳入质子治疗计划中仍没有明确的共识，大多数中心仍将质子的 RBE 统一设为 1.1[20]。

三、质子立体定向放射外科技术

固定和图像引导

有效的固定对于保证靶区的精确定位至关重要。与光子 SRS 相比，质子 SRS 的设置误差对剂量分布的影响更大，因为布拉格峰对靶区附近组织的深度和密度的变化非常敏感。用于质子 SRS 的固定装置经过特殊设计，可以限制粒子的散射。例如马萨诸塞州总医院（MGH）改进

的 Gill-Thomas-Cosman 框架就是为脑肿瘤的质子治疗开发的固定化框架，该框架包括圆形的碳纤维枕骨支撑、低密度垫子和固定在立体定向颅环上的牙模（图 13-5A）。这种装置用于治疗没有延伸到颅底的颅内病灶，但需要患者有良好的牙列，以进行可重复的良好固定。不使用牙齿固定的替代固定装置，在设计时即需考虑质子治疗的敏感性，同时利用热塑面罩和定制枕垫使体位的固定变得舒适和可重复[21]。

现在许多新建的质子治疗平台都集成了锥束 CT 和自动定位系统[22]。然而，这些进展是近期才出现的，一些老的质子中心仍继续使用颅骨基准标记对患者的位置进行严格地三角测量，以确保给予精确的治疗（图 13-5B）。放置基准标志物可由神经外科医生 15～20min 在门诊完成，且并发症极少。

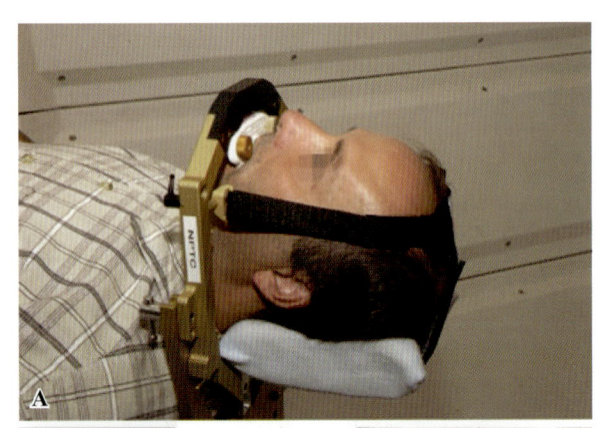

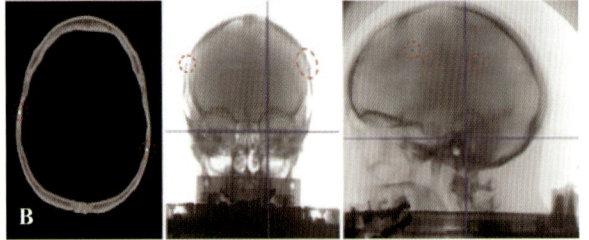

▲ 图 13-5 质子治疗的固定和定位

A. 改良的 Gill-Thomas-Cosman 面罩通过固定患者前额的魔术贴绑带和可紧贴患者牙齿的定制牙托，实现了可重复的无创固定；B. 通过微创手术将基准点放置到颅骨外板深处。CT（左）展示了定位良好的基准点（红圆圈）。治疗前的 kV 成像（中，右）通过对齐基准点（红圆圈）来设置等中心点，精度为 ±0.5mm

四、剂量学注意事项

由于颅内肿瘤通常位于重要结构附近，因此最佳的放射治疗计划可能需要不完全覆盖靶区或超过正常组织的限制。为此，许多学术团队评估了哪种方式——光子抑或质子能最大限度地覆盖颅内靶区，同时将正常组织毒性降至最低。Bolsi 等同时对 12 例患者（脑膜瘤 5 例、听神经瘤 5 例、垂体腺瘤 2 例）制定三维适形光子放疗、调强放疗、立体定向弧形光子治疗、点扫描质子治疗和被动散射质子治疗的计划。所有计划的靶区覆盖良好，但是使用质子的治疗计划对脑干、眼睛和正常大脑组织的平均照射剂量明显降低[23]。Freund 等对 13 例计划分次放疗的儿童 CNS 肿瘤患者，分别采用容积弧形调强放射治疗（volumetric modulated arc therapy，VMAT）、被动散射质子（passively scattered protons，PSP）治疗和调强质子（IMPT）治疗进行比较。与 VMAT 相比，PSP 和 IMPT 的脑最大剂量明显增加，接受低剂量照射的脑体积明显减少，脑坏死的预测风险降低[24]。

质子束剂量学

PBS 系统多用于治疗不规则体积的病灶，但脑转移瘤通常是球形的小病灶，因此可以用简单的调强技术来处理。单散射系统对不需要横向光束扩散的小病灶非常适用，笔形质子束穿过低原子序数材料，以实现所需的布拉格峰回拉，虽然合成场的剂量分布不均匀，但中心部分剂量基本一致，可以精准治疗小靶点。与更复杂的扫描技术和双散射系统相比，单散射系统可以设计成更小的有效源直径和更大的等中心距离，从而在浅层产生更窄的横向半影。Safai 等还指出，对于在水中深度 < 14cm 的病灶（即大多数颅内病灶），准直散射束的横向半影较笔形质子束更锐利，即使是 3mm 的 PBS 束斑也是如此。例如，对于在水中 4cm 深的靶区，PBS（光斑大小为 3mm）80%～20% 的横向半影为 1cm，而同样条件下准

直光束约为 3mm [25]。还有人发现，在 PBS 平台上增加一个准直器可以显著增加深度＜11cm 的水中横向半影[26]。著者指出，这些观察结果不能广泛应用，因为质子束大小的配适参数高度依赖各单位系统的具体情况。

五、临床应用

（一）颅内良性病变

由于良好的剂量分布，质子治疗设备在立体定向放射外科中应用广泛。质子是治疗颅内良性病变的优先选择，因为患者通常预后极好，须优先考虑正常脑组织的剂量限制。MGH 发表了数个病例系列研究，详细介绍了他们在治疗前庭神经鞘瘤[27]、垂体腺瘤[28, 29] 和动静脉畸形[30, 31] 时使用质子 SRS 的经验。有关质子 SRS 治疗详细、全面的临床讨论见下文[32]。

（二）质子 SRS 在脑转移瘤中的应用

关于质子立体定向放射外科治疗脑转移瘤的数据有限。MGH 发表了迄今为止唯一的系列研究，报道了他们在 1991—2016 年为 370 名患者治疗 815 次脑转移瘤的经验[33]。纳入患者的中位年龄为 61 岁，大多数患者功能状态良好，2/3 的患者 KPS 评分＞80 分。原发肿瘤组织来源中，非小细胞肺癌患者占多数（34%），其次是黑色素瘤（28%）和乳腺癌（17%）。约 50% 患者没有颅外转移灶，约 50% 患者为单个转移。

患者在哈佛回旋加速器实验室接受治疗，直至 2001 年位于麻省理工学院主校区的弗朗西斯·H. 伯尔质子中心（Francis H.Burr Proton Center）竣工。根据临床情况不同，患者使用不同的技术进行固定（如上所述）。所有患者均接受头颅基准标志物的放置，以确保直角 X 线的准确设置。靶区体积为 0.02～23.3cm³（平均 1.6cm³，中位数 0.6cm³），剂量范围为 8～28Gy［平均 17.3Gy，中位数为 18Gy（RBE）]。

中位随访时间为 9.2 个月，肿瘤治疗结果与光子 SRS 系列研究的结果相当。6 个月和 12 个月的局部复发率分别为 4.3% 和 8.5%，6 个月和 12 个月的远处 CNS 转移率分别为 39% 和 48%，中位总生存期为 12.4 个月。治疗耐受性良好，2 级以上急性不良反应发生率仅为 11%，1 年内病理证实的放射性坏死发生率为 3.6%。作者对有 3～4 处脑转移瘤的 10 例患者进行了回顾性分析，比较了质子与光子 SRS 技术的剂量分布。发现与光子相比，质子治疗时正常脑组织照射剂量达到 4Gy 的体积明显更小。图 13-6 显示了一名患者的类似比较，该患者最初接受质子 SRS 治疗，后来重新设计计划后使用高密度 MLC VMAT 治疗。

六、重离子 SRS 在脑转移瘤中的应用

鉴于重离子具有更好的剂量学和放射生物学特性，人们对使用重离子治疗某些肿瘤的兴趣与日俱增。欧洲和亚洲有 11 个使用重离子（如碳离子）疗法的治疗中心，还有几个目前正在建设中[34]。与质子相比，碳离子具有更锐利的横向半影，并且在其布拉格峰内具有更高的 RBE。这些优点使碳离子疗法（carbon ion therapy，CIT）适用于治疗紧邻关键结构的放射抵抗性肿瘤[35]。海德堡离子束治疗中心对中/低级别颅底软骨肉瘤患者进行的回顾性研究显示，3 年和 4 年的局部控制率分别为 96% 和 90%[36]，优于接受质子治疗的患者[37, 38]。然而，据我们所知，目前发表的用 CIT 或其他重离子治疗脑转移患者的系列研究还很少。虽然技术上可行，但可能并不实用，因为 CIT 平台少，而且相比其他放射外科平台优势并不明显。

七、讨论

一些医生对常规使用质子 SRS 治疗脑转

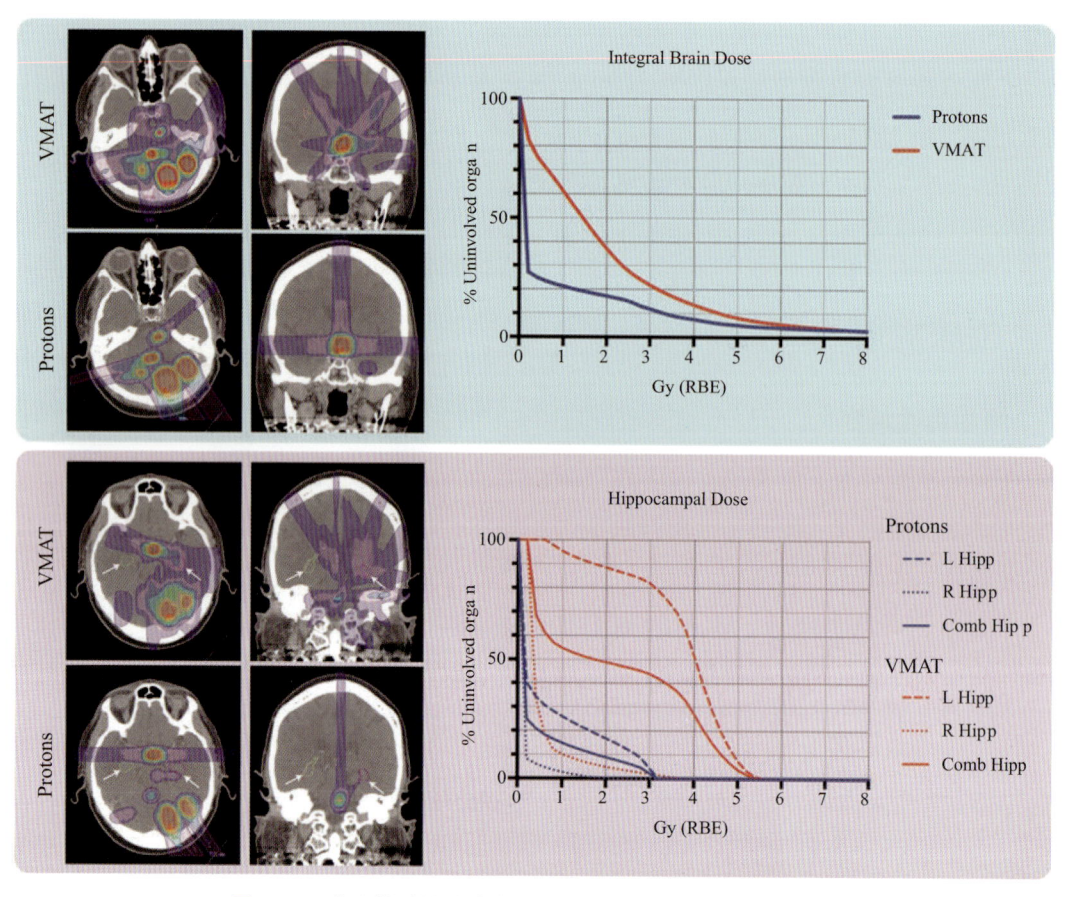

▲ 图 13-6 多发性脑转移瘤患者质子 SRS 与 VMAT-SRS 的比较

蓝框显示 VMAT 计划（上）和质子计划（下）剂量分布的代表性层面；DVH（右）显示质子计划相较于光子，在照射野之外接受低剂量照射的脑组织剂量更低（平均剂量为 0.96Gy vs. 2.03Gy）；紫框显示 VMAT 计划（上）和质子计划（下）剂量分布的代表性层面，海马用白色箭头标记；DVH（右）显示质子计划较 VMAT 计划在左侧海马（平均剂量分别为 0.68Gy vs. 3.75Gy）、右侧海马（平均剂量分别为 0.07Gy vs.0.54Gy）和双侧海马（平均剂量分别为 0.39Gy vs. 2.22Gy）产生较低的剂量。值得注意的是，无论是质子计划还是 VMAT 计划都没有特别优化以避开海马区

译者注：图中表述为专业词不需要翻译

移瘤表示担忧。针对上文介绍的哈佛经验，Kirkpatrick 等重申，与使用光子 SRS 治疗脑转移瘤相比，质子的局部控制和颅内进展并没有改善，考虑到质子治疗患者接受了与光子类似的剂量，甚至更温和的剂量，这是一个可预见的结果[39]。他们进一步指出，对于质子治疗减少的总剂量能否转化为神经认知的改善，尤其是与脑转移相关的不良预后，还缺乏数据支持；同时产生类似治疗结果，质子 SRS 的成本比光子 SRS 高得多。

本章著者认为，目前没有足够的数据证明在脑转移瘤治疗中应常规推荐质子 SRS 而不是光子 SRS。在大多数情况下，采用 VMAT 的光子技术仅利用一个或多个等中心点，同时、高效地针对多个转移瘤进行高度适形的放射治疗。由于许多这样的平台通常具有锥束 CT 的图像引导和体表跟踪系统，因此不需要额外的侵入性固定或基准标记。

尽管光子在剂量给予和图像引导治疗方面有所改进，仍有一些特殊的脑转移瘤病例适合质子治疗。对于大的或不规则的靶区，PBT 有剂量学优势[40]，并且可以减少靶区周围关键结构的损害[41]。因此，对于某些肿瘤位置欠佳，光子 SRS 不能安全给予剂量的患者，质子 SRS 可能有助于脑转移瘤的消融治疗。

系统治疗的进展延长了许多脑转移瘤患者的生存时间。Sperduto 等最近更新了非小细胞肺癌的疾病特异性分级预后评估（disease specific-grade prognostic assessment，DS-GPA）。*ALK* 突变或 *EGFR* 突变的腺癌患者（包括一些脑转移瘤＞4 个的患者）预后最好（DS-GPA 3.5～4），中位生存期为 47 个月[42]。*HER2* 阳性脑转移瘤患者预后良好，中位生存期为 27 个月[43]。随着靶向治疗的新进展，转移性患者伴有"有利突变"的越来越多，即使发生脑转移，他们仍能与癌症共存多年。对于这类患者，探索质子 SRS 减少全脑剂量能否转化为神经认知功能的改善非常有意义。

过量的全脑剂量可能会对受累病变外的正常脑组织产生有害影响。在生理条件下，在 30s 的心脏传输时间内，大脑接受约 16% 的心输出量[44]。Yovino 等为了量化恶性胶质瘤放射治疗过程中循环淋巴细胞的辐射剂量，通过仔细建模，计算出循环淋巴细胞的平均辐射剂量约为 2Gy 时能杀死 50% 暴露的淋巴细胞；99% 的淋巴细胞接受＞ 0.5Gy 的辐射，预计能杀死至少 10% 的暴露淋巴细胞[45]。Huang 等对 183 例高级别恶性胶质瘤患者进行了 Logistic 回归分析，发现 V25Gy 与急性重型淋巴细胞减少症（acute severe lymphopenia，ASL）的发生显著相关[46, 47]。这项研究和其他相关研究也描述了 ASL 与较差的总体生存率相关[48]。值得注意的是，在接受分次放疗的脑胶质瘤患者中，正常脑组织的总辐射剂量远远高于接受光子 SRS 治疗的脑转移瘤患者的剂量。然而，随着免疫疗法在转移性患者中的治疗作用不断增强，对于放射治疗如何影响免疫系统的认知变得越来越重要。

综上所述，质子 SRS 是治疗脑转移瘤的一种安全有效的方法。虽然目前还没有证据表明常规使用质子 SRS 治疗优于光子 SRS，但质子对于大病灶的治疗安全性更好，对于有多个小病灶的转移瘤患者，最终的全脑剂量也更低。因此仍需要进一步的研究来确定这种较低的全脑剂量能否转化为更好的神经认知结果，或更好地保护患者的抗癌免疫力。

> **要　点**
>
> - 质子治疗相较于光子放疗具有剂量学优势。不同于在穿透深度的整个光束路径上沉积剂量的光子，质子在特定深度停止，在狭窄的布拉格峰射程末尾沉积大部分剂量。这会导致沉积在靶区远端的出口剂量很小。
> - 鉴于先进的光子 SRS 平台可及性更好，并且提供的高度适形放疗基本能满足临床需求，因此本章的作者不建议常规使用质子 SRS 来治疗脑转移瘤。
> - 质子 SRS 是脑转移瘤一种安全有效的治疗方法，与光子 SRS 相比，具有相似的疗效且正常组织毒性更低。
> - 只有在需要消融治疗，但光子 SRS 不能达到预期要求的情况下，方可优先选择质子 SRS。
> - 还需进一步研究以明确质子 SRS 较低的出射剂量能否更好地保护抗肿瘤免疫，或者保护预后良好患者的长期神经认知功能。

参考文献

[1] Newhauser WD, Zhang R. The physics of proton therapy. Phys Med Biol. 2015;60(8):R155–209.

[2] Almond PR, Biggs PJ, Coursey BM, Hanson WF, Huq MS, Nath R, et al. AAPM's TG-51 protocol for clinical reference dosimetry of high-energy photon and electron beams. Med Phys. 1999;26(9):1847–70.

[3] Willers H, Allen A, Grosshans D, McMahon SJ, von Neubeck C, Wiese C, et al. Toward A variable RBE for proton beam therapy.

Radiother Oncol. 2018;128(1):68–75.

[4] Bortfeld T. An analytical approximation of the Bragg curve for therapeutic proton beams. Med Phys. 1997;24(12):2024–33.

[5] Wilson RR. Radiological use of fast protons. Radiology. 1946;47(5):487–91.

[6] Larsson B. Pre-therapeutic physical experiments with high energy protons. Br J Radiol. 1961;34:143–51.

[7] Paganetti H. Proton therapy physics. Boca Raton: CRC Press; 2016.

[8] Trofimov A, Bortfeld T. Optimization of beam parameters and treatment planning for intensity modulated proton therapy. Technol Cancer Res Treat. 2003;2(5):437–44.

[9] Madani I, Lomax AJ, Albertini F, Trnkova P, Weber DC. Dose-painting intensity-modulated proton therapy for intermediate- and high-risk meningioma. Radiat Oncol. 2015;10:72.

[10] Paganetti H. Range uncertainties in proton therapy and the role of Monte Carlo simulations. Phys Med Biol. 2012;57(11):R99–117.

[11] Giantsoudi D, Grassberger C, Craft D, Niemierko A, Trofimov A, Paganetti H. Linear energy transfer-guided optimization in intensity modulated proton therapy: feasibility study and clinical potential. Int J Radiat Oncol Biol Phys. 2013;87(1):216–22.

[12] Brownstein JM, Wisdom AJ, Castle KD, Mowery YM, Guida P, Lee CL, et al. Characterizing the potency and impact of carbon ion therapy in a primary mouse model of soft tissue sarcoma. Mol Cancer Ther. 2018;17(4):858–68.

[13] Durante M, Loeffler JS. Charged particles in radiation oncology. Nat Rev Clin Oncol. 2009;7(1):37–43.

[14] International Atomic Energy Agency. Dose reporting in ion beam therapy. Vienna: International Atomic Energy Agency; 2007.

[15] Paganetti H, Niemierko A, Ancukiewicz M, Gerweck LE, Goitein M, Loeffler JS, et al. Relative biological effectiveness (RBE) values for proton beam therapy. Int J Radiat Oncol Biol Phys. 2002;53(2):407–21.

[16] Paganetti H. Relative biological effectiveness (RBE) values for proton beam therapy. Variations as a function of biological endpoint, dose, and linear energy transfer. Phys Med Biol. 2014;59(22):R419–72.

[17] Peeler CR, Mirkovic D, Titt U, Blanchard P, Gunther JR, Mahajan A, et al. Clinical evidence of variable proton biological effectiveness in pediatric patients treated for ependymoma. Radiother Oncol. 2016;121(3):395–401.

[18] Hall EJ, Giaccia AJ. Radiobiology for the radiologist. Philadelphia: Wolters Kluwer Health/Lippincott Williams & Wilkins; 2012.

[19] Fontana AO, Augsburger MA, Grosse N, Guckenberger M, Lomax AJ, Sartori AA, et al. Differential DNA repair pathway choice in cancer cells after proton- and photon-irradiation. Radiother Oncol. 2015;116(3):374–80.

[20] McMahon SJ, Paganetti H, Prise KM. LET-weighted doses effectively reduce biological variability in proton radiotherapy planning. Phys Med Biol. 2018;63(22):225009.

[21] Yerramilli D, Bussière MR, Loeffler JS, Shih HA. Proton beam therapy (for CNS tumors). In: Chang EL, Brown PD, Lo SS, Sahgal A, Suh JH, editors. Adult CNS radiation oncology: principles and practice. Cham: Springer International Publishing; 2018. p. 709–22.

[22] Hua C, Yao W, Kidani T, Tomida K, Ozawa S, Nishimura T, et al. A robotic C-arm cone beam CT system for image-guided proton therapy: design and performance. Br J Radiol. 2017;90(1079):20170266.

[23] Bolsi A, Fogliata A, Cozzi L. Radiotherapy of small intracranial tumours with different advanced techniques using photon and proton beams: a treatment planning study. Radiother Oncol. 2003;68(1):1–14.

[24] Freund D, Zhang R, Sanders M, Newhauser W. Predictive risk of radiation induced cerebral necrosis in pediatric brain cancer patients after VMAT versus proton therapy. Cancers. 2015;7(2):617–30.

[25] Safai S, Bortfeld T, Engelsman M. Comparison between the lateral penumbra of a collimated double-scattered beam and uncollimated scanning beam in proton radiotherapy. Phys Med Biol. 2008;53(6):1729–50.

[26] Winterhalter C, Lomax A, Oxley D, Weber DC, Safai S. A study of lateral fall-off (penumbra) optimisation for pencil beam scanning (PBS) proton therapy. Phys Med Biol. 2018;63(2):025022.

[27] Weber DC, Chan AW, Bussiere MR, Harsh IVGR, Ancukiewicz M, Barker IIFG, et al. Proton beam radiosurgery for vestibular schwannoma: tumor control and cranial nerve toxicity. Neurosurgery. 2003;53(3):577–88.

[28] Wattson DA, Tanguturi SK, Spiegel DY, Niemierko A, Biller BMK, Nachtigall LB, et al. Outcomes of proton therapy for patients with functional pituitary adenomas. Int J Radiat Oncol Biol Phys. 2014;90(3):532–9.

[29] Petit JH, Biller BM, Yock TI, Swearingen B, Coen JJ, Chapman P, et al. Proton stereotactic radiotherapy for persistent adrenocorticotropin-producing adenomas. J Clin Endocrinol Metab. 2008;93(2):393–9.

[30] Hattangadi-Gluth JA, Chapman PH, Kim D, Niemierko A, Bussière MR, Stringham A, et al. Single-fraction proton beam stereotactic radiosurgery for cerebral arteriovenous malformations. Int J Radiat Oncol Biol Phys. 2014;89(2):338–46.

[31] Hattangadi JA, Chapman PH, Bussière MR, Niemierko A, Ogilvy CS, Rowell A, et al. Planned two-fraction proton beam stereotactic radiosurgery for high-risk inoperable cerebral arteriovenous malformations. Int J Radiat Oncol Biol Phys. 2012;83(2):533–41.

[32] Shih HA, Chapman PH, Loeffler JS. Proton beam radiosurgery: clinical experience. In: Lozano AM, Gildenberg PL, Tasker RR, editors. Textbook of stereotactic and functional neurosurgery. Berlin, Heidelberg: Springer Berlin Heidelberg; 2009. p. 1131–7.

[33] Atkins KM, Pashtan IM, Bussiere MR, Kang KH, Niemierko

A, Daly JE, et al. Proton stereotactic radiosurgery for brain metastases: a single-institution analysis of 370 patients. Int J Radiat Oncol Biol Phys. 2018;101(4):820–9.

[34] Particle Therapy Co-operative Group. Particle therapy facilities in clinical operation. 2018. Available from: https://www.ptcog.ch/index.php/ facilities-in-operation.

[35] Durante M, Loeffler JS. Charged particles in radiation oncology. Nat Rev Clin Oncol. 2010;7(1):37–43.

[36] Schulz-Ertner D, Nikoghosyan A, Hof H, Didinger B, Combs SE, Jakel O, et al. Carbon ion radiotherapy of skull base chondrosarcomas. Int J Radiat Oncol Biol Phys. 2007;67(1):171–7.

[37] Ares C, Hug EB, Lomax AJ, Bolsi A, Timmermann B, Rutz HP, et al. Effectiveness and safety of spot scanning proton radiation therapy for chordomas and chondrosarcomas of the skull base: first long-term report. Int J Radiat Oncol Biol Phys. 2009;75(4):1111–8.

[38] Mizoe JE. Review of carbon ion radiotherapy for skull base tumors (especially chordomas). Rep Pract Oncol Radiother. 2016;21(4):356–60.

[39] Kirkpatrick JP, Laack NN, Halasz LM, Minniti G, Chan MD. Proton therapy for brain metastases: a question of value. Int J Radiat Oncol Biol Phys. 2018;101(4):830–2.

[40] Fossati P, Vavassori A, Deantonio L, Ferrara E, Krengli M, Orecchia R. Review of photon and proton radiotherapy for skull base tumours. Rep Pract Oncol Radiother. 2016;21(4):336–55.

[41] Adeberg S, Harrabi S, Bougatf N, Verma V, Windisch P, Bernhardt D, et al. Dosimetric comparison of proton radiation therapy, volumetric modulated arc therapy, and three-dimensional conformal radiotherapy based on intracranial tumor location. Cancers. 2018;10(11):401.

[42] Sperduto PW, Yang TJ, Beal K, Pan H, Brown PD, Bangdiwala A, et al. Estimating survival in patients with lung cancer and brain metastases: an update of the graded prognostic assessment for lung cancer using molecular markers (Lung-molGPA). JAMA Oncol. 2017;3(6):827–31.

[43] Sperduto PW, Kased N, Roberge D, Xu Z, Shanley R, Luo X, et al. Effect of tumor subtype on survival and the graded prognostic assessment for patients with breast cancer and brain metastases. Int J Radiat Oncol Biol Phys. 2012;82(5):2111–7.

[44] Ganong WF. Review of medical physiology. 21st ed. Boston: McGraw-Hill; 2003.

[45] Yovino S, Kleinberg L, Grossman SA, Narayanan M, Ford E. The etiology of treatment-related lymphopenia in patients with malignant gliomas: modeling radiation dose to circulating lymphocytes explains clinical observations and suggests methods of modifying the impact of radiation on immune cells. Cancer Investig. 2013;31(2):140–4.

[46] Petr J, Platzek I, Hofheinz F, Mutsaerts H, Asllani I, van Osch MJP, et al. Photon vs. proton radiochemotherapy: effects on brain tissue volume and perfusion. Radiother Oncol. 2018;128(1):121–7.

[47] Huang J, DeWees TA, Badiyan SN, Speirs CK, Mullen DF, Fergus S, et al. Clinical and dosimetric predictors of acute severe lymphopenia during radiation therapy and concurrent temozolomide for high-grade glioma. Int J Radiat Oncol Biol Phys. 2015;92(5):1000–7.

[48] Vaios EJ, Nahed BV, Muzikansky A, Fathi AT, Dietrich J. Bone marrow response as a potential biomarker of outcomes in glioblastoma patients. J Neurosurg. 2017;127(1):132–8.

第 14 章 特殊类型脑转移瘤的治疗
Special Topics in Brain Metastases Management

James Byrne　Kevin S. Oh　Nancy Wang　著
张莹莹　龙艺文　朱　红　译
伍海军　校

一、颅底转移瘤

(一) 病例介绍

病例 1

一名 71 岁 IV 期直肠癌女性患者，临床表现为逐渐加重的复视、右侧上睑下垂、右眼视物模糊和双眼不共轭。头部 CT 示右前鞍突溶骨性破坏。脑部 MRI 也证实有一分叶状的肿块，压迫了视神经管内的视神经和位于眶上裂内的第 Ⅲ 对脑神经。

(二) 概述

颅底转移十分罕见，仅能在约 4% 的癌症患者中发现[1]。这些转移瘤早期可能没有临床症状，但当转移瘤增大到引起疼痛或是压迫脑神经及血管系统时可出现症状。常见的是易出现骨转移的肿瘤，包括前列腺癌、乳腺癌、淋巴瘤、肾癌和肺癌[2]。

(三) 循证基础

1. 诊断

大多数颅底转移瘤没有症状，最常见的症状是脑神经功能障碍，约 21% 的患者会出现[3]。其中以动眼神经、三叉神经或舌下神经受压或受损最为多见。脑神经功能障碍及邻近颅底孔隙和鼻窦的血管受压可分别引起不同的综合征，包括眼眶综合征、鞍旁综合征、颅中窝综合征、颈静脉孔综合征和枕髁综合征[4]。表 14-1 总结了每种综合征的体征和症状。

表 14-1　颅底转移的临床表现

部　位	症　状	体　征
眼眶	• 眶上疼痛 • 复视	• 上睑下垂 • 眼肌麻痹 • 伴/不伴面部麻木 • 伴/不伴视力下降 • 伴/不伴眶周肿胀
鞍旁（蝶鞍座、岩尖）	• 额部疼痛 • 复视	• 眼肌麻痹 • 面部麻木（第 Ⅵ 对脑神经） • 眶周肿胀
颅中窝（岩嵴）	• 面部麻木 • 感觉异常 • 非典型面部疼痛	• 面部麻木（第 Ⅶ、Ⅷ 对脑神经） • 外展麻痹（前嵴） • 面瘫（后嵴）
颈静脉孔	• 枕部疼痛 • 声音嘶哑 • 吞咽困难	• 脑神经麻痹（第 Ⅸ、Ⅹ、Ⅺ 对脑神经）
枕髁	• 枕部疼痛 • 构音障碍	• 脑神经麻痹（第 Ⅻ 对脑神经）

经 Springer Nature 许可转载，引自 Laigle-Donadey 等[1]

颅底转移瘤的诊断需要具有合适分辨率的影像学检查，包括覆盖乳突、颞骨和整个颅底的头颅平扫 CT，以及颅脑特别是增强的 MRI T_1 加权图像。例如，在 CT 上可显示占位性病变伴骨破坏（图 14-1），在 MRI 上可显示增强的肿块及其累及的邻近脑神经、硬脑膜或脑实质，以及通过颅底孔道侵犯的咀嚼肌间隙或鼻旁窦的图像（图 14-2）[5]。影像学检查对于确定下一步的治疗及识别放疗或外科治疗的关键结构至关重要。若需要对转移病灶进行病理确诊，则尽可能使用内窥镜活检或其他微创技术。

2. 治疗

颅底转移瘤的治疗可能需要放疗、手术和全身治疗相结合的综合治疗。对于需要缓解疼痛或减轻神经功能障碍的患者，放射治疗是主要的治疗方法[6, 7]。放射治疗后的神经功能改善率与神经症状出现后治疗是否及时密切相关。部分患者可采用外科手术治疗。神经血管结构受累的病灶，使外科手术为避免严重并发症并获得完整切缘的尝试变得复杂化；但对于某些辐射抵抗的组织类型，与单纯放射治疗相比，手术能获得更加显著的治疗效果。对于无症状、无生命威胁不需要紧急做局部治疗的患者，全身治疗或监测可能是合适的选择。

3. 颅底转移瘤的放射治疗

Svare 等[8] 报道，约 70% 的前列腺癌颅底转移患者接受了放疗。放射治疗能很好地缓解疼痛并改善神经功能[6, 7]。影响照射剂量和分割方案的因素有很多，包括病灶的大小和与关键结构的邻近程度。

（1）常规分割光子放射治疗：颅底转移瘤主要的放射治疗方式是常规剂量分割模式的光子照射。常规剂量分割模式的放疗能显著缓解大多数患者的症状。一项来自纪念斯隆凯特琳癌症中心的回顾性分析显示，43 名颅底转移患者中有 37 名

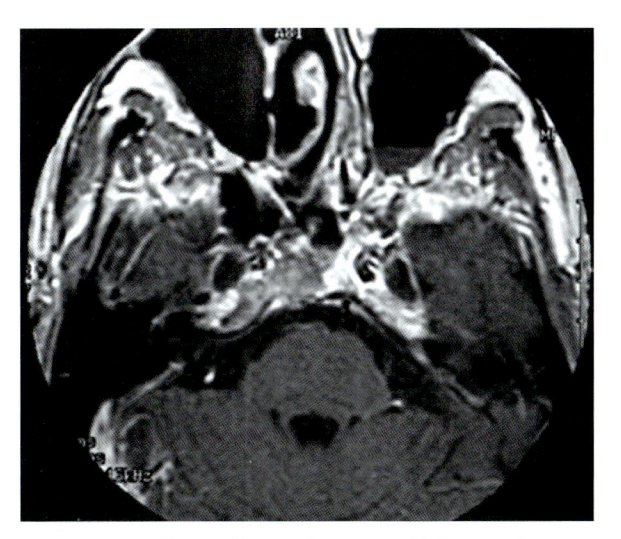

▲ 图 14-2 增强（钆对比剂）后的轴位 T_1 加权 MRI 显示强化病变侵犯斜坡和蝶窦后部，邻近 Meckel 腔未受侵犯

经 Springer Nature 许可转载，引自 Laigle-Donadey 等[1]

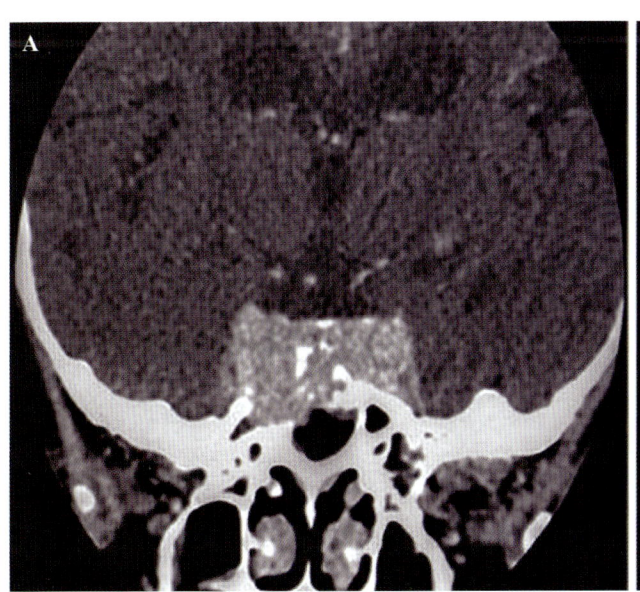

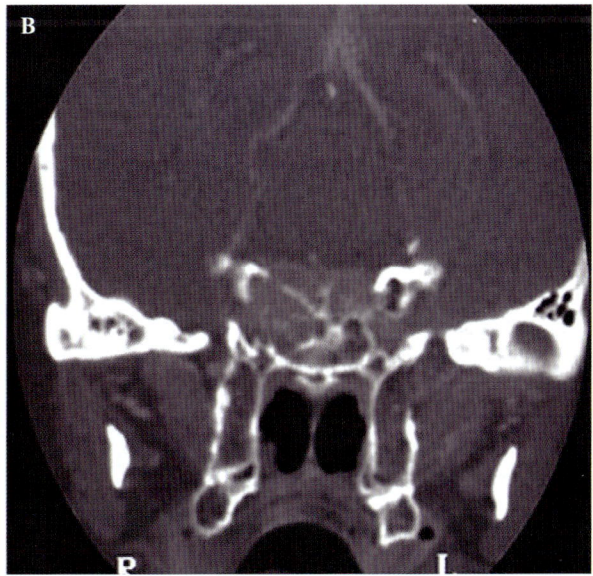

▲ 图 14-1 增强的冠状位 CT 重建图：软组织窗（A）和骨窗（B）显示明显强化、轮廓清晰的肿块侵入蝶骨体，并有明显的骨质破坏

经 Springer Nature 许可转载，引自 Laigle-Donadey 等[1]

在常规分割放疗后症状缓解，其中 7 名患者的脑神经症状完全消失[9]。另一项回顾性研究评估了去势抵抗的前列腺癌颅底转移瘤的放疗疗效，大多数患者放疗后达到了完全或部分临床缓解。不幸的是，2/3 的患者在治疗后 3 个月内仍因转移性疾病死亡。多个研究均强调了患者在确诊后应尽快接受放射治疗，以提高症状缓解的可能性[10, 11]。以往颅底转移瘤主要采用左右对穿野或三野的普通放疗技术[11]。然而，现代成像技术能够更好地勾画骨病变，调强放射治疗（intensity-modulated radiation therapy，IMRT）已经被广泛应用于颅底转移瘤，它能将非靶结构（如视器、垂体和神经认知中枢）的放射剂量降至最低[12]。

（2）立体定向放射放疗：立体定向放射外科治疗（SRS）在颅底转移瘤的治疗中显示出了良好的前景。在小型回顾性研究报道中，SRS 显示出较高的局部控制率（67%~95%）[13, 14]和较低的并发症发生率（6%）[13]，同时也能很好地缓解症状。此外，另一项涉及立体定向放射治疗（stereotactic radiotherapy，SRT）（剂量 44Gy/5 次）的研究显示，在累及颅底的局部晚期或复发性头颈部恶性肿瘤患者中，即使既往接受过放疗，其不良反应发生率也较低（3 级发生率 15%，4 级及以上发生率 0%）[15]。此外，使用伽马刀（Gamma Knife，GK）放射外科治疗颅底转移瘤导致三叉神经痛的患者，60% 的患者在 6 个月时疼痛消失，40% 的患者因无疼痛而停止服用镇痛药[16]。因此，采用适当的固定方法和机载成像，SRS 成为一种颅底转移瘤可选择的治疗方法。

（四）争议

传统分割的放疗剂量选择目前仍存在争议。在比较单次分割（如 8Gy/1 次）和多次分割（如 4Gy/6 次）方案时，有多个随机试验显示出相似的短期止痛效果[17, 18]。然而，有关颅底转移瘤剂量选择的数据则仅限于回顾性研究。有报道称，与标准剂量（30Gy/10 次）相比，使用更高剂量（36Gy）可以提高神经功能恢复率，这种获益可能是组织学功能和放射敏感性差异的结果[19, 20]。而 SRS 或放射治疗联合全身治疗（如免疫治疗）等综合治疗模式的有效性和安全性尚需前瞻性研究来评估。

（五）结论和建议

癌症患者出现新发的脑神经症状或颅面部疼痛时应高度怀疑颅底转移，这对于提高早期诊断率是重要的。早期治疗是改善潜在致残症候的关键。姑息治疗的主要手段是放射治疗。症状出现后尽快进行放射治疗，可以显著缓解疼痛和脑神经症状。SRS 是另一种有效的放疗形式，但受限于病变的大小和邻近的关键结构（如视神经通路）。仅少数患者进行手术切除。

> **要　点**
> - 颅底转移瘤最常见的临床表现是脑神经受损症状。
> - 放射治疗是颅底转移瘤最主要的治疗手段。
> - 早期治疗对于改善潜在致残症状和最大限度地减轻症状至关重要。
> - 尚无 I 类证据来指导如何对颅底转移瘤进行放射治疗。

二、脉络膜转移瘤

（一）病例介绍

病例 2

一位 69 岁 ER+/PR+/HER2- 的 IV 期乳腺癌患者，最初主诉为视物模糊，随后出现左眼闪光感。她两年前的最后一次检查结果都在正常范围内。眼科医生检查后诊断为左侧脉络膜转移瘤：病变大小约 16mm×15mm，贴近视盘和黄斑中心。她的右眼视力为 20/20，左眼视力为 20/70，是进行保留眼球治疗的合适人选。

第 14 章 特殊类型脑转移瘤的治疗
Special Topics in Brain Metastases Management

（二）概述

脉络膜转移瘤虽然罕见，但却是最常见的眼内恶性肿瘤。患者经常出现视物模糊、飞蚊症、幻视或疼痛[21, 22]。15%～20% 的乳腺癌患者在常规分期过程或眼科检查中发现脉络膜转移[23]。其发病率稳步上升，很可能是由于早期诊断的技术进步和血行转移的肿瘤患者生存率的提高。在利物浦眼科肿瘤中心的一系列研究中，发现多达 1/3 的[21]肿瘤患者血行转移的首发表现是脉络膜转移。脉络膜转移最常见的原发肿瘤来源为乳腺癌和肺癌[22, 23]。源于乳腺癌的转移通常为双侧或多灶性，而源于肺癌的转移通常为单侧和单灶性[22, 23]。

（三）循证基础

1. 诊断

早期发现脉络膜转移对视力下降的保护或逆转至关重要。脉络膜转移瘤的诊断需要配合多种检测方法来确定疾病的严重程度和治疗方案，如吲哚菁绿血管造影、光学相干断层扫描（optical coherence tomography，OCT）、光谱域（spectral domain）-OCT、眼底检查（图 14-3）、超声检查等。部分情况还可能需要通过脉络膜肿瘤活检以获取病理组织学的确诊[24]。此外，很大一部分脉络膜转移患者也会出现眼外转移[25]。因为合并脑转移的风险很高，脉络膜转移的病例推荐行头部 MRI，尤其原发病是肺癌和乳腺癌的患者（在某些研究中脑转移率分别为 32% 和 62%）[26, 27]。

2. 治疗

脉络膜转移瘤可导致视力丧失，最终丧失生活自理能力。治疗的主要目标是预防或逆转视觉功能损害。避免眼球摘除是一个首要的目标，因为眼球摘除会带来身体功能和心理障碍。一般来说，早期及时的治疗可以阻止不可逆的失明。由

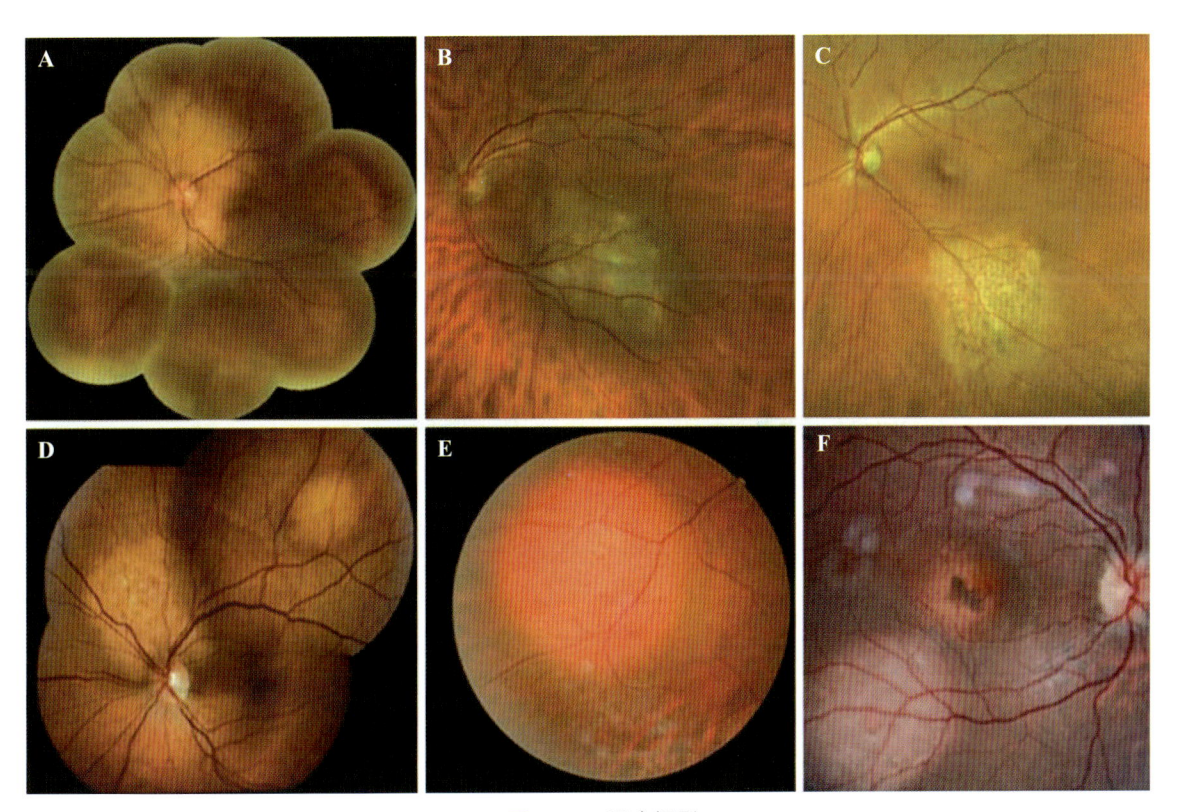

▲ 图 14-3 眼底摄影

A. 肺癌：淡黄色；B. 乳腺癌：小叶乳白色；C. 前列腺癌：无色素性肿块；D. 肾癌：颞部橙色肿块伴另一淡黄色乳头旁肿块；E. 肺类癌：橙色；F. 甲状腺肿瘤：凹陷的橙色肿块并与下方另一个白色肿块相连。经 Elsevier 许可转载，引自 Mathis 等[24]

175

于起效快、有效率高，放射治疗是目前脉络膜转移瘤的主要治疗手段[24]。全身治疗和局部治疗相结合可以在取得局部控制的同时减少全身临床症状的恶化。

3. 脉络膜转移瘤的放射治疗

放射治疗因放射技术、剂量、分割方式和靶区的不同而有很多种选择。治疗脉络膜转移瘤的主要技术包括光子放疗、质子放疗和敷贴近距离照射治疗。在光子放疗中，分次常规 3D 适形放疗、分次 IMRT 和 SRS/SRT 是主要的模式类别[24]。这些技术的选择取决于局部病灶的大小和侵犯范围、是否接近黄斑、病变的数量、预后和护理目标。每种放疗方式都有独特的技术考量因素，包括剂量和分割方式、适形度、治疗时间和技术的可及性。表 14-2 显示了标准分割剂量下的正常组织耐受剂量，所有这些因素都必须在风险收益分析中加以考虑，正常组织可以更好地耐受较小的分割剂量，且不良反应随分割剂量和总剂量的递增而增加。多数脉络膜转移瘤可通过标准的姑息性分割剂量（如 3Gy/10 次）得到控制。从既往的治疗情况来看，放疗抵抗的肿瘤（如黑色素瘤和肾癌）可能需要更高的分割剂量才能获益，但可能导致黄斑受损增加[28]。

（1）放疗计划：治疗计划的体位摆放和固定方法取决于放射治疗的方式。多数情况下，患者的头部是用个体化的热塑面罩或硬质面罩来固定的。为提高摆位的重复性，患者被要求闭上眼睛，保持眼球向下或直视方向。勾画靶区时，需要融合高分辨率 MRI 和平面眼底图像（如果有）（图 14-4）到计划 CT 图像中。在单侧受累的情况下，可以采用三维适形技术，例如楔形对穿野或非共面照射野。如果双侧受累或高度怀疑有对侧微转移（如同时合并多发性脑转移），可使用平行对穿侧野。通常 GTV 外扩 5mm 为 CTV，并根据固定方法的不同，CTV 再外扩 0~5mm 得到 PTV[29]。放疗计划过程则根据放疗模式的不同，有不同的射束和设野方式的组合。

（2）立体定向放疗：SRS 在脉络膜转移瘤治

表 14-2 眼眶放疗的危及器官限量

组织	标准分割的剂量限制	备注
晶状体	晶状体平均剂量 < 0.5Gy 可避免晶状体混浊 晶状体平均剂量 < 5~8Gy 可避免白内障	放疗诱发白内障一般发生在照射后 1~3 年
角膜	角膜最大剂量 < 40~60Gy 可避免角膜炎症、溃疡或水肿 穿孔罕见，仅发生剂量在 60Gy 以上	
泪腺	接受 30Gy 照射的泪腺体积 < 50%	
视网膜	接受 45Gy 照射的视网膜体积 < 50%	严重的视网膜病变通常发生在放疗后 3 个月~3 年，具体取决于剂量和其他身体状况
视神经	视神经最大剂量 < 55 Gy	放射诱发的视神经病变发生在治疗后 3 个月~8 年，并在 18 个月达到峰值
视交叉	视交叉最大剂量 < 55Gy	视交叉是后位的，通常在脉络膜转移瘤的治疗中能获得较好的保护

经 Elsevier 许可转载，引自 Mathis 等[24]，标准分割 = 每次 1.8~2.0Gy

疗中的研究数据似乎很有前景，但仅限于少数病例报道。在一组 10 例患者的研究中[29]，SRS（12~20Gy）使所有患者的肿瘤得到了长期控制，且 10 例患者中有 5 例出现肿瘤完全缓解，但只有 4 例患者视力稳定或改善，未发现晚期放疗毒性。另一项研究显示，使用伽马刀（15~25Gy）治疗脉络膜转移瘤没有发现急性并发症，但其样本量同样非常有限（仅 7 名患者）。SRS 的局限性包括治疗时间长、眼球跟踪和眼球完全固定困难，这些可通过麻醉性眼球阻滞和眼外肌缝合固定限制眼球运动来加以克服[30]。

（3）质子放疗：脉络膜转移瘤的质子放射治疗仅能在全球有限的几个中心进行。麻省总医院的研究者对 77 名脉络膜转移瘤患者的回顾性分析显示，在平均 7.7 个月的随访中，局部控制率

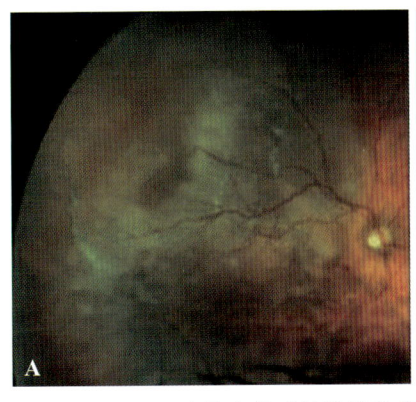

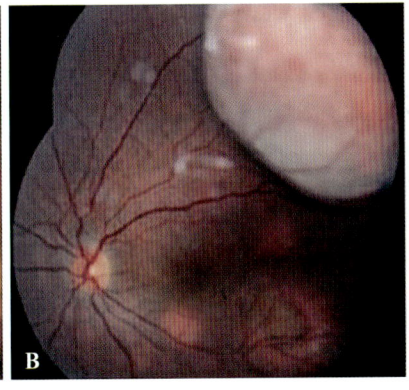

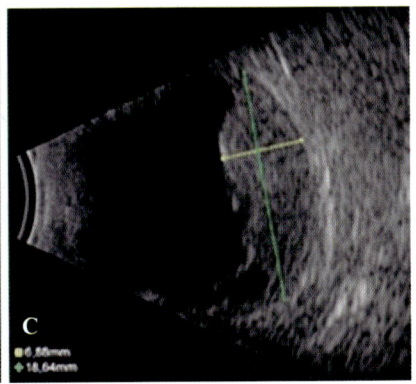

▲ 图 14-4 大体积的脉络膜转移瘤（A）鼻咽癌脉络膜转移的视网膜摄影；（B，C）神经内分泌肿瘤脉络膜转移的视网膜摄影和相应的超声检查

黄色标记；厚度（高度）；绿色标记；直径（底部）。经 Elsevier 许可转载，引自 Mathis 等 [24]

为 94%。38% 的患者视力改善或稳定，31% 的患者发生了治疗相关不良事件 [31]。这些已发表的研究大多数是采用被动散射质子治疗技术，而关于笔形束质子治疗的数据很少。此外，对位于眼球后极的肿瘤，质子放疗技术保护黄斑的能力有限。因此对于黄斑附近的肿瘤，我们更倾向于使用较小的分割剂量以保护正常组织。在治疗前，在肿瘤周围放置基准点并依此进行跟踪，有助于靶区勾画和追踪。此外，红外线摄像机可以在患者眼球移动改变视线时立即阻断质子束以更好地保护正常组织 [24]。

(4) 敷贴近距离照射：敷贴近距离治疗需要在肿瘤附近放置具有一定半衰期的放射性同位素敷贴，它通常被缝合在肿瘤附近的巩膜上，并一直保持在适当的位置，直到释放的剂量达到治疗剂量为止（通常是 2～4 天）。最常用的同位素是低剂量率的 I-125。在病例数最多的几项研究中，一项入组了 36 名患者的临床研究显示：敷贴近距离放射治疗使所有患者都出现了肿瘤退缩，在接受 45～70Gy 剂量范围的患者中，完全缓解率为 94%。同时他们强调这种放疗方式的并发症发生率较低，最常见的并发症是视网膜病变、视神经病变和白内障 [32]。总体而言，尽管比外照射更具侵入性，敷贴近距离治疗是一个很好的治疗选择，但只有少数特定的机构能提供该治疗。

(5) 放射治疗后遗症：放射治疗的早期并发症包括放射性皮炎、局灶性脱发、结膜炎和干眼症。晚期并发症可能在治疗后数月至数年发生，包括持续结膜炎、干眼症、白内障、激素失衡、视力下降以及正常脑组织损害。而根据预后的不同，疾病控制与并发症需相互平衡，特别是在长期存活的患者中。放射性黄斑损伤通常在治疗后 2 年达到高峰，因而不良反应应结合整体预后来考虑。不论是外照射还是近距离放疗，避开黄斑和视神经盘对于保存视力至关重要 [33]，而能否实现避开黄斑和视神经盘则取决于其与肿瘤病灶之间的距离远近。

（四）争议

由于脉络膜转移瘤的罕见性以及跨中心获得治疗的机会有限，使相关研究工作面临很大的挑战。至今没有前瞻性随机试验比较不同放疗方式的疗效和不良反应，因此尚不清楚治疗脉络膜转移瘤的最佳放射治疗方式。

（五）结论和建议

放射治疗是脉络膜转移瘤的主要治疗手段。放射治疗可以单独使用，也可以与全身治疗联合，特别是在发生广泛转移的情况下更需要联合全身治疗。多种放射治疗技术都可用于脉络膜转移瘤的治疗，包括常规分割放射治疗、SRS、质子治疗和敷贴近距离放射治疗。

> **要　点**
> - 脉络膜转移瘤通常因出现视物模糊、飞蚊症、幻视或疼痛而被诊断。
> - 放射治疗是脉络膜转移瘤的主要治疗手段。
> - 主要的放射治疗方式包括常规分割放射治疗、SRS、质子放射治疗和敷贴近距离放射治疗。
> - 目前尚不清楚脉络膜转移瘤的最佳放射治疗方式。

三、脑干转移瘤

（一）病例介绍

病例 3

一位 60 岁右乳浸润性导管癌的女性患者，临床分期为 Ⅱ 期（$T_2N_0M_0$），*ER/PR* 阴性，*HER2* 阳性。在临床试验中接受了新辅助 T-DM1 和帕妥珠单抗治疗，随后接受了右乳切除术和前哨淋巴结活检。病理显示病理完全缓解，前哨淋巴结无转移（0/3）。患者继续接受 4 个周期的紫杉醇联合赫赛汀和帕妥珠单抗的辅助治疗，之后每 3 周接受一次赫赛汀维持治疗，为期 1 年。治疗结束 1 年后，患者出现头痛和右下肢无力的症状。头部 MRI 可见脑桥部的囊性边缘强的肿块，如图 14-5 所示。

（二）概述

脑干转移瘤仅占所有脑转移病例的 5%，这反映了脑部各区域相对血流的分布情况。脑干转移瘤的进展通常会导致迅速且无法挽救的神经性死亡，而脑干转移瘤的治疗也面临着独特的挑战。尽管有大量关于 SRS 治疗脑转移的随机临床研究数据，但对于脑干转移的患者，通常由于担心常用的 SRS 剂量超过脑干耐受量而被排除在这些试验之外[34-36]。就放射治疗而言，脑干周边的剂量限制使得无论是采用单一分割放疗、大分割放疗还是常规分割放疗，都无法实现消融剂量的安全递送，寻找既有效又安全的最低剂量是临床医生不可避免的挑战。手术治疗对于脑干转移瘤来说既不能作为首要治疗，也不能用作挽救治

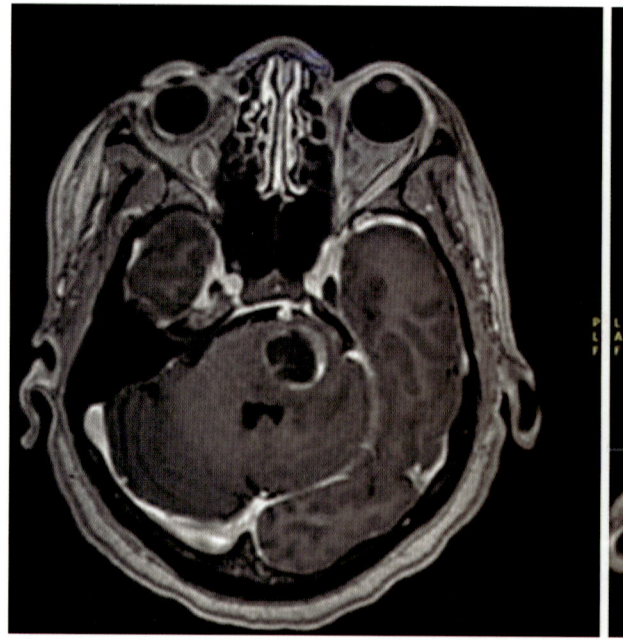

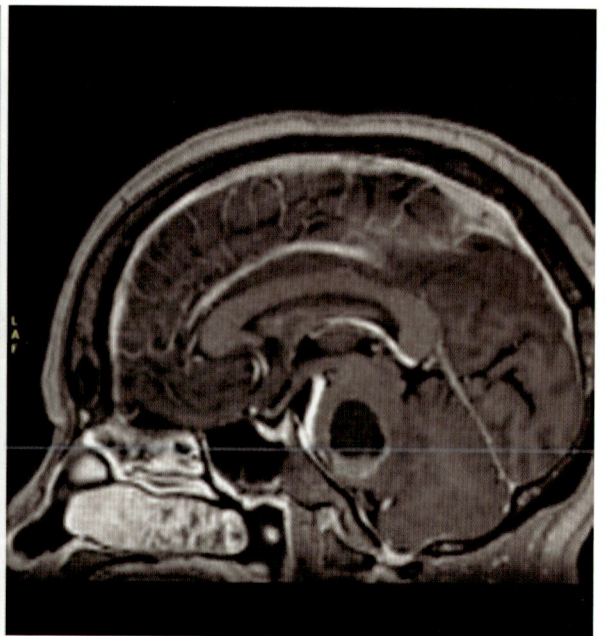

▲ 图 14-5　冠状位和矢状位 T_1 增强序列显示囊性脑干病变，沿下方和左侧均有结节状强化

疗。脑干转移的进展通常会导致快速且不可治愈的神经系统疾病死亡。

（三）循证基础

1. 单次立体定向放射外科治疗

几个小型单中心研究报道了单次 SRS 治疗脑干转移瘤的结果[37-47]。如表 14-3 所示，该系列中的大多数研究采用了基于伽马刀的放射外科治疗，入组人数小于 50 名。局部控制率为 75%～95%，中位剂量一般为单次 13～16Gy。尽管不同研究报道的方法不一致，放射外科治疗相关并发症发生率一般不到 10%。其中几项研究显示肿瘤体积较大[37, 40, 42, 43]或放疗抵抗的病理类型，如黑色素瘤或肾癌[37, 39]的局控相对较差。Trifiletti 等通过国际伽马刀研究基金会（International Gamma Knife Research Foundation）发布了最大的汇集数据分析，其中包括 547 例接受伽马刀治疗的脑干转移瘤患者。患者的中位边缘剂量为 16Gy（规定为 50% 等剂量水平），12 个月局部控制率为 81.8%，总生存率为 32.7%。严重的放射外科治疗相关毒性（≥ 3 级）发生率为 7.4%[48]。

在选择脑干转移瘤病灶的放射治疗剂量和分割方式时，安全性是首要考虑因素。《临床正常组

表 14-3 脑干转移瘤的单一机构系列放射外科治疗

作者	年份	数量	SRS 模式	平均剂量（范围）	局控率	中位生存时间（个月）	毒性反应
Hatiboglu 等	2011	60	LINAC	15Gy（8～18）	76%（粗算率）	4	20% SRS 相关并发症
Hussain 等	2007	22	GK	16Gy（14～23）	100%（粗算率）	8.5	5% SRS 术后偏瘫
Kased 等	2008	42	GK	16Gy（10～19.8）	77%（1年局控率）	9	9.5% SRS 相关并发症
Kawabe 等	2012	200	GK	18Gy（12～25）	82%（2年局控率）	6	1 例死亡和 6 例无症状放射学瘤周改变
Kilburn 等	2014	44	GK	18Gy（10～22）	74%（1年局控率）	6	9% SRS 相关并发症
Koyfman 等	2010	43	GK	15Gy（9.6～24）	85%（1年局控率）	5.8	未观察到 3～4 级毒性
Lin 等	2012	45	LINAC	14Gy（10～17）	88%（1年局控率）	11.6	两年内并发症发生率为 4.7%
Lorenzoni 等	2009	25	GK	20Gy（15～24）	95%（粗算率）	11.1	未记录到有 SRS 引起的并发症
Peterso 等	2014	41	GK	17Gy	91%（粗算率）	22% 达到 12 个月	1 例患者治疗后死于出血
Sengoz 等	2013	44	GK	16Gy（10～20）	96%（粗算率）	8	4% 的肿瘤周围有无症状的 X 线改变
Shuto 等	2003	25	GK	平均 13 Gy（8～18）	77%（粗算率）	4.9	8% 的放射损伤

SRS. 立体定向放疗；LINAC. 直线加速器放疗；GK. 伽马刀放疗

织效应定量分析》（QUANTEC）指南汇编了包括脑干在内的各种神经结构耐受剂量的可用数据。作为这项工作的一部分，Mayo 等汇编了采用不同分割方式[49]的脑干照射耐受剂量的可用安全性数据。根据现有的数据，其结论是若采用传统的分割模式，整个脑干可以接受 54Gy 的照射且毒性风险小；较小的体积（最多 10ml）可以以 2Gy 或更小的分割剂量照射至 59Gy，神经病变或坏死的风险不到 5%。而可用的单次放射外科治疗耐受剂量的安全数据仅限于 5 项研究，且其剂量和处方剂量参考点都存在一定变化区间。对于单次 SRS 治疗，当剂量＞ 12Gy 时，脑干的毒性风险增加。然而，随着单次 SRS 治疗脑干转移病灶经验的积累，发现转移灶的特点是挤压占位而不是直接浸润脑干实质。因此，只要靶区位于大体病变范围内，就有可能对其进行更高剂量的 SRS。Foote 等报道了一项规模最大的研究，包括 149 例前庭神经鞘瘤患者，采用 10~22.5Gy[50]基于 LINAC 的 SRS 治疗。单因素分析显示，Dmax ≥ 17.5Gy 和 12.5Gy 分别是发生面神经病变和任何脑神经病变的重要危险因素，因而得出结论，外周剂量≥ 15Gy 时，神经并发症显著增加。

2. 大分割立体定向方案

许多机构，特别是那些使用直线加速器的中心，选择使用大分割的策略来治疗脑干转移瘤。大分割放射治疗是指每日剂量≥ 4Gy 的治疗，常与立体定向放射治疗（stereotactic body radiation therapy，SBRT）技术联合使用。常见的方案包括 8Gy/3 次和 6Gy/5 次。这些剂量和分割方式是基于使用线性平方模型（L-Q 模型）建立的安全曲线模型来计算"nBED2/2"的，nBED2/2 是假设 α∶β 为 2，换算成 2Gy 每分次剂量的等效生物剂量。应该注意的是，在高分次剂量的前提下，该模型的可靠性是有争议的。Clark 等回顾了 77 例接受了 7Gy/6 次（90% 等剂量线）放射治疗的良 / 恶性脑转移肿瘤患者，20 例脑膜瘤患者中有 4 例出现脑干并发症[51]。采用线性平方模型计算，假设 α∶β 为 2.5Gy，并发症与 BED ＞ 70Gy 相关。

（四）未来发展方向

更有效、更持久的脑转移瘤系统治疗的出现可能会减少脑转移瘤对放射治疗的需要，特别是在脑干等高危部位。例如，在黑色素瘤中，对伊匹木单抗单药、PD-1 抑制药单药或伊匹木单抗与纳武利尤单抗联合使用的颅内反应率分别高达 10%~25%、25%~35% 和 55%，这些反应通常是持久的[52-54]。在有驱动基因突变的患者中，已有多种可用的靶向药物，其 CNS 穿透率和颅内反应率一般＜ 60%~70%。这些药物包括用于 *EGFR* 突变的非小细胞肺癌（nonsmall-cell lung cancer，NSCLC）治疗的厄洛替尼和奥希替尼，用于治疗 NSCLC *ALK* 突变的阿来替尼，以及用于治疗黑色素瘤 *BRAF* 突变的各种 *BRAF/MEK* 抑制药。但对靶向药物反应的持久性受到耐药的限制。因此，放射治疗在脑干转移瘤初始治疗或挽救治疗中的作用需要重新定义。此外，免疫疗法和靶向药物可能通过增加放射性坏死的风险或延长疾病的自然病程而增加高剂量放射带来的毒性风险。

（五）结论和建议

脑干是颅内转移性疾病的罕见部位。由于手术难度大，放射治疗仍然是主要的治疗手段。已发表的有关脑干转移瘤单次放射外科治疗的文献仅限于小的、单中心的回顾性研究和汇集分析。总体而言，根据这些有限的资料，单次剂量为 13~24Gy 时，局部控制率为 75%~95%，与治疗相关的并发症概率一般＜ 10%。为了提高安全性，通常采用大分次剂量方案，但至今对于最佳分割方案尚无共识。最后，在免疫治疗和靶向药物治疗的背景下，越来越多的系统治疗选择和对放射脑性坏死风险增加的担忧可能会导致临床医生对放射治疗变得越来越保守。

第 14 章 特殊类型脑转移瘤的治疗
Special Topics in Brain Metastases Management

> **要 点**
> - 脑干是临床上脑转移的高危部位,需要更保守的治疗方法。
> - 目前治疗的主要手段是放射治疗,可配合 SRS、大分割或常规分割放疗。大多数可用的数据都是在 SRS 的背景下进行的。
> - 最近兴起的对颅内治疗有效的全身治疗方法,如免疫检查点抑制药和 TKI 靶向药物,可能会减少对脑干转移瘤进行放射治疗的必要。

腺癌,转移病灶累及骨、肝和肺,临床表现为右臂无力。自 4 年前确诊以来,患者接受了多种系统治疗,目前使用环磷酰胺/阿霉素化疗。本次就诊前患者在数周内出现了不断加重的意识模糊。MRI 显示多发性出血性脑转移瘤,包括以右侧颞部硬脑膜为主的转移瘤并延伸至颅骨,伴有水肿和占位效应(图 14-6)。

(二)概述

除了转移到脑实质或脑脊液,肿瘤细胞还可能转移至硬脑膜。这可能与肿瘤可延伸至硬膜外或硬膜下间隙有关,多达 1/3 的患者可见实质内直接侵犯[55]。硬脑膜转移与脑实质内或颅骨转移常同时发生。单纯发生硬脑膜转移相对少见,根据尸检报告其发病率为 9%~14%[4]。硬脑膜转移多见于乳腺癌、前列腺癌、肺癌和血液系统恶性肿瘤(如粒细胞性肉瘤),常见于疾病晚期,预后不良。它主要通过直接侵犯(特别是在颅骨转移的情况下)或血行播散发生。

四、硬脑膜转移瘤

(一)病例介绍

病例 4

一名 58 岁男性,诊断为右腮腺转移性导管

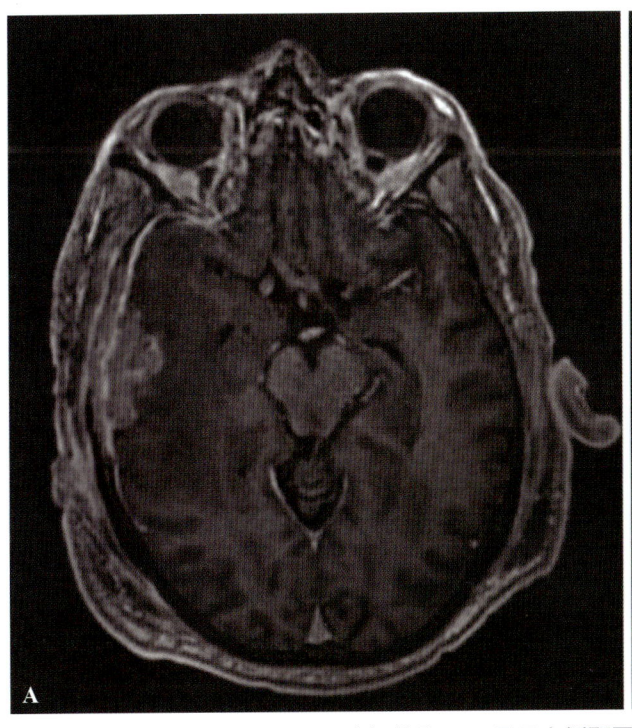

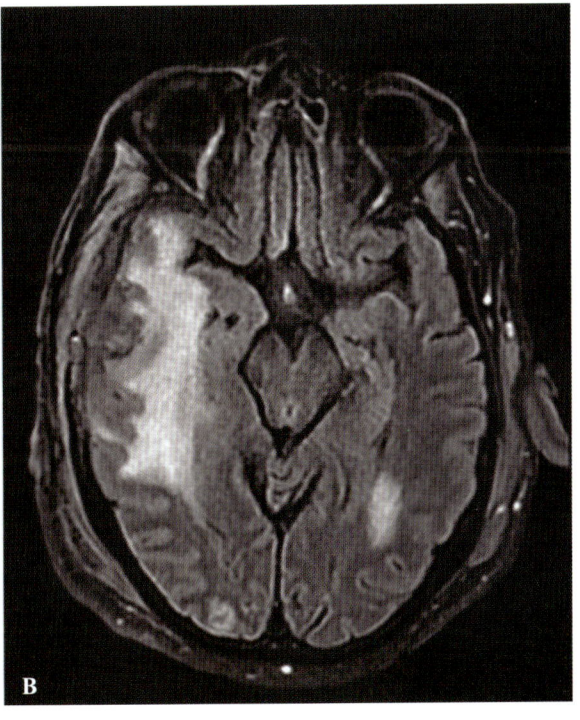

▲ 图 14-6 脑部增强 MRI 显示右侧颞区硬脑膜病变,呈不规则、不均匀强化
右侧额颞部硬脑膜增厚并延伸至邻近颅骨。周围明显水肿和局部占位效应导致左侧中线移位(B)。左侧颞枕叶和右侧枕叶 T₂/FLAIR 高信号区与(A)中显示不清楚的实质内病变相对应

其预后与脑实质内转移瘤类似，主要死因是系统性进展，中位总生存期约为6个月[55, 56]。一项对122例硬脑膜转移瘤患者的回顾性研究发现，低KPS评分和肺癌来源是[55]预后差的因素。而血液恶性肿瘤，乳腺癌和前列腺癌的转移，以及孤立的硬脑膜转移瘤是有利的预后因素[56]。尽管有多种可用的治疗方法，包括手术、放疗和全身治疗，但硬脑膜转移瘤仍经常导致严重的神经功能障碍和死亡。

（三）循证基础

1. 诊断

钆剂增强MRI是诊断硬脑膜转移瘤首选的影像学检查，并且可提供有关脑实质外起源的线索，包括存在硬脑膜鼠尾征、脑脊液裂、蛛网膜下腔血管移位和颅顶反应性改变等。与原发硬膜外或硬膜下转移不同（硬膜外或硬膜下转移灶的外观为新月形），硬脑膜转移灶通常呈双凸或透镜状强化[55]，可见邻近的血管源性水肿或占位效应。血管结构损害可导致梗死或实质内出血。硬脑膜转移瘤也可能与硬膜下血肿有关。硬脑膜强化肿块的鉴别诊断包括肿瘤性（如脑膜瘤、神经鞘瘤、血管外皮细胞瘤和淋巴瘤）和非肿瘤性（如结节病、脓胸和伴有骨损伤情况下的骨髓炎）。

临床症状取决于病灶的部位，而且通常为非特异性。发生在硬脑膜的转移瘤通常是偶然通过筛查或复查影像而被诊断。对脑实质的直接挤压或水肿可导致头痛和其他颅内压增高的征象。颅底的病变通常表现为脑神经受损症状，还可能会出现癫痫发作和局灶性神经功能障碍，如无力等。

2. 治疗

硬脑膜转移瘤的治疗方式包括手术、放疗和化疗。尽管数据大多来自回顾性研究，对于仅有疼痛症状且不需要紧急减压的硬脑膜转移瘤患者，放射治疗在提供局部控制和缓解症状方面起着重要作用。放射治疗通常是分次的，比如30Gy/10次[57]，但对于放疗抵抗的肿瘤类型，可以考虑更高的等效生物剂量。高度适形放疗技术被用来保护未受累脑组织，对于邻近关键结构的病灶，如颅底病变，应考虑立体定向或图像引导放疗。一项回顾性研究显示，SRS可用于远离关键组织的较小病灶，前列腺癌硬脑膜转移的局部控制率高达85%[58]。脑膜转移瘤放疗常用的处方剂量为15～24Gy，而对于最大直径超过3cm的病灶，可考虑采用大分割立体定向放射治疗（如9Gy/3次或6Gy/5次）。手术切除仍然是病理诊断的标准，并且能够迅速缓解占位效应或水肿导致的症状。如果有不完全切除或脑实质侵犯的证据，建议进行术后辅助放疗。

由于硬脑膜转移瘤位于血脑屏障之外，全身治疗可能有效。药物的选择应取决于原发肿瘤病理类型、肿瘤的分子特征和全身疾病的状态。经筛查发现的无症状病变且存在治疗靶点突变时，可考虑系统治疗，如黑色素瘤中的*BRAF*基因、肺癌中的*EGFR/ALK*基因和乳腺癌中的*HER2*基因。化疗可改善无进展生存率，但回顾性数据显示，其并不能延长总生存[55]。皮质类固醇可用于治疗症状性水肿，抗惊厥药仅用于有癫痫发作病史的患者。

（四）存在的问题

关于硬脑膜转移瘤的治疗数据很少，即使是回顾性研究也通常排除了没有同时合并脑实质内转移的硬脑膜转移患者。更多情况下，硬脑膜转移被归类到CNS转移瘤或软脑膜转移瘤中，而将此研究结果直接应用于孤立的硬脑膜转移瘤是有争议的。在靶向治疗和免疫治疗时代，需要更多的研究来确定靶向或免疫治疗与手术和放射治疗的疗效比较，尤其是对小的、无症状的病变。

（五）结论和建议

硬脑膜转移瘤十分罕见，但常与脑实质或颅骨转移同时发生。预后不良，并可导致严重的并发症。如果体积小且无症状，则可在接受积极全身治疗的前提下密切监测。对于仅有疼痛症状且不需要紧急减压的硬脑膜转移瘤的患者，无论是常规分割放疗、大分割放疗或是放射外科治疗都是标准的治疗方法。而对于伴有明显水肿或者有占位效应的大肿块，则推荐选择手术切除联合术后放疗。

> **要　点**
> - 硬脑膜转移瘤通常在偶然情况下被发现，且常与脑实质转移或颅骨转移同时发生。
> - 肿块占位效应和水肿通常会导致头痛、脑神经损伤、癫痫发作和局灶性功能缺失等症状，这些症状取决于肿块位置。
> - 对于仅有疼痛症状且不需要紧急减压的硬脑膜转移瘤患者，放射治疗是标准的治疗方法。
> - 对于肿块或水肿引起的较大的、症状性病变，可能需要手术切除，必要时可以利用手术进行病理确诊。
> - 由于硬脑膜转移瘤位于血脑屏障外，对于小的、无症状的硬脑膜转移瘤，全身治疗可能是有效的。

五、软脑膜病

（一）病例介绍

病例 5

一位 79 岁的女性，数月前出现步态不稳和跌倒的症状并进行性加重。脑部 MRI 显示以基底为主的广泛性软脑膜强化和脑积水。患者接受了腰椎穿刺，结果显示脑脊液压力正常，总蛋白升高，8 个有核细胞，葡萄糖正常，细胞学阴性。全身 PET/CT 扫描显示双肺嗜 FDG 的结节。患者接受了肺结节的穿刺活检，显示为分化良好的神经内分泌肿瘤。随后做了脑室-腹腔分流术以改善步态不稳症状。

（二）概述

软脑膜病（leptomeningeal disease，LMD），也被称为癌性脑膜炎或软脑膜癌病，通常由肿瘤细胞血源性播撒到脑脊液（cerebral spinal fluid，CSF）中引起。它发生在 5%～8% 的实体瘤患者和 5%～15% 的血液系统恶性肿瘤患者中[59]。转移到软脑膜的最常见的实体肿瘤是肺癌、乳腺癌和恶性黑色素瘤。尽管对治疗的反应因病理类型不同而有所差别，软脑膜病预后极差，平均生存期普遍 < 2～4 个月。

（三）循证基础

1. 诊断

LMD 的临床表现是非特异性的，通常取决于受累部位。常见的表现包括癫痫、脑神经功能障碍（特别是复视、面部下垂、听力改变）和脊神经功能障碍（包括神经根性疼痛、肠/膀胱功能障碍、四肢无力）。脑脊液回收功能受损时，可导致颅内压升高，引起头痛和搏动性耳鸣。由于症状的非特异性，遇到相关临床症状时应高度怀疑脑膜转移的可能。诊断评估应包括颅脑和全脊柱的增强（MRI）及腰椎细胞学穿刺检查。MRI 常显示不规则及结节性软脑膜强化（图 14-7）。如果临床高度怀疑，MRI 异常即可诊断。腰椎穿刺可发现脑脊液淋巴细胞增多、蛋白升高和低血糖症。流式细胞术能够增加恶性血液病患者脑脊液评估的敏感性[60]。免疫功能低下的癌症患者应注意排除感染性脑膜炎或脑炎的可能。

2. 治疗

由于缺乏前瞻性的随机临床试验数据，LMD 的最佳治疗方法尚未明确。当腰穿示脑脊液压力升高或有颅内压升高的体征和症状时，应考虑行姑息性脑室-腹腔分流术。支持鞘内和全身化疗的数据主要来自回顾性临床研究。在 LMD 中进行的 6 个随机临床试验都集中于鞘内治疗（intrathecal therapy，IT），药物包括甲氨蝶呤、阿糖胞苷、脂质体阿糖胞苷和三胺硫磷[61-66]。只有一项研究比较了鞘内化疗与未进行鞘内治疗的疗效，结果发现在乳腺癌患者中，接受甲氨蝶呤鞘内注射和未接受鞘内注射治疗的患者相比，其生存率或神经系统症状缓解率没有差异[65]。但鞘

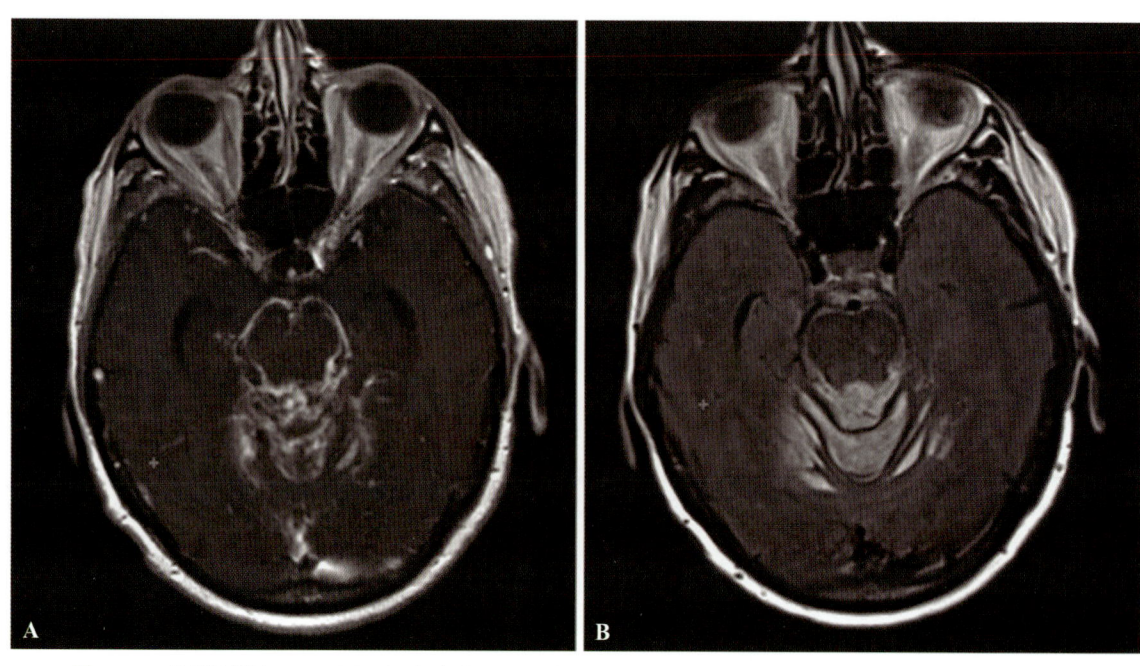

▲ 图 14-7　钆增强脑部 MRI 显示沿小脑叶和周围脑池强化（A），同时相邻的脑沟也出现高 FLAIR 信号（B）

内化疗通常会增加治疗相关的神经毒性，特别是无菌性脑膜炎。需要指出的是，这些研究通常排除了体力状态评分低或病情太重而不能治疗的患者，而这部分患者占到了就诊患者的很大比例。虽然血脑屏障（blood–brain barrier，BBB）透过率低是系统治疗的一个问题，但在 LMD 的情况下，BBB 可能已被破坏，许多化疗药物被证明在脑脊液中达到了治疗水平。与鞘内治疗不同的是，系统治疗不依赖于脑脊液流动，且能够渗透入巨大的结节性病变。使用的药物应以最初的组织学病理类型为指导，已报道有效的化疗方案包括大剂量甲氨蝶呤、大剂量阿糖胞苷、卡培他滨、三胺硫磷、大剂量依托泊苷和替莫唑胺[59]。总体而言，全身化疗与鞘内化疗的作用取决于最初的组织学病理类型，鞘内治疗在淋巴瘤和乳腺癌患者中没有有价值研究。

全脑放射治疗（WBRT）是常用的放射治疗方法，其作用主要是姑息性的。对乳腺癌和肺癌患者进行的回顾性研究表明，尽管放射治疗可能诱导症状迅速缓解，但患者的生存率没有改善[67, 68]。尽管全脑全脊髓都被认为是可能受累的靶区，但由于骨髓和神经毒性较重，通常情况下不推荐对整个神经轴进行放射治疗，仅对具有高度放射敏感性的肿瘤（如精原细胞瘤、白血病或淋巴瘤）进行全脑全脊髓放疗。累及野照射可用于治疗大脑或脊柱中体积较大、有症状的疾病部位。常规 WBRT 的总剂量为 30Gy/10 次[69]，脑膜间隙应注意包括在放疗靶区中。对于预后较差或不太可能耐受治疗的患者，可考虑采用 20Gy（4Gy/5 次）的大分割方案。一组回顾性研究表明，在非小细胞肺癌中，具有良好的体力状态的患者，出现 LMD 时间越晚，以及没有并发脑实质内转移是对 WBRT 良好反应的预测因素[70]。值得注意的是，当放疗与某些化疗药物特别是甲氨蝶呤联合使用时，患白质脑病的风险会增加。小而孤立的软脑膜转移病灶可以通过 SRS 达到姑息治疗目的，从而避免 WBRT 相关的后遗症。最近一项对 16 名接受 SRS 治疗的局灶性 LMD 患者的回顾性研究表明，自 SRS 治疗之日起，中位精准总生存期为 10 个月[71]，其中 7 例患者在中位时间为 7 个月时发生远处 LMD。

（四）未来发展方向

许多恶性肿瘤的靶向治疗已经取得了重大进

展，包括针对黑色素瘤的 BRAF/MEK 抑制药，针对 EGFR/ALK 突变肺癌的酪氨酸激酶抑制药，以及针对 HER2 阳性乳腺癌的抗 HER2 靶向治疗。许多较新的靶向药物可以穿透 BBB，并已被证实对 LMD 有一定的疗效。其中知名度最高的是治疗 EGFR 突变肺腺癌的奥希替尼[72]。多项评估免疫检查点抑制药（博利珠单抗、伊匹单抗联合纳武利尤单抗）治疗 LMD 疗效的临床研究也正在进行中，初步结果令人振奋[73]。

赖于原发肿瘤的组织病理学类型。近年来，靶向药物和免疫疗法的应用在 LMD 中初步显示出了令人振奋的疗效。WBRT 和累及野放疗能迅速改善症状但并未显示出对生存的改善。

（五）结论和建议

LMD 是恶性肿瘤的严重并发症，几乎没有有效的治疗方法。脑神经和脊神经功能障碍及头痛是常见的临床症状，钆增强 MRI 和脑脊液检查对诊断有很大帮助。治疗的重点是缓解症状，支持鞘内化疗和全身化疗的数据是混杂的，且依

> **要 点**
> - 软脑膜转移预后差，由于临床表现无特异性，遇到相关临床症状时应高度怀疑脑膜转移的可能。
> - 放射治疗的目标是缓解症状，包括全脑放射治疗或针对大肿块、有症状的疾病部位的累及野放疗。
> - 小而孤立的软脑膜转移病灶可以通过立体定向放射外科治疗达到姑息治疗目的，从而避免 WBRT 相关的后遗症。

参考文献

[1] Laigle-Donadey F, Taillibert S, Martin-Duverneuil N, Hildebrand J, Delattre JY. Skull-base metastases. J Neurooncol. 2005;75(1):63–9.

[2] Gupta SR, Zdonczyk DE, Rubino FA. Cranial neuropathy in systemic malignancy in a VA population. Neurology. 1990;40(6):997–9.

[3] Mitsuya K, Nakasu Y, Horiguchi S, Harada H, Nishimura T, Yuen S, et al. Metastatic skull tumors: MRI features and a new conventional classification. J Neurooncol. 2011;104(1):239–45.

[4] Harrison RA, Nam JY, Weathers SP, DeMonte F. Intracranial dural, calvarial, and skull base metastases. Handb Clin Neurol. 2018;149:205–25.

[5] Maroldi R, Farina D, Battaglia G, Maculotti P, Nicolai P, Chiesa A. MR of malignant nasosinusal neoplasms. Frequently asked questions. Eur J Radiol. 1997;24(3):181–90.

[6] McAvoy CE, Kamalarajab S, Best R, Rankin S, Bryars J, Nelson K. Bilateral third and unilateral sixth nerve palsies as early presenting signs of metastatic prostatic carcinoma. Eye (Lond). 2002;16(6):749–53.

[7] Moris G, Roig C, Misiego M, Alvarez A, Berciano J, Pascual J. The distinctive headache of the occipital condyle syndrome: a report of four cases. Headache. 1998;38(4):308–11.

[8] Svare A, Fossa SD, Heier MS. Cranial nerve dysfunction in metastatic cancer of the prostate. Br J Urol. 1988;61(5):441–4.

[9] Greenberg HS, Deck MD, Vikram B, Chu FC, Posner JB. Metastasis to the base of the skull: clinical findings in 43 patients. Neurology. 1981;31(5):530–7.

[10] McDermott RS, Anderson PR, Greenberg RE, Milestone BN, Hudes GR. Cranial nerve deficits in patients with metastatic prostate carcinoma: clinical features and treatment outcomes. Cancer. 2004;101(7):1639–43.

[11] Vikram B, Chu FC. Radiation therapy for metastases to the base of the skull. Radiology. 1979;130(2):465–8.

[12] Fossati P, Vavassori A, Deantonio L, Ferrara E, Krengli M, Orecchia R. Review of photon and proton radiotherapy for skull base tumours. Rep Pract Oncol Radiother. 2016;21(4):336–55.

[13] Iwai Y, Yamanaka K. Gamma Knife radiosurgery for skull base metastasis and invasion. Stereotact Funct Neurosurg. 1999;72(Suppl 1):81–7.

[14] Miller RC, Foote RL, Coffey RJ, Gorman DA, Earle JD, Schomberg PJ, et al. The role of stereotactic radiosurgery in the treatment of malignant skull base tumors. Int J Radiat Oncol Biol Phys. 1997;39(5):977–81.

[15] Xu KM, Quan K, Clump DA, Ferris RL, Heron DE. Stereotactic ablative radiosurgery for locally advanced or recurrent skull base malignancies with prior external beam radiation therapy. Front Oncol. 2015;5:65.

[16] Phan J, Pollard C, Brown PD, Guha-Thakurta N, Garden AS, Rosenthal DI, et al. Stereotactic radiosurgery for trigeminal pain secondary to recurrent malignant skull base tumors. J

Neurosurg. 2018;130(3):812–21.
[17] Chow E, Harris K, Fan G, Tsao M, Sze WM. Palliative radiotherapy trials for bone metastases: a systematic review. J Clin Oncol. 2007;25(11):1423–36.
[18] Steenland E, Leer JW, van Houwelingen H, Post WJ, van den Hout WB, Kievit J, et al. The effect of a single fraction compared to multiple fractions on painful bone metastases: a global analysis of the Dutch Bone Metastasis Study. Radiother Oncol. 1999;52(2):101–9.
[19] Posner JB. Cancer involving cranial and peripheral nerves. In: Davis F, editor. Neurologic complications of cancer. Philadelphia: F.A. Davis Co.; 1995. p. 172–84.
[20] Ransom DT, Dinapoli RP, Richardson RL. Cranial nerve lesions due to base of the skull metastases in prostate carcinoma. Cancer. 1990;65(3):586–9.
[21] Konstantinidis L, Rospond-Kubiak I, Zeolite I, Heimann H, Groenewald C, Coupland SE, et al. Management of patients with uveal metastases at the Liverpool Ocular Oncology Centre. Br J Ophthalmol. 2014;98(1):92–8.
[22] Shields CL, Shields JA, Gross NE, Schwartz GP, Lally SE. Survey of 520 eyes with uveal metastases. Ophthalmology. 1997;104(8):1265–76.
[23] Demirci H, Shields CL, Chao AN, Shields JA. Uveal metastasis from breast cancer in 264 patients. Am J Ophthalmol. 2003;136(2):264–71.
[24] Mathis T, Jardel P, Loria O, Delaunay B, Nguyen AM, Lanza F, et al. New concepts in the diagnosis and management of choroidal metastases. Prog Retin Eye Res. 2019;68:144–76.
[25] Jardel P, Sauerwein W, Olivier T, Bensoussan E, Maschi C, Lanza F, et al. Management of choroidal metastases. Cancer Treat Rev. 2014;40(10):1119–28.
[26] Amer R, Pe'er J, Chowers I, Anteby I. Treatment options in the management of choroidal metastases. Ophthalmologica. 2004;218(6):372–7.
[27] Kreusel KM, Bechrakis NE, Wiegel T, Krause L, Foerster MH. Incidence and clinical characteristics of symptomatic choroidal metastasis from lung cancer. Acta Ophthalmol. 2008;86(5):515–9.
[28] Caujolle JP, Mammar H, Chamorey E, Pinon F, Herault J, Gastaud P. Proton beam radiotherapy for uveal melanomas at nice teaching hospital: 16 years' experience. Int J Radiat Oncol Biol Phys. 2010;78(1):98–103.
[29] Bellmann C, Fuss M, Holz FG, Debus J, Rohrschneider K, Volcker HE, et al. Stereotactic radiation therapy for malignant choroidal tumors: preliminary, short-term results. Ophthalmology. 2000;107(2):358–65.
[30] Cho KR, Lee KM, Han G, Kang SW, Lee JI. Gamma knife radiosurgery for cancer metastasized to the ocular choroid. J Korean Neurosurg Soc. 2018;61(1):60–5.
[31] Kamran SC, Collier JM, Lane AM, Kim I, Niemierko A, Chen YL, et al. Outcomes of proton therapy for the treatment of uveal metastases. Int J Radiat Oncol Biol Phys. 2014;90(5):1044–50.
[32] Shields CL, Shields JA, De Potter P, Quaranta M, Freire J, Brady LW, et al. Plaque radiotherapy for the management of uveal metastasis. Arch Ophthalmol. 1997;115(2):203–9.
[33] Rudoler SB, Shields CL, Corn BW, De Potter P, Hyslop T, Curran WJ Jr, et al. Functional vision is improved in the majority of patients treated with external-beam radiotherapy for choroid metastases: a multivariate analysis of 188 patients. J Clin Oncol. 1997;15(3):1244–51.
[34] Kocher M, Soffietti R, Abacioglu U, Villa S, Fauchon F, Baumert BG, et al. Adjuvant whole-brain radiotherapy versus observation after radiosurgery or surgical resection of one to three cerebral metastases: results of the EORTC 22952-26001 study. J Clin Oncol. 2011;29(2):134–41.
[35] O'Neill BP, Iturria NJ, Link MJ, Pollock BE, Ballman KV, O'Fallon JR. A comparison of surgical resection and stereotactic radiosurgery in the treatment of solitary brain metastases. Int J Radiat Oncol Biol Phys. 2003;55(5):1169–76.
[36] Shaw E, Scott C, Souhami L, Dinapoli R, Kline R, Loeffler J, et al. Single dose radiosurgical treatment of recurrent previously irradiated primary brain tumors and brain metastases: final report of RTOG protocol 90-05. Int J Radiat Oncol Biol Phys. 2000;47(2):291–8.
[37] Hatiboglu MA, Chang EL, Suki D, Sawaya R, Wildrick DM, Weinberg JS. Outcomes and prognostic factors for patients with brainstem metastases undergoing stereotactic radiosurgery. Neurosurgery. 2011;69(4):796–806; discussion.
[38] Hussain A, Brown PD, Stafford SL, Pollock BE. Stereotactic radiosurgery for brainstem metastases: survival, tumor control, and patient outcomes. Int J Radiat Oncol Biol Phys. 2007;67(2):521–4.
[39] Kased N, Huang K, Nakamura JL, Sahgal A, Larson DA, McDermott MW, et al. Gamma knife radiosurgery for brainstem metastases: the UCSF experience. J Neurooncol. 2008;86(2):195–205.
[40] Kawabe T, Yamamoto M, Sato Y, Barfod BE, Urakawa Y, Kasuya H, et al. Gamma Knife surgery for patients with brainstem metastases. J Neurosurg. 2012;117(Suppl):23–30.
[41] Kilburn JM, Ellis TL, Lovato JF, Urbanic JJ, Bourland JD, Munley MT, et al. Local control and toxicity outcomes in brainstem metastases treated with single fraction radiosurgery: is there a volume threshold for toxicity? J Neurooncol. 2014;117(1):167–74.
[42] Koyfman SA, Tendulkar RD, Chao ST, Vogelbaum MA, Barnett GH, Angelov L, et al. Stereotactic radiosurgery for single brainstem metastases: the cleveland clinic experience. Int J Radiat Oncol Biol Phys. 2010;78(2):409–14.
[43] Lin CS, Selch MT, Lee SP, Wu JK, Xiao F, Hong DS, et al. Accelerator-based stereotactic radiosurgery for brainstem metastases. Neurosurgery. 2012;70(4):953–8; discussion 8.
[44] Lorenzoni JG, Devriendt D, Massager N, Desmedt F, Simon S, Van Houtte P, et al. Brain stem metastases treated with radiosurgery: prognostic factors of survival and life expectancy estimation. Surg Neurol. 2009;71(2):188–95; discussion 95, 95–6.
[45] Peterson HE, Larson EW, Fairbanks RK, MacKay AR, Lamoreaux WT, Call JA, et al. Gamma knife treatment of

[46] Sengoz M, Kabalay IA, Tezcanli E, Peker S, Pamir N. Treatment of brainstem metastases with gammaknife radiosurgery. J Neurooncol. 2013;113(1):33–8.

[47] Shuto T, Fujino H, Asada H, Inomori S, Nagano H. Gamma knife radiosurgery for metastatic tumours in the brain stem. Acta Neurochir. 2003;145(9):755–60.

[48] Trifiletti DM, Lee CC, Kano H, Cohen J, JanopaulNaylor J, Alonso-Basanta M, et al. Stereotactic radiosurgery for brainstem metastases: an international cooperative study to define response and toxicity. Int J Radiat Oncol Biol Phys. 2016;96(2):280–8.

[49] Mayo C, Yorke E, Merchant TE. Radiation associated brainstem injury. Int J Radiat Oncol Biol Phys. 2010;76(3 Suppl):S36–41.

[50] Foote KD, Friedman WA, Buatti JM, Meeks SL, Bova FJ, Kubilis PS. Analysis of risk factors associated with radiosurgery for vestibular schwannoma. J Neurosurg. 2001;95(3):440–9.

[51] Clark BG, Souhami L, Pla C, Al-Amro AS, Bahary JP, Villemure JG, et al. The integral biologically effective dose to predict brain stem toxicity of hypofractionated stereotactic radiotherapy. Int J Radiat Oncol Biol Phys. 1998;40(3):667–75.

[52] Kluger HM, Chiang V, Mahajan A, Zito CR, Sznol M, Tran T, et al. Long-term survival of patients with melanoma with active brain metastases treated with pembrolizumab on a phase II trial. J Clin Oncol. 2019;37(1):52–60.

[53] Long GV, Atkinson V, Lo S, Sandhu S, Guminski AD, Brown MP, et al. Combination nivolumab and ipilimumab or nivolumab alone in melanoma brain metastases: a multicentre randomised phase 2 study. Lancet Oncol. 2018;19(5):672–81.

[54] Margolin K, Ernstoff MS, Hamid O, Lawrence D, McDermott D, Puzanov I, et al. Ipilimumab in patients with melanoma and brain metastases: an open-label, phase 2 trial. Lancet Oncol. 2012;13(5):459–65.

[55] Nayak L, Abrey LE, Iwamoto FM. Intracranial dural metastases. Cancer. 2009;115(9):1947–53.

[56] Laigle-Donadey F, Taillibert S, Mokhtari K, Hildebrand J, Delattre JY. Dural metastases. J Neurooncol. 2005;75(1):57–61.

[57] Newton HB. Skull and dural metastases. In: Schiff D, Kesari S, Wen PY, editors. Cancer neurology in clinical practice. Totowa: Humana Press; 2008. p. 145–61.

[58] Flannery T, Kano H, Niranjan A, Monaco EA, Flickinger JC, Lunsford LD, et al. Stereotactic radiosurgery as a therapeutic strategy for intracranial metastatic prostate carcinoma. J Neurooncol. 2010;96(3):369–74.

[59] Wang N, Bertalan MS, Brastianos PK. Leptomeningeal metastasis from systemic cancer: review and update on management. Cancer. 2018;124(1):21–35.

[60] Bromberg JE, Breems DA, Kraan J, Bikker G, van der Holt B, Smitt PS, et al. CSF flow cytometry greatly improves diagnostic accuracy in CNS hematologic malignancies. Neurology. 2007;68(20):1674–9.

[61] Hitchins RN, Bell DR, Woods RL, Levi JA. A prospective randomized trial of single-agent versus combination chemotherapy in meningeal carcinomatosis. J Clin Oncol. 1987;5(10):1655–62.

[62] Grossman SA, Finkelstein DM, Ruckdeschel JC, Trump DL, Moynihan T, Ettinger DS. Randomized prospective comparison of intraventricular methotrexate and thiotepa in patients with previously untreated neoplastic meningitis. Eastern Cooperative Oncology Group. J Clin Oncol. 1993;11(3):561–9.

[63] Glantz MJ, Jaeckle KA, Chamberlain MC, Phuphanich S, Recht L, Swinnen LJ, et al. A randomized controlled trial comparing intrathecal sustained-release cytarabine (DepoCyt) to intrathecal methotrexate in patients with neoplastic meningitis from solid tumors. Clin Cancer Res. 1999;5(11):3394–402.

[64] Glantz MJ, LaFollette S, Jaeckle KA, Shapiro W, Swinnen L, Rozental JR, et al. Randomized trial of a slow-release versus a standard formulation of cytarabine for the intrathecal treatment of lymphomatous meningitis. J Clin Oncol. 1999;17(10):3110–6.

[65] Boogerd W, van den Bent MJ, Koehler PJ, Heimans JJ, van der Sande JJ, Aaronson NK, et al. The relevance of intraventricular chemotherapy for leptomeningeal metastasis in breast cancer: a randomised study. Eur J Cancer. 2004;40(18):2726–33.

[66] Shapiro WR, Schmid M, Glantz M, Miller JJ. A randomized phase III/IV study to determine benefit and safety of cytarabine liposome injection for treatment of neoplastic meningitis. J Clin Oncol. 2006;24(18_suppl):1528.

[67] Morris PG, Reiner AS, Szenberg OR, Clarke JL, Panageas KS, Perez HR, et al. Leptomeningeal metastasis from non-small cell lung cancer: survival and the impact of whole brain radiotherapy. J Thorac Oncol. 2012;7(2):382–5.

[68] Gani C, Müller AC, Eckert F, Schroeder C, Bender B, Pantazis G, et al. Outcome after whole brain radiotherapy alone in intracranial leptomeningeal carcinomatosis from solid tumors. Strahlenther Onkol. 2012;188(2):148–53.

[69] Souchon R, Feyer P, Thomssen C, Fehm T, Diel I, Nitz U, et al. Clinical recommendations of DEGRO and AGO on preferred standard palliative radiotherapy of bone and cerebral metastases, metastatic spinal cord compression, and leptomeningeal carcinomatosis in breast cancer. Breast Care (Basel). 2010;5(6):401–7.

[70] Ozdemir Y, Yildirim BA, Topkan E. Whole brain radiotherapy in management of non-small-cell lung carcinoma associated leptomeningeal carcinomatosis: evaluation of prognostic factors. J Neurooncol. 2016;129(2):329–35.

[71] Wolf A, Donahue B, Silverman JS, Chachoua A, Lee JK, Kondziolka D. Stereotactic radiosurgery for focal leptomeningeal disease in patients with brain metastases. J Neurooncol. 2017;134(1):139–43.

[72] Yang JC-H, Cho BC, Kim D-W, Kim S-W, Lee J-S, Su W-C, et al. Osimertinib for patients (pts) with leptomeningeal metastases (LM) from EGFRmutant non-small cell lung cancer (NSCLC): updated results from the BLOOM study. J Clin Oncol. 2017;35(15_suppl):2020.

[73] Brastianos PK, Prakadan S, Alvarez-Breckenridge C, Lee EQ, Tolaney SM, Nayak L, et al. Phase II study of pembrolizumab in leptomeningeal carcinomatosis. J Clin Oncol. 2018;36(15_suppl):2007.

第 15 章 补救治疗 / 再放疗 / 再治疗
Salvage/Reirradiation/Retreatment

David Roberge 著
凡 丹 译
伍海军 校

一、病例介绍

(一) 病例 1

67 岁肺腺癌患者（无 *EGFR* 或 *ALK* 突变），初诊时分期为 $T_2N_2M_1$（参考 AJCC 第 8 版分期），可见左顶叶孤立脑转移瘤。患者的 GPA 评分为 3 分，预期中位总生存期为 26.5 个月[1]。

2014 年 7 月（图 15-1A），针对患者头部病灶行放射外科治疗（单次照射 21Gy），并于术后同年对其胸部病灶行同步放化疗。

2015 年 5 月（图 15-1C 和 D），患者出现颅内新发转移灶（治疗前头部 MRI 的 FLAIR 序列显示为毫米级病变（图 15-1B）并行第二次放射外科治疗。此后，患者于 2015 年 12 月和 2016 年 7 月分别给予颅内另外出现的 2 个新发转移灶的放射外科治疗。

治疗后病情稳定，直至 2016 年 11 月左侧枕叶病灶再次增大，患者接受了开颅手术切除颅内病灶（图 15-1F 和 H）。术后病理诊断为腺癌，再次予以针对瘤床的辅助放射外科治疗（图 15-1H）。

尽管后续进行了放射外科治疗以及 WBRT，患者的硬脑膜复发灶仍然持续进展（图 15-1I 和 K）。2018 年，患者死于无法控制的颅内转移，总生存期为 44 个月。

(二) 病例 2

2018 年初，一名 54 岁的亚洲男性因肺腺癌伴广泛转移就诊，可见骨转移和恶性胸腔积液。患者检查发现颅内广泛转移，但除轻微头痛外并无局部神经症状。颅内病灶多达 10 个以上，其中 3 个超过 20mm，一个位于脑干（图 15-2A）。*ALK* 基因试剂盒荧光原位杂交检测提示 *2p23 ALK* 基因异位。患者的功能状态评分为 90%，GPA 评分为 3 分，预期中位总生存期为 26.5 个月。

经口服阿来替尼（Alectinib）靶向治疗后，患者胸腔内外的病灶均有显著缩小（图 15-2B）。但治疗 8 个月后，患者右侧顶叶 1 个转移灶从 6mm 迅速增大至 16mm（图 15-2C）。针对该处病灶，患者接受了放射外科治疗（单次照射 20Gy）和酪氨酸激酶抑制药维持治疗。患者存活至今，且从就诊开始 9 个月来均无神经系统异常症状。

(三) 病例 3

2016 年夏，一名 68 岁的老年患者因步态异常就诊。影像学检查显示患者左侧额叶有一大小为 31mm 的转移灶，伴严重的血管源性水肿且中线稍有移位（图 15-3A）。全身 FDG PET 检查可见左肺病灶及纵隔淋巴结代谢活跃。患者的 GPA 评分为 2 分，预期中位总生存期为 13.7 个月。

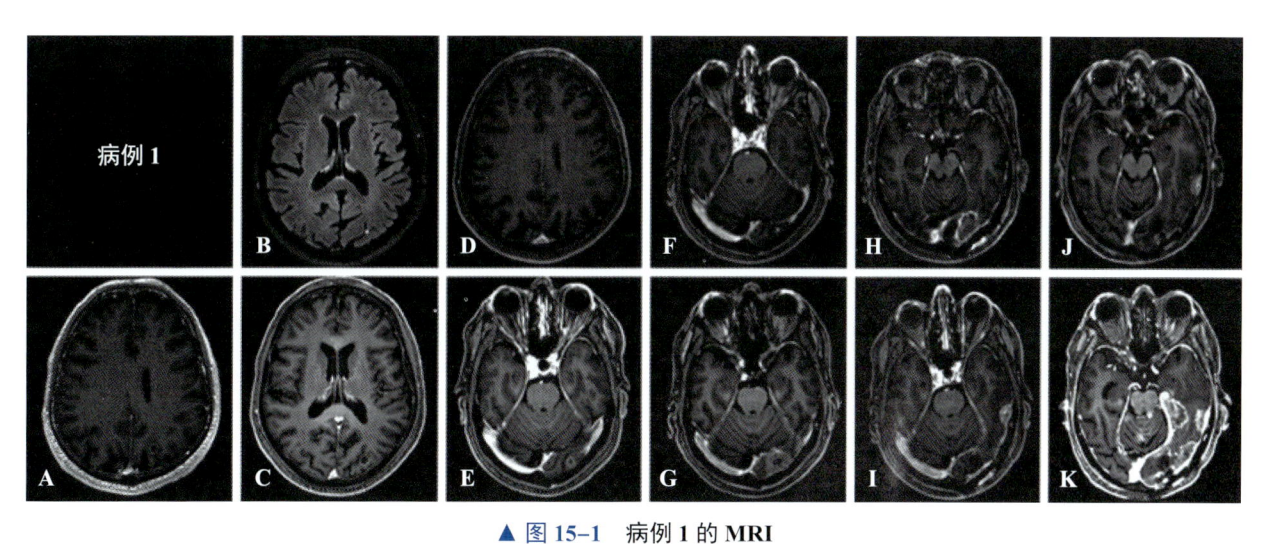

▲ 图 15-1 病例 1 的 MRI
A. 初始转移灶；B 至 E. 后续转移灶；F. 治疗效果；G. 枕叶局部复发；H. 手术切除后；J 和 K. 硬脑膜复发

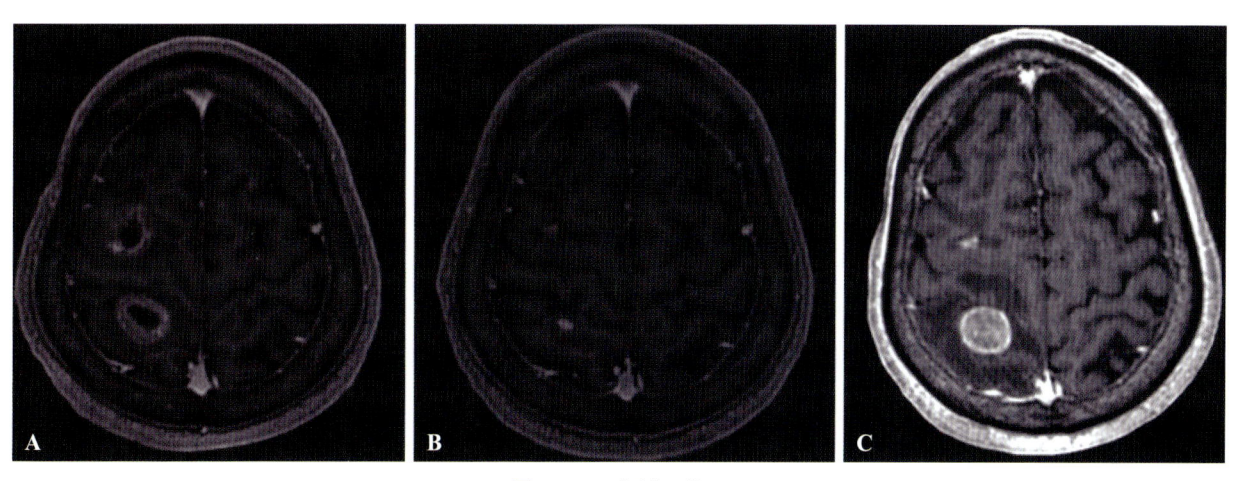

▲ 图 15-2 病例 2 的 MRI
A. 治疗前；B. 靶向治疗后；C. 寡病灶进展

由于其功能状态评分低于 70%，不适合接受开颅手术。患者接受了单次的放射外科治疗，剂量减少至 15Gy。

经细胞毒性化疗后，患者的头部转移灶明显缩小，但 1 年后再次呈结节状增大（图 15-3B）且出现右侧顶叶的新发转移灶（图 15-3C），影像学提示原有病灶部位的 $T_2/T_1 > 0.6$。患者在第一次 SRS 治疗后 1 年后再次接受了放射外科治疗，原有病灶予以单次 15Gy 照射，新发转移灶予以单次 21Gy 照射。

术后改为免疫单药治疗维持，患者的颅内外病灶均得到控制，总生存期已达 29 个月（图 15-3D）。

二、概述

随着脑转移患者生存率的提高，新的靶向治疗的发现以及 WBRT 的应用逐渐减少，复发脑转移瘤的治疗比以往任何时候都更加普遍和复杂。

非小细胞肺癌（nonsmall-cell lung，NSCLC）仍然是最易发生脑转移的原发恶性肿瘤，其生存数据也显示出脑转移患者疗效的提高。在过去的 20 年间，NSCLC 脑转移患者的中位总生存期从 7 个月提高至 12 个月[1]，而 WBRT 的使用率则从 40% 下降至约 20%[2]，这两个数据说明针对脑转移瘤的治疗手段已越来越多。

除此之外，各项治疗的临床应用也在发生变

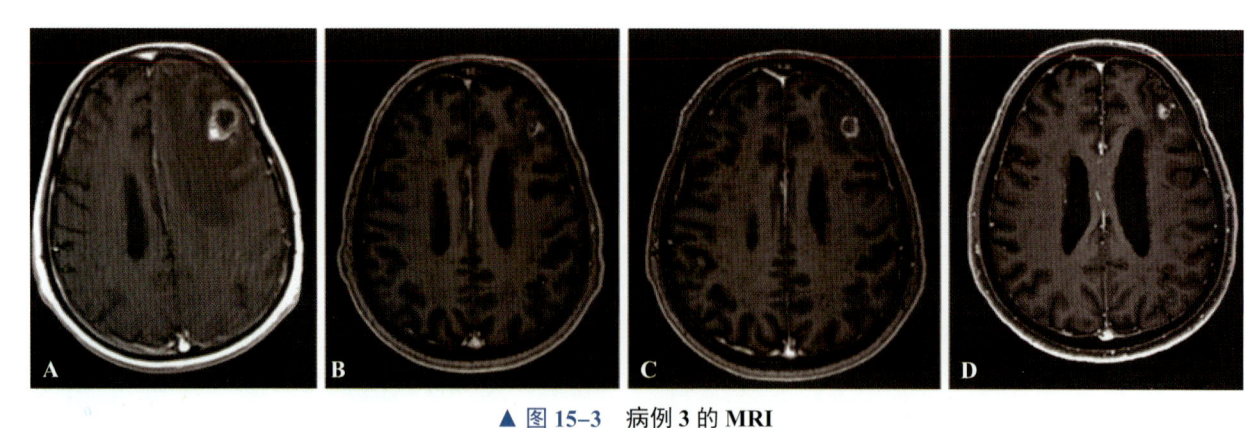

▲ 图 15-3 病例 3 的 MRI
A. 治疗前；B. 初始治疗后；C. 新发转移灶；D. 二次放射外科治疗后

化。比如，术后辅助放射外科治疗明显增加硬脑膜的复发率[3]，肿瘤的分子学特点也更加复杂，正如 ALK 或 EGFR 突变的 NSCLC 患者可选择特有的靶向治疗且预后较好一样，ROS1 和 BRAF 突变的发现也为部分患者提供了新的靶向治疗选择。

目前仍然缺乏高级别证据来指导各类复发性脑转移瘤的治疗，许多治疗决策仅基于初始治疗的研究数据。而由于复发性脑转移患者病情的复杂多样性，目前也暂无广泛适用的随机临床试验。

三、循证基础

（一）脑转移瘤复发的诊断

脑转移的复发常表现为新发脑实质病变、硬脑膜病变、原有病灶的增大/复发及软脑膜种植转移。复发灶通常是经影像学发现的无症状病灶，有症状时常为脑膜转移和大病灶治疗后进展。

脑转移的复发非常常见。既往接受过放射外科的患者中约 50% 在 1 年内发生远处脑转移[4]，而颅内大病灶接受 15Gy 单次照射的患者，约 50% 出现局部复发[5]。手术切除和对瘤床进行放射外科治疗的局部复发率相近[6]。对于部分患者而言，这些风险将进一步降低初始颅内控制率。

脑转移瘤的生长速度可能与原发肿瘤的组织学类型有关。黑色素瘤转移灶的平均增长速度较快，最常见的 NSCLC 的转移灶中位倍增时间约为 2 个月[7]。

决定 MRI 复查频率时应评估肿瘤失败的风险和病灶的预期增长速度，但临床实际中大部分患者遵循标准的影像学随访原则，即每 2~3 个月复查一次增强 MRI。随访频率随无进展期的延长而逐渐下降。

新转移灶的诊断往往较为直观，一般无须行除增强 MRI 以外的诊断性检查。相对来说，放射外科治疗后的病灶进展更加复杂，通常需要和放射性坏死相鉴别。除影像学差异以外，两者很难有其他的鉴别方法。有些机构在 SPECT、PET、MR 光谱、MR 灌注成像或延迟增强溢出成像（delayed contrast extravasation imaging，TRAM）[8-10] 等高级诊断手段方面非常专业。对于没有这些诊断技术的机构，可以通过 MRI 影像上简单的 T_2 像肿块影与 T_1 像增强的面积的比值来帮助判断病变性质。较低的比值（＜0.3）通常提示为放射性坏死[11]。在临床工作中，仅有小部分患者会接受开颅手术明确诊断，而大部分患者可通过耐心的针对既往治疗方式的评估，从而得出最有可能的诊断。

除了头部影像学检查、定期的脑脊液监测以及可疑软脑膜病变的脊柱 MRI 检查，及时进行患者颅外病变的分期并评估是否存在可用来治疗的突变位点也非常重要。许多患者在初诊时往往没有进行基因学检查，而基因突变也可能随治疗的进行而发生改变。此外，初诊的标本有时不够用于后续的基因检测或者患者可能已经选择了针对新的基因突变的治疗方法。若单纯为取得基因学检测的标本，不推荐进行脑组织的活检，此时可重新对原发灶进行活检或者进行血液学分析。比如血清中 *EGFR T790M* 突变就具有高特异性，由于奥希替尼现在普遍应用于缺乏特异性20外显子突变的患者，该检查可用于减少其不必要的应用[12]。

（二）颅内新发转移灶的治疗

脑转移的二线治疗尚未成为随机临床试验的主要研究内容。仅在某些药物试验和旨在降低WBRT毒性的临床试验中纳入了少量的脑转移病例[13,14]，但并未对复发脑转移患者的最佳治疗手段或治疗顺序提供具体指导。

对于前期未接受 WBRT 的患者，其治疗方案制定的依据是前期临床试验的结果。数量较少的小转移灶通常接受 SRS，而广泛的转移灶更倾向于接受挽救性 WBRT。回顾性研究指出这些患者的预后与脑转移瘤初始治疗后的相一致。除脑转移瘤数量以外，选择 SRS 或者 WBRT 治疗时还需将患者和疾病本身的相关因素列入考量，肿瘤的总体积以及新病灶出现的速度可能比单纯计算病灶数量更有意义[15,16]。

对于前期已接受过 WBRT 治疗的患者，应用挽救性 SRS 治疗数量较多的转移灶时需要考虑患者的耐受性。但无论是针对转移灶行单次 SRS 的初步安全性剂量数据，还是 RTOG 剂量学指南（31～40mm 的病灶予以 15Gy 照射，21～30mm 的病灶予以 18Gy 照射，1～20mm 的病灶予以 24Gy 照射）推荐的照射剂量，均来自一项所有患者既往均接受过头部放疗（WBRT 或适形放疗）的 Ⅰ 期临床试验[17]。因此，尽管接受过 WBRT 后行再程放疗可能会增加不良反应的发生率，仍然不需要降低挽救性 SRS 的照射剂量。回顾性研究数据显示，若患者不适合 SRS，再次行 WBRT 也是安全可行的。再程的 WBRT 通常予以较低的总剂量和单次照射剂量，常为 20Gy/10 次[18]。尽管尚无研究将 HA-WBRT 和美金刚应用于再程 WBRT 的患者，但可能的情况下应用这些保护手段也是合理的。当总剂量较低时（如 20Gy/10 次），也可应用容积调强放疗差异化增大大体肿瘤靶区的照射剂量[19]。

和脑实质转移灶一样，软脑膜复发的治疗和初次治疗基本类似，但相关的循证医学证据比脑实质转移更为少见。可根据具体情况选择以下任一治疗或将其结合进行治疗。

- 放射外科治疗。
- 针对有症状的病灶进行放疗。
- 全脑放疗。
- 鞘内或脑室内注射治疗。
- 系统性治疗。
- 支持治疗。

瘤床复发的治疗一直充满挑战。前期的回顾性研究数据发现在脑实质复发灶中，局部治疗可作为 WBRT 的替代治疗手段[3]，但目前仍缺乏该方面的研究数据。

四、诊断与治疗

图 15-4 所示为脑转移复发的治疗流程，反映了各种复发情况下治疗的复杂性。也正是由于其复杂性并且缺乏高级别的循证医学证据，这些建议与实际的临床决策判断可能存在一定的偏差。总的来说，对于数目、增长速度或总体积等较局限的新发病灶，通常予以 SRS 治疗；而对于更为广泛的病灶，若有疗效较好的药物可选择系统治疗，若无合适的药物则选择 WBRT 或支持治疗。

对于合适的患者也可采用其他的治疗手段。颅内病灶进展且有症状但其他病灶控制良好时可选择开颅手术治疗，*HER2* 阳性的软脑膜转移的患者可选择鞘内注射曲妥珠单抗（赫赛汀）[20]，

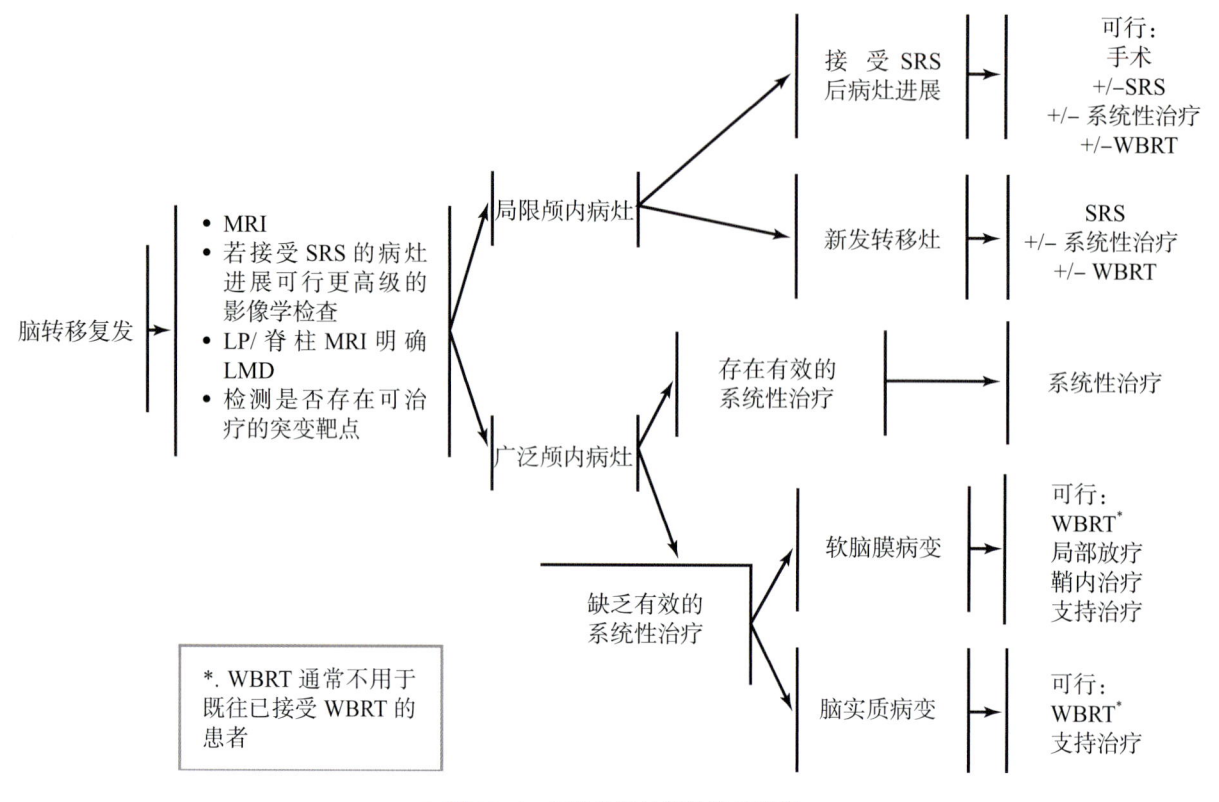

▲ 图 15-4 复发性脑转移的治疗流程

局部姑息性放疗可用于缓解脑神经麻痹；而广泛颅后窝病变的患者即使既往接受过 WBRT，也可行部分脑组织的再程放疗[21]。

这里提出的治疗流程，以及本章"指南"部分里的指南推荐，均未解决治疗后颅内持续存在的寡转移灶或颅内寡复发灶的问题。病例 2 中的患者在接受酪氨酸激酶治疗广泛的转移灶后仅颅内单发病灶进展，此时后续应该如何治疗。尽管只治疗进展病灶是合理的，但仍缺乏循证数据支持。更难确定的是，除了少量转移灶以外的所有病灶完全消失时，采取观察是否更为谨慎。

（一）再程放射外科

复发性脑转移的再程 SRS 与脑转移初次 SRS 在治疗流程上具有相似性。但鉴于患者多年前可能已有多处病灶接受了治疗，为了避免不必要的重复治疗或遗漏新发病灶，可将既往的计划图像和靶区与本次影像相融合，并标明每个可见病灶是本次治疗的 GTV 还是既往治疗的靶区。

再程 SRS 的剂量尚无标准的指南建议，需要考虑的因素很多，包括和初次治疗的间隔时间、既往是否接受 WBRT 等，再程治疗的剂量可能相近或稍低于初次治疗的剂量。对于大部分小病灶而言，再程 SRS 可选择单次分割照射；尽管分割方式是否可提高治疗有效率仍有待考证，但多次分割照射更常用于较大病灶的治疗[22]。

（二）挽救性全脑放疗

无论患者既往是否接受过 WBRT，行挽救性 WBRT 治疗时均应避免照射海马区。目前对仅避免照射部分海马是否获益知之甚少，但保护优势侧海马不接受照射可能也是有利的。其他需要保护的正常结构包括眼、晶体、视交叉、视神经、中耳以及内耳。

保护区结构的最大照射剂量应尽可能控制在 16Gy 以下，并将尽可能多的靶区剂量控制在 9Gy 以下[23]。放疗计划最好使用容积适形调强技术。视器的勾画有助于减少剂量热点，双眼、晶体以及听觉器官等结构的勾画也将使剂量减至最低。大部分 WBRT 的分割次数为 5 次，这样可使海马区的照射剂量减少 1/3。

当给予第二个疗程的 WBRT 时，通常会适当减低照射总剂量，通常为 20Gy/10 次。这种情况下，可对可见转移灶及外扩边界予以局部加量（保守加量至 30Gy），海马区也可以很大程度上得到保护。

五、治疗的不确定性

脑转移瘤的治疗仍然存在许多不确定性。在许多肿瘤中，WBRT（和第二个疗程的 SRS 相比）的适应证仍然是临床的难点。WBRT 的选择是否应基于新转移灶的数量、出现转移的速度、病灶的总体积或者患者的体能状态？而避免照射海马区和美金刚的预防性使用在降低 WBRT 认知毒性的同时，也使 WBRT 的适用指征变得更加复杂[13, 24]。尽管目前仍缺乏前瞻性的研究证据，当新的转移瘤数目以每月一个以上的速度出现时可考虑进行 WBRT。

对于可接受系统治疗脑转移的肿瘤而言，选择再程放疗还是系统治疗的临床试验也值得进一步探讨（表 15-1）。这类肿瘤大多指 *HER2* 阳性乳腺癌、*ALK/EGFR/ROS1* 突变的非小细胞肺癌、适合免疫治疗的黑色素瘤以及越来越多的 *BRAF* 突变肿瘤。一项被广泛引用的回顾性研究指出，系统治疗联合放疗的预后要优于单纯系统治疗[25]。然而，该研究除了受到回顾性研究常见的偏倚影响之外，并未说明治疗时机、患者生活质量是否改善或结论与更新、更有效的药物是否相关的问题。

六、未来研究方向

随着晚期肿瘤患者预后的逐步改善，越来越多的脑转移患者需要接受挽救治疗。但无论是大于 5 个转移灶的患者还是接受过手术切除的患者，SRS 和 WBRT 更常见于脑转移的初始治疗[6, 24]。由于初诊时接受 WBRT 的患者数较少，因此可以设计 WBRT 在复发脑转移中应用的临床试验。

如前所述，对于有突变靶点或接受免疫治疗的患者，系统治疗在脑转移瘤中的作用日益凸显。如何证明放疗联合有效的系统治疗可带来更多的临床获益以及如何优化两者的结合方式是未来值得研究的方向。对于接受免疫治疗的患者，治疗的顺序可能很重要。当放疗分次插入每周期的免疫治疗中时可能更易观察到常说不常见的远隔效应。尽管目前证据指出大多数系统治疗联合 SRS 是安全的，但随着更多新药的投入使用，两者联合可能带来的不良反应仍然需要不断的被研究证实[26]。

迄今为止，脑转移的治疗仍聚焦于手术、放疗以及日益增多的系统治疗药物，而新型的物理

表 15-1 复发性脑转移的系统性治疗实例

肿瘤类型	药 物	影像学缓解率	反应持续时间（个月）
HER2 阳性乳腺癌	阿来替尼 + 卡培他滨	49%[31]	5.5
ALK 突变非小细胞肺癌	克唑替尼，色瑞替尼，阿来替尼，布加替尼	44%（95%CI 33%～55%）[32]	14.6（范围为 8～22）
EGFR 突变非小细胞肺癌	奥希替尼	91%[14]	无（中位随访时间 12.4 个月）
黑色素瘤	纳武利尤单抗 + 伊匹木单抗	55%[33]	无（中位随访时间 14 个月）
BRAF 突变黑色素瘤	达拉非尼 + 曲美替尼	43%[34]	5.8
BRAF 突变非小细胞肺癌	达拉非尼	33%[35]	5.5

治疗方法［尤其是交流电场的形式（所谓的肿瘤电场治疗）］可能会打破现有的格局。肿瘤电场治疗（tumor treating fields，TTF）是一种抗有丝分裂的治疗，已被证实在 CNS 肿瘤中具有一定的临床抗肿瘤活性。一项Ⅲ期临床试验正在研究辅助 TTF 在非小细胞肺癌脑转移患者中的应用，研究纳入患者的新发脑转移瘤均可接受 SRS。若该研究得出阳性结论，那么 SRS 可能将局限于脑转移的初始治疗，而 TTF 可能将成为肺癌患者脑转移复发的治疗手段。

七、治疗指南

正如前文所述，脑转移患者具有很大的异质性，因此很难仅仅依据指南做出具体的临床决策，此外，患者既往接受的其他治疗也使问题变得更加复杂。鉴于部分指南未将脑转移复发的治疗内容汇总，本节将包含了复发性颅内转移相关内容的治疗指南总结如下。

（一）国家综合癌症网络（National Comprehensive Cancer Network，NCCN）指南

2019 年的 NCCN 指南（https://www.nccn.org/professionals/physician_gls/pdf/cns.pdf）为治疗后复发的局限或广泛脑转移提供了总指南。

对于已接受治疗的局部脑转移复发病灶，可再次行局部治疗（手术、单次或多次分割的 SRS）；对于更多的脑转移复发灶，既往未接受 WBRT 时可考虑行 WBRT。

对于远处颅内复发病灶，可根据脑转移病灶的数目和大小选择 WBRT（既往未接受过 WBRT）、手术和局部放疗。

对于相比初治时更广泛的脑转移病灶和无法接受有效系统性治疗的颅外病变进展的患者，选择支持治疗。

以上各种情况均可以考虑全身治疗，且复发患者可选的药物更多，尤其是对于肺癌、乳腺癌和黑色素瘤患者。某些传统的细胞毒性药物（例如拓扑替康应用于小细胞癌）也可用于脑转移的治疗，但大多情况下为靶向药物或免疫治疗。无论是卡培他滨/阿来替尼还是奥希替尼，新型药物都可提高诊治 CNS 病变的疗效。

（二）美国神经外科医师协会（American Association of Neurological Surgeons，AANS）指南[27]

发表于 2009 年的 AANS 指南指出复发性脑转移瘤的治疗仍然缺乏高质量的循证医学证据，并且其后 10 年无明显进展："由于复发/进展性脑转移瘤推荐明确治疗的证据不足，应根据患者的功能状态、疾病范围、转移灶体积和数量、复发或进展位于原发部位还是非原发部位、既往治疗、肿瘤类型等进行个体化治疗，并且鼓励患者参与临床试验的研究。基于以上原则，可根据患者自身情况选择以下治疗：不接受进一步治疗（支持治疗），再程放疗［WBRT 和（或）SRS］，手术（切除或部分切除）或化疗。"

（三）美国临床肿瘤学会（American Society of Clinical Oncology，ASCO）指南[28]

ASCO 于 2018 年更新了 *HER2* 阳性乳腺癌和脑转移瘤的治疗指南。指南对于颅内进展性病变的治疗推荐较为广泛，无论是否接受过放疗，可选的治疗手段包括 SRS、手术、WBRT 或系统治疗。对于广泛复发的患者，最佳支持治疗可作为治疗选择。

（四）欧洲神经肿瘤学会（European Association of Neuro-Oncology，EANO）指南

2017 年 EANO 指南明确提出了对于复发脑转移的治疗建议以及系统治疗的原则[29]。明确了手术在鉴别放射性坏死和肿瘤进展中所起的作用，以及对特定患者（年轻、体能状态较好、全身疾病可控）可手术病灶的局部挽救治疗中的潜在作用。此外，指南中也提及了既往接受 SRS 或 WBRT 后再行 SRS 的可能。

对于药物治疗有如下几点建议。

- 化疗敏感肿瘤（如小细胞肺癌或乳腺癌）的脑转移，尤其是病灶较小或无症状时，初始治疗可选择常规的化疗。
- 目前尚无针对任何实体瘤脑转移的靶向药物。
- 携带 EGFR 突变或 ALK 基因重排的 NSCLC 脑转移患者可从特定的 TKI 药物中获益。
- HER2 阳性乳腺癌伴 CNS 转移的患者应持续予以 HER2 抑制药治疗。
- HER2 阳性乳腺癌脑转移患者可从拉帕替尼联合或不联合卡培他滨中获益。
- 黑色素瘤脑转移患者可从伊匹木单抗或 BRAF 抑制药中获益。
- 肾细胞癌脑转移患者可从多靶点 TKI 中获益，尤其是舒尼替尼。
- 脑转移放疗期间可暂停新型系统治疗药物以降低不可预期的毒性。

指南中还指出，唯一一项关于舒尼替尼的前瞻性临床试验报道的原发性肾细胞癌颅内转移的客观缓解率为 0%（16 例可评估病例）[30]。

八、结论与建议

综上所述，复发性脑转移瘤的治疗非常复杂，其合理的治疗选择往往不止一种。

总之，最重要的是需要认识到许多患者可以通过治疗延长生存，让患者参与到治疗决策的制定中，同时及时了解全身治疗及临床试验的最新进展。尽可能成立脑转移多学科团队以共同探讨治疗相关问题。

参考文献

[1] Sperduto PW, Yang TJ, Beal K, Pan H, Brown PD, Bangdiwala A, et al. Estimating survival in patients with lung cancer and brain metastases: an update of the graded prognostic assessment for lung cancer using molecular markers (Lung-molGPA). JAMA Oncol. 2017;3(6):827–31.

[2] Sperduto PW, Yang TJ, Beal K, Pan H, Brown PD, Bangdiwala A, et al. The effect of gene alterations and tyrosine kinase inhibition on survival and cause of death in patients with adenocarcinoma of the lung and brain metastases. Int J Radiat Oncol Biol Phys. 2016;96(2):406–13.

[3] Prabhu RS, Soltys SG, Turner BE, Marcrom S, Fiveash JB, Foreman PM, et al. Timing, presentation, and patterns of failure of leptomeningeal disease after surgical resection and radiosurgery for brain metastases: a multi-institutional analysis. J Clin Oncol. 2018;36(15_suppl):2070.

[4] Prabhu RS, Press RH, Boselli DM, Miller KR, Lankford SP, McCammon RJ, et al. External validity of two nomograms for predicting distant brain failure after radiosurgery for brain metastases in a biinstitutional independent patient cohort. J Neurooncol. 2018;137(1):147–54.

[5] de Azevedo Santos TR, Tundisi CF, Ramos H, Maia MA, Pellizzon AC, Silva ML, et al. Local control after radiosurgery for brain metastases: predictive factors and implications for clinical decision. Radiat Oncol. 2015;10:63.

[6] Roberge D, Brown P. SRS versus WBRT for resected brain metastases – Authors' reply. Lancet Oncol. 2017;18(10):e560.

[7] Yoo H, Nam BH, Yang HS, Shin SH, Lee JS, Lee SH. Growth rates of metastatic brain tumors in nonsmall cell lung cancer. Cancer. 2008;113(5):1043–7.

[8] Lohmann P, Kocher M, Ceccon G, Bauer EK, Stoffels G, Viswanathan S, et al. Combined FET PET/MRI radiomics differentiates radiation injury from recurrent brain metastasis. Neuroimage Clin. 2018;20:537–42.

[9] Zach L, Guez D, Last D, Daniels D, Grober Y, Nissim O, et al. Delayed contrast extravasation MRI: a new paradigm in neuro-oncology. Neuro Oncol. 2015;17(3):457–65.

[10] Chuang MT, Liu YS, Tsai YS, Chen YC, Wang CK. Differentiating radiation-induced necrosis from recurrent brain tumor using MR perfusion and spectroscopy: a meta-analysis. PLoS One. 2016;11(1):e0141438.

[11] Dequesada IM, Quisling RG, Yachnis A, Friedman WA. Can standard magnetic resonance imaging reliably distinguish recurrent tumor from radiation necrosis after radiosurgery for brain metastases? A radiographic-pathological study. Neurosurgery. 2008;63(5):898–903; discussion 4.

[12] Sim WC, Loh CH, Toh GL, Lim CW, Chopra A, Chang AYC, et al. Non-invasive detection of actionable mutations in advanced non-small-cell lung cancer using targeted sequencing of circulating tumor DNA. Lung Cancer. 2018;124:154–9.

[13] Brown PD, Pugh S, Laack NN, Wefel JS, Khuntia D, Meyers C, et al. Memantine for the prevention of cognitive dysfunction in patients receiving whole-brain radiotherapy: a randomized,

[14] Reungwetwattana T, Nakagawa K, Cho BC, Cobo M, Cho EK, Bertolini A, et al. CNS response to osimertinib versus standard epidermal growth factor receptor tyrosine kinase inhibitors in patients with untreated EGFR-mutated advanced non-small-cell lung cancer. J Clin Oncol. 2018:JCO2018783118. https://doi.org/10.1200/JCO.2018.78.3118.

[15] Farris M, McTyre ER, Cramer CK, Hughes R, Randolph DM 2nd, Ayala-Peacock DN, et al. Brain metastasis velocity: a novel prognostic metric predictive of overall survival and freedom from whole-brain radiation therapy after distant brain failure following upfront radiosurgery alone. Int J Radiat Oncol Biol Phys. 2017;98(1):131–41.

[16] Hirshman BR, Wilson B, Ali MA, Proudfoot JA, Koiso T, Nagano O, et al. Superior prognostic value of cumulative intracranial tumor volume relative to largest intracranial tumor volume for stereotactic radiosurgery-treated brain metastasis patients. Neurosurgery. 2018;82(4):473–80.

[17] Shaw E, Scott C, Souhami L, Dinapoli R, Bahary JP, Kline R, et al. Radiosurgery for the treatment of previously irradiated recurrent primary brain tumors and brain metastases: initial report of radiation therapy oncology group protocol (90-05). Int J Radiat Oncol Biol Phys. 1996;34(3):647–54.

[18] Guo S, Balagamwala EH, Reddy C, Elson P, Suh JH, Chao ST. Clinical and radiographic outcomes from repeat whole-brain radiation therapy for brain metastases in the age of stereotactic radiosurgery. Am J Clin Oncol. 2016;39(3):288–93.

[19] Hsu F, Carolan H, Nichol A, Cao F, Nuraney N, Lee R, et al. Whole brain radiotherapy with hippocampal avoidance and simultaneous integrated boost for 1–3 brain metastases: a feasibility study using volumetric modulated arc therapy. Int J Radiat Oncol Biol Phys. 2010;76(5):1480–5.

[20] Ferrario C, Davidson A, Bouganim N, Aloyz R, Panasci LC. Intrathecal trastuzumab and thiotepa for leptomeningeal spread of breast cancer. Ann Oncol. 2009;20(4):792–5.

[21] Choi JH. Outcomes following re-irradiation for symptomatic brain metastasis. J Cancer Sci Ther. 2015;7(10):308–11.

[22] Rana N, Pendyala P, Cleary RK, Luo G, Zhao Z, Chambless LB, et al. Long-term outcomes after salvage stereotactic radiosurgery (SRS) following infield failure of initial SRS for brain metastases. Front Oncol. 2017;7:279.

[23] Gondi V, Pugh SL, Tome WA, Caine C, Corn B, Kanner A, et al. Preservation of memory with conformal avoidance of the hippocampal neural stemcell compartment during whole-brain radiotherapy for brain metastases (RTOG 0933): a phase II multiinstitutional trial. J Clin Oncol. 2014;32(34):3810–6.

[24] Roberge D, Brown PD, Whitton A, O'Callaghan C, Leis A, Greenspoon J, et al. The future is nowprospective study of radiosurgery for more than 4 brain metastases to start in 2018! Front Oncol. 2018;8:380.

[25] Magnuson WJ, Lester-Coll NH, Wu AJ, Yang TJ, Lockney NA, Gerber NK, et al. Management of brain metastases in tyrosine kinase inhibitor-naive epidermal growth factor receptor-mutant non-small-cell lung cancer: a retrospective multi-institutional analysis. J Clin Oncol. 2017;35(10):1070–7.

[26] Kim JM, Miller JA, Kotecha R, Xiao R, Juloori A, Ward MC, et al. The risk of radiation necrosis following stereotactic radiosurgery with concurrent systemic therapies. J Neurooncol. 2017;133(2):357–68.

[27] Robinson PD, Kalkanis SN, Linskey ME, Santaguida PL. Methodology used to develop the AANS/CNS management of brain metastases evidence-based clinical practice parameter guidelines. J Neurooncol. 2010;96(1):11–6.

[28] Ramakrishna N, Temin S, Chandarlapaty S, Crews JR, Davidson NE, Esteva FJ, et al. Recommendations on disease management for patients with advanced human epidermal growth factor receptor 2-positive breast cancer and brain metastases: ASCO clinical practice guideline update. J Clin Oncol. 2018;36(27):2804–7.

[29] Soffietti R, Abacioglu U, Baumert B, Combs SE, Kinhult S, Kros JM, et al. Diagnosis and treatment of brain metastases from solid tumors: guidelines from the European Association of Neuro-Oncology (EANO). Neuro Oncol. 2017;19(2):162–74.

[30] Chevreau C, Ravaud A, Escudier B, Amela E, Delva R, Rolland F, et al. A phase II trial of sunitinib in patients with renal cell cancer and untreated brain metastases. Clin Genitourin Cancer. 2014;12(1):50–4.

[31] Freedman RA, Gelman RS, Melisko ME, Anders CK, Moy B, Blackwell KL, et al. TBCRC 022: phase II trial of neratinib + capecitabine for patients (Pts) with human epidermal growth factor receptor 2 (HER2+) breast cancer brain metastases (BCBM). J Clin Oncol. 2017;35(15_suppl):1005.

[32] Petrelli F, Lazzari C, Ardito R, Borgonovo K, Bulotta A, Conti B, et al. Efficacy of ALK inhibitors on NSCLC brain metastases: a systematic review and pooled analysis of 21 studies. PLoS One. 2018;13(7):e0201425.

[33] Tawbi HA, Forsyth PA, Algazi A, Hamid O, Hodi FS, Moschos SJ, et al. Combined nivolumab and ipilimumab in melanoma metastatic to the brain. N Engl J Med. 2018;379(8):722–30.

[34] Geukes Foppen MH, Boogerd W, Blank CU, van Thienen JV, Haanen JB, Brandsma D. Clinical and radiological response of BRAF inhibition and MEK inhibition in patients with brain metastases from BRAF-mutated melanoma. Melanoma Res. 2018;28(2):126–33.

[35] Planchard D, Kim TM, Mazieres J, Quoix E, Riely G, Barlesi F, et al. Dabrafenib in patients with BRAF(V600E)-positive advanced non-smallcell lung cancer: a single-arm, multicentre, openlabel, phase 2 trial. Lancet Oncol. 2016;17(5):642–50.

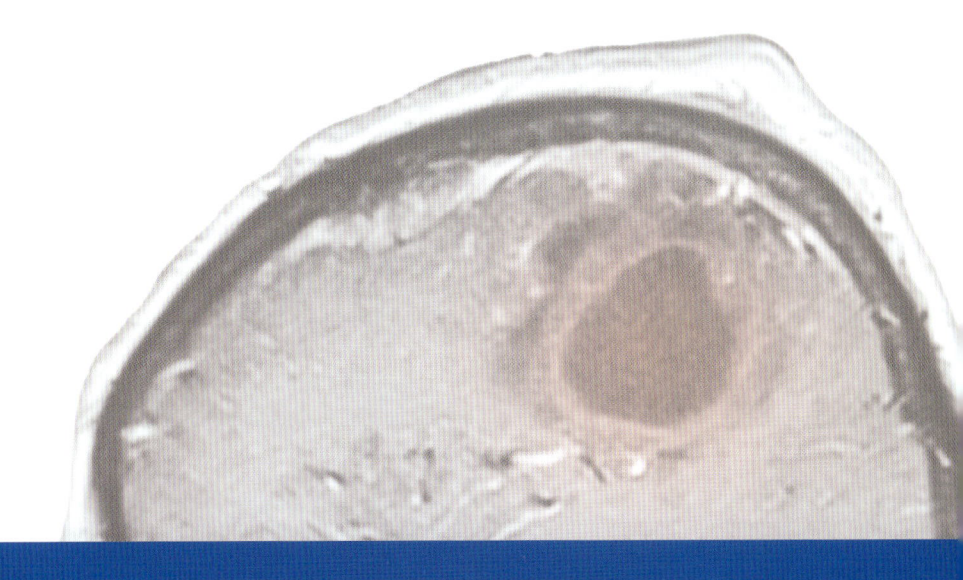

技术篇
治疗计划与实施技术
Technical: Treatment Planning and Delivery

第 16 章	常用的放射外科技术	198
第 17 章	多发性脑转移瘤的单中心治疗计划	213
第 18 章	脑转移瘤治疗中的耐受剂量	241
第 19 章	放射外科计划的质量评估	255
第 20 章	无头架放射外科的图像引导技术（包括体表成像）	267
第 21 章	放射外科治疗的安全程序和检查清单	277
第 22 章	小野放疗的质量保证	288
第 23 章	保护海马的全脑放疗技术	297

第 16 章 常用的放射外科技术
General Techniques for Radiosurgery

Mark Ruschin　Arjun Sahgal　Lijun Ma　Lei Wang　Ermias Gete　Alan Nichol　著
刘渊渊　张子健　译
杨　振　校

一、病例介绍

某患者，肺癌，无脑部放疗史，一般状况良好，脑部有 17 个转移灶，直径为 3mm～1.8cm（图 16-1）。拟采用立体定向放射外科（stereotactic Radiosurgery, SRS），选用何种技术最优呢？

在决定使用哪种 SRS 技术治疗多发性脑转移时，需要考虑技术（剂量学）、医保（财务）等多方面的因素。从剂量学的角度看，在保证靶区剂量高度适形的同时，使正常组织所受剂量最小化是优先考虑的因素。对于给定的计划系统和技术，各靶区之间的剂量会相互作用，从而影响每个靶区周围剂量的紧致度。除了计划质量外，治疗时的剂量学和机械精度也是治疗成功的关键。因此相关人员应知晓多发性脑转移瘤治疗相关的质量保证（quality assurance, QA）建议和指南，并付诸实践，这对治疗也至关重要。

本章概述了 SRS 技术的几种主要类型，每种技术涉及技术介绍、基于回顾性证据的剂量学优缺点以及最优化的质量保证和实践的指南及建议。

二、主要技术概述

三类最先进的 SRS 治疗设备，包括伽马刀（GK, Elekta AB, Stockholm, Sweden）、基于自动

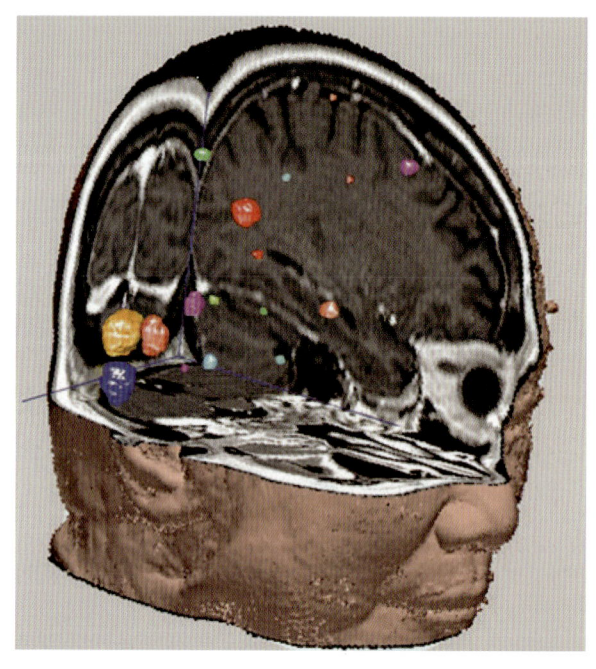

▲ 图 16-1　一位 17 个脑转移瘤患者的头部三维重建

机械臂多叶准直器（Multi-leaf collimator, MLC）的 X 波段射波刀系统（CK, Accuray, Sunnyvale, US）、基于高分辨率（HD）MLC 的 S 波段直线加速器（linac）系统。

（一）伽马刀（GK）SRS 系统

2006 年，GK 经历了一次革新式的设计，GK Perfexion（PFX）机型问世，它的治疗区域更大，具有固定的准直器头盔和相应的电驱动放射源[1]。此外，放射源被分为八个部分（称为"扇区"），这有助于在同一个等中心使用可变的准直器尺

寸。患者定位系统也完全重新设计，改由机器自动驱动。

2015 年，GK 厂商对其做了最新的技术改进，推出了一个名为 GK Icon（GKI）的新系统，如图 16-2 所示，该系统集成了机载立体定向锥束 CT（cone-beam CT，CBCT）图像引导系统。这种改进主要是为了给无框架 SRS 和多次分割（2～5 次治疗，每次剂量 ≥ 5Gy）的 GK 治疗提供图像引导支持[2, 3]。

众所周知，^{60}Co 能谱由两种不同能量的伽马射线（能量 1.17 MeV 和 1.33 MeV）构成，GK 的射束输出因子和侧向剂量分布已由蒙特卡罗方法计算确定，并通过不同的测量方法进行了验证[4]。通过简单地调整处方等剂量水平，基于框架的 GK-SRS 可以精确地对 1mm 的小病灶（包括脑组织内功能紊乱的局部区域，如三叉神经痛和顽固性震颤）进行定位治疗。

当前系统的工作流程出现了一个新的变化，即基于诊断 MRI 的预计划能力。一旦患者使用框架模拟定位，那么预计划的图像就可以配准到立体定向计划 CT 或 MRI 图像上，预计划也将叠加到相应的立体定向参考坐标上。该参考坐标系可以相对于预先计划的图像集进行旋转，然后可以根据患者在参考坐标系的实际定位来调整枪的位置。GK 的治疗床只能平移，不能在 6 个自由度（6DOF）内运动以补偿旋转误差。好在由于 192 束射线同时聚焦于等中心，因此单个枪的剂量分布对于较小的平移或旋转误差并不敏感，这也是该方法成功的关键。因此，平移或旋转误差可以通过对枪的位置做简单的数学变换来精确校正。对于 GKI，在线自适应定位检测和实时 3D 剂量评估可借助于 CBCT 影像和治疗前的再计划予以实现。未来 GKI 的临床数据将为明确立体定向 CBCT 用于小病灶和低分割大病灶的准确性提供支持。

（二）射波刀（CK）

射波刀（CyberKnife，CK）是一种安装在机械臂上的 X 波段紧凑型 6MV 直线加速器[5-7]。机械臂能够按照预定路径在 6 个自由度移动，允许等中心和非等中心治疗。在射线照射的每个位置或节点，机械臂还可以通过倾斜直线加速器，使多束射线指向靶区。因此，在 CK 治疗中，以节点为中心比等中心照射更常见。这有助于治疗多发性脑转移瘤，任何地方的病灶都可能通过机械臂运动路径上的一个给定节点进行治疗。CK 治疗的另一个显著特征是，靶区定位中小于 1cm 的平移和（或）1°～2° 的旋转都可以通过操纵机械臂来快速补偿，无须对患者重新定位或重新摆位[7, 8]。

在射束准直方面，原来的 CK 系统配备了直径从 0.5～6cm 的可拆卸物理锥型筒。为了方便准直器的快速切换，引入了 Iris 准直器系统，在治疗过程中可以自动调整锥型筒的直径[9]。Iris 准直器采用上下两组共 12 片钨铜合金片，形成一个正 12 边形的射野，用于模拟锥形野。该多边形射野最大尺寸与物理锥形准直器类似，为 0.5～6cm。为了减少输出因子测量中的不确定性，Iris 准直器射野的尺寸通常限定为 ≥ 7mm。由于 Iris 准直器具有改变射束孔径的能力，因此默认情况下，会为其规划一条自动路径。

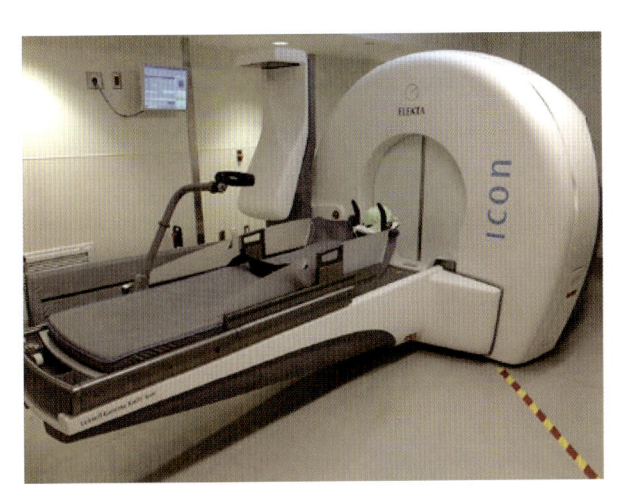

▲ 图 16-2 **Sunnybrook Odette 癌症中心的伽马刀 Icon 系统**

该装置配备了一个可伸缩的 90 kV 的 CBCT 装置，该 CBCT 坐标与立体定向治疗坐标匹配，且可达亚毫米精度。图示为处于回缩位置的 CBCT 臂对于最新的 CK M6 型，已经可以使用一个可互换的多叶准直器（multi-leaf collimator，MLC）系统。MLC 系统由 26 对 MLC 叶片组成，在源轴距为 80cm 位置叶片宽度为 3.85mm，因此源轴距为 80cm 时的最大矩形野尺寸为 10cm×11.5cm。为了保持与 Iris 准直器相似的剂量学可靠性，最小的 MLC 野限制在 0.8cm×0.8cm 左右。MLC 叶片透射率为 0.5%，每片叶片由 9.0cm 厚的钨制成。大多数基于 MLC 的 CK 治疗都是针对较大的病灶设计的，旨在提高治疗的效率。该 MLC 系统还支持常规分次的 CK 治疗。根据病变的位置和治疗分割方案（常规、单次或低分割治疗），目前用户可以灵活选择物理锥形筒、Iris 多页准直器或者 MLC 进行治疗。为了尽量减少治疗中准直器切换的停机时间，已经研制出一种准直器自动更换器（图 16-3）。关于在线靶区定位，CK 主要通过一对立体 X 线成像仪来检测靶区并实现和机头的几何匹配。

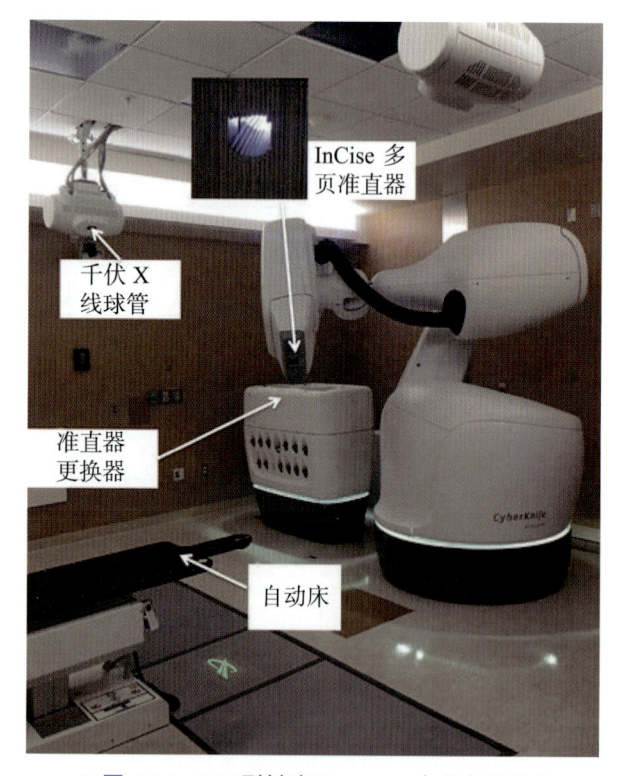

▲ 图 16-3 M6 型射波刀，MLC 安装在机头上
准直器更换器位于主机旁。图中所示的天花板上安装了两个立体 X 线源

（三）直线加速器

直线加速器放射手术治疗脑转移瘤的方法，始于锥形准直器和头架的应用，该方法中，每个等中心只治疗一个病灶。考虑到超过三个病灶的多数患者难以耐受长时间的治疗，因此起初这种方法仅用于治疗寡转移病灶。随着高分辨率 MLC 的引入，使这项技术变得更加高效。同时，随着用于摆位验证的成像技术的提高，以及可校正六个自由度的治疗床的出现，无框架 SRS 成为可能。新型直线加速器具有更高的剂量率和无均整器（flattening-filter free，FFF）模式，缩短了整体治疗时间，让许多患者可以一次治疗更多的转移灶。每个等中心治疗一个病灶的方式保证了很高的精度，从而可以采用很窄的治疗边界，这是因为等中心位于每个转移灶的中心，摆位的旋转误差对剂量的影响很小。这种方法的缺点是治疗时间与转移灶的数目成正比。

具备了机载图像引导系统、六维床、快速射束调制器、FFF 功能的新一代数控直线加速器（图 16-4），和具备容积调强治疗（volumetric modulated arc therapy，VMAT）功能的先进治疗计划软件，使单一等中心同步治疗多个颅内病灶成为可能。

对于多转移瘤的计划，治疗时间随着调制程度和 MU 的增加而增加，但如果把 15 个转移瘤的患者与 3 个转移瘤的患者进行相比，增加的时间并没有实质性的意义。出束时间短带来的好处是患者的舒适度和工作效率。这种技术的一个重要问题是对摆位精度的高要求，即使是微小的旋转不确定性也会随着等中心和转移瘤之间距离的增加而放大。对于靠近颅骨且远离等中心的脑转移瘤而言，1°的旋转不确定性可导致 2mm 的平移不确定性[10]。当转移瘤聚集在一起时，等中心可以放在簇内以尽量减少这种影响。然而，当转移瘤广泛分布于脑内，并且采用多个治疗床位置进行治疗时，这种情况必须通过计划靶区（planning target volume，PTV）边界来处理，因

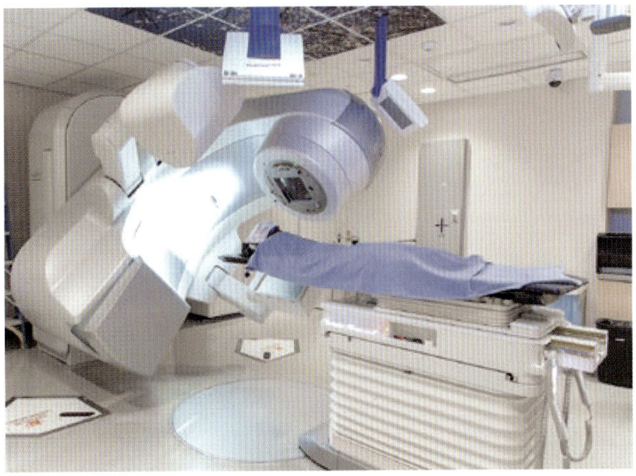

第 16 章 常用的放射外科技术
General Techniques for Radiosurgery

▲ 图 16-4 安装有 ExacTRAC 摆位验证设备的 Truebeam STX 直线加速器

此每个放疗机构必须在放疗流程中确定自己的最佳 PTV 边界。有一种降低放射性坏死风险的策略，即使用可变边界，也就是边界大小随靶区距等中心距离的增加而增加[11]。

在基于直线加速器的 SRS 中，通常采用旋转动态适形（dynamic conformal arc，DCA）放疗或 VMAT 的非共面弧来实现高度的剂量适形性[12, 13]。这种非共面弧通过多个治疗床位置及加速器机架和 MLC 的运动来实现。为了在整个治疗过程中始终达到所需的剂量和几何精度，保持直线加速器的机械和剂量精度是非常重要[14]的。

Varian 的 TrueBeam（2010）直线加速器以及 PerfectPitch（2013）治疗床的引入极大地改变了 SRS 的应用形式，特别在多发性脑转移瘤的 SRS 治疗方面[15]。TrueBeam 是新一代的直线加速器，其先进的控制系统使其能够在出束的同时保证每个自由度上的高精度运动[16]。在 FFF 模式下，TrueBeam 可以在等中心产生剂量率高达 24Gy/min 的射束，从而缩短治疗时间，而其高分辨率多叶准直器（high-definition multileaf collimator，HDMLC）可以生成高度适形的剂量分布[17]。直线加速器的机载影像系统和 PerfectPtich 6 维治疗床与直线加速器的整体操作完全集成，允许在治疗前对患者进行可靠且精确的定位[18]。Elekta 为立体定向应用也推出了一种设计类似的直线加速器 Versa HD[19]。

三、循证基础

SRS 治疗计划研究表明，尽管 PFX、直线加速器和 CK 在治疗方式和计划策略上有很大差异，但是对单靶 SRS 而言，剂量跌落特征具有相似性。物理特征方面，PFX 在头脚方向有着陡峭的剂量跌落（半影），4mm 枪的半影为 1.6mm（20%～80%）。在其他方向，现代治疗模态也报道了类似的半影，CK 5mm 直径射野半影为 2.2mm、PFX 半影为 2.8mm（轴向）、6 MV 直线加速器 MLC 形成的窄射野半影为 2.5～3mm。如何将这些半影转换到一个综合计划是一个复杂的问题，这涉及枪（PFX）或射束单元（beamlets）的叠加，特别是对于多个靶区。一般来说，对单个射束，文献支持所有的模态具有类似的剂量跌落。对多发性脑转移瘤，多项研究比较了不同治疗模态的治疗效果[20-26]，CK 比传统的基于直线加速器的治疗方法更具优势；CK 组与 GK 组相比，外周正常脑剂量稍高[20, 22, 24, 27]。这种差异和临床结果的潜在关系尚不清楚。实践中，需要检查每一个病灶的外周剂量及全脑剂量，以确保治疗安全。

由于多靶区治疗是一项复杂的技术，在尚不明确哪种方式更具剂量学或临床优势的情况下，应重点确保投照的可靠性和精准性。这里涉及 SRS 的三个问题：①计划考量；②小野剂量学；③定位精度。

四、治疗计划考量

（一）伽马刀

设计 GK SRS 计划基本上是一个手动过程，用户在每个单独的靶区中放置等中心（或"枪"），并选择适当的准直器设置、权重和处方等剂量水平，以获得适形剂量分布。较大的靶区通常需要多个等中心，但添加额外的低权重等中心几乎没有时间损失，因为治疗床能自动准确地移动到每

201

个等中心位置。对于分散的多个靶区，一个靶区对另一个靶区几乎没有剂量贡献。对于间距较近的靶区，必须考虑剂量外展，靶区之间距离越近，剂量外展就越具有挑战性。一般来说，由于GK的剂量快速跌落，每个靶区周围的剂量分布很好地隔开。图 16-5 给出的病例和图 16-1 相同，在几个横断面上显示了等剂量线。

由于每个靶区是按顺序治疗的，多发性转移瘤的总治疗时间可能很长。减少患者时间负担的一种方法是将转移瘤分组成更小的簇，并增加治疗天数。随着 Icon 系统以及基于面罩的固定，目前这已经成为可能。对于上述病例，治疗分为4天：第 1 天（77min）+ 第 2 天（86min）+ 第 3 天（44min）+ 第 4 天（37min）=4h/4d 的治疗时间。这种方法的一个放射生物学优势是，正常组织剂量相当于分割治疗，而每个靶区仍然受到完整的 SRS 处方，另一个优点是，能够进行靶区低分割和单分割的联合[28]。应该注意到，治疗这17 个靶区格外具有挑战性，因为大、小靶区处方剂量各不相同，距离又近。

（二）射波刀

针对多发性脑转移瘤的治疗，病灶大小通常决定了使用何种准直器。如果靶区的尺寸很小（<1cm），那么物理锥形准直器较常用，以锐化外围剂量分布。最近的一项研究表明，对于小尺寸病灶，基于 MLC 的治疗计划通常比基于锥形准直器的治疗计划适形性差[29]。对于直径≥ 1cm 的病灶，为了提高治疗效率，首选 Iris 准直器或者 MLC 系统。如果存在大小不等的脑部病灶，则通常最多使用 3 种尺寸的锥形准直器，以避免在治疗期间频繁更换准直器。不同大小脑转移瘤的同时存在也对治疗计划提出了挑战。如果其中一些靶区指定了相同的剂量，则可将其分组并设计为复合靶区，采用与单一靶区治疗计划相同的方法。然而，如果靶区的大小不同，那么处方剂量水平可能会因靶区不同而明显不同。随着靶区数量和大小的增加，靶区间剂量相互影响效应也可能发生显著变化[8, 9]。

在治疗计划优化过程中，需要仔细设置剂量 - 体积限制。正常组织的成形结构，例如围绕单个靶区的同心壳结构，通常用于改善剂量一致性和靶区周围的剂量梯度。此外，降低每个节点的最大 MU 可防止在有限数量的方向上照射过高的剂量，从而在更大的角度范围上产生更多的射束。

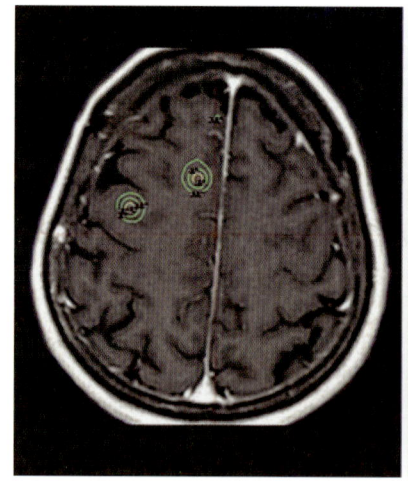

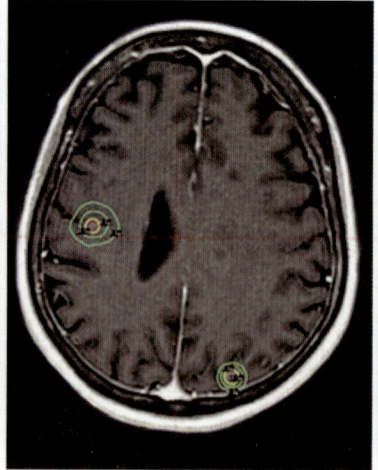

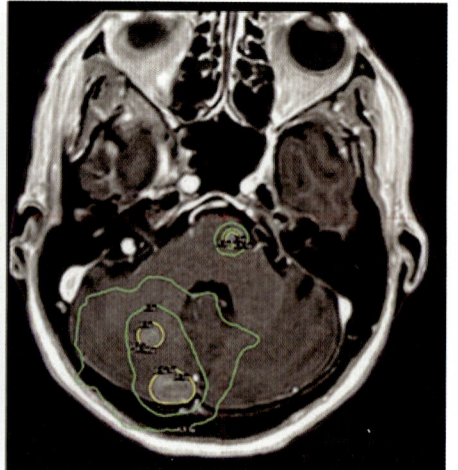

▲ 图 16-5 伽马刀治疗计划的横断面样例

黄色等剂量线为处方剂量（除一例脑干病灶为 15Gy 外，其他病灶为 18Gy）。外部绿色等剂量线为 9Gy 和 4.5Gy（即 50% 和 25%）。图中可见的小靶区（3～4mm）剂量的相互作用可以忽略不计。对于最右边相邻的较大靶区（> 2cm），50% 和 25% 等剂量线可以同时包含这两个靶区，却避开了几厘米开外的较小靶区当治疗大量的脑部病灶（$n>5$）时，一种所谓的两步法可以最小化靶区的剂量相互影响效应[30]。第一步，用户可以将大小相似的靶区组合在一起计划。第二步，不同靶区组的相对权重被迭代优化以产生一个综合的治疗计划。研究表明，两步法可以增强外周的剂量跌落，并改善正常脑组织在治疗中的损伤[30]。最新的 CK 计划系统 Precision 1.1 已经实现了在几个治疗阶段对多个脑转移瘤进行分组和优化的功能。图 16-6 所示的病例中，对 4 个 < 1.0cm 的脑转移瘤进行了计划设计。计划设计总共用时约 1h，总治疗时间估计需要 59min。

（三）直线加速器

使用直线加速器进行 SRS 计划设计和实施的方法可以宽泛地分为两类，即多等中心和单等中心。传统上，使用多个等中心，每个靶区定位在等中心，并像 CK 一样按顺序治疗。对于每个等中心/靶区，通常使用一系列 3~6 个非共面弧来获得具有陡峭剂量梯度的适形计划（图 16-7）。过去 SRS 使用锥形准直器，通过选择不同的直径来匹配不同大小地靶区。随着 MLC 的引入，各大治疗中心开始首先研究旋转适形技术，接着研究旋转动态适形技术，其中 MLC 开口形状随机架角度变化，以匹配靶区的投影形状。

然而，最近由于 MLC 的应用，人们对单等中心方法治疗多个靶区产生了浓厚的兴趣。首先，研究了通过 MLC 实现的偏中心动态适形野，射野的形状随着不同机架角度下的靶区形状的变化而变化。最近，有治疗中心正在使用 VMAT 方法，计划系统的逆向优化程序生成经过强度调制的射野，以获得适形剂量并控制正常组织剂量。

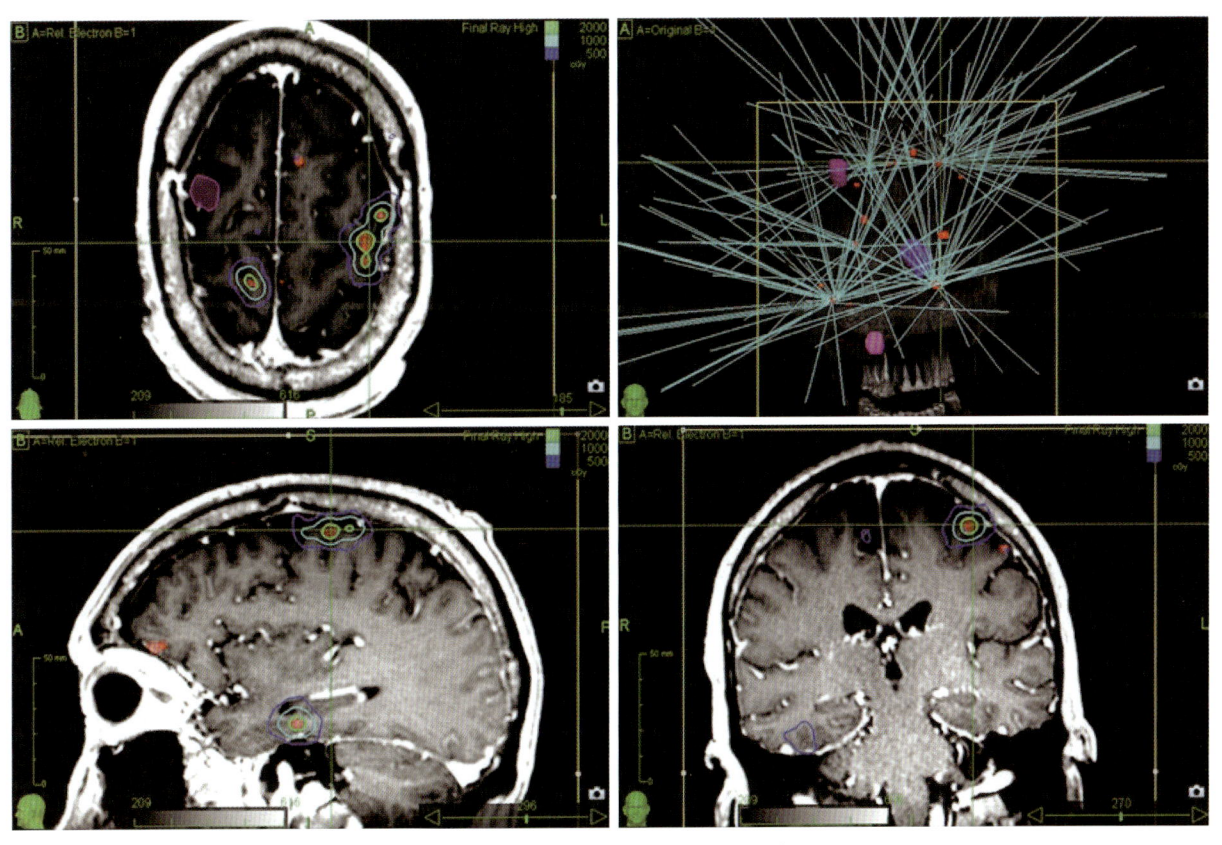

▲ 图 16-6　CK 治疗 4 个脑转移瘤

对于该病例，所有病灶的处方剂量为 20Gy，归一在最大剂量的 70% 等剂量面上，10Gy 和 5Gy 等剂量线也示于图中。需要注意到当靶区彼此接近时，低水平等剂量线会融合在一起。该病例采用了由 7.5mm 锥形准直器形成的共 178 束射束，四个病灶的预计治疗时间为 59min

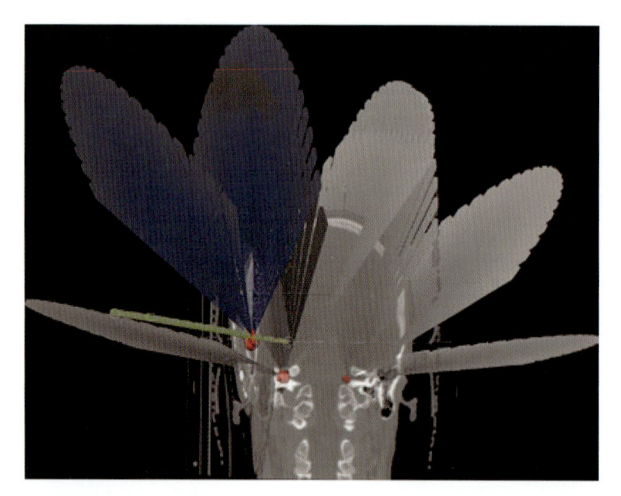

▲ 图 16-7　多等中心旋转动态适形计划治疗 3 个脑转移瘤

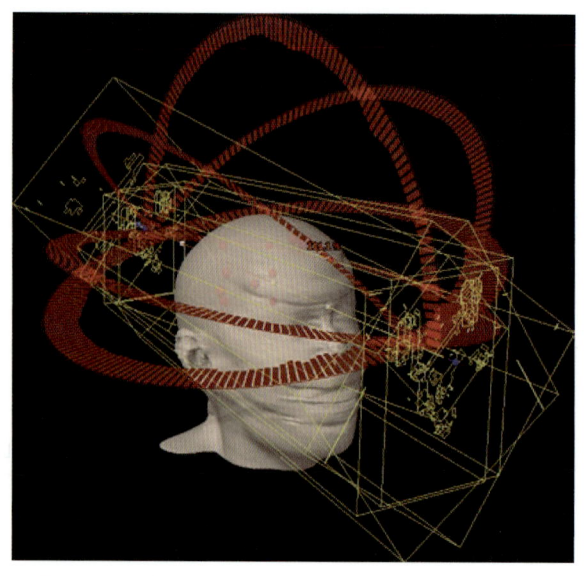

▲ 图 16-8　采用单等中心为 9 个脑转移瘤设计的容积旋转调强放疗计划

这样，如果等中心位于头部的中心位置，只需使用数个弧（通常为非共面），就可以优化得到一个经过调制的 VMAT 计划，从而可以在尽可能短的治疗时间内治疗所有靶区，如图 16-8 所示。

五、小野剂量学

由于辐射源的遮挡、侧向电子不平衡及探测器对光子野的扰动等因素，小光子野的剂量学极具有挑战性[31]。2007 年 Doblado 等证实了小野剂量测量中探测器选择的重要性[32]。他们发现了不同探测器对 < 3.0cm 射野的响应差异，当使用不合适的探测器如大体积电离室时，对 < 10mm 的极小射野，偏差会超过 50%。因此需要特别注意如何精确测量 SRS 计划系统（treatment planning systems，TPS）调试所需的剂量学指标，并且这项工作只能由专业的物理师完成。过去十年里，针对小野测量的探测器开发一直在稳步发展[33-35]。

目前，AAPM TG51 协议[36] 及其更新版[37]，以及 IAEA TRS-398 [38] 构成了临床参考剂量测量的基本体系。这些技术规程需要的参考条件为 10cm×10cm 射野大小，100cm 源轴距或源皮距离等，但像射波刀这样的放疗设备并不能实现这个条件。这种情况下，建议使用所谓的特定机器参考野（MSR 野），这是一个由特定装置提供的最接近参考条件的中间固定野[39]。MSR 野与参考野及参考条件（即探测器的校准条件）的差异越大，射线质的潜在差异和探测器响应变化就会越大。对于一个合格的医学物理师，其职责首先要确保为给定的 MSR 野使用大小合适的探测器，其次是确保应用适当的射线质校正因子来修正 MSR 和参考野/条件的差异。

目前，专门针对小野参考剂量学的全面的技术规程[39, 40] 已经推出，探测器尺寸和侧向带电粒子失衡等因素的影响可以通过引入校正因子来修正。如果遵循小野剂量学规程的相关规定并注意探测器的选择，小野剂量学参数的测量精度可小于 2%[39]。

（一）伽马刀

应用参考剂量学规程最大的挑战来自伽马刀。由于对每个单独的放射源进行校准并不现实且作用有限，因此合适的 MSR 野应通过最大直径准直器头盔（如对于 GK Icon 为 16mm）来实现，并将所有放射源处在照射状态。应该慎重考虑探测器的选择，以平衡小体积探测器的灵敏度和准确度。

（二）射波刀

射波刀的质量保证（quality assurance，QA）测试除了特定机器的 QA 测试（譬如保证毫米定位精度的自动 QA 测试），还有针对多发转移瘤治疗的特定患者的 QA 测试，这种测试可在内嵌有基准点的固体水模体或头部模体中执行。可进行点剂量验证和二维等剂量胶片测量，以验证实际的剂量分布与治疗计划系统预测的剂量分布是否一致。建议使用独立的软件进行治疗计划的机器跳数（monitor unit，MU）检查，可利用商用软件（如 MUcheck、Oncology Data System、OK，USA）在治疗实施之前对射束路径和相关的 MU 设置进行验证。对于射波刀，直径为 60mm 的固定准直器（距离放射源 80cm）提供了一个相对平坦和均匀的射野，通常建议将其作为 MSR 野。

（三）直线加速器

基于 VMAT 的单等中心技术治疗多发性转移瘤独具挑战性。除了 TPS 调试所必需的基本剂量测量外，还需要经验参数来模拟 VMAT 实施中使用的动态辐射野。例如，Varian Eclipse 的 AAA 算法需要一个称为剂量学叶片间隙（dosimetric leaf gap，DLG）的参数，用于 MLC 圆形端面的建模。在射束调试期间，通过将测量值与 TPS 的计算值进行比较，以迭代方式对这些参数进行微调。

单等中心 VMAT 计划的剂量学验证测量非常复杂，这是因为要在偏轴位置进行测量，且等效野尺寸较小。日常用于传统 VMAT 计划剂量验证的探测器阵列不适合 SRS 剂量测量，因为采样不足导致肿瘤所在位置处仅产生一两个测量点。通常点剂量的测量使用小型固态探测器，通过对模体进行多次定位来测量每个靶区的剂量。虽然用胶片进行绝对剂量测量容易受系统误差影响，但高空间分辨率使其在验证 SRS 投照的空间精度方面非常有价值（图 16-9）。一旦 TPS 调试完毕并投入使用，就可以用一些简便方法进行特定患者的剂量验证，如使用直线加速器的电子射野影像系统进行基于通量的测量，或使用蒙特卡罗方法进行独立的剂量计算。

与商业治疗计划系统采用的剂量算法不同，蒙特卡罗方法根据基本的物理原理计算剂量，被称为剂量计算的金标准，特别适用于复杂输运的剂量计算[39]。在加拿大不列颠哥伦比亚省温哥华市肿瘤医院，一个基于 EGSnrc 代码[41]自开发的蒙特卡罗剂量验证系统已用于复杂 VMAT 的独立剂量计算。图 16-10 的示例对比了 Eclipse AAA 算法和蒙特卡罗算法计算的剂量分布，这是一个多发脑转移瘤 SRS VMAT 计划，采用了 5 个非共面弧。

六、定位精度

（一）伽马刀

传统上，Leksell 立体定向框架是 GK-SRS 的标志，它通过外科方式安装在患者头部，保证刚性固定并提供定位坐标系。最近，在 GK Icon 系统上集成了 CBCT 图像引导装置，使无框架 SRS 成为可能。然而，无论是框架还是面罩，GK 的主要优点是聚焦的机械精度高。最新的 GK Icon 型号中，准直器头盔是固定的，所有 192 束射束同时会聚在焦点处。此外，据报道，患者定位系统在治疗区域内的精度 < 0.3mm[42]。

（二）射波刀

为了可视化小的脑转移瘤，首先需要采集薄层计划 CT，由此生成高分辨率的二维数字重建影像（digitally reconstructed radiographs，DRR）作为配准的参考影像。计划 CT 的层厚通常设置为 1.0mm，以获得足够的 DRR 分辨率，并将靶区定位的系统不确定性降至最低。证据表明颅内任何位置的病灶，其定位精度可达 0.3mm[7, 43]。由于患者采用面罩固定，因此建议治疗期间每隔 30~45s 进行一次成像，以便及时跟踪和验证每

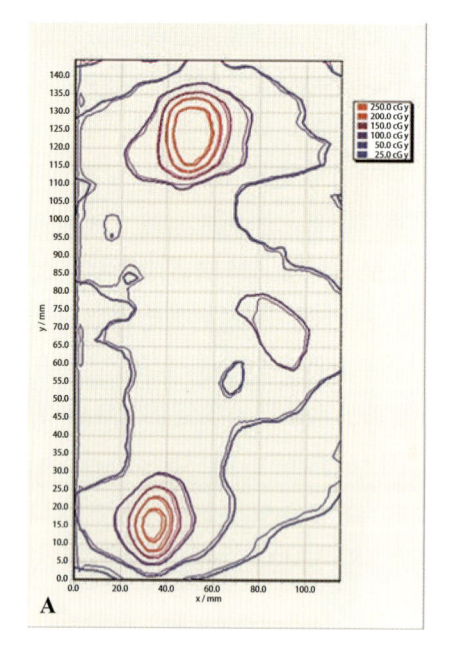

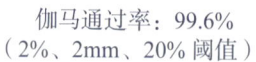

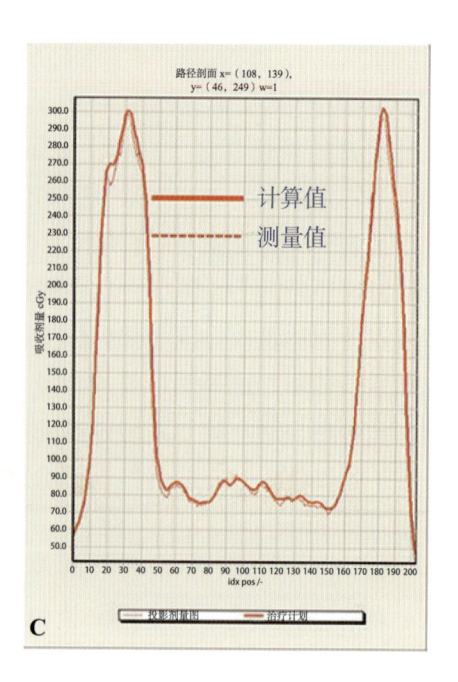

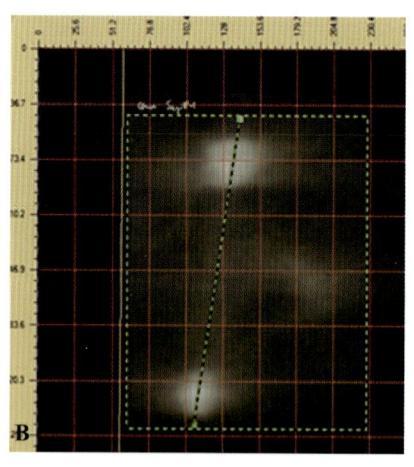

▲ 图 16-9 A. 多发性脑转移瘤单等中心非共面 VMAT 计划的等剂量分布与胶片测量的比较；B. 胶片测量；C. 图（B）所示的直线上，测量和计算的剂量分布对比（未发表）

个病灶的位置。频繁成像对于小的脑转移瘤尤其重要，因为 1~2mm 的位移可能导致射束完全脱靶。利用头部模体和自显影胶片进行端到端测试，一般情况下最大定位误差 < 1mm。

（三）直线加速器

直线加速器的机械精度受机架头部重量（导致下垂）、治疗床晃动以及 MLC 叶片位置校准的影响。TG-142 要求 SRS 装置的等中心精度 < 1mm [14]。

Winston Lutz（WL）试验[44]是测量机架、准直器、MLC 和治疗床对等中心精度综合影响的标准方法。该测试使用安装在治疗床上的金属滚珠轴承（ball bearing，BB），将其与直线加速器等中心精确对准，然后在不同的机架、治疗床和准直器位置拍摄一系列 MLC 小野的射野影像，从而测量 BB 与射野的对准情况。除了标准的 WL 测试，还需要对整个治疗床旋转范围内的旋转精度（三个旋转自由度方向）进行量化，因为这些因素会影响偏中心靶区的定位精度。研究表明，TrueBeam 治疗床的角度精度在 0.1°以内[45]。

除了等中心精度测试外，患者定位过程中的所有环节（OBI、六维治疗床和患者固定）还需通过非可见靶区测试来验证和定期监测，该测试可利用仿真头模来完成。非可见靶区测试模拟了

第 16 章 常用的放射外科技术
General Techniques for Radiosurgery

Eclipse　　　　　　　蒙特卡罗

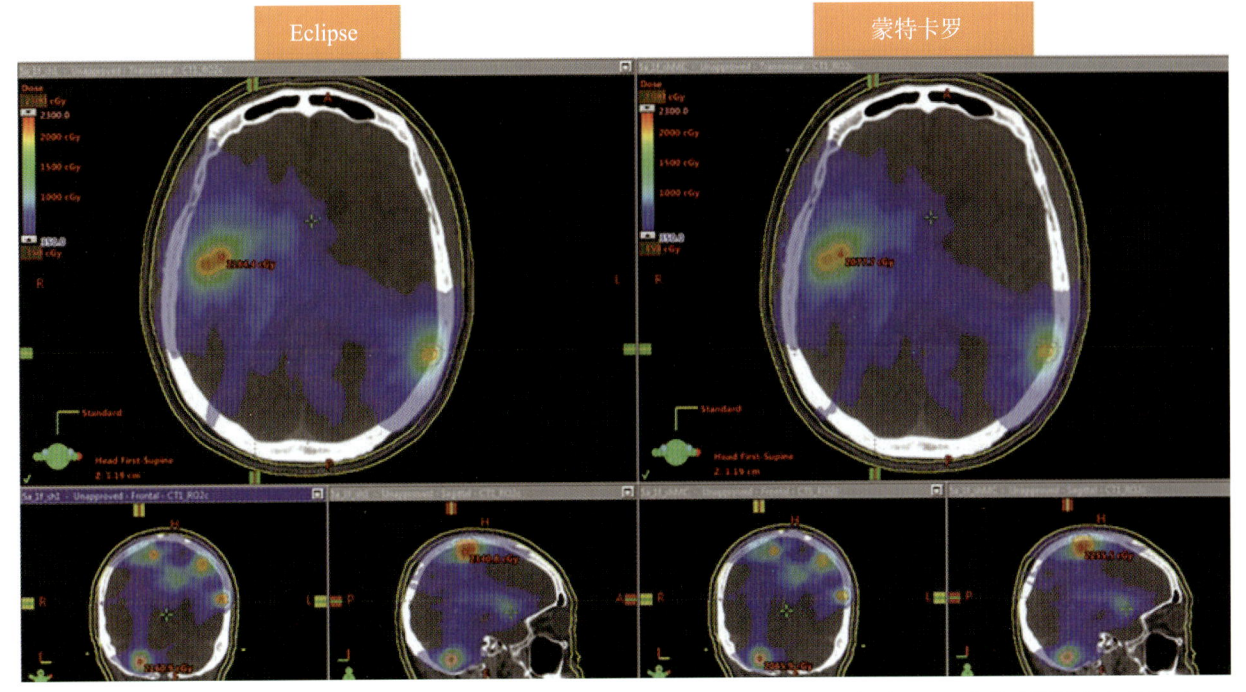

▲ 图 16-10　Eclipse AAA 算法和蒙特卡罗算法计算的剂量分布对比，这是一个采用了五个非共面弧的多发脑转移瘤 SRS VMAT 计划（未发表）

从 CT 模拟到治疗实施的整个图像引导放射治疗（image-guided radiotherapy，IGRT）的工作流程，用来量化靶区定位的系统不确定性。通常，该测试用于等中心靶区。

随着单等中心 SRS 技术在多发转移瘤治疗中的应用，有必要测量偏中心靶区计划的定位精度。在加拿大不列颠哥伦比亚省温哥华市肿瘤医院，单等中心多靶区计划的靶区准确性利用仿真头模来测试。在这个测试中，六个放射显像的标记被置于模体的不同位置，使用有多个开口的射野照射每个靶区。图 16-11 给出了照射六个靶区的侧位射野的 DRR 与相应的射野影像的对比。通过比较 DRR 与射野影像，可以量化患者定位系统在偏中心不同位置处的准确度。

七、不确定性领域和发展趋势

就临床结果而言，还没有任何确凿的证据支持一种技术胜过另一种技术。在提高效率或疗效方面，有以下 7 个研究方向。

（一）伽马刀

伽马刀治疗多发性转移瘤往往需要很长时间。然而，当前 Icon 系统提供的灵活性，可以将治疗划分为多个时段去完成。这可能会有放射生物学优势，因为单个肿瘤在一次治疗中即可受照全部放射外科剂量，而整个大脑的正常组织接受的却是分次照射剂量[28]。针对多发转移瘤患者，结合先进的自动计划技术，包括治疗床连续运动路径优化，更快速和更加个体化的计划正在 GammaKnife 平台上不断推出[46-48]。

（二）射波刀

对于多发性脑转移瘤的 CK 治疗，患者采用热塑面罩固定，主要使用非共面非等中心射束。与以前的 CK 型号相比，最新的 CK M6 系统大大扩展了射束角度，特别是后方向。InCise MLC 系统的引入提高了大病灶（如 > 1cm）的治疗效率。就像插图中病例展示的那样，脑转移瘤大小为数毫米到数厘米，因此进一步改进高分辨率

207

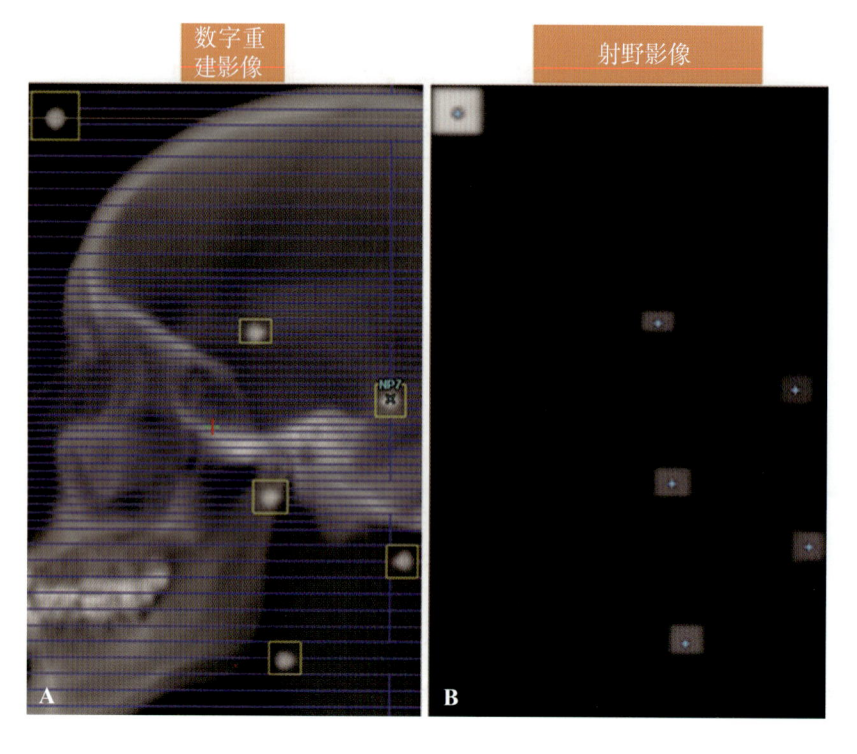

图 16-11　侧位射野图像
A. 数字重建影像；B. 通过仿真头模非可见靶区测试获得的射野影像。这是一个单等中心、多发转移瘤计划，等中心位于 3# 靶区的中心。射野影像上的蓝色星星显示了 BB 的中心（未发表）

MLC 系统，譬如减小叶片宽度和提高叶片定位精度，将扩大其在小病灶治疗中的应用范围。另一个方向是发展多功能的质量保证工具和流程，以便同时满足目前 CK 系统的三套准直器的质控要求。

（三）直线加速器

单等中心治疗多发性转移瘤的一个优点是治疗速度快。然而，对于多发（5+）脑转移病例，若要使用传统 VMAT 技术实现高质量的 SRS 计划，可能需要从计划算法、剂量成形结构、计划技巧、计算资源、避让结构和计划时间等方面予以考虑。这给放疗医师和剂量师带来了挑战，可能让接受单等中心治疗的患者并不一定能从中受益。可喜的是，针对改进此类患者计划质量的相关方法已经商业实现了，并正在应用于临床。

（四）Elements™

BrainLAB 是 SRS 硬件和软件的重要供应商。他们开发了一套正交 X 线影像系统和一套六维治疗床（ExacTRAC）™，前者可以在任何治疗床角度进行摆位验证，后者用于校正平移和旋转位置误差。多年来，他们一直在为基于传统直线加速器的 SRS 提供专用软件，应用该软件，需要将等中心放置在每个转移瘤的中心。新版的 Elements Cranial SRS™ 软件使用轻度调制的动态旋转适形技术，可以采用单一等中心对多个转移瘤进行治疗。计划技术方面的创新包括：优化每个弧的准直器角度；在不同的治疗床角度治疗转移瘤集合的不同子集；限制叶片开口的宽度，使得仅单个转移瘤位于叶片开口中。使用 Elements 对 10 例多发性脑转移瘤患者进行计划设计，每个患者同时采用的 VMAT-SRS、多等中心动态旋转和单等中心动态旋转技术设计三个计划，计划对比表明，Elements 计划改善了梯度指数和 V12，适形指数与其他三种技术相似[49]。

（五）HyperArc™

为了优化单等中心多转移瘤 SRS，瓦里安医疗系统公司开发了一种专用的 VMAT 算法，称为 HyperArc，它使用准直器角度优化来提高计划的质量。有项研究比较了 15 例患者用 VMAT-SRS、射波刀和 HyperArc-SRS 技术设计的计划，结果显示 VMAT 和 HyperArc 治疗时间更短，但在 Paddick 适形指数或梯度指数方面没有显著差异[50]。另外两项针对 20 个或者更多病灶的单等中心、多发转移瘤病例的计划研究表明，HyperArc SRS 在适形指数和梯度指数方面比传统 VMAT SRS 有统计学意义的改善[51, 52]。

（六）新概念

治疗过程中 MLC 准直器角度的动态变化是一个活跃的研究领域。通过将这个额外的自由度添加到多发转移瘤单等中心动态旋转适形计划中，在不牺牲计划质量的情况下，计划实施所需的 MU 可以减少 50%[53]。

（七）MLC

目前，瓦里安立体定向 MLC 是根据单靶区立体定向放疗和同中心靶区常规放疗目的而优化的。中心 8cm 的射野内，叶片宽度为 2.5mm。然而，对于采用单等中心治疗多发转移瘤的情况，对大脑外围的病灶，更多的剂量是通过 5mm 的叶片调制的，因此这些病灶的剂量分布质量将降低。解决方法之一是认真选择几个等中心，病灶就不会超出高分辨率叶片的范围[54]。然而，这增加了计划时间和治疗时间。一个硬件解决方案是增加多叶准直器中心窄叶片的数量、速度和精度，这将改善单等中心、多转移瘤 SRS 的剂量学效果。Elekta Versa HD 有 160 片 MLC 叶片，叶片宽度为 5mm[19]。

八、指南

无论采用何种技术，一个有效的 SRS 治疗流程离不开一个完整、持续的 QA 规程，以确保治疗装置的相应指标符合设备制造商的推荐，并在国际国内指南以及推荐所规定的临床允许范围内[14, 55–58]。

CK M6 系统的 QA 任务需遵循 TG135 指南，以及 AAPM-RSS 医学物理实践指南[59]中规定的最低设备容差水平，涉及机械检查、辐射特性检查、影像/跟踪系统检查以及准直器检查[60]。

为了确保亚毫米的定位准确度，需对应用于 SRS 的窄束射线的投照准确度和精度进行很好的量化并定期检测。对基于 MLC 的多发转移瘤的偏中心治疗，可能需要专门的 QA 设备验证在机架、准直器和治疗床的整个运动范围的布野准确度[61, 62]。建议对治疗实施的准确度进行端到端测试，尽可能覆盖从 MRI 到靶区勾画，再到治疗实施的整个工作流程。

根据最近的 TRS-483 报道，推荐使用机器特定的参考（machine-specific reference，MSR）野作为参考条件[39]。微分探测器在小野和 MSR 野条件下的响应差异须考虑使用蒙特卡罗计算进行校正。此外，在小野相对剂量学中，探测器和射野的对准及其放置的方向也很重要。

> **要 点**
> - 治疗脑转移瘤的 SRS 技术在持续发展。
> - 现有技术都有优缺点，在技术选择的时候应予以考虑。
> - 随着脑转移患者数量的增加及患者寿命的延长，治疗效率可能成为一个高度优先项。
> - 另一方面，尽管厂商让治疗流程变得简化和自动化，但仍不能低估技术的复杂性。
> - 随着时间的推移，各种技术变得更加一致和精确，对物理基础的基本理解变得越来越重要。

参考文献

[1] Lindquist C, Paddick I. The Leksell Gamma Knife Perfexion and comparisons with its predecessors. Neurosurgery. 2007;61(3 Suppl):130–40; discussion 40-1.

[2] Zeverino M, Jaccard M, Patin D, Ryckx N, Marguet M, Tuleasca C, et al. Commissioning of the Leksell Gamma Knife® Icon™. Med Phys. 2017;44(2):355–63.

[3] Sarfehnia A, Ruschin M, Chugh B, Yeboah C, Becker N, Cho YB, et al. Performance characterization of an integrated cone-beam CT system for dedicated gamma radiosurgery. Med Phys. 2018;45(9):4179–90.

[4] Pappas EP, Moutsatsos A, Pantelis E, Zoros E, Georgiou E, Torrens M, et al. On the development of a comprehensive MC simulation model for the Gamma Knife Perfexion radiosurgery unit. Phys Med Biol. 2016;61(3):1182–203.

[5] Adler JR Jr, Murphy MJ, Chang SD, Hancock SL. Image-guided robotic radiosurgery. Neurosurgery. 1999;44(6):1299–306; discussion 306-7.

[6] Andrews DW, Bednarz G, Evans JJ, Downes B. A review of 3 current radiosurgery systems. Surg Neurol. 2006;66(6):559–64.

[7] Chang SD, Main W, Martin DP, Gibbs IC, Heilbrun MP. An analysis of the accuracy of the CyberKnife: a robotic frameless stereotactic radiosurgical system. Neurosurgery. 2003;52(1):140–6; discussion 6-7.

[8] Yu C, Main W, Taylor D, Kuduvalli G, Apuzzo ML, Adler JR Jr. An anthropomorphic phantom study of the accuracy of Cyberknife spinal radiosurgery. Neurosurgery. 2004;55(5):1138–49.

[9] van de Water S, Hoogeman MS, Breedveld S, Nuyttens JJ, Schaart DR, Heijmen BJ. Variable circular collimator in robotic radiosurgery: a time-efficient alternative to a mini-multileaf collimator? Int J Radiat Oncol Biol Phys. 2011;81(3):863–70.

[10] Winey B, Bussiere M. Geometric and dosimetric uncertainties in intracranial stereotactic treatments for multiple nonisocentric lesions. J Appl Clin Med Phys. 2014;15(3):122–32.

[11] Chang J. Incorporating the rotational setup uncertainty into the planning target volume margin expansion for the single isocenter for multiple targets technique. Pract Radiat Oncol. 2018;8(6):475–83.

[12] Otto K. Volumetric modulated arc therapy: IMRT in a single gantry arc. Med Phys. 2008;35(1):310–7.

[13] Solberg TD, Boedeker KL, Fogg R, Selch MT, DeSalles AA. Dynamic arc radiosurgery field shaping: a comparison with static field conformal and noncoplanar circular arcs. Int J Radiat Oncol Biol Phys. 2001;49(5):1481–91.

[14] Klein EE, Hanley J, Bayouth J, Yin FF, Simon W, Dresser S, et al. Task Group 142 report: quality assurance of medical accelerators. Med Phys. 2009;36(9):4197–212.

[15] Schmidhalter D, Fix MK, Wyss M, Schaer N, Munro P, Scheib S, et al. Evaluation of a new six degrees of freedom couch for radiation therapy. Med Phys. 2013;40(11):111710.

[16] Scorsetti M, Alongi F, Castiglioni S, Clivio A, Fogliata A, Lobefalo F, et al. Feasibility and early clinical assessment of flattening filter free (FFF) based stereotactic body radiotherapy (SBRT) treatments. Radiat Oncol. 2011;6:113.

[17] Dhabaan A, Elder E, Schreibmann E, Crocker I, Curran WJ, Oyesiku NM, et al. Dosimetric performance of the new high-definition multileaf collimator for intracranial stereotactic radiosurgery. J Appl Clin Med Phys. 2010;11(3):3040.

[18] Zhang Q, Driewer J, Wang S, Li S, Zhu X, Zheng D, et al. Accuracy evaluation of a six-degree-offreedom couch using cone beam CT and IsoCal phantom with an in-house algorithm. Med Phys. 2017;44(8):3888–98.

[19] Thompson CM, Weston SJ, Cosgrove VC, Thwaites DI. A dosimetric characterization of a novel linear accelerator collimator. Med Phys. 2014;41(3):031713.

[20] Ma L, Nichol A, Hossain S, Wang B, Petti P, Vellani R, et al. Variable dose interplay effects across radiosurgical apparatus in treating multiple brain metastases. Int J Comput Assist Radiol Surg. 2014;9(6):1079–86.

[21] Slosarek K, Bekman B, Wendykier J, Grzadziel A, Fogliata A, Cozzi L. In silico assessment of the dosi metric quality of a novel, automated radiation treatment planning strategy for linac-based radiosurgery of multiple brain metastases and a comparison with robotic methods. Radiat Oncol. 2018;13(1):41.

[22] Zhang I, Antone J, Li J, Saha S, Riegel AC, Vijeh L, et al. Hippocampal-sparing and target volume coverage in treating 3 to 10 brain metastases: a comparison of Gamma Knife, single-isocenter VMAT, CyberKnife, and TomoTherapy stereotactic radiosurgery. Pract Radiat Oncol. 2017;7(3):183–9.

[23] Ma L, Petti P, Wang B, Descovich M, Chuang C, Barani IJ, et al. Apparatus dependence of normal brain tissue dose in stereotactic radiosurgery for multiple brain metastases. J Neurosurg. 2011;114(6):1580–4.

[24] Sio TT, Jang S, Lee SW, Curran B, Pyakuryal AP, Sternick ES. Comparing gamma knife and cyberknife in patients with brain metastases. J Appl Clin Med Phys. 2014;15(1):4095.

[25] Thomas EM, Popple RA, Wu X, Clark GM, Markert JM, Guthrie BL, et al. Comparison of plan quality and delivery time between volumetric arc therapy (RapidArc) and Gamma Knife radiosurgery for multiple cranial metastases. Neurosurgery. 2014;75(4):409–17; discussion 17-8.

[26] Potrebko PS, Keller A, All S, Sejpal S, Pepe J, Saigal K, et al. GammaKnife versus VMAT radiosurgery plan quality for many brain metastases. J Appl Clin Med Phys. 2018;19(6):159–65.

[27] Eaton DJ, Lee J, Paddick I. Stereotactic radiosurgery for multiple brain metastases: results of multicenter benchmark planning studies. Pract Radiat Oncol. 2018;8(4):e212–e20.

[28] Kelly DA. Treatment of multiple brain metastases with a

divide-and-conquer spatial fractionation radiosurgery approach. Med Hypotheses. 2014;83(4):425–8.

[29] Jang SY, Lalonde R, Ozhasoglu C, Burton S, Heron D, Huq MS. Dosimetric comparison between cone/ Iris-based and InCise MLC-based CyberKnife plans for single and multiple brain metastases. J Appl Clin Med Phys. 2016;17(5):184–99.

[30] Ma L, Sahgal A, Hwang A, Hu W, Descovich M, Chuang C, et al. A two-step optimization method for improving multiple brain lesion treatments with robotic radiosurgery. Technol Cancer Res Treat. 2011;10(4):331–8.

[31] Das IJ, Ding GX, Ahnesjö A. Small fields: nonequilibrium radiation dosimetry. Med Phys. 2008;35(1):206–15.

[32] Sánchez-Doblado F, Hartmann GH, Pena J, Roselló JV, Russiello G, Gonzalez-Castaño DM. A new method for output factor determination in MLC shaped narrow beams. Phys Med. 2007;23(2):58–66.

[33] Lárraga-Gutiérrez JM, Ballesteros-Zebadúa P, Rodríguez-Ponce M, García-Garduño OA, de la Cruz OO. Properties of a commercial PTW-60019 synthetic diamond detector for the dosimetry of small radiotherapy beams. Phys Med Biol. 2015;60(2):905–24.

[34] De Coste V, Francescon P, Marinelli M, Masi L, Paganini L, Pimpinella M, et al. Is the PTW 60019 microDiamond a suitable candidate for small field reference dosimetry? Phys Med Biol. 2017;62(17):7036–55.

[35] Carrasco P, Jornet N, Jordi O, Lizondo M, LatorreMusoll A, Eudaldo T, et al. Characterization of the Exradin W1 scintillator for use in radiotherapy. Med Phys. 2015;42(1):297–304.

[36] Almond PR, Biggs PJ, Coursey BM, Hanson WF, Huq MS, Nath R, et al. AAPM's TG-51 protocol for clinical reference dosimetry of high-energy photon and electron beams. Med Phys. 1999;26(9):1847–70.

[37] McEwen M, DeWerd L, Ibbott G, Followill D, Rogers DW, Seltzer S, et al. Addendum to the AAPM's TG-51 protocol for clinical reference dosimetry of highenergy photon beams. Med Phys. 2014;41(4):041501.

[38] Andreo P, Huq MS, Westermark M, Song H, Tilikidis A, DeWerd L, et al. Protocols for the dosimetry of high-energy photon and electron beams: a comparison of the IAEA TRS-398 and previous international codes of practice. International Atomic Energy Agency. Phys Med Biol. 2002;47(17):3033–53.

[39] Vatnisky S, Meghzifene A, Christaki K, Palmans H, Andrew P, Saiful Huq M, et al. IAEA TRS-483. Dosimetry of small fields used in external beam radiotherapy: an international code of practice for reference and relative dose determination. International Atomic Energy Agency. 2017.

[40] Alfonso R, Andreo P, Capote R, Huq MS, Kilby W, Kjäll P, et al. A new formalism for reference dosimetry of small and nonstandard fields. Med Phys. 2008;35(11):5179–86.

[41] Rogers DWO, Kawrakow I, Seuntjens JP, Walters BRB, Mainegra-Hing E. NRC user codes for EGSnrc. National Research Council Canada. Institute for National Measurement Standards.

[42] Ma L, Chiu J, Hoye J, McGuiness C, Perez-Andujar A. Quality assurance of stereotactic alignment and patient positioning mechanical accuracy for robotized Gamma Knife radiosurgery. Phys Med Biol. 2014;59(23):N221–6.

[43] Okamoto H, Hamada M, Sakamoto E, Wakita A, Nakamura S, Kato T, et al. Log-file analysis of accuracy of beam localization for brain tumor treatment by CyberKnife. Pract Radiat Oncol. 2016;6(6): e361–e7.

[44] Lutz W, Winston KR, Maleki N. A system for stereotactic radiosurgery with a linear accelerator. Int J Radiat Oncol Biol Phys. 1988;14(2):373–81.

[45] Wilson B, Gete E. Machine-specific quality assurance procedure for stereotactic treatments with dynamic couch rotations. Med Phys. 2017;44(12):6529–37.

[46] Cevik M, Shirvani Ghomi P, Aleman D, Lee Y, Berdyshev A, Nordstrom H, et al. Modeling and comparison of alternative approaches for sector duration optimization in a dedicated radiosurgery system. Phys Med Biol. 2018;63(15):155009.

[47] Ghobadi K, Ghaffari HR, Aleman DM, Jaffray DA, Ruschin M. Automated treatment planning for a dedicated multi-source intracranial radiosurgery treatment unit using projected gradient and grassfire algorithms. Med Phys. 2012;39(6):3134–41.

[48] Vandewouw MM, Aleman DM, Jaffray DA. Robotic path finding in inverse treatment planning for stereotactic radiosurgery with continuous dose delivery. Med Phys. 2016;43(8):4545.

[49] Gevaert T, Steenbeke F, Pellegri L, Engels B, Christian N, Hoornaert MT, et al. Evaluation of a dedicated brain metastases treatment planning optimization for radiosurgery: a new treatment paradigm? Radiat Oncol. 2016;11:13.

[50] Slosarek K, Bekman B, Wendykier J, Grządziel A, Fogliata A, Cozzi L. In silico assessment of the dosimetric quality of a novel, automated radiation treatment planning strategy for linac-based radiosurgery of multiple brain metastases and a comparison with robotic methods. Radiat Oncol. 2018;13(1):41.

[51] Ruggieri R, Naccarato S, Mazzola R, Ricchetti F, Corradini S, Fiorentino A, et al. Linac-based VMAT radiosurgery for multiple brain lesions: comparison between a conventional multi-isocenter approach and a new dedicated mono-isocenter technique. Radiat Oncol. 2018;13(1):38.

[52] Ohira S, Ueda Y, Akino Y, Hashimoto M, Masaoka A, Hirata T, et al. HyperArc VMAT planning for single and multiple brain metastases stereotactic radiosurgery: a new treatment planning approach. Radiat Oncol. 2018;13(1):13.

[53] MacDonald RL, Thomas CG, Syme A. Dynamic collimator trajectory algorithm for multiple metastases dynamic conformal arc treatment planning. Med Phys. 2018;45(1):5–17.

[54] Ballangrud Å, Kuo LC, Happersett L, Lim SB, Beal K, Yamada Y, et al. Institutional experience with SRS VMAT planning for multiple cranial metastases. J Appl Clin Med Phys. 2018;19(2):176–83.

[55] Benedict SH, Yenice KM, Followill D, Galvin JM, Hinson W, Kavanagh B, et al. Stereotactic body radiation therapy: the report of AAPM Task Group 101. Med Phys. 2010;37(8):4078–101.

[56] Kirkby C, Ghasroddashti E, Angers CP, Zeng G, Barnett E. COMP report: CPQR technical quality control guideline for medical linear accelerators and multileaf collimators. J Appl Clin Med Phys. 2018;19(2):22–8.

[57] Vandervoort E, Patrocinio H, Chow T, Soisson E, Nadeau DB. COMP report: CPQR technical quality control guidelines for CyberKnife ((R)) technology. J Appl Clin Med Phys. 2018;19(2):29–34.

[58] Berndt A, van Prooijen M, Guillot M. COMP report: CPQR technical quality control guidelines for Gamma Knife radiosurgery. J Appl Clin Med Phys. 2018;19:365.

[59] Halvorsen PH, Cirino E, Das IJ, Garrett JA, Yang J, Yin F, Fairobent LA. AAPM-RSS medical physics practice guideline 9.a. for SRS-SBRT. J Appl Clin Med Phys. 2017;18:10–21.

[60] Dieterich S, Cavedon C, Chuang CF, Cohen AB, Garrett JA, Lee CL, et al. Report of AAPM TG 135: quality assurance for robotic radiosurgery. Med Phys. 2011;38(6):2914–36.

[61] Gao J, Liu X. Off-Isocenter Winston-Lutz tEST for stereotactic radiosurgery/stereotactic body radiotherapy. Int J Med Phys. 2016;5:154–61.

[62] Du W, Gao S, Wang X, Kudchadker RJ. Quantifying the gantry sag on linear accelerators and introducing an MLC-based compensation strategy. Med Phys. 2012;39(4):2156–62.

第 17 章 多发性脑转移瘤的单中心治疗计划
Single-Isocenter, Multiple Metastasis Treatment Planning

Evan M.Thomas　Richard A. Popple　Elizabeth Covington　John B. Fiveash　**著**
刘渊渊　张子健　**译**
曹　瑛　**校**

一、多发性脑转移瘤治疗的研究背景及历史

在过去，出现肿瘤转移的患者预后非常差，尤其是当肿瘤转移到大脑时，一个非常小的转移灶也可能使患者致残。然而，近年来，随着系统治疗的进展，特别是免疫治疗和分子靶向治疗，显著改善了晚期恶性肿瘤患者的预后，并提高了生存期。事实上，导致大多数脑转移的三种原发性恶性肿瘤（肺癌、乳腺癌和黑色素瘤）的系统治疗方面取得了较大的进展。相比于颅内病灶，新一代的药物对颅外病灶效果更明显，使用这些药物治疗的患者生存期更长，故发生脑转移的可能性更大。

在多发性脑转移瘤的患者中，立体定向放射外科已经逐渐成为可靠的主流放疗技术，多个随机试验表明 SRS 在保护认知方面优于 WBRT，而且能够实施 SRS 技术的机构也在逐步增加。Modh 等[1]回顾了 2004—2014 年脑转移瘤患者的 SRS 与 WBRT 的利用率对比，接受 SRS 的患者比例从 2004 年的 7% 增长到 2014 年的 37%。2017 年，NCCN 脑转移瘤指南只推荐对有 1~3 个转移瘤的患者使用 SRS。截至 2019 年版[2]，该指南仍将患者归类为有限脑转移和广泛脑转移患者，但将 SRS 作为两组患者的治疗选择之一，以及作为有限脑转移患者的首要治疗选择。

这些因素让神经肿瘤学家、神经外科医生和放射肿瘤学家更加确信 SRS 能够在一个疗程内治疗更多脑转移病灶。在本章中，我们将回顾多发脑转移瘤治疗历史和发展，然后讨论和展示最先进的单中心放疗技术。

二、多发性脑转移瘤的单中心治疗技术

（一）起源

随着多叶准直器（multi-leaf collimator, MLC）和调强放射治疗（intensity modulated radiation therapy, IMRT）的出现，放射肿瘤学家逐步意识到用一个等中心同时治疗多个靶点的潜力，不需要为每个靶区都使用单独的等中心和射野。关于治疗大脑中多个靶区的单一等中心的计划设计工作最早发表于 1996 年，由 Peacock 计划系统完成的[3]，但该技术在一段时间内并没有被广泛使用。虽然马里兰大学的 Cedric Yu[4] 同时开发了一种 IMRT 旋转算法，但其计算能力和软件平台都不够先进，无法广泛集成该技术。在 2008 年，Karl Otto 提出了一种改进算法，能够优化最佳通量图，匹配机架旋转和多叶准直器运动，即容积旋转调强放射治疗（volumetric modulated arc therapy, VMAT）[5]。与此同时，摩尔定律预测的 CPU 可用速度呈指数级增长，使得 VMAT 优化和剂量计算所需的时间能够充分满足临床需求，

VMAT 很快被用于单靶区放射治疗计划。因为利用单一等中心治疗多个病灶的潜在效率提高，所以迅速吸引了大批研究者将 VMAT 技术应用在多个病灶上[6, 7]。2009 年，Mayo 等描述了他们最初使用 RapidArc™ VMAT 进行颅内放射外科的经验，包括治疗一名有两个转移灶的患者，以及关于"同时治疗多个病灶的能力将对多发性转移患者的治疗模式产生重大影响"的预测。

2010 年，阿拉巴马大学伯明翰分校（UAB）的 Clark 等[8] 发表了第一篇完整的论文，论证了 VMAT 技术在单中心多发性脑转移放射外科中的剂量学和执行的可行性。2012 年，Clark 等出版了一类关于该技术的解决方案，并以其原始和更新的形式分发给世界各地的数百个机构，其中许多机构目前仍在使用该方法。该技术最初是在 Eclipse™（Varian Medical Systems，Palo Alto，CA）治疗计划系统上开发的，并在其他平台上进行了不同程度的改造，包括 Pinnacle™（Phillips，Amsterdam，荷兰）[9] 和 Raystation（Ray Search Laboratories，Stockholm，瑞典）[10]，取得了不同程度的成功。

此后，利用单中心的 VMAT 技术治疗多发性转移瘤得到迅速发展，特别是在没有专用放射外科平台的中心。然而，直到 2014 年，对于多发性脑转移瘤患者，大多数神经外科医生和放射肿瘤学家仍然认为，基于伽马刀的多中心计划优于基于直线加速器的 SRS 技术（包括单中心 VMAT 技术）。由 Ma 等[11, 12] 在 Novalis Tx™（Varian Medical Systems，Palo Alto，USA）平台上发表的基于少病例的剂量学比较显示，伽马刀治疗在剂量梯度和低剂量体积方面明显优于单中心 VMAT 技术。然而，在 2014 年，阿拉巴马大学伯明翰分校（UAB）的 Thomas 等发表了一个病例更多、更全面的基于伽马刀和单中心 VMAT 技术的比较，这项工作表明，在 28 例多达 9 个脑转移瘤的病例中，设计良好的单中心 VMAT 计划与伽马刀计划在所有评价指标中质量相当，包括中低等剂量的溢出范围，如图 17-1 所示。这些不同的研究结果表明了在 VMAT 计划设计时技术细节处理的重要性。

（二）单中心治疗计划的优点

单中心治疗计划的主要优点是治疗效率[13]。众所周知，共面射野的设计将导致在轴向平面上的剂量溢出，即使是单个靶区也会出现这种情况。利用伽马刀治疗则不会出现这个问题，因为它能利用几乎整个 4π 空间的上半部分的射野角度。但是，每增加一个靶区，至少需要一个新的等中心和额外的射野，对于形状较大或复杂的靶区则需要几个射野，治疗几个以上的肿瘤可能需要几个小时。而对于单中心 VMAT 计划，治疗时间通常不取决于肿瘤的数量，除非添加额外的弧。

对于基于机架的直线加速器的多中心放射外科计划，无论是利用锥状准直器，还是动态适形弧治疗，想要获得一个剂量分布较优的计划，除了来自轴向平面的射野，还需要至少一个非共面角度的射野。因此，对于每个靶区，至少需要一次平移床或旋转床。

对于使用锥体的 CyberKnife™（Accuray Inc，Sunnyvale，USA）SRS 计划，剂量分布较优的计划至少需要有几个节点，每个靶区通常有更多的节点，具有 > 200 节点的多发性转移放射外科计划[14] 很常见。一些更新的 CyberKnife™ 配置了一个小型的 MLC（Incise™，Accuray Inc）（而不是锥形准直器），在理论上可以减少多发性转移放射外科计划所需的射野角度，但目前只有关于剂量学的可行性研究[15]，尚未发表临床研究。

单中心的 VMAT 计划只需要初始的移床就能精确地实现患者摆位，然后 1～3 个床旋转就能实现非轴向弧角照射，无须考虑靶区数量。当使用非均整照射模式（flattening filter-free，FFF）下高剂量率照射时，治疗效率非常高。在 Varian 直线加速器 Edge™ 和 TrueBeam STx™ 平台上可以使用自带的 FFF 治疗模式，6MV 和 10MV 光束的剂量率分别为 1400MU/min 和 2400MU/min。

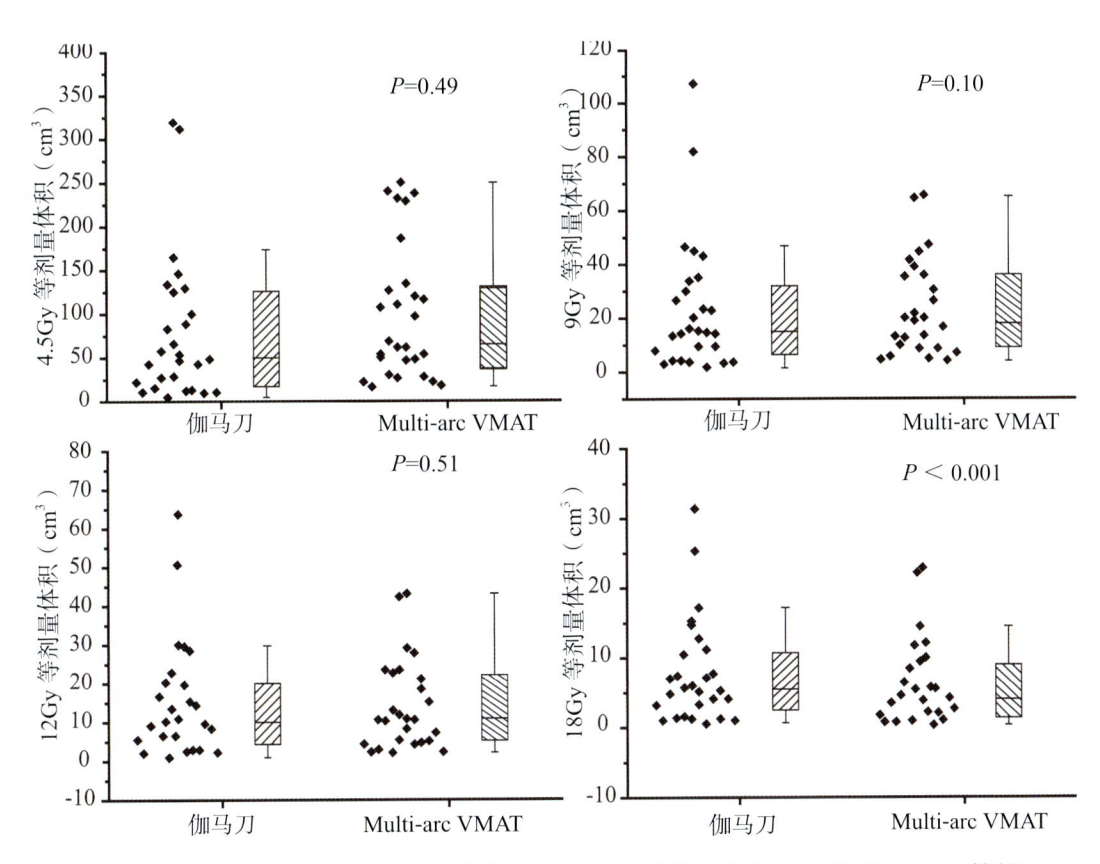

第 17 章 多发性脑转移瘤的单中心治疗计划
Single-Isocenter, Multiple Metastasis Treatment Planning

▲ 图 17-1 伽马刀和 VMAT 放射外科计划在治疗多发性脑转移瘤的病例比较：4.5Gy 等剂量体积、9Gy 等剂量体积、12Gy 等剂量体积和 18Gy 等剂量体积

经 Oxford University Press 许可转载，引自 Thomas 等[13]

Elekta 直线加速器中，Versa HD™ 是目前唯一配有 FFF 照射模式的机型，具有同样的高剂量率照射能力。

射野调制程度（给定射野的 MLC 模式和 MU 计数）决定了每个射野的最终 MU 计数和计划 MU 总计数。但一般来说，大多数 360°的射野在 FFF 模式下的照射时间为 1~2min，大多数 180°的射野只需要 30~60s。每个射野所需的时间取决于给定计划中所需的射野数量，以及每次治疗是否需要进入治疗室调整床。

在我们的机构（UAB），所有颅内 SRS 计划都是在 FFF 模式下、能量为 10 MV、剂量率为 2400MU/min 的条件下进行单中心照射。总照射时间为 1~4min，大多数计划的总治疗时间为 10~20min，主要取决于所使用的射野数（2~4），同时也与患者摆位的重合度、光学体表监测系统检测到的运动情况有关。一旦检测到患者运动都会提示治疗师停止治疗，将床恢复到 0°，并重复锥形束 CT（CBCT）进行位置校准。图 17-2 显示了一例 8 个转移瘤患者的治疗过程。从第一个 kV 图像开始的总治疗时间约为 13min。

最小化照射时间可以减少患者的焦虑，增加患者治疗的舒适度和满意度，最大限度地减少由于患者运动而导致治疗中断的可能性[16, 17]，并减少患者在多分次 SRS 计划中不遵守顺序治疗的可能性。

（三）单中心计划的潜在隐患

对于任何提供颅内放射外科的中心来说，单中心相对于多中心计划的治疗效率是显而易见的。然而，放射外科团队需要了解其中的缺陷，并制定预防措施和工作流程，以减小风险。

首先，因为患者摆位没对准射野中心，无论是平移还是旋转引起的几何误差，这将导致一个

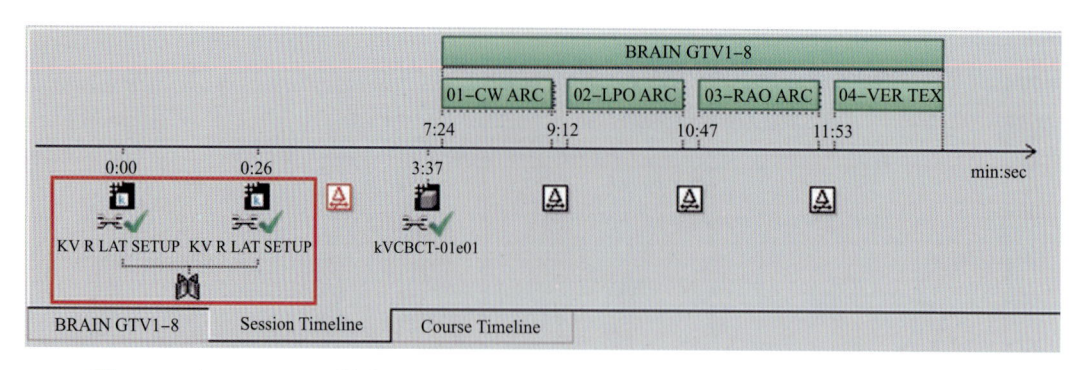

▲ 图 17-2 在 10MV FFF 模式下，采用 Varian Edge 单中心 SRS 技术治疗 8 个转移瘤的患者计划投照流程

或多个靶区的剂量不足，以及正常组织的过量照射。对于邻近靶区的危及器官，轻微的位置误差也可能导致该器官意外地暴露在高剂量区域，导致严重的并发症。多项工作特别研究了单中心多靶区放射外科计划中旋转误差的风险、发生频率和剂量学后果，Roper 等[18]进行了彻底的剂量学分析，对包含 2 个靶区的 50 个 SRS 计划模拟沿所有轴旋转误差为 0.5°、1.0° 和 2.0° 时，对靶区的 D95%（95% 的 PTV 所受剂量）的影响。研究发现，靶区 D95% 随着旋转程度增大和靶区到等中心的距离增加而成比例地下降。如图 17-3A 所示散点图，显示了 D95% 与旋转误差及靶区中心到等中心距离的关系。图 17-3B 所示，当旋转误差为 2.0° 时，剂量云图和 DVH 图。

管理和预防位置错误和（或）不确定性的技术有多种，可以粗略地分为精确的位置摆位、运动预防、运动监测和运动缓解措施。虽然本文在其他地方进行了详细讨论，但由于不确定性对单中心治疗的影响较大，这里进行了概述。当然，最重要和强制性的步骤是通过在初始摆位期间进行适当的成像和治疗床位置调整，最大限度地消除所有的位置误差（平移和旋转）。幸运的是，从定位 CT 扫描到治疗时，颅内放射外科的靶区很少发生变化。此外，现代放射外科平台上的 CBCT 可提供骨性解剖标志，用于 CBCT 和定位 CT 之间的自动和手动配准。计划设计者和治疗师应该注意可能出现的解剖变化，比如囊腔、快速增长的肿瘤（如来自侵袭性肺鳞状细胞癌的转移）和不断变化的水肿（恶化或改善），对于这些情况，可以给 CTV 添加一个外扩值。

一旦在初始摆位中消除了位置不确定性，下一步则是固定患者，以防止治疗过程中的运动。多年来的黄金标准一直是将立体框架用大头钉固定在头骨上，但随着聚合物的持续改进促进了更多可塑、无侵入性固定装置的研发。Babic[19]等对基于框架或无框架的固定方法的 SRS 和 FSRT 患者进行 CBCT 扫描，分析运动情况，SRS 患者固定使用了 Cosman-Roberts-Wells（CRW）框架（IntegraRadionics, Burlington, MA, USA）或非侵入性 PinPoint 系统（AktinaMedical, Congers, NY, USA）；而 FSRT 患者固定使用了非侵入性 Gill-ThomasCosman（GTC）可再定位框架（IntegraRadionics, Burlington, MA, USA）或非侵入性 PinPoint 系统、Uniframe 面膜（WFR/AquaplastCorp, Avondale, PA, USA）或 Orfit 面罩（OrfitIndustries, Wijnegem, Belgium）。对于 SRS 患者，PinPoint 系统的平均三维运动（定义为治疗前后 CBCT 的差值）为 0.45 ± 0.33mm，CRW 侵袭性框架为 0.30 ± 0.21mm。所有固定方法的治疗中运动情况如图 17-4 所示。

管理位置误差影响的近一步措施是对治疗分次间的运动进行监测，目前已有多种分次间运动监测方法成功应用在单中心 SRS 平台上。最简单的方法是由治疗师和医师通过视频监视器对患者进行连续的视觉检查。虽然可以看到大幅度的运动，但通过视频监视器的视觉检查不太可能精准地识别出有临床意义的运动。如果没有达到亚毫

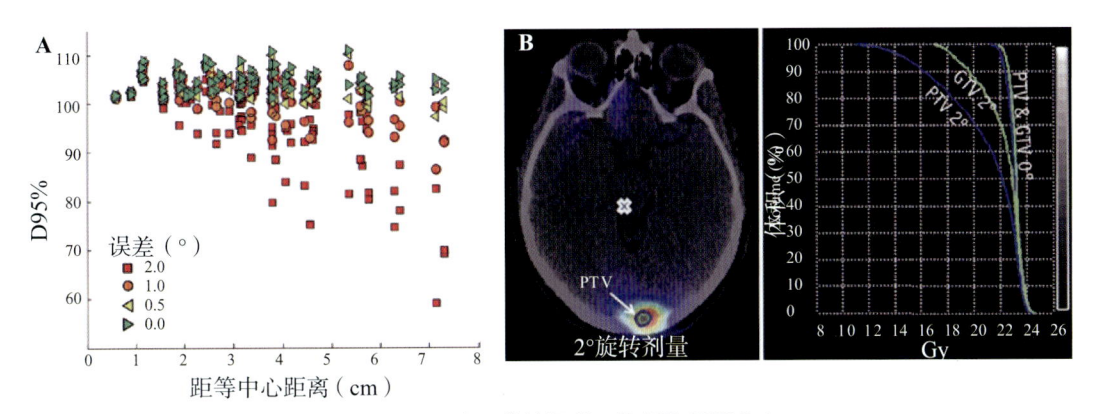

第 17 章　多发性脑转移瘤的单中心治疗计划
Single-Isocenter, Multiple Metastasis Treatment Planning

▲ 图 17-3　由于旋转误差而降低靶区覆盖率

A. 以 PTV 到等中心的距离为横坐标、以 D95% 为纵坐标绘图，不同旋转误差的 D95% 分布如图所示，D95% 和 V95 理想值均是 100%；B. 在距等中心 7.3cm 处、旋转误差为 2.0° 时，0.78cm³ 的 PTV 的靶区覆盖率大幅下降，未显示位于不同平面上的其他 PTV。图中十字叉为该横断面的等中心位置，剂量体积直方图显示了旋转误差为 0.0° 和 2.0° 时 GTV 和 PTV 剂量覆盖情况。经 Elserevier 许可转载，引自 Roper 等[18]

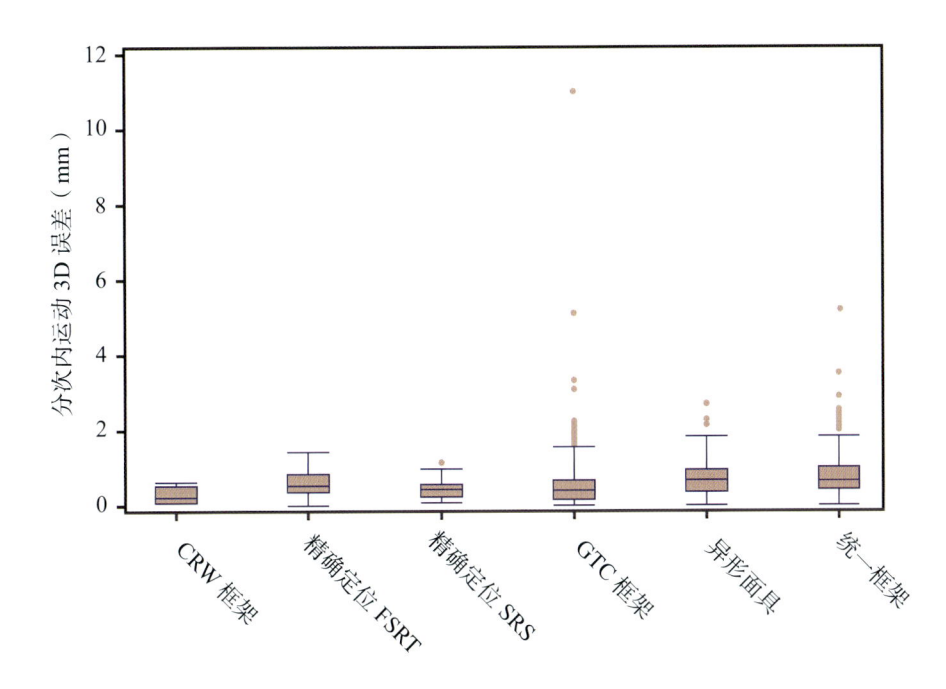

◀ 图 17-4　几种侵入式和非侵入式固定装置的治疗前后 CBCT 所计算的三维矢量误差比较

经知识共享授权许可转载，引自 Babic S 等[19]

米精度的解决方案，著者不建议使用该方法。治疗过程中运动监测的常见技术是治疗期间进行连续的 kV 成像和体表成像。前者由 ExacTrac™（BrainLab，慕尼黑，德国）和 CyberKnife™ 系统使用，在治疗过程中使用从多个角度获得的 kV 图像与治疗计划 CT 进行配准，以检测位移。体表成像技术，如 AlignRT™（VisionRT，伦敦，英国）或 IDENTIFY（HumediQ/Varian MedialSystems，PaloAlto，CA）系统中所使用的技术，使用多个摄像头生成参考体表的实时三维网格，然后监视体表变化。另外一种如 BrainLab，使用热成像相机生成三维体表热轮廓线，并对其进行变化监测。在较短的治疗时间内，通过治疗中的运动监测，< 5% 的患者需要重新定位或再次 CBCT 扫描。在 UAB，从治疗开始到结束的中位运动范围约为 0.3mm（体表成像测量的实时增量）[20]。

位置不确定性的最终解决方法是靶区外扩。当没有足够可靠的固定装置和监测方法时，可以通过增加 PTV 外扩范围来治疗。增加靶区外扩

217

范围可能会牺牲计划质量，这将在本章后面进一步讨论。

（四）岛屿封锁现象（island blocking）

在大多数 VMAT 优化算法中，每个准直器叶片对的内侧方向与靶区的侧边对齐，很容易获得沿整个弧段每个叶片的位置。当一对靶区与准直器叶片的方向共线对齐，且给定的叶片对两个靶区（而不是只有一个靶区）同时打开时，就会出现"island blocking"现象，这导致了两个靶区之间的正常组织接受了非必要照射。图 17-5 所示例子就是在一个有 8 个转移瘤的患者中发生的上述情况。

计划设计者们逐渐意识到这一现象，更新的优化算法在很大程度上缓解了该现象。当遇到这种情况时，无法使用最新软件的计划者可能需要采用其他技术。Yuan 等[21] 对这一现象和解决方法进行了详细的讨论。

下文列出了可采用的方法，稍后将详细讨论。

- 额外的非共面弧。
- 准直器角度调整 / 优化。
- 增加成本函数中对正常脑组织的优先级（权重）。
- 增加邻近靶区之间的剂量限制结构"壁"。

（五）单中心多发性转移计划采用的技术

目前，所有的单中心多发性转移技术只能应用于配备多叶准直器的机架式直线加速器，且只能在允许执行非共面射野的平台上使用。在没有非共面治疗能力的平台上也逐步展开了单中心技术治疗脑转移的研究，如 Tomo 治疗系统和最新的 MR 直线加速器［MRIdian（Viewray Technologies，Oakwood Village，United States）和 Unity（Elekta）］，但是，如图 17-6 所示（来自 Clark 等的单中心可行性论文），局限于轴向平面的共面计划（VMAT 或 IMRT）质量明显低于非共面计划[22]。

我们认为，设计高质量的单中心多发性转移放射外科计划，必须具备以下先决条件。

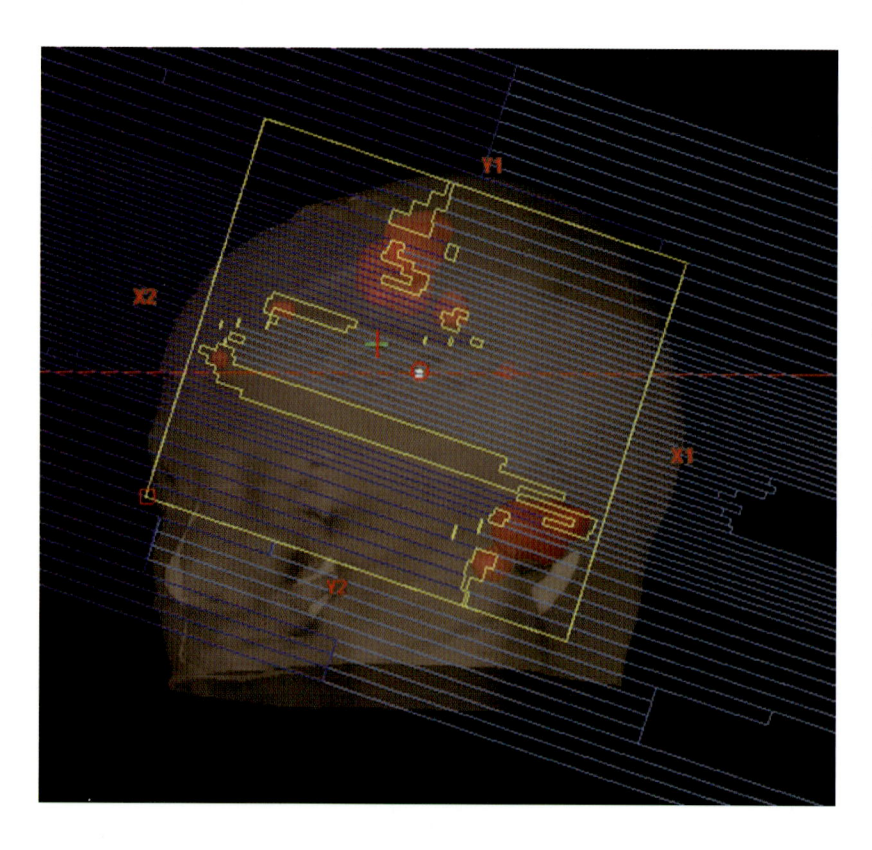

◀ 图 17-5 在两个靶区之间打开的一对多叶准直器叶片所形成的"岛屿封锁"现象，位于两个靶区之间的正常组织获得不必要的照射

本例所示是一例有 8 个转移病灶的患者，可在治疗计划中增加非共面射束，或在两个靶区之间的设置限制剂量的结构"壁"来缓解这种现象

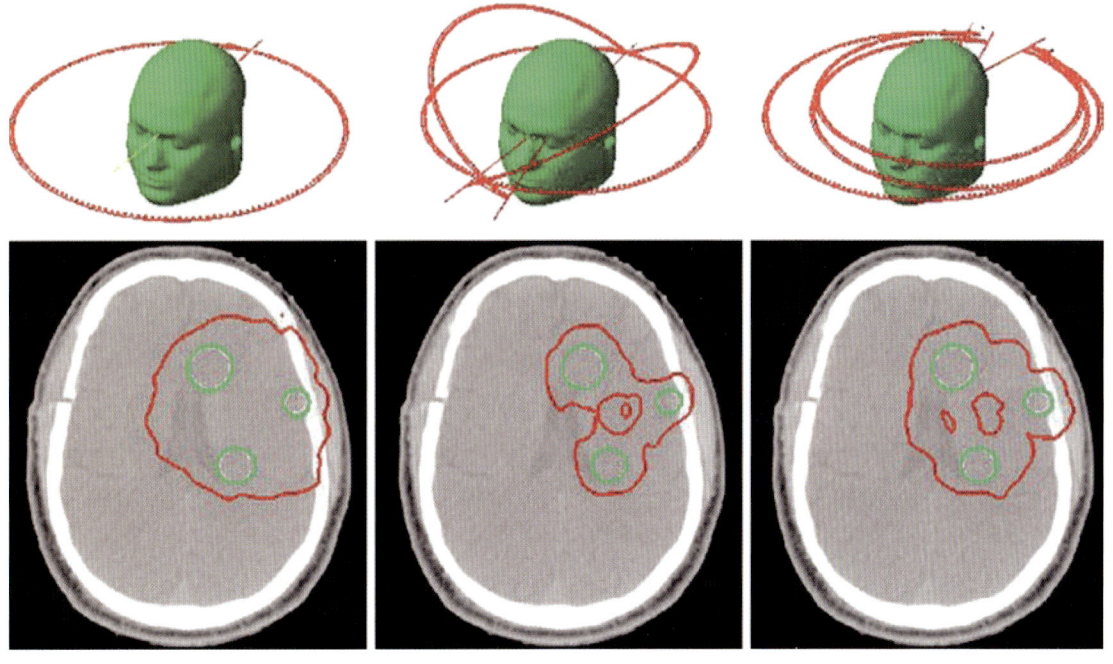

第 17 章 多发性脑转移瘤的单中心治疗计划
Single-Isocenter, Multiple Metastasis Treatment Planning

▲ 图 17-6 共面与非共面计划的质量对比

三种计划的弧形射野形状和同一平面的等剂量线分布如图所示（3 个病灶相隔 3cm），（左）单弧 / 单中心，（中）三弧 / 单中心，及（右）三弧 / 三中心。白色为靶区体积；绿色为 100% 等剂量线；红色为 50% 等剂量线。经 Elsevier 许可转载，引自 Clark 等[8]

- 现代基于机架的直线加速器，必须具备 6MV 以上能量的光子束，以及精确的输出因子。
- 多叶准直器中心投影宽度＜ 5mm。
- 治疗床能够旋转 90°实现非共面照射。

三、IMRS

调强放射外科（intensity-modulated radiosurgery，IMRS）是指在颅内放射外科中使用一组静态的调强射野。90 年代，随着多叶准直器的发展和应用，使其能够产生更适形的治疗计划，人们对其在颅内靶区的应用产生了浓厚的兴趣，该技术被广泛用于分次治疗较大的、孤立的颅内靶区，但早期 MLC 的中心叶片较宽，限制了该技术在靶区＜ 1cm 的多发性脑转移计划中的广泛应用。尽管如此，一些中心确实使用单中心技术来治疗多发性脑转移，但这种方法很快就被放弃，而倾向于采用非共面的 VMAT 技术，因为其良好的剂量分布和高效性。

四、VMAT

如前所述，Clark 等[22] 阐明了一种治疗多个颅内靶区的 VMAT 技术，著者机构用其单次治疗多达 27 个转移瘤[23]。

这里概述了计划方法，附录 17-1 为读者提供了最新的计划设计流程。计划包括 2~4 个 VMAT 弧（一个 360°轴向弧，和最多 3 个 180°非共面半弧，床角分别为 45°、90°和 315°（IEC 坐标系统）。除机架进行角度旋转之外，准直器角度也可以进行旋转，进一步调整每个弧的准直器角度有利于消除或减少"岛屿封锁"现象，减少对正常组织过量照射。为实现这一目的，多个研究人员独立开发了脚本技术，以优化铅门和准直器设置。Yuan 等在 10 个靶区计划中，通过使用铅门跟随（加速器的初级和次级铅门形成的孔径与 MLC 形成边界一致）、优化准直器角度，和增加低剂量约束条件的权重来改善靶区的剂量分布，减少对正常组织的照射，如图 17-7 所示[24-26]。

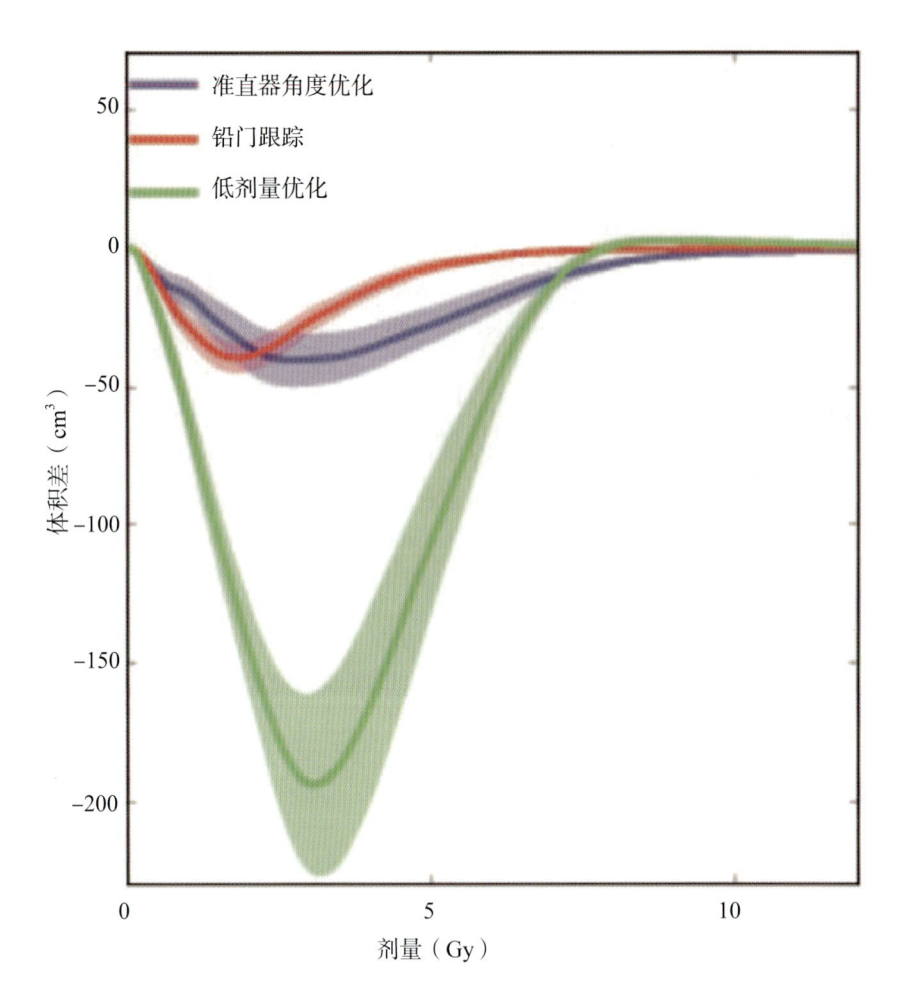

◀ 图 17-7 各参数下的正常大脑组织剂量体积直方图的平均差值

负数表示准直器角度优化、铅门跟随或者低剂量约束条件减小给定剂量下正常脑组织的体积。带宽表示 95% CI。蓝色、红色和绿色的线条分别表示准直器角度优化、铅门跟随和低剂量约束条件

大多数治疗计划软件的逆向优化设置了一个正常的组织目标条件（normal tissue objective，NTO），其目的是限制处方剂量照射到未指定为靶区的正常组织中，通常有"自动""手动"或"自定义"的 NTO，"自动" NTO 有默认的优先级（权重），非靶区组织在优化器中被罚分。在很大程度上，经典的 NTO 功能适用于被正常组织包围的靶区或相邻的靶区，但 NTO 不适用于多发转移的 SRS 计划，靶区之间需要有陡峭的剂量梯度，靶区之间的距离有时不到 1cm。有效解决方案是在优化过程使用辅助结构实现每个靶区周围剂量快速跌落。Clark 等利用治疗计划软件的布尔运算符轮廓功能，在每个靶区周围构建了嵌套同心环，靶区周围的每个连续环结构罚分的剂量水平依次降低，以实现靶区周围剂量各向同性快速降低（除非该靶区附近存在另一个靶区或危及器官），概念如图 17-8 所示。

基于约束的逆向优化计划的剂量衰减只会惩罚最大环对应的最低等剂量水平。剂量分布取决于靶区数量和大小，一些等剂量曲线将不会在靶区周围呈离散的量化状态，而是彼此毗连。如果需要考虑的溢出剂量低于环结构中的罚分剂量，计划者就必须设置额外的环或约束条件限制低剂量溢出，比如限制剂量 – 体积阈值或正常脑组织的平均剂量。剂量分布取决于具体的优化算法、靶区数、体积和分布，目前尚未发现限制低剂量溢出的最有效方法。图 17-9 显示了一例 5 个转移瘤的例子，用单中心 VMAT 治疗，并使用不同的剂量限制条件进行比较。

多发性脑转移病例的单中心治疗计划设计的最终步骤是剂量归一化。在多中心计划［Gamma 刀（GK）或 Linac］中，对于每个单独的靶区，可以对每个等中心进行单独的归一化。对于多中心计划，特别是伽马刀计划，每个靶区通常被归

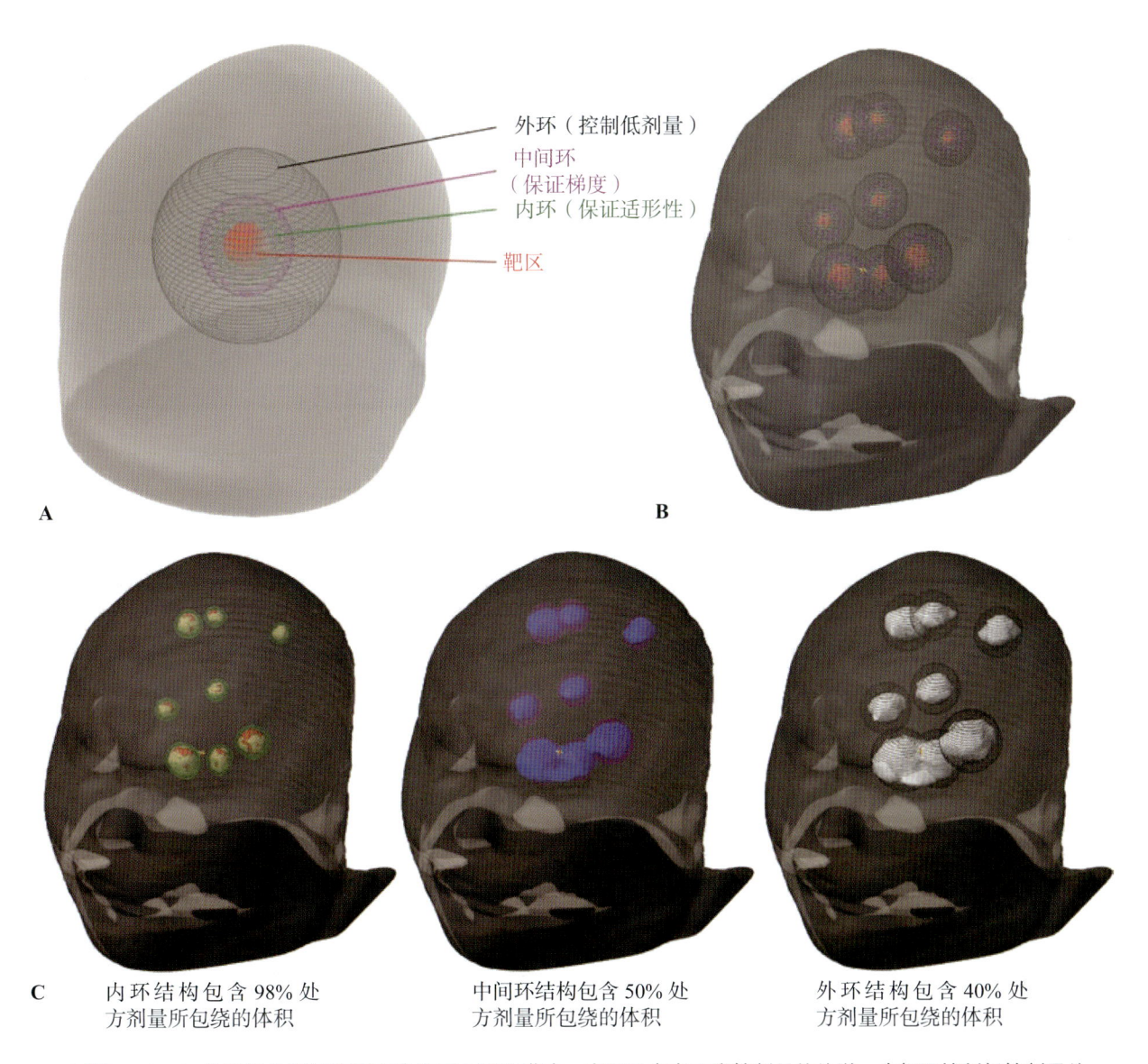

第 17 章 多发性脑转移瘤的单中心治疗计划
Single-Isocenter, Multiple Metastasis Treatment Planning

▲ 图 17-8　A. 关于罚分剂量连续下降的同心环的描述。内环重点在于高等剂量的外溢。中间环控制低等剂量外溢。可以另外加环以控制相应的剂量分布。B. 同心环应用于 8 个转移瘤患者的示例。C. 每个环及其在单中心计划中所限制的等剂量水平的说明

一化为给定的处方等剂量线。对于给定尺寸的准直器，如不堵塞准直器孔，通量差异可以忽略不计。众所周知，最佳梯度和等剂量线相关，因此命中靶区最简单的方式是做相应的剂量归一（如 4mmGK 准直器一般用 50% 等剂量线归一）。然而，在单中心 VMAT 计划中，只能在全局执行一次归一化，因此，计划设计人员必须考虑归一化通量将如何影响每个靶区的覆盖范围。在归一化之前，如果一个靶区相对于其余靶区过度覆盖，则该靶区在归一化后仍将被过度覆盖，这会加重该靶区周围的低、中度等剂量溢出，并使附近的危及器官得过高的剂量照射。图 17-10 显示了一个既平衡正常组织又保证了每个靶区整体获得处方剂量或接近处方剂量的例子。

五、VMAT 计划中其他该考虑的情况

1. 剂量桥接（bridging）

如果等剂量线存在有临床意义的"桥接"现

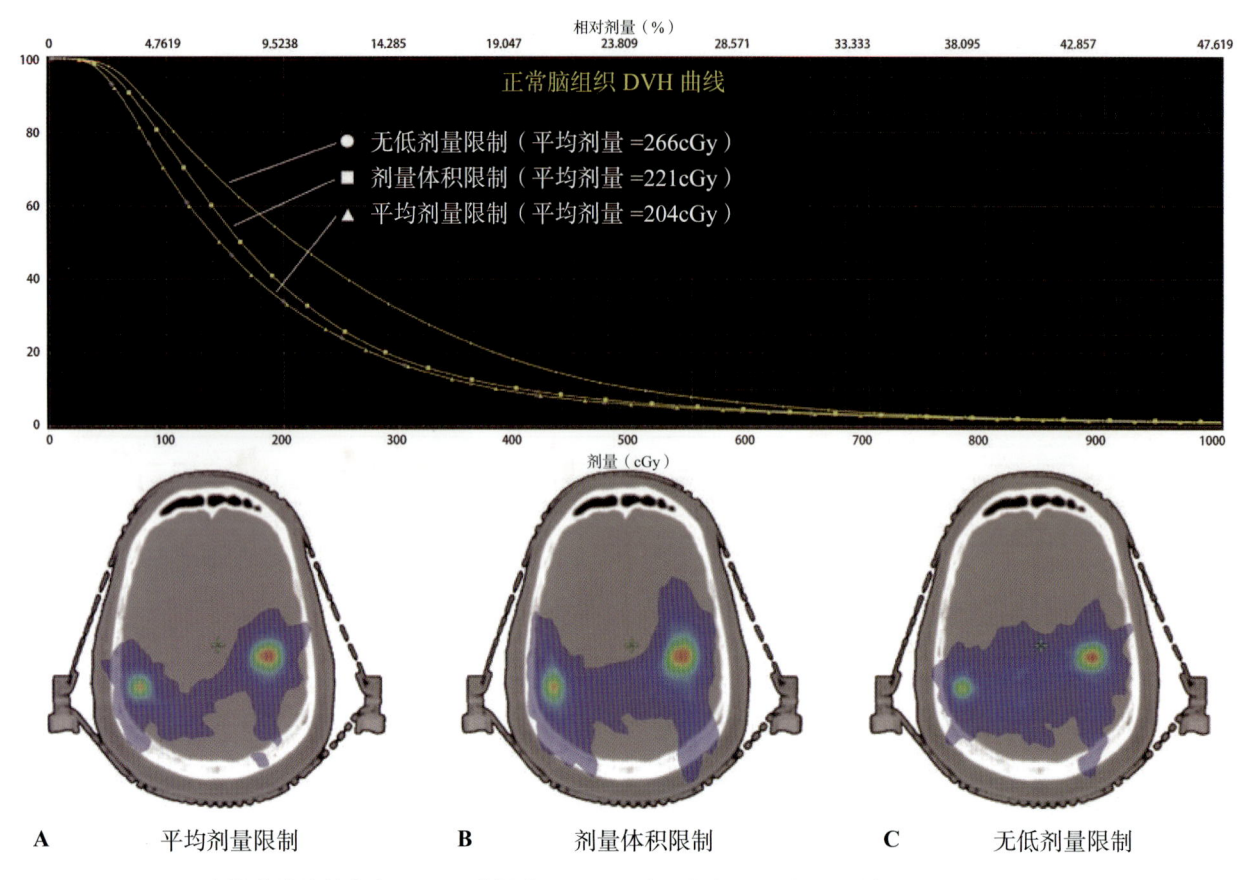

| A | 平均剂量限制 | B | 剂量体积限制 | C | 无低剂量限制 |

▲ 图 17-9 5个转移灶的单中心 VMAT 病例演示，（A）对正常脑组织采用平均剂量限制、（B）剂量 – 体积限制和（C）不采用低剂量限制的方案，3.33Gy 等剂量线溢出情况比较

象（如12Gy等剂量线相连），计划就可能需要重新优化，利用某种方法断开该衔接的等剂量线，以减少接受该剂量的正常组织体积。从射束方向观查看每个弧段可以确定两个靶区之间是否存在"岛屿封锁"现象。如果存在，可以调整准直器角度解决剂量桥接问题；如果该方法不行，可以考虑勾画"剂量断开"结构（图17-11），即当不希望剂量衔接时，在两个靶区之间绘制盘状或壁状的剂量断开结构，然后，对该结构给予更低剂量的重点罚分，强制优化器获得满足给定优化目标的通量图。

2. 限制热点/异质性

单中心 VMAT 放射外科计划中一个仍有争议的话题是是否应该限制靶区内的剂量不均匀性（热点）。从事伽马刀治疗的神经外科医生和放射肿瘤学家几乎从不限制热点，只要求产生最佳剂量跌落的处方等剂量线，这通常导致在靶区的中心有约 200% 的处方剂量的热点。相反，现代放射外科计划平台中的逆向优化计划，靶区最大剂量很少超过 170% 的处方剂量。然而，一些放射肿瘤学家认为，放射外科计划的最大剂量应该 < 110% 的处方剂量（类似于常规分割治疗的剂量限制）。我们坚决反对这种观点，因为限制靶区内的热点将把剂量推到靶区之外，导致中、低等剂量线溢出，该现象如图 17-12 所示。

如果 PTV 遍布大量正常组织中时，才应该限制剂量热点，但是在脑转移的放射外科计划中，尤其是热点位于恶性或缺氧的转移灶中，则不应该限制热点。

六、单中心动态适形弧计划

另一种最近开发的单个等中心治疗多发性脑转移的技术是单中心动态适形弧（single-isocenter

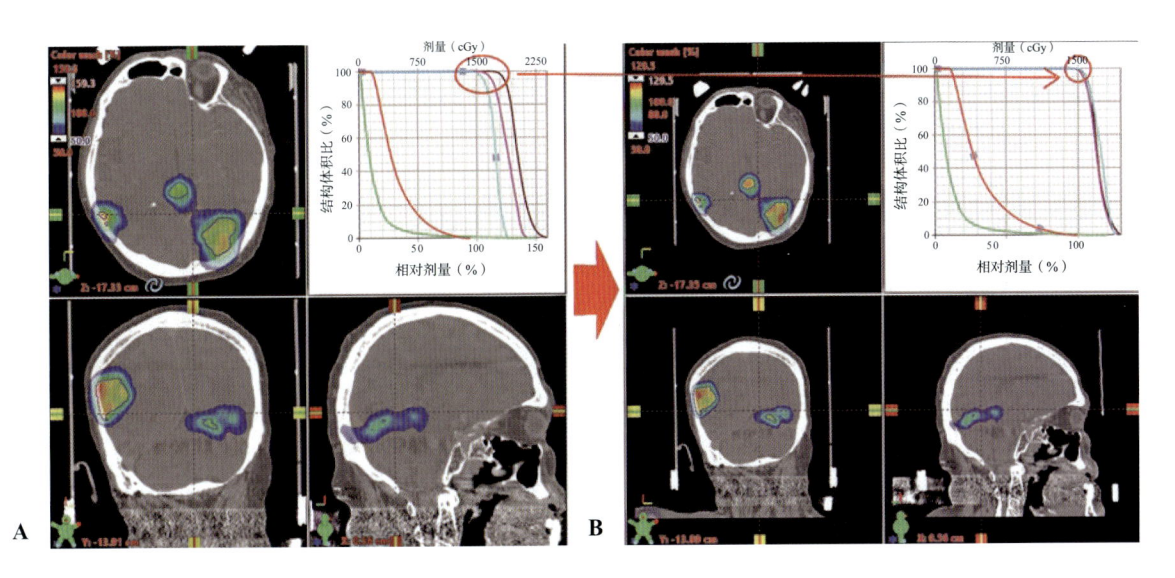

靶区 DVH 未均匀覆盖和均匀 DVH 覆盖的
3 个转移灶病例的计划质量

处方剂量 =15Gy		
	未均匀覆盖的 DVH	均匀性覆盖的 DVH
RTOG 适形指数（左枕叶）	1.37	1.04
RTOG 适形指数（中脑）	1.18	1.09
RTOG 适形指数（右枕叶）	1.64	1.10
整个计划的 RTOG 适形指数	1.43	1.06
正常脑组织被 12Gy 等剂量线所包绕的体积	36.3cm^3	22.1cm^3
正常脑组织平均剂量	188cGy	164cGy
正常脑组织接受 25% 处方剂量的体积	358cm^3	277cm^3

▲ 图 17-10　3 个转移灶病例的计划比较

A. 未均匀覆盖的 DVH；B. 均匀性覆盖的 DVH；C. 该表显示了靶区剂量均匀覆盖后，计划质量的显著改善

dynamic conformal arc，SIDCA）技术。亨利·福特医院的 Huang 等 [27] 于 2014 年描述了 SIDCA 技术。在单中心 DCA 计划中，每个单独的靶区由一组适形弧照射，MLC 的形状适形靶区结构，每次只允许一组 MLC 叶片对治疗一个给定的病灶。当给定的治疗床和准直角导致两个靶区共享一个叶片对时，则叶片对将只适形一个靶区，并用额外的弧来治疗另一个转移灶。在这种情况下，SIDCA 很好地避免了"岛屿封锁"现象。虽然使用单个等中心，但射野与其他靶区、

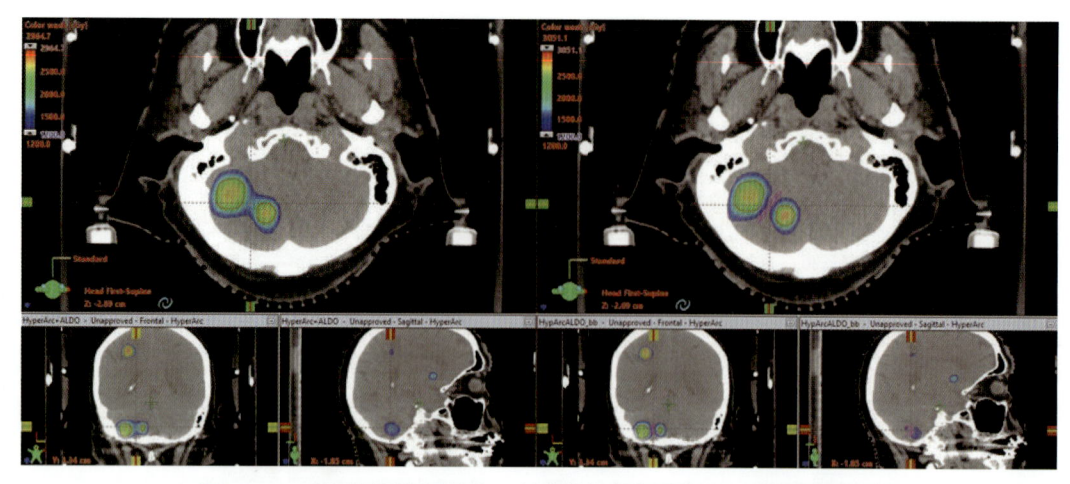

▲ 图 17-11 利用剂量断开结构，以降低相邻靶区间 12Gy 剂量线的桥接

无均匀性限制　　　　　　　　　　均匀性限制（最大剂量＜处方剂量的 120%）

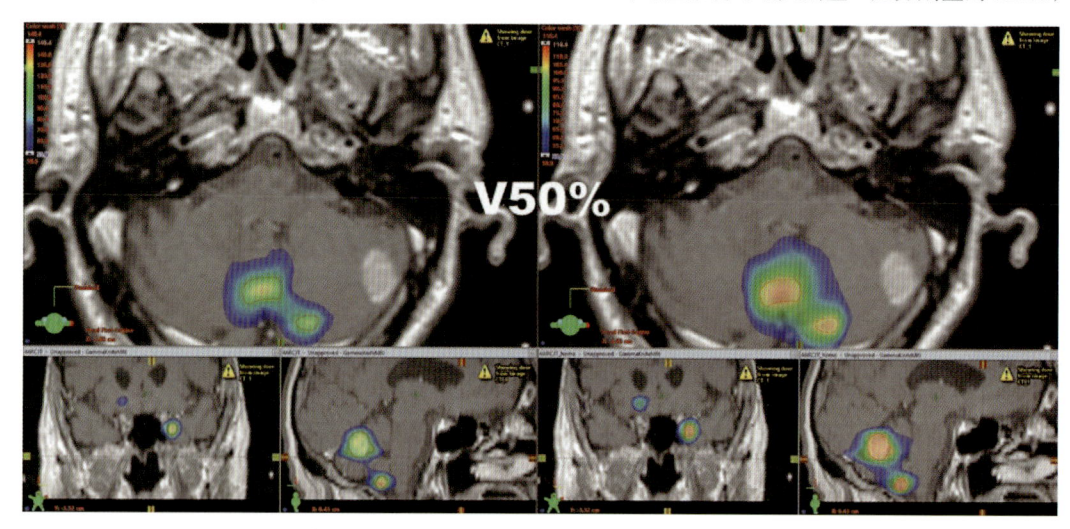

▲ 图 17-12 限制热点会降低计划质量

图中所示为 8 个脑肿瘤病例的 SRS 计划，显示的是 50% 等剂量线的剂量云图，未对热点进行限制如左图所示，对热点进行了限制如右图所示。对于这个例子，控制热点使得 50% 等剂量线包绕的体积增加了 87%，同时正常脑组织的平均剂量增加了 27%

其他射野相互独立，所以仍可以对每个病灶进行单独归一。图 17-13 展示了一例有 8 个转移瘤病例的 SIDCA 计划的弧形几何形状和准直器设置。

动态适形弧计划大部分是进行正向优化的，因此与 VMAT 计划相比，其计算强度小，计算速度更快；同时，因为计划设计中，可调整的关键变量是每个靶区的准直器角、出束弧的角度和处方归一化值（很容易找到这些值的最优解），所以不同计划者设计的计划差异性较小。

七、多发性转移瘤自动治疗计划方案

（一）Multiple Metastasis Elements（MME）™

（MME）™ 是 BrainLab 在 iPlan™ 平台专门为单中心适形弧治疗设计的一个治疗计划软件模块。图 17-13 展示了 MME 计划的典型模式。该软件旨在评估一组勾画好的肿瘤结构，并自动产生一个正向优化的非共面弧及准直器角度，该准直器角度适用于单中心动态适形弧计划。如图所示，在扫弧过程中，所有肿瘤都被照射，除非一个或多个肿瘤与准直器角共线对齐，在这种情况下，只有一个靶区由该叶片对治疗，该弧逆向旋转以治疗另外的共线靶区，解决"岛屿封锁"问题，但降低了效率。

（二）HyperArc

HyperArc™（瓦里安）是 Eclipse 平台内的一个治疗计划软件模块，旨在简化和自动化设计单中心 VMAT 计划治疗多发性脑转移瘤。类似于 MME，一旦指定靶区，HyperArc 模块将在靶区几何中心设置一个等中心，并向计划者提供 2～5 个非共面部分弧（图 17-14），以提高计划质量，同时也允许扫弧时自动移动床。为了确保无碰撞治疗，HyperArc 需要使用 Encompass™（Qfix，Avondale，PA）固定系统。由于 VMAT 是一种逆向的旋转调强放疗，优化后需要进行全网格剂量计算，优化和计算需要 5～30min，时间长短取决于正在进行优化的工作站所选择的计算网格的分辨率和硬件能力。后文病例章节会展示一个 HyperArc 的计划。

（三）单中心治疗计划比较

BrainLab 的 MME 模块和 Varian 的 HyperArc 软件都是自动设计单中心 VMAT 计划，并不断为多个脑转移瘤病例生成高质量的放射外科计划，这种自动化的 VMAT 技术消除了计划设计者间的差异性。两家不同单位对多发性脑转移瘤病

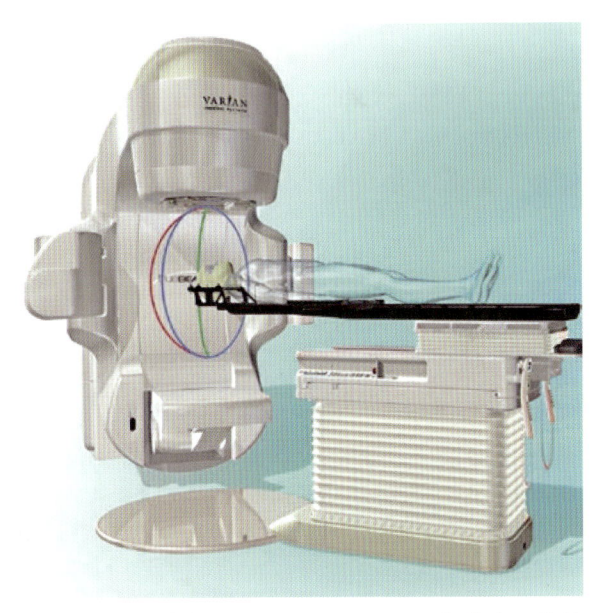

▲ 图 17-14 描述 HyperArc VMAT SRS 治疗中可能使用的弧角

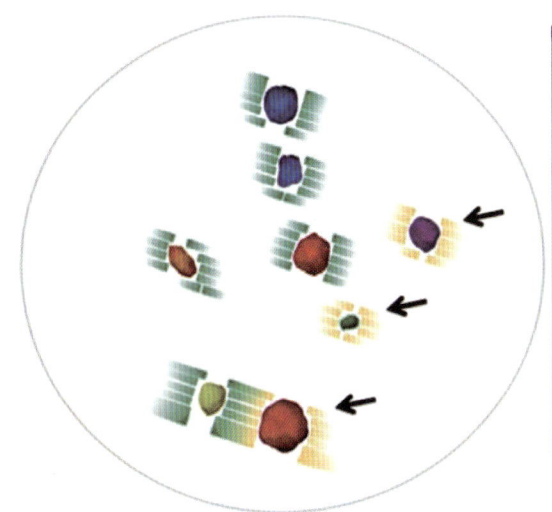

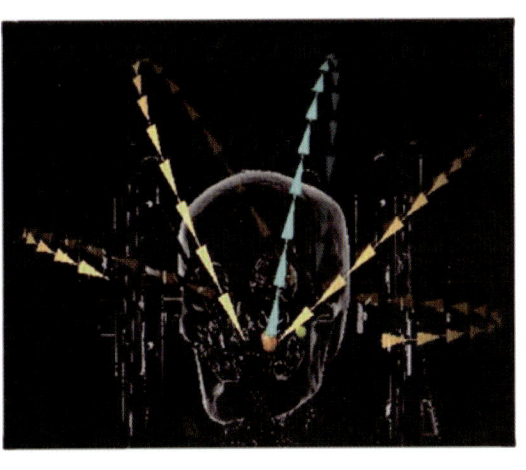

▲ 图 17-13 单中心动态适形弧计划

在这个例子中，8 个转移瘤均由多叶准直器适形照射（左）。所有转移灶由一组多弧计划照射，箭所示 3 个转移灶由本例中"逆向"弧照射，本例中共 5 个"正向"弧，5 个"逆向"弧（右）。经开源访问协议创新条款允许，在未修改前提下转载自 Mori 等 [28]

例进行了病例对比和质量评估。罗格斯大学、托马斯杰斐逊大学和宾夕法尼亚大学进行了多家单位的病例比较，包括伽马刀、手动 VMAT 计划，HyperArc 和 MME 设计的多发性转移 SRS 病例，结果表明 HyperArc 和手动 VMAT 计划的一致性优于伽马刀和 MME 计划（除了 < 1cm 的靶区，这种情况下计划质量与伽马刀相似）。较低的等效剂量溢出体积差异如图 17-15 所示。在他们的研究中，与 MME 相比，HyperArc 在脑平均剂量、V12Gy、V6Gy 和 V3Gy 表现更优。但 MME 计划仍优于手动 VMAT 计划。本研究也比较了梯度指数，但是，由于各组计划一致性较差，很难解释梯度指数的差异。

另一项在托马斯·杰斐逊大学和伯明翰的大学阿拉巴马大学之间多机构的研究，比较了由专业剂量师设计的 MME（V1.5）与 Eclipse 中手动 VMAT 计划。这项研究发现，VMAT 计划表现出优越的一致性，以及较低的中等剂量溢出（V12Gy），但 MME 计划在剂量溢出体积上表现更佳，等剂量曲线和 DVH 如图 17-16 所示。在这两项研究中，基于计算机优化的技术（手动 VMAT、HyperArc）相比三维适形弧技术产生了更好的适形计划。

> **要 点**
> - 单中心治疗计划设计和实施大大改变了多发性转移瘤放射外科的前景。
> - 以前，高质量的放射外科需要多个等中心，无论是基于伽马刀的多弧治疗，还是基于直线加速器锥型束的动态适形弧治疗。现在，与多个等中心方法相比，从业者可以使用单中心计划同时治疗尽可能多的靶区，且在保证计划质量的前提下不会增加额外的照射时间。
> - 现代 FFF 投照平台，单次放射外科可以在 10~20min 内进行，不仅提高了治疗效率、改善了患者体验，而且优化了临床放射肿

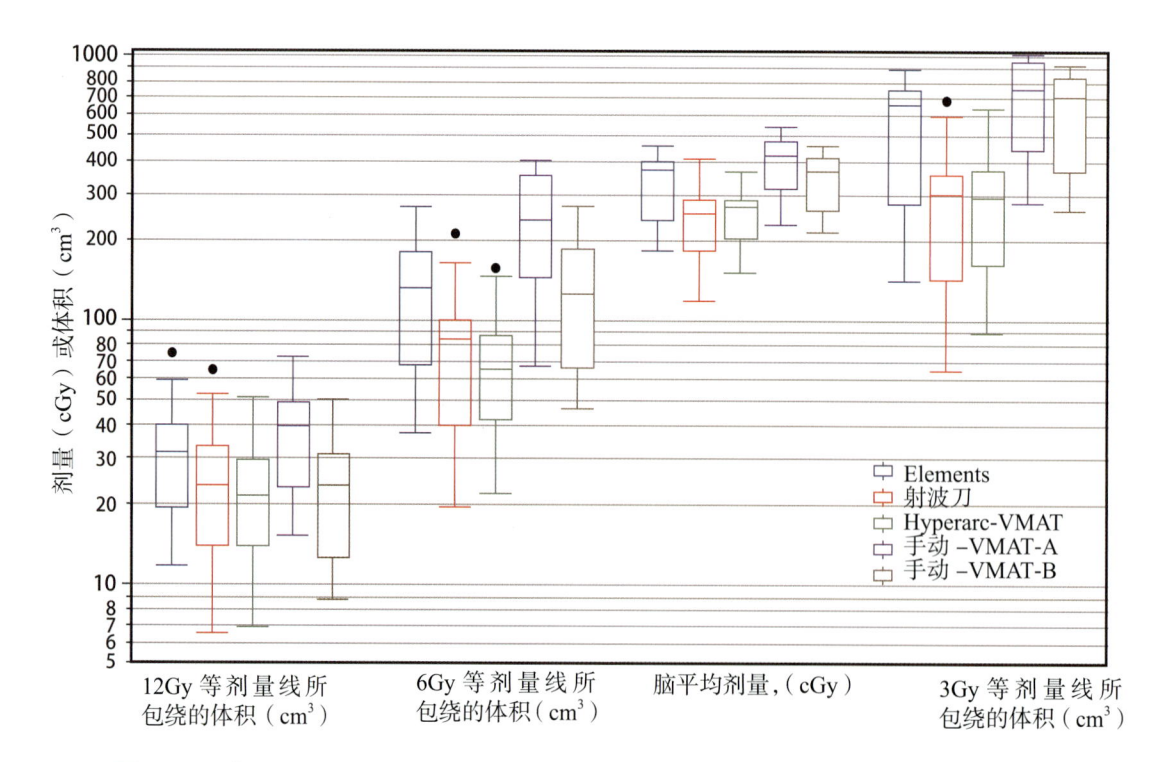

▲ 图 17-15 伽马刀，BrainLab 的 MME，Varian 的 HyperArc 和手动 VMAT 计划治疗多发性脑转移瘤的中等和低剂量溢出体积对比
经开源访问协议创新条款允许，在未修改前提下转载自 Vergalasova I 等[29]

第 17 章　多发性脑转移瘤的单中心治疗计划
Single-Isocenter, Multiple Metastasis Treatment Planning

瘤学家、神经外科医生和医学物理师的工作流程，提高了工作效率。这使得单中心治疗比其他放射外科方法更具成本效益。
- 当患者摆位不精准，增加了远离等中心的靶区剂量不足、危及器官过度照射的风险。放射外科团队在临床工作流程中，必须时刻注意患者的摆位流程和分次间运动管理过程。

八、病例介绍

某患者，颅内 8 个转移瘤，需进行单次放射外科，每个肿瘤的处方剂量是 21Gy。治疗机型为 TrueBeam STx，具有 10MV FFF 模式，同时配备了 HD-MLC，其中心叶片机械宽度 2.5mm，可以使用 VMAT 或 SIDCA 技术进行 SRS 治疗。每种计划情况怎样？计划质量如何？出束时间是多少？

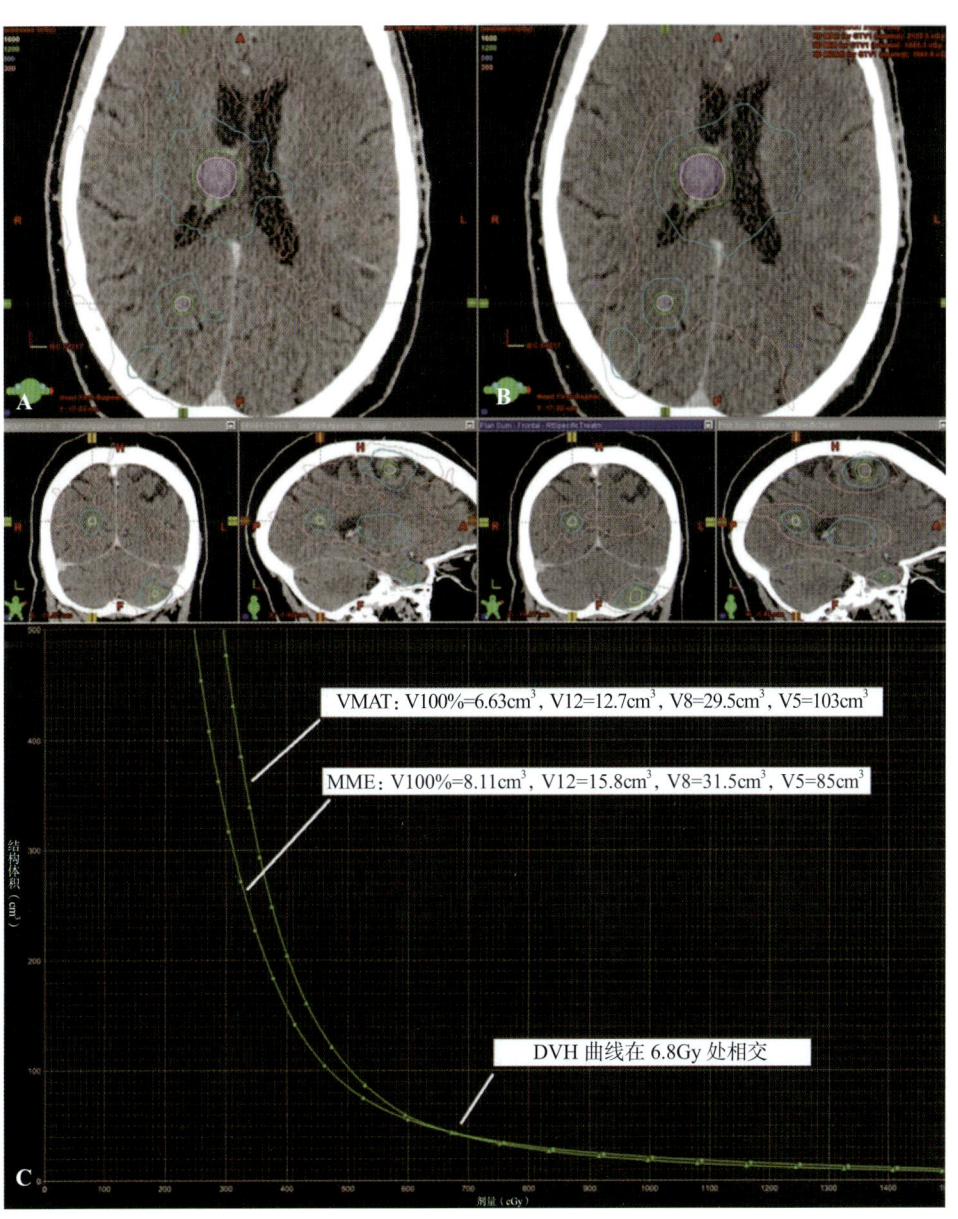

▲ 图 17-16　轴状、矢状和冠状位 CT 上的剂量分布比较

A. VMAT 计划；B. MME 计划。本例为 5 个脑转移瘤的患者，其总 PTV 体积为 6.24cm³，处方剂量为 16Gy。C. 本例中每个计划的正常脑组织的 DVH 分布，DVH 线在 6.8Gy 处相交

227

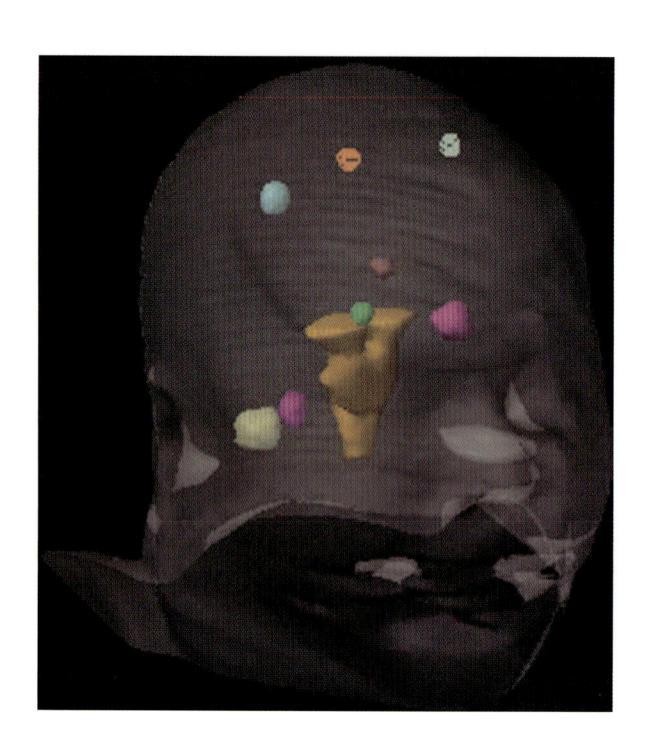

（一）VMAT（RapidArc）

1. 使用布尔函数可以创建所有靶区的复合结构（请确保所有的靶区都被指定为高分辨率的靶区）。

2. 在复合 GTV 周围创建一个外扩范围，创建至少三个复合 GTV 的调节环（shell）结构（如附录 17-1，1（5）所述）。从外环开始，使用抠除（Crop）或布尔（Boolean）函数从它周围的较大环中删除中间的体积（包括内环中的 GTV）。

3. 通过将"复合 GTV"从大脑结构中裁剪出来，创建一个正常大脑结构。

4. 根据附录 17-1，2（1），使用两个或两个以上圆弧创建射野的几何形状。对于这个有 8 个

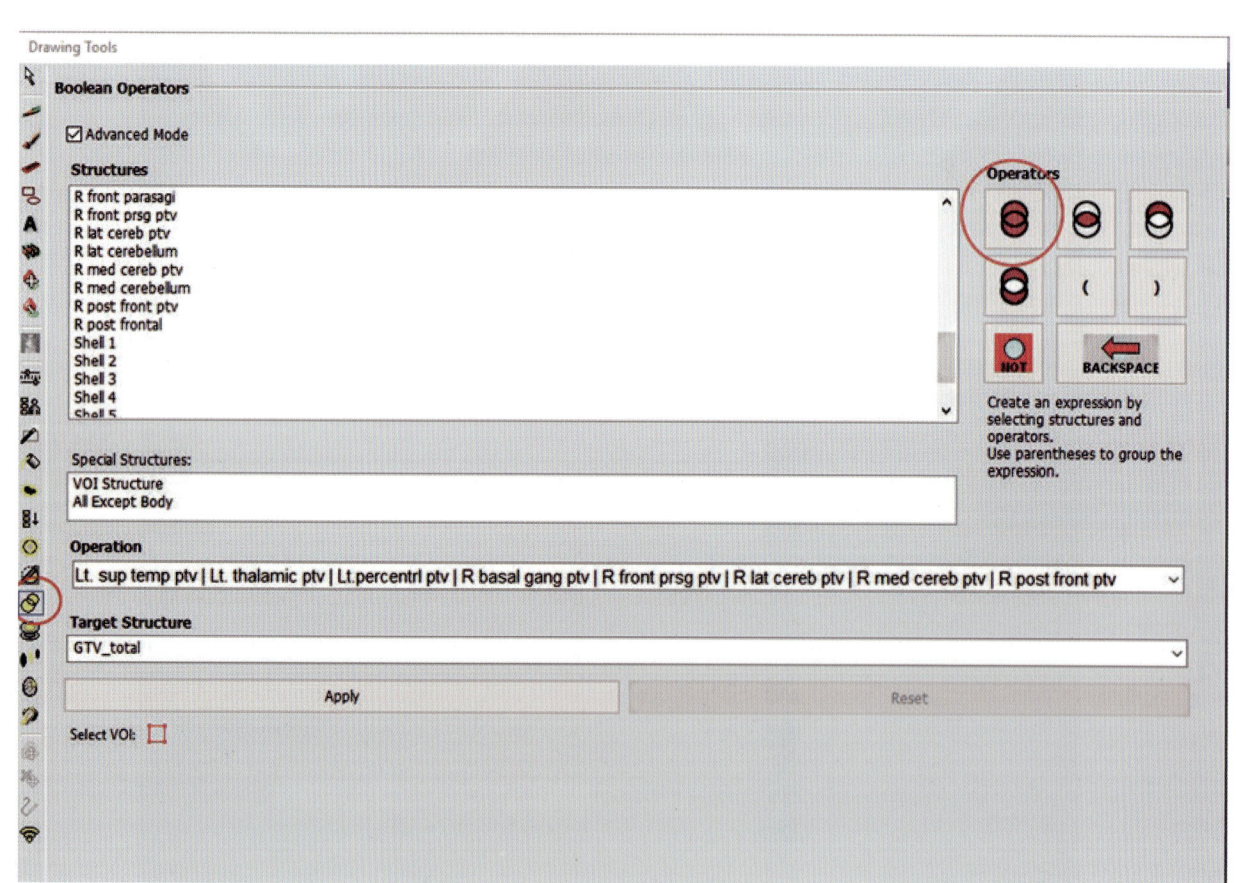

转移瘤的病例，我们选择了4个弧。（请注意，在下图中，每个控制点处的红条长度表示该点处的通量）

5. 确保将计算网格设置为高分辨率（0.1~0.125cm）。为每个靶区指定下限值，为每个环指定剂量上限值，以及对正常脑组织指定剂量上限或平均剂量限值。

6. 在优化过程中，调整靶区约束条件的优先级（权重），使靶区覆盖范围在所有靶区之间是一致的（附录17-1，3（6）②a）

7. 归一化到所需的剂量覆盖水平。我们倾向于这种归一方式：100%的处方剂量覆盖99%的靶区体积。

8. 根据所需的指标来评估计划。

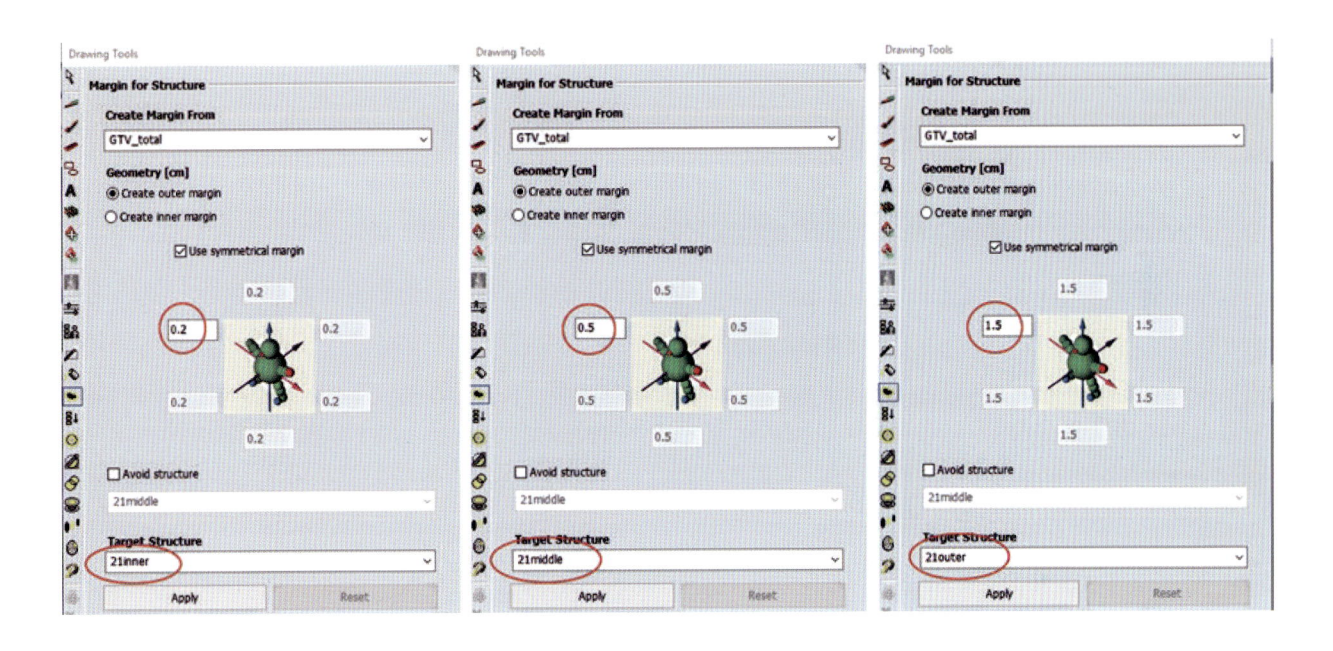

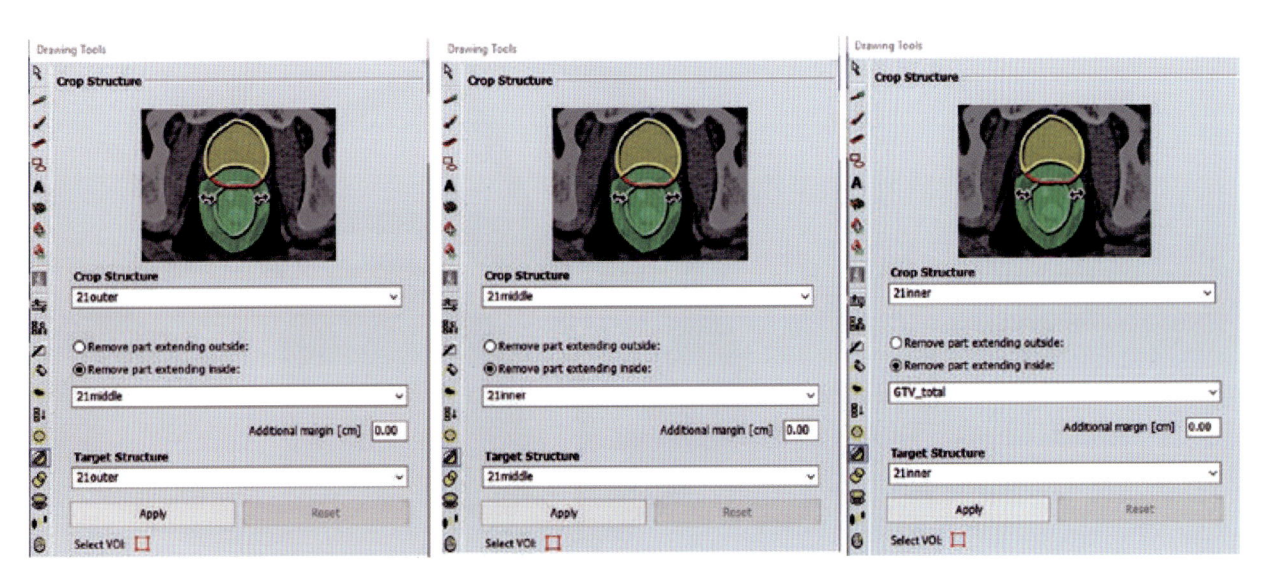

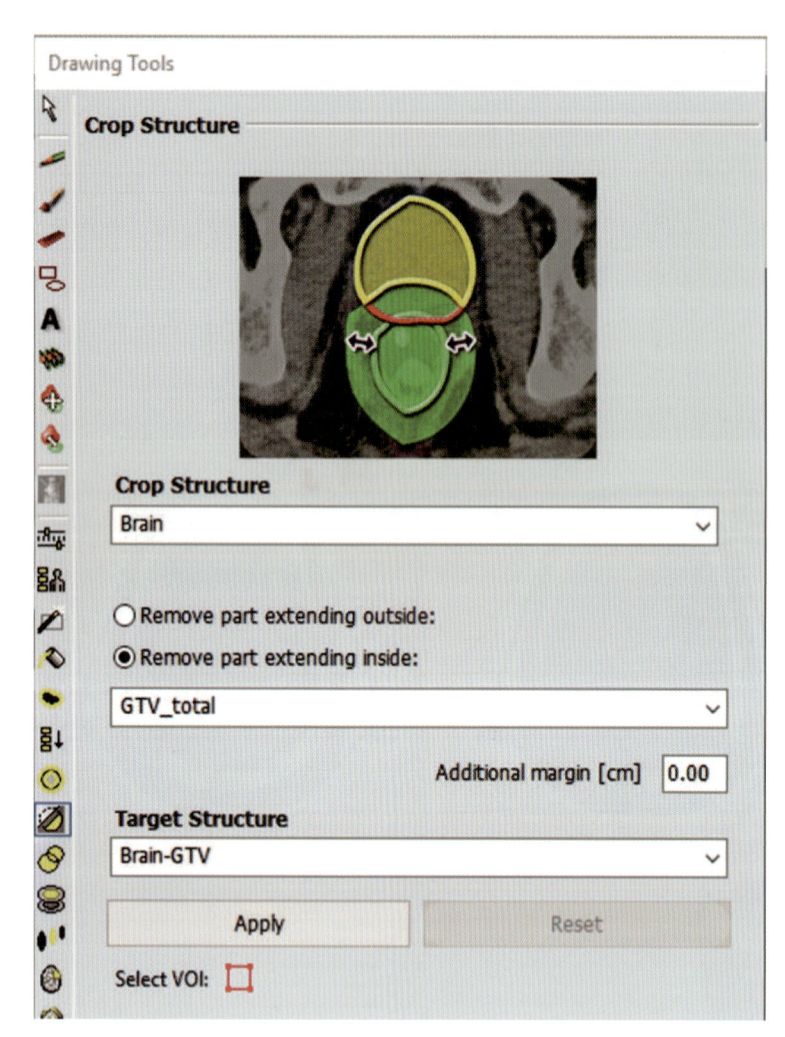

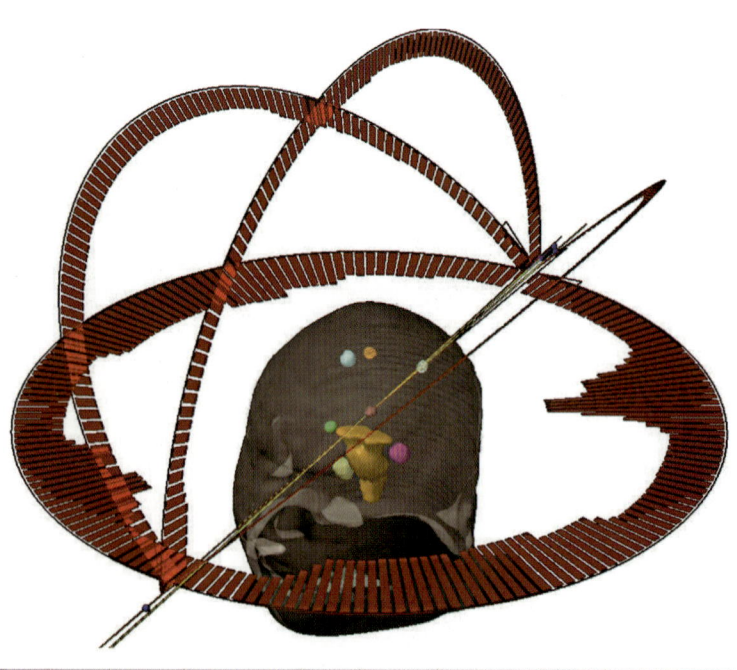

脑转移瘤放射治疗学：基于病例的研究
Radiotherapy in Managing Brain Metastases: A Case-Based Approach

230

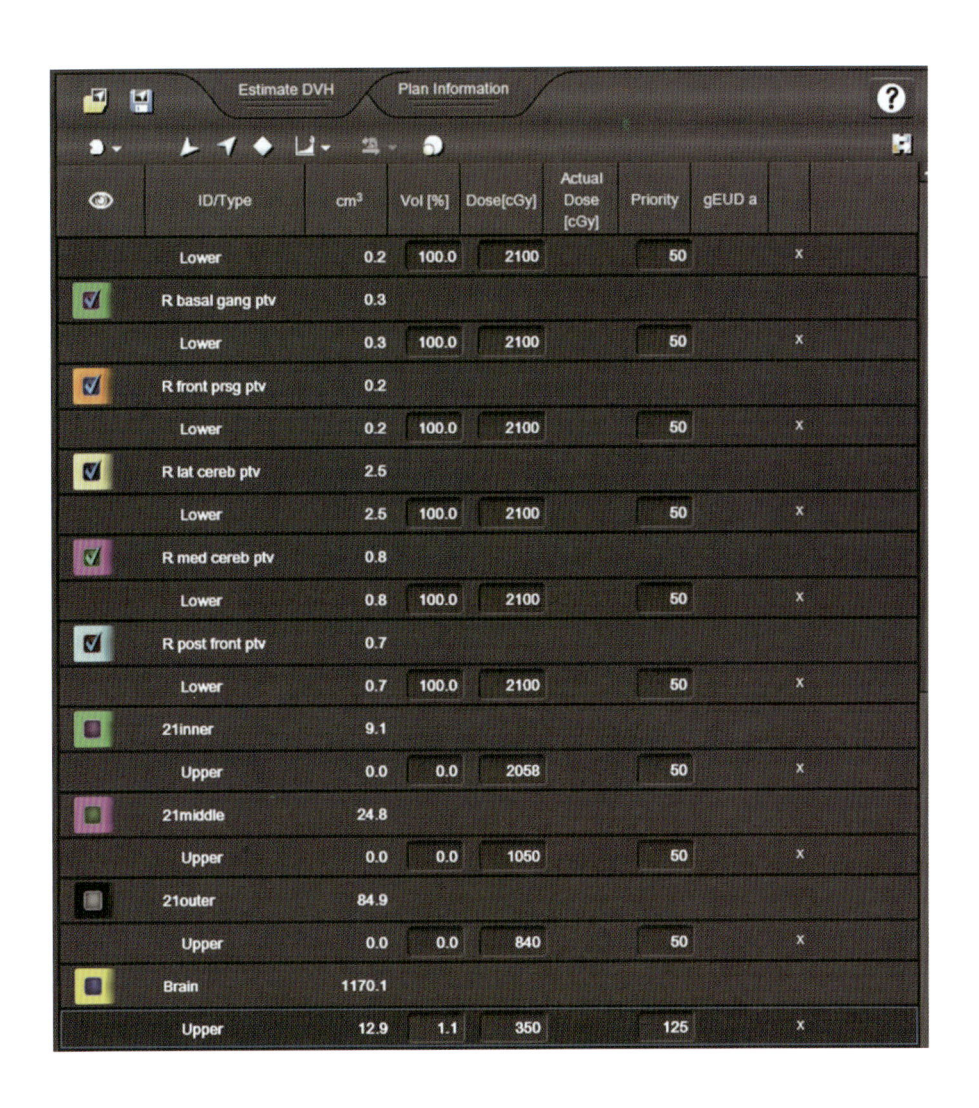

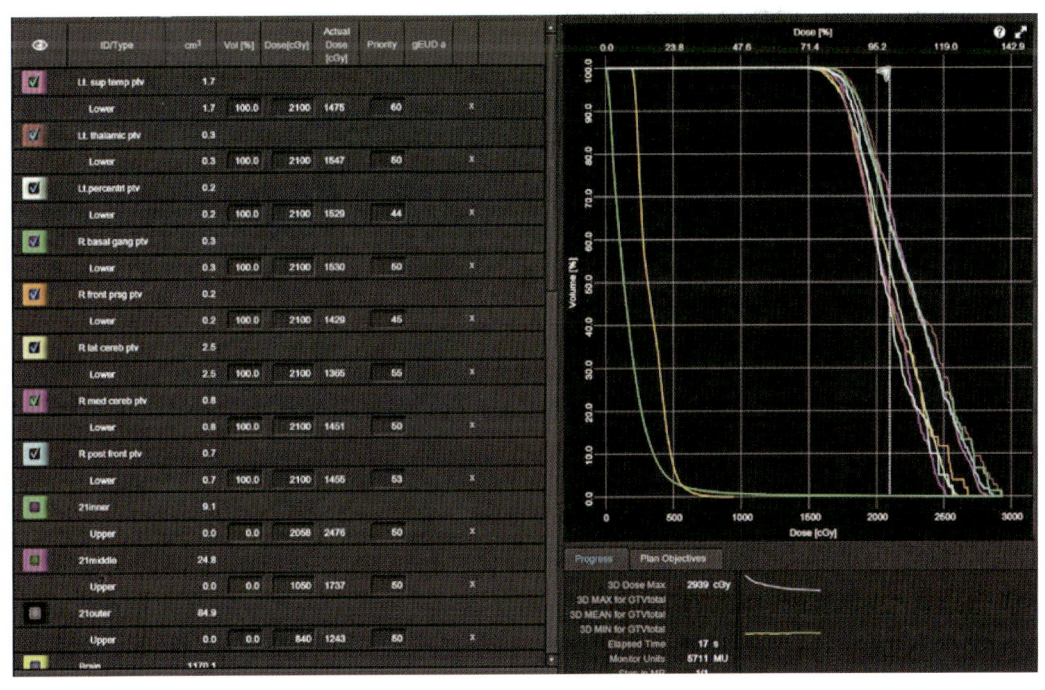

第 17 章　多发性脑转移瘤的单中心治疗计划
Single-Isocenter, Multiple Metastasis Treatment Planning

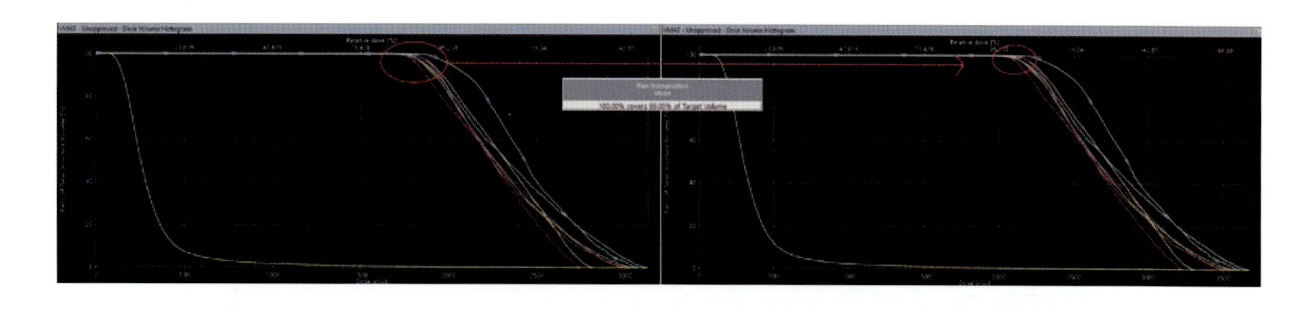

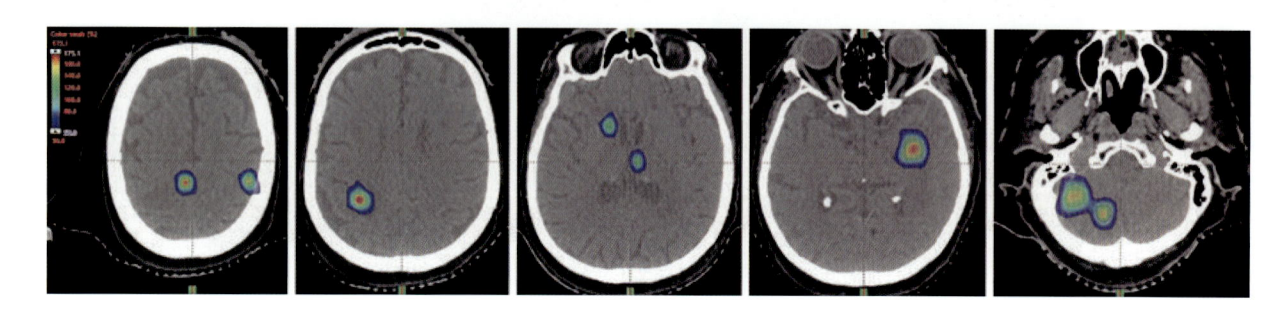

（二）VMAT（HyperArc）

1. 对于 HyperArc 计划，不需要调整结构。一旦勾画完靶区，将添加 HyperArc 计划，指定靶区处方并选择所需的射野。

2. SRS NTO（正常组织目标）取代了调节结构的功能，而 ALDO（自动低剂量目标）则自动使多个结构之间的靶区覆盖范围均匀化。

3. 在剂量计算后，通常需要进行归一化，一般归一化前后剂量分布差异不大，但如果优化过程中成本函数中包含了较高的 OAR 优先级（权重），则归一前后剂量分布变化较大。我们的做法通常是将 100% 的处方剂量覆盖 99% 的复合靶体积，但如果其中一个靶区相对其他靶区剂量覆盖不足，计划者不必重新设计计划，可将覆盖最少的靶区作为归一化靶区，来确保每个靶区都得到足够的剂量覆盖。

4. 归一化后，最后一步是计划检查和质量评价指标计算。除了评估靶区覆盖率，还包括适形度、R50（V50%/V100%），放射性坏死风险指标（单分次计划中，12Gy 所包绕的最大的连续区域），以及相邻靶区之间的任何高到中等剂量线的衔接。HyperArc 可显示 RTOG CI、Paddick CI、Paddick GI 和 ICRU 剂量不均匀性指数。

附录 17-1

1. 伯明翰阿拉巴马大学针对单中心 VMAT 放射外科更新的计划设计流程（V.2019）勾画

(1) 勾画所有的正常的结构，包括大脑、视神经和脑干。

(2) 勾画每个 GTV 并标记为 GTV1、GTV2、GTV3 等。

(3) 使用布尔运算符，创建一个 GTV_total；例如，针对三个靶区"GTV_total"="GTV1"∪("GTV2"∪"GTV3")。

*注意：本指南的以前版本错误地使用了布尔运算符∩，而不是∪。

(4) 使用布尔运算符，为正常的大脑组织等创建一个结构，如"BRAIN"去除"GTV_TOTAL"。

(5) 创建围绕靶区体积的环结构作为限制结构。

① 以递进的方式创建不同环结构，并使用如下函数绘制"结构外放"。

a. "内环"=GTV_total + 0.2cm。

b. "中间环"=GTV_total + 0.5cm。

c. "外环"=GTV_total + 1.5cm。

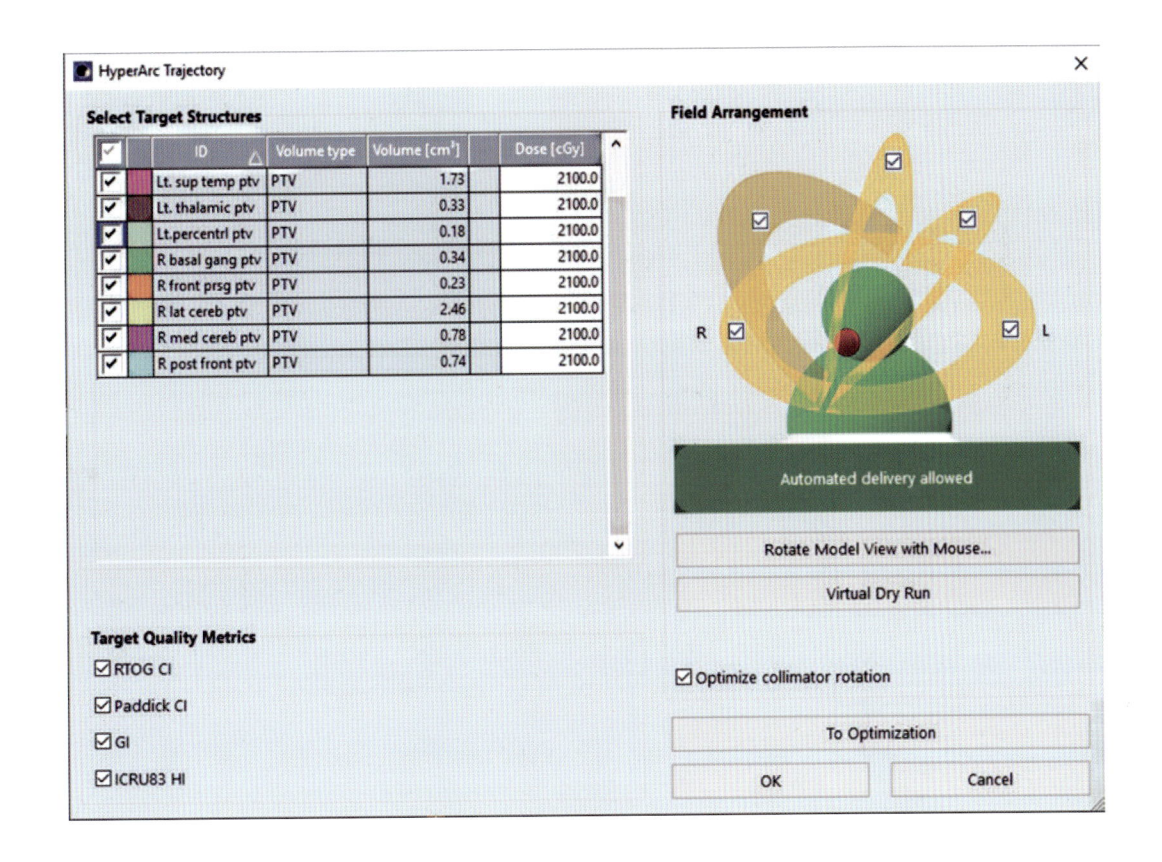

d. 下面列出了原始技术中的外环尺寸，但我们发现环越小计划质量更优。

- "内环"=GTV_total + 0.5cm。
- "中间环"=GTV_total + 1.0cm。
- "外环"=GTV_total + 3.0cm。

② 布尔运算："外环"＝"外环"－"中间环"；

③ 布尔运算："中间环"＝"中间环"－"内环"；

④ 布尔运算："内环"＝"内环"－"GTV_total"；

⑤ 使用布尔运算裁剪体外的任何控制结构。

(6) 如果一个计划包含多个处方，为了获得最佳剂量分布，每个处方级别应有单独的 GTV_total 和外环结构集（如 GTV_total_18、外环_18、中环_18 和内环_18 等）。

(7) 如果计划中包含邻近的靶区，则可能会发生剂量"桥接"现象。这是指在给定的等剂量水平下，两个靶区的剂量线相连接。这种情况只会在中至高等剂量水平中出现（如单次处方剂量为 18Gy 的计划中，＞9Gy 的剂量线相连接）。为了减轻这种现象，在两个剂量"桥接"的靶区之间创建一个结构，并为之添加一个优化条件：该结构的最大剂量低于所关注的剂量水平 –1Gy（若关注 9Gy 的剂量水平，该结构的剂量约束上限设置为受到 8Gy 照射的结构体积为 0）。如果这样做不能减轻"桥接"现象，则增加该结构的优先级（权重）或降低约束条件中的剂量限值。

(8) 对于 DVH 计算的适形指数，使用"结构外放"函数创建评估结构，就像前文表述一样，"GTV1_eval"=GTV1 + 1cm，"GTV2_eval"=GTV2 + 1cm。对于单个靶区，无须这样操作；BODY 结构的处方等剂量体积可用于适形度计算，或者 Eclipse 将在剂量统计信息表格中自动计算 RTOG CI。

(9) 为了获得最大精度（或为了进一步提高小靶区的计划质量），在每个靶区结构上单击右键，并选择"高分辨率"。在"外照射计划"窗口中，选择"计算模型"，单击相应体积剂量算法旁边的"编辑"，然后将剂量网格分辨率从 0.25cm 更改为 0.1cm。（请注意，这将显著增加计算所需的时间，Acuros 算法相比其他算法时间增加的幅度

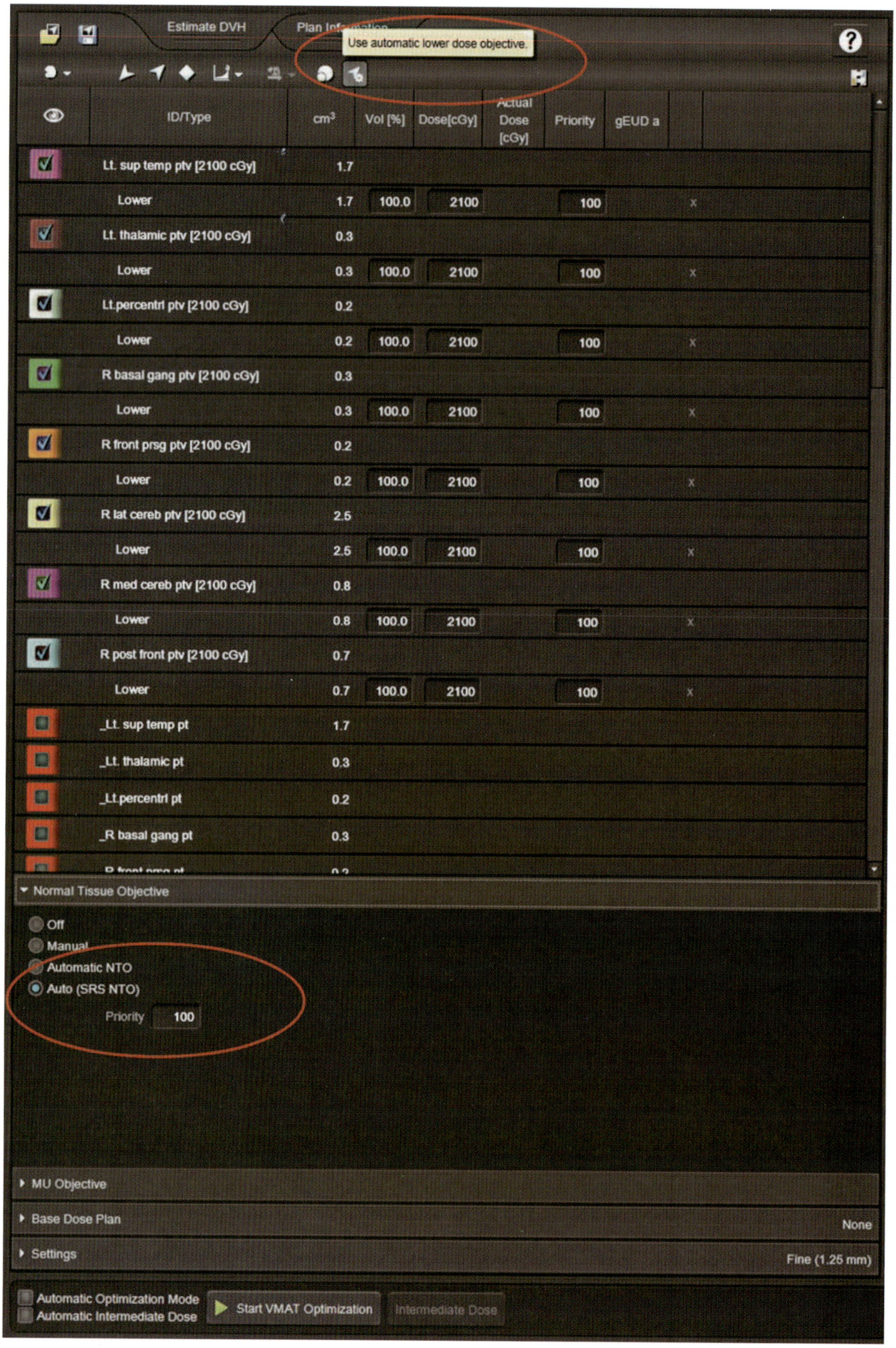
Estimate DVH
Use automatic lower dose objective.
ID/Type
cm³
Vol [%]
Dose[cGy]
Actual Dose [cGy]
Priority
gEUD a
Lt. sup temp ptv [2100 cGy] 1.7
Lower 1.7 100.0 2100 100
Lt. thalamic ptv [2100 cGy] 0.3
Lower 0.3 100.0 2100 100
Lt.percentrl ptv [2100 cGy] 0.2
Lower 0.2 100.0 2100 100
R basal gang ptv [2100 cGy] 0.3
Lower 0.3 100.0 2100 100
R front prsg ptv [2100 cGy] 0.2
Lower 0.2 100.0 2100 100
R lat cereb ptv [2100 cGy] 2.5
Lower 2.5 100.0 2100 100
R med cereb ptv [2100 cGy] 0.8
Lower 0.8 100.0 2100 100
R post front ptv [2100 cGy] 0.7
Lower 0.7 100.0 2100 100
_Lt. sup temp pt 1.7
_Lt. thalamic pt 0.3
_Lt.percentrl pt 0.2
_R basal gang pt 0.3
Normal Tissue Objective
Off
Manual
Automatic NTO
Auto (SRS NTO)
Priority 100
MU Objective
Base Dose Plan
None
Settings
Fine (1.25 mm)
Automatic Optimization Mode
Automatic Intermediate Dose
Start VMAT Optimization
Intermediate Dose

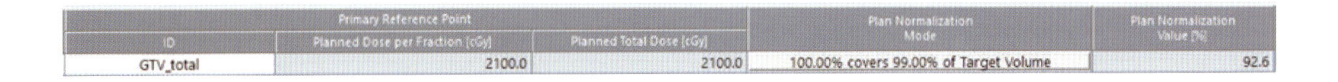

第 17 章　多发性脑转移瘤的单中心治疗计划
Single-Isocenter, Multiple Metastasis Treatment Planning

更小）。

2. 等中心和射野分布

(1) 考虑如下的弧（arc）形射野如下（图17-17）（最优照射顺序）。

(2) 通过右键单击射野并选择"将一组射野与结构（GTV_total）对齐"，将等中心放置在 GTV_total 的几何中心。如果这使得等中心离一个大靶区太近，以至于一个小靶区不在射野覆盖的范围内，则可手动调整等中心，使所有靶区都在射野内。

3. 计划优化和归一化

(1) 如果可以，请启用铅门跟随功能。

(2) 每个单独的 GTV（不是复合 GTV）接收较低的剂量目标：100% 的靶区体积接收 100% 的处方剂量；默认优先级（权重）=50（可以根据计划者的偏好调整到 100，并按类似的比例调整其他优先级）。

(3) 计划中最优先的结构应该获得最高的优化优先级；归一化将按比例调整剂量，以实现足够的靶区覆盖。

(4) 对于无关键 OAR 的计划应尽量减少低剂量溢出到正常组织，每个限制结构均设置以下剂量上限。

① 内环：0 体积接受 98% 的处方剂量；权重 = 50。

② 中间环：0 体积接受处方剂量的 50%；去

弧 号	靶 区	弧长（°）	床旋转角度（°）	准直器角度（°）	电弧方向	机架角度（°）	停止角度（°）
1	1	360	0	45	CW	181	179
2	1	360	0	45	CW	181	179
	2	180	315/45/90[a]	45	CCW	180	0
3	1	360	0	45	CW	181	179
	2	180	315	45	CCW	180	0
	3	180	45	315	CCW	0	180
4	1	360	0	45	CW	181	179
	2	180	315	45	CCW	179	0
	3	180	45	315	CCW	0	181
	4	360	90	45	CW	181	0

a. 对这些弧选择 315° 或 45° 而非 90° 床旋转，将使其出射剂量溢出头部而不是沉积在体内。请注意，一些加速器可能默认的床位置为 180° 而不是 0°

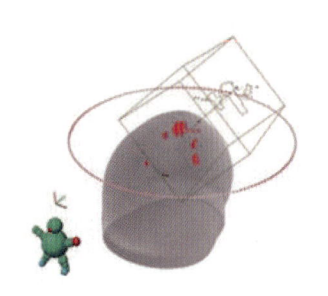

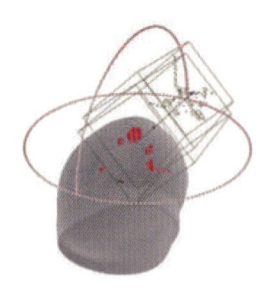

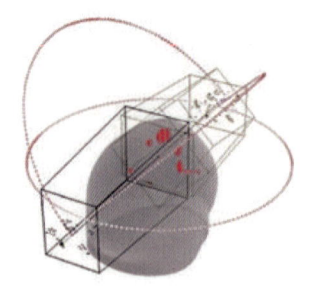

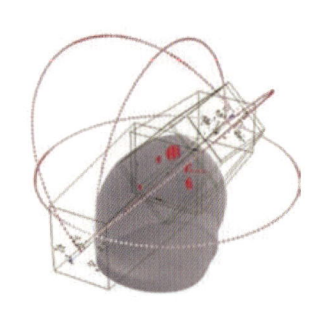

▲ 图 17-17　一个、两个、三个和四个弧的几何分布情况

权重 =50。

③ 外环：0 体积接受处方剂量的 40%；权重 = 50。

④ 正常大脑组织：1% 结构接受 1/6 的处方剂量；优先级 =125（根据我们的经验，这通常是健康组织 DVH 曲线的拐点）。

a. 请注意，将优先级加权到较高的值将会导致更低的计划归一化值（因此也会导致更高程度的归一化）。如果该值使您对后面计算的 MU 级别感到不满意，则可以降低此优化目标的优先级。

b. 同时注意，这些优先级值表征正在优化的数学表达式中的加权系数，它们是成比例的。

(5) 如果邻近的敏感正常结构在限制结构内（例如脑干、视神经、交叉神经等），则可能需要设置额外的剂量约束条件，如果不在附近，限制结构可严格限制这些器官的剂量。例如，如果脑干与外环重叠，请考虑以下附加的剂量约束条件 - 脑干：0 体积接受 800cGy 的剂量，优先级 = 75。优先级必须≥限制结构的优先级，否则优化算法不会优先考虑危及器官。

(6) 对于处方相同的多个靶区计划，当处方剂量均匀覆盖在所有靶区上时，低剂量线溢出将最小化。这是因为对计划进行全局归一化，而不是像伽马刀计划独立地针对每个靶区进行归一化。

① 理想情况下，当靶区剂量均匀覆盖时，所有靶区的 DVH 曲线在处方剂量处重合（图 17-18）。

a. 注意：靶区覆盖均匀性不要与计划均匀性混淆（尽量减少肿瘤体积内的热点）。

② 我们发现，通过在第一级的第一步暂停优化并等待优化达到稳定状态（通过优化线形图中每个结构的水平线表示）可以提高计划质量。根据需要增加或降低每个结构的代价函数的优先级，以实现均匀的靶区覆盖范围。一旦达到此要求，从第一级开始暂停优化。

a. 如果计划完成，DVH 显示了非均匀的剂量覆盖，则可以重新启动优化并"继续先前的优化"。优化将在最后的状态重新开始，代价函数的优先级也可以调整，实现所需的均匀覆盖。

(7) 对计划进行归一化。将 100% 的处方覆盖到 99%~100% 的 GTV_total，并确保每个靶区都得到适当的剂量覆盖。

(8) 对于不同靶区具有不同处方的计划，为确保每个靶区得到足够的剂量覆盖，但不过度覆盖，可能需要进行额外操作。

① 在初始优化过程中，暂停多级分辨率优化的第一级或第二级，并选择一个靶区作为锚靶区（anchor）。

② 调整每个靶区的优化约束条件，使优化 DVH 曲线指示的靶区剂量与锚靶区剂量的相对差异，与对应靶区处方剂量的相对差异相同。

a. 例如，靶区 A 的处方剂量为 18Gy，靶区 B 为 24Gy（∆=6Gy 或 25%）。靶区 A 被指定为锚靶区。如果在优化的初始阶段，靶区 A 的 DVH 曲线表示 12Gy 覆盖 100% 体积，则调整靶区 B 的优化约束权重，使其曲线指示 16 Gy（原稿为

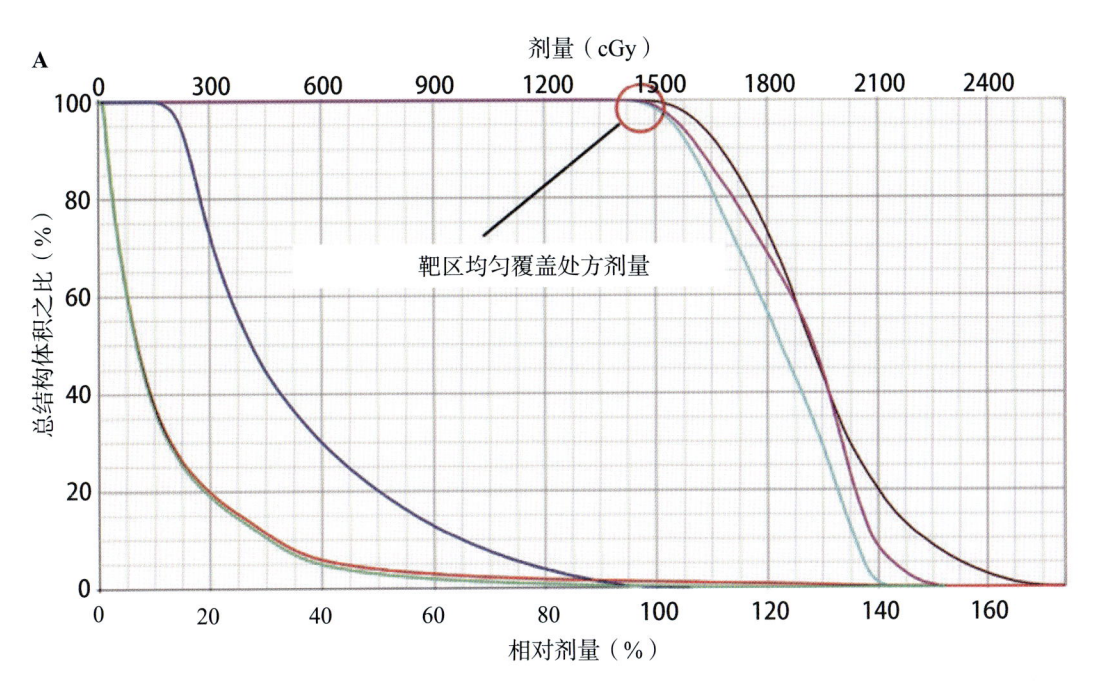

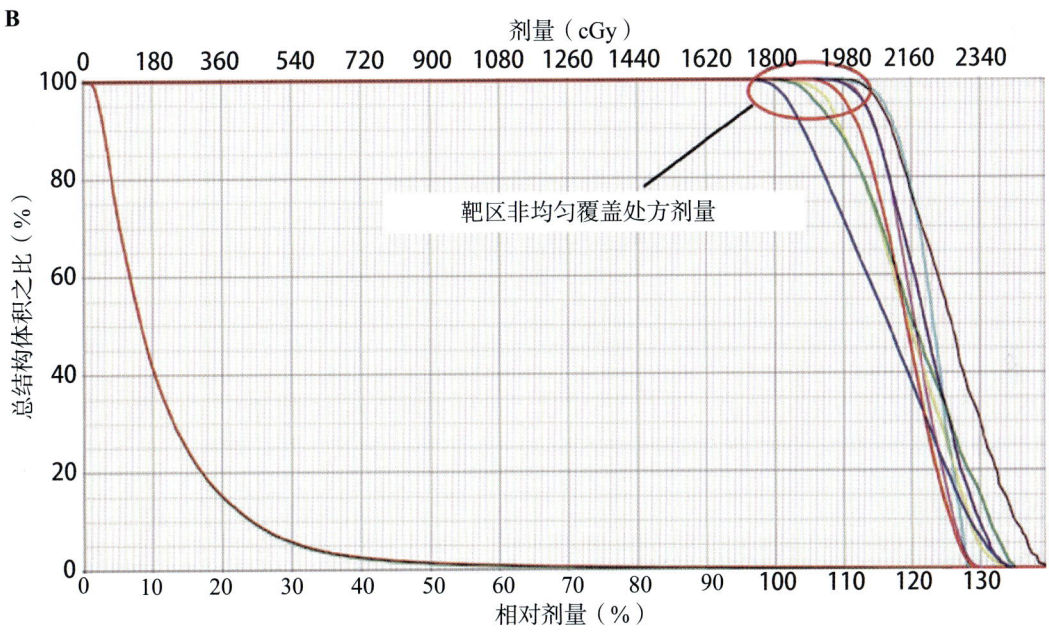

▲ 图 17-18 100% 处方剂量均匀覆盖（A）非均匀覆盖（B）

15Gy，译者此处更正为 16Gy）覆盖 100% 体积。因此，当优化后的计划进行归一化后，每个靶区应该有 100% 的处方剂量覆盖率。

4. 计划评价

(1) 利用评估结构计算各靶区的适形度指标（conformity index，CI）。

①确保 100% 等剂量线不延伸到评估结构之外（如果是，计划质量欠佳）及不与另一个靶区的 100% 等剂量线重叠。② RTOG CI = 评估结构的 100% 等剂量线除以靶区的体积，如 GTV1 CI=GTV1_eval 的 100% 等剂量线体积除以 GTV1 的体积。通过 Eclipse 治疗计划软件也可以计算 CI，但如果计划包含多个靶区，则当前软件版本将不能准确计算 CI；在这种情况下，可以通过从每个评估结构中提取处方体积来获得单个靶区 100% 等剂量线包绕的体积。

(2) 评估高-中剂量的跌落。

①计划的帕迪克(paddick)梯度指数(gradient index，GI)或者计划的 R50%。

a. GI=50% 等剂量线包绕的体积（V50%）除以 100% 处方等剂量线的体积（prescription isodose line，PIV）。

b. R50%=50% 等剂量线包绕的体积（V）除以总靶区体积（GTV_total）。

c. 请注意，Eclipse 计算梯度与上述计算的梯度不同。

d. 还应注意，Paddick GI 不能用来准确地比较不同适形度计划间的剂量衰减，因为不同的适形指数表示不同的 100% 处方等剂量体积。

②为了比较不同适形度的两个放射外科计划之间的高、中等剂量跌落，我们建议比较。

a. AUC-DVH：感兴趣区域内 DVH 曲线下的面积（如 9～18Gy）。这很容易做到，通过设置足够精细的剂量分辨率（如 1cGy）以 EXCEL 的格式导出 DVH，并利用梯形规则进行数值积分。

b. R50%=50% 等剂量线包绕的体积（V50%）除以总靶区体积（GTV_total）。

参考文献

[1] Modh A, Burmeister C, Elshaikh M, Siddiqui F, Siddiqui S, Shah M. Radiation utilization trends in the treatment of brain metastases from non-small cell lung cancer. Int J Radiat Oncol Biol Phys. 2017;99(2):E94.

[2] Network NCC. Central Nervous System Cancers (Version 1.2019) [03/15/2019]. Available from: https://www.nccn.org/professionals/physician_gls/ pdf/cns.pdf.

[3] Woo SY, Grant WH III, Bellezza D, Grossman R, Gildenberg P, Carpenter LS, et al. A comparison of intensity modulated conformal therapy with a conventional external beam stereotactic radiosurgery system for the treatment of single and multiple intracranial lesions. Int J Radiat Oncol Biol Phys. 1996;35(3):593–7.

[4] Yu CX. Intensity-modulated arc therapy with dynamic multileaf collimation: an alternative to tomotherapy. Phys Med Biol. 1995;40(9):1435–49.

[5] Otto K. Volumetric modulated arc therapy: IMRT in a single gantry arc. Med Phys. 2008;35(1):310–7.

[6] Lagerwaard F, Verbakel W, van der Hoorn E, Slotman B, Senan S. Volumetric modulated arc therapy (RapidArc) for rapid, non-invasive stereotactic radiosurgery of multiple brain metastases. Int J Radiat Oncol Biol Phys. 2008;72(1):S530.

[7] Kang J, Ford EC, Smith K, Wong J, McNutt TR. A method for optimizing LINAC treatment geometry for volumetric modulated arc therapy of multiple brain metastases. Med Phys. 2010;37(8):4146–54.

[8] Clark GM, Popple RA, Young PE, Fiveash JB. Feasibility of single-isocenter volumetric modulated arc radiosurgery for treatment of multiple brain metastases. Int J Radiat Oncol Biol Phys. 2010;76(1):296–302.

[9] McDonald D, Schuler J, Takacs I, Peng J, Jenrette J, Vanek K. Comparison of radiation dose spillage from the Gamma Knife Perfexion with that from volumetric modulated arc radiosurgery during treatment of multiple brain metastases in a single fraction. J Neurosurg. 2014;121(Suppl 2):51–9.

[10] Han EY, Kim G-Y, Rebueno N, Yeboa DN, Briere TM. End-to-end testing of automatic plan optimization using RayStation scripting for hypofractionated multimetastatic brain stereotactic radiosurgery. Med Dosim. 2019;44(4):e44–50.

[11] Ma L, Nichol A, Hossain S, Wang B, Petti P, Vellani R, et al. Variable dose interplay effects across radiosurgical apparatus in treating multiple brain metastases. Int J Comput Assist Radiol Surg. 2014;9(6):1079–86.

[12] Ma L, Petti P, Wang B, Descovich M, Chuang C, Barani IJ, et al. Apparatus dependence of normal brain tissue dose in stereotactic radiosurgery for multiple brain metastases. J Neurosurg. 2011;114(6):1580–4.

[13] Thomas EM, Popple RA, Wu X, Clark GM, Markert JM, Guthrie BL, et al. Comparison of plan quality and delivery time between volumetric arc therapy (RapidArc) and Gamma Knife radiosurgery for multiple cranial metastases. Neurosurgery. 2014;75(4):409–18.

[14] Jang SY, Lalonde R, Ozhasoglu C, Burton S, Heron D, Huq MS. Dosimetric comparison between cone/ Iris-based and InCise MLC-based CyberKnife plans for single and multiple brain metastases. J Appl Clin Med Phys. 2016;17(5):184–99.

[15] Ermiş E, Blatti-Moreno M, Leiser D, Cihoric N, Schmidhalter D, Henzen D, et al. Dose analysis of InCise 2 multi leaf collimator and IRIS-based stereotactic radiotherapy plans for brain and liver tumors. Biomed Phys Eng Express. 2019;5(3):035007.

[16] Hoogeman MS, Nuyttens JJ, Levendag PC, Heijmen BJ. Time dependence of intrafraction patient motion assessed by repeat stereoscopic imaging. Int J Radiat Oncol Biol Phys. 2008;70(2):609–18.

[17] Kim J, Hsia A, Xu Z, Ryu S. Motion likelihood over spine

radiosurgery treatments—an intrafraction motion analysis. Int J Radiat Oncol Biol Phys. 2017;99(2):E678.

[18] Roper J, Chanyavanich V, Betzel G, Switchenko J, Dhabaan A. Single-isocenter multiple-target stereotactic radiosurgery: risk of compromised coverage. Int J Radiat Oncol Biol Phys. 2015;93(3):540–6.

[19] Babic S, Lee Y, Ruschin M, Lochray F, Lightstone A, Atenafu E, et al. To frame or not to frame? Conebeam CT-based analysis of head immobilization devices specific to linac-based stereotactic radiosurgery and radiotherapy. J Appl Clin Med Phys. 2018;19(2):111–20.

[20] Covington EL, Fiveash JB, Wu X, Brezovich I, Willey CD, Riley K, et al. Optical surface guidance for submillimeter monitoring of patient position during frameless stereotactic radiotherapy. J Appl Clin Med Phys. 2019;20(6):91–8.

[21] Yuan Y, Thomas EM, Clark GM, Fiveash JB, Popple RA, editors. Factors influencing normal brain dose for single-isocenter multi-target radiosurgery. AAPM 55th annual meeting & exhibition; 2013 Aug 4–8; Indianapolis, IN.

[22] Clark GM, Popple RA, Prendergast BM, Spencer SA, Thomas EM, Stewart JG, et al. Plan quality and treatment planning technique for single isocenter cranial radiosurgery with volumetric modulated arc therapy. Pract Radiat Oncol. 2012;2(4):306–13.

[23] Thomas EM FC-G, Dempsey K, Riley K, Fiveash JB, Popple RA, Bredel M. Treatment of 27 brain metastases with single-isocenter VMAT radiosurgery: a case report. 13th international stereotactic radiosurgery society congress; Montreaux, Switzerland, 2017.

[24] Yuan Y, Thomas EM, Clark GA, Markert JM, Fiveash JB, Popple RA. Evaluation of multiple factors affecting normal brain dose in single-isocenter multiple target radiosurgery. J Radiosurg SBRT. 2018;5(2):131–44.

[25] Wu Q, Snyder KC, Liu C, Huang Y, Zhao B, Chetty IJ, et al. Optimization of treatment geometry to reduce normal brain dose in radiosurgery of multiple brain metastases with single–Isocenter volumetric modulated arc therapy. Sci Rep. 2016;6:34511.

[26] Huang Y, Yue H, Wang M, Li S, Zhang J, Liu Z, et al. Fully automated searching for the optimal VMAT jaw settings based on Eclipse Scripting Application Programming Interface (ESAPI) and RapidPlan knowledge-based planning. J Appl Clin Med Phys. 2018;19(3):177–82.

[27] Huang Y, Chin K, Robbins JR, Kim J, Li H, Amro H, et al. Radiosurgery of multiple brain metastases with single-isocenter dynamic conformal arcs (SIDCA). Radiother Oncol. 2014;112(1):128–32.

[28] Mori Y, Kaneda N, Hagiwara M, Ishiguchi T. Dosimetric study of automatic brain metastases planning in comparison with conventional multi-isocenter dynamic conformal arc therapy and gamma knife radiosurgery for multiple brain metastases. Cureus. 2016;8(11):e882.

[29] Vergalasova I, Liu H, Alonso-Basanta M, Dong L, Li J, Nie K, et al. Multi-institutional dosimetric evaluation of modern day stereotactic radiosurgery (SRS) treatment options for multiple brain metastases. Front Oncol. 2019;9:483.

第 18 章 脑转移瘤治疗中的耐受剂量
Dose Tolerances in Brain Metastasis Management

Giuseppe Minniti　Claudia Scaringi　Barbara Tolu　著
梁　瞻　译
胡永梅　张子健　校

一、概述

近年来，随着全脑放射治疗（whole-brain radiation therapy，WBRT）向立体定向放射手术（stereotactic radiosurgery，SRS）的转变，脑转移瘤患者的临床治疗发生了重大变化。目前，对于少量（最多 5 个）脑转移瘤的患者，推荐单独使用 SRS，其疗效已在随机试验中得到证实。这些试验结果显示 1 年的局部控制率约为 75% 或以上，生存获益与使用 SRS+WBRT 观察到的相似，但长期神经毒性风险较低[1-4]。

根据美国肿瘤放射治疗协作组织（RTOG）90-05 指南[5]，对于小于 20mm 的病灶可照射最多 24Gy 的剂量；对于 21～30mm 的病灶，可照射 18Gy；31～40mm 的病灶可照射 15Gy。研究表明，尽管对大于 2～3cm 的肿瘤，单次大剂量 SRS 在提供有效、安全剂量照射的能力方面有限，但其在控制肿瘤生长和保护正常组织方面均表现为有效。

由于高剂量的单次 SRS 会带来更高的神经并发症风险，在过去的几年，多分次 SRS（名义上 2～5 个分次数），也称为大分割 SRS、分次 SRS、多剂量 SRS、多分期 SRS 或大分割立体定向放射治疗，已被用来替代单次 SRS，其目的是平衡肿瘤的控制与正常脑组织的毒性，尤其是对于较大的病灶和对那些邻近或位于大脑关键区域的病灶。几项回顾性研究报道，分 3～5 次共给予 24～35Gy 的剂量，1 年的局部控制率为 70%～90%，正常脑组织损伤的风险相对较低，为 2%～10%[6-12]。

线性二次方程（linear-quadratic，LQ）模型通常用于比较给定特定剂量的不同分次方案的生物等效剂量（biologically effective Dose，BED），其公式为 BED=D[1+d/(α/β)][13]，特定值（α/β）、总剂量（D）和单次剂量（d）[14]；然而，它应用于 8～10Gy 以上的剂量，如用于多分次 SRS，仍然存有争议。因此，创建了不同的模型。Joiner 等[15]提出了线性二次立方模型，其中 BED 的计算方法是在线性二次模型的公式中增加一项与剂量的立方成比例的项；根据该模型，对于较大的病灶，分 3 次照射，单次剂量 8.5～9Gy（相当于 20～22Gy 的单分次照射），与同等体积使用 15～18Gy 的单分次照射组相比，具有更高的疗效和更低的放射性坏死风险。

在临床实践中，SRS 的关键目标是最大限度地减少辐射对大脑正常组织的损伤。对于单分次和多分次 SRS 而言，脑组织剂量限制结构包括以下几种：例如脑干、脑神经、耳蜗以及运动和感觉皮层。在本章中，我们总结了当前有关颅脑 SRS 的放射耐受性的临床证据，讨论了剂量、体积、分次和其他相关临床病理变量的影响。

二、循证基础

SRS 在脑转移瘤的治疗中起着重要作用，但同时它与病灶周围正常组织发生放射损伤的风险有关。因此，量化放射损伤风险至关重要，以便能降低与放射治疗相关的毒性。在下面的临床病例中（病例 1），一名乳腺癌患者因颅内转移而接受了 SRS 治疗。4 个＜ 2cm 的病灶接受单分次 SRS 治疗，1 个＞ 3cm 的病灶采用多分次 SRS 治疗。根据上述考虑，剂量和分次的选择主要是基于最小化神经毒性的风险。

SRS 治疗的正常组织的剂量耐受限值的建议来自于 2010 年发表的 QUANTEC 指南[16-19]，该指南由美国医学物理协会（American Association of Physics in Medicine，AAPM）的"临床正常组织效应的定量分析"或美国放射肿瘤学会（American Society of Therapeutic Radiology and Oncology，ASTRO）发表。QUANTEC 指南基本上对现有关于正常组织的辐射剂量 / 体积 / 结果的文献进行了评论，就脑部 SRS，给出了 16 个解剖部位和辐射类型的正常组织毒性的剂量 – 体积限制的建议。然而，关于多分次 SRS 的耐受剂量的数据相当有限，且剂量限制的数据仍然未得到验证。表 18-1 和表 18-2 总结了单分次 SRS 和多分次 SRS 的正常组织剂量限制。

三、中枢神经系统的正常组织剂量限制

（一）正常脑实质

在脑部的 SRS 治疗中，正常组织的毒性似乎是与受照剂量、体积及与敏感脑组织接近程度有关的函数。评估脑部放射性并发症的终点通常是脑部发生放射性坏死，这与多达 1/3 的患者出现不同程度的神经功能缺损有关[16-23]。其他评估终点还包括使用类固醇，维持一般状态和保留神经认知功能[2, 4]。与放射性脑坏死发生的相关因素有辐射剂量、靶区体积和受到不同剂量照射的正常脑组织体积。

放射性坏死的诊断具有挑战性[24]。包括活检在内的外科探查是放射性坏死或肿瘤进展组织学确认的金标准。常规 MRI 成像显示，放射性坏死区域在 T_2 加权序列中表现为白质高信号，在 T_1 加权序列中表现为肿瘤增强或占位性增强病灶，并伴有中心区域坏死，然而这些特征的预测值很低[25]。将"常规"与先进的 MRI 成像技术（例如扩散加权成像，磁共振波谱和磁共振灌

表 18-1 单分次 SRS 的正常组织剂量限制

器 官	放疗类型	剂量（毒性发生率 %）	剂量体积参数	毒性反应	参考文献
脑	单分次 SRS	V12＜ 5~10cm³（＜ 20）	当 V12 ＞ 10cm³ 时，剂量曲线快速上升	有症状的坏死	QUANTEC[16, 17, 21, 22, 33]
脑干	单分次 SRS	D_{max}＜ 12.5Gy（＜ 5）	脑干 1/3 剂量的风险 12.5Gy（1%）、14.2Gy（13%）、16Gy（61%）和 17.5Gy（94%）	永久性神经缺损或坏死	QUANTEC[36]
视神经 /视交叉	单分次 SRS	D_{max}＜ 8Gy（＜ 3），D_{max}8~12Gy（＜ 10），D_{max}＞ 12Gy（＞ 10）	V12＜ 2~4mm³ 低风险	视神经病变	QUANTEC[18, 43, 44]
脊髓	单分次 SRS	D_{max}＜ 13Gy（＜ 1）		脊髓病	QUANTEC[19]
海绵窦脑神经	单分次 SRS	D_{max}16~18Gy（＜ 4）		永久性脑神经缺损	QUANTEC[40, 41]

表 18-2 未经验证的多分次 SRS 的正常组织剂量限制

器 官	放疗类型	剂量（毒性发生率 %）	剂量体积参数	毒性反应	参考文献
脑	3 分次 SRS	27Gy 分 3 次照射（5～10）	V18 ≤ 30.2ml，5% V18 > 30.2ml，14%	有症状的坏死	QUANTEC [6, 7]
脑干	3 分次 SRS， 5 分次 SRS	18Gy（6Gy/ 次）< 1ml（< 3%） 26Gy（5.2Gy/ 次）< 1ml（< 3%）	D_{max} 23Gy（7.67Gy/ 次） D_{max} 31Gy（6.2Gy/ 次）	永久性神经缺损或坏死	QUANTEC [39]
视神经 / 视交叉	3 分次 SRS， 5 分次 SRS	15Gy（5Gy/ 次）< 0.2ml（< 3%）， 20Gy（4Gy/ 次）< 0.2ml（< 3%）	D_{max} 19.5Gy（6.5Gy/ 次） D_{max} 25Gy（5Gy/ 次）	视神经病变	QUANTEC [39, 50]
耳蜗	3 分次 SRS， 5 分次 SRS		D_{max} 20Gy（6.67Gy/ 次） D_{max} 25Gy（5Gy/ 次）	失聪	QUANTEC [39]
脊髓	3 分次 SRS， 5 分次 SRS	18Gy（6Gy/ 次）< 0.25ml（< 1%）， 22.5Gy（4.5Gy/ 次）< 0.25ml（< 1%）	D_{max} 22.5Gy（6.67Gy/ 次） D_{max} 30Gy（6Gy/ 次）	脊髓病	QUANTEC [19, 39]

注成像）相结合，可能有助于区分肿瘤进展与放射性坏死 [26, 27]。除了先进的磁共振成像技术外，正电子断层扫描（positronemission tomography，PET），尤其是使用氨基酸类似物，例如 ^{11}C 蛋氨酸（MET）、^{18}F 氟乙基酪氨酸（fluoroethyl-tyrosine，FET），以及最近的 ^{18}F 氟 - 二羟基苯丙氨酸（F-DOPA），也是一种很有前景的技术，具有很高的灵敏度和特异性，可用于 SRS 治疗后放射性坏死和复发的鉴别诊断 [28-31]。因此，在已发表的各项研究中报道的放射性脑坏死发生率的不同，至少在一定程度上反映了各项评估技术在诊断时的准确性差异。

RTOG 90-05 试验是一项关于复发性脑转移和原发性肿瘤的 SRS 剂量递增研究，患者先前接受过全脑或部分脑照射，研究发现晚期毒性导致的不可逆严重神经系统症状，对受照 24Gy、< 2cm 的病灶，发生率为 10%；对受照 18Gy、2.1～3cm 病灶，发生率为 14%，对于那些 3.1～4cm，接受 15Gy 照射的群体，其发生率为 20% [5]。在另一项 RTOG 试验（RTOG 95-08）中，纳入了 333 名随机接受 SRS+WBRT 或 WBRT 治疗的脑转移瘤患者，治疗使用 RTOG 90-05 中制定的剂量限制，3% 和 6% 的患者中观察到 3 级和 4 级急性和晚期毒性 [32]。

在一些已发表的研究中，接受 10Gy（V10）或 12Gy（V12）的正常脑体积 [17, 21, 22, 33] 是辐射导致放射性坏死的一个常见的独立预测因素。根据对这些结果的回顾，QUANTEC 建议表明，V12 为 5～10cm^3 的患者发生有症状的放射性坏死风险高达 20%。Blonigen 等在 63 例患者（单分次 SRS，共 173 处脑转移瘤）的研究中 [21] 发现 V10 > 14.5cm^3 和 V12 > 10.8cm^3 时，放射性坏死的风险高达 68.8%，V10 < 0.68cm^3 和 V12 < 0.5cm^3 时无放射性坏死病例。在 2006 年 9 月至 2010 年 1 月期间，罗马大学圣安德里亚医院对 206 例患者进行了单分次 SRS 治疗，共 310 处转移灶，单个患者颅内 1～4 个转移灶，其中 V12 < 3.3cm^3 时 1 年放射性坏死率为 0%，V12：3.3～5.9cm^3 时为 16%，V12：6.0～10.9cm^3 时为 24%，V12 > 10.9cm^3 时为 51% [22]。

这些发现对临床实践具有重要意义。当将 RTOG 推荐的放射手术治疗剂量应用于直径分别为 2cm、3cm 和 4cm 的球形病灶（相应体积为 4.3cm^3、14.1cm^3 和 33.4cm^3）时，计算出的 V12 分别约为 21cm^3、57cm^3 和 101cm^3，导致放射性坏死的风险很高。此外，随着 V12 的增加超过 5～10cm^3，神经系统并发症迅速增加，这表明将大体肿瘤体积（gross tumor volume，GTV）外放 1~2mm 边界产生计划靶区（planning target volume，PTV）可能导致无法接受的放射坏死风险，即使在治疗小病变时也是如此；一般来说，在 8mm 和 15mm 的 GTV 边缘外放至 PTV 时，外放距离分别增加 1mm 和 2mm，靶体积均将增加一倍。这意味着 1.5cm³ 的 GTV 到 PTV 的外放范围分别为 0mm、1mm、2mm，生成的 PTV 体积分别为 1.5cm³、2.1cm³ 和 2.8cm³，接受单次剂量 24Gy 的照射时，V12 分别为 3.8cm³、7.7cm³ 和 11.4cm³，可能导致放射性坏死的风险显著增加。

单次大剂量 SRS 将导致不可接受的严重神经毒性风险，故多分次 SRS 通常用于脑转移瘤的治疗。几项研究报道显示，使用 3~5 分次数，共 24~35Gy 的照射剂量，发生有症状的放射性坏死的风险相对较低，在 2%~10% 范围内[6-12]；然而，很少有研究系统地报道低分割方案（6~9Gy 范围内的小分次剂量方案）的正常组织剂量限制。Minniti 等[6]报道了 289 例脑转移瘤患者（转移灶大于 2.0cm）的临床结果，患者在 2008 年至 2014 年期间在罗马大学萨皮琴察分校接受单次 SRS（16~18Gy）或多分次 SRS（3×9Gy）治疗。多分次和单次的 SRS 在 12 个月后的累积局部控制率分别为 90% 和 77%（$P=0.01$），放射性脑坏死的风险分别为 18% 和 9%（$P=0.01$）。对于接受多分次的 SRS 患者，接受 18Gy 剂量照射的正常脑组织体积（V18）是预测脑坏死的最重要指标；V18 ≤ 30cm³ 的发病率为 5%，V18 > 30cm³ 的发病率为 14%（$P=0.04$）。根据四分位数的分布，对于 V18 < 22.8cm³、22.8~30.2cm³、30.3~41.2cm³ 和 > 41.2cm³，12 个月时发生放射性脑坏死的风险分别为 0%、6%、13% 和 24%。

（二）脑干

脑干由中脑，脑桥和延髓组成。对于单次 SRS，脑干最大剂量为 12~14Gy 时，神经系统并发症发生率 < 5%，> 15Gy 时神经系统并发症发生率会显著增加[34-38]。在 QUANTEC 对与辐射相关的脑干毒性的回顾中，Mayo 等[36]计算了脑干部分体积照射剂量为 12.5Gy、14.2Gy、16Gy 和 17.5Gy 时，正常组织并发症发生的风险分别为 1%、13%、61% 和 94%，当将相同剂量照射到很小的体积（< 1%）时，并发症的风险可能会降低。在一项大型回顾性研究中，对接受 SRS 治疗的 547 例患者的 596 个脑转移瘤进行了研究，他们的中位边缘剂量为 16Gy，1 年局控率为 81.8%[38]。44 名患者（7.4%）进行治疗后会在随访过程中的任何时间点发生 3 级~4 级毒性。SRS 治疗后发生严重毒性的概率与肿瘤体积增加，边界剂量增加和之前已进行 WBRT 相关（分别为 $P < 0.001$、$P=0.049$ 和 $P=0.002$）。目前，关于单次 SRS 对脑干剂量 – 体积效应的影响尚无定论。虽然在治疗脑干转移瘤时，单次照射至小体积脑干的剂量可达 20Gy，且并发症发生率较低，但在常规临床实践中，应谨慎向脑干照射大于 16Gy 的剂量。

对于脑干的多分次 SRS，几乎没有相关正常组织的剂量限值。一般来说，当用 3 或 5 分次 SRS 治疗的病变接受的最大点剂量为 23Gy 和 31Gy，并且 < 1cm³ 的脑干体积最大剂量为 18Gy 和 26Gy 时，预计永久性神经功能缺损的风险 < 3%[36, 40]（表 18-2）。由于大多数数据是使用各种放射生物学模型从脑干毒性的等效应曲线推断得出的，因此应谨慎使用剂量 – 体积指标来预测多分次 SRS 对脑干的毒性。

（三）视觉通路和其他颅底结构

在 SRS 治疗脑转移瘤时，视神经和视交叉可能会接受大量辐射，特别是对于病灶位于颅底的患者，视觉通路通常是剂量限制结构。视神经和视交叉很细（直径 < 5mm），最好使用薄层（≤ 2mm）T_1 或 T_2 加权 MRI 显示效果最佳。辐射诱发的视神经病变（radiation-induced optic neuropathy，RION）的主要终点是视觉损害，由视力和视野大小/范围来定义。

视神经和视交叉对单分次 SRS 的耐受性还

不清楚。在一些研究中发现，对于视神经前路接受最大剂量为 8~10Gy 和 12~15Gy 的患者，RION 的风险高达 2% 和 > 10%[40-44]；但是，当将 10~12Gy 的剂量只照射到视神经通路的一小部分（2~4mm³）时，这种风险似乎很低[43]。关于海绵窦脑神经的耐受性知之甚少。一系列针对原发性颅底肿瘤的 SRS 研究称，剂量在 13~18Gy 范围内，脑神经损害的发生率为 1%~6%[40, 41]。尽管无法确定单次 SRS 后海绵窦脑神经的精确耐受剂量，但来自多项研究的数据支持这样一种概念，即海绵窦中受照射量达 16~18Gy 与低毒性相关。

关于视觉神经通路对多分次 SRS 的耐受性的证据有限[39, 45]。回顾性的分析了一些视觉通路附近的颅底肿瘤或脑转移瘤研究[45-50]，分 3 次接受 21Gy 或分 5 次接受 25Gy 的患者中不到 1% 的有严重的视力障碍；但在大多数研究中，没有提供详细的剂量。罗马大学圣安德里亚医院对 34 例患者观察，患者因颅底转移受压或紧贴视神经和视交叉，接受多分次 SRS（5×5Gy）治疗，中位随访时间为 13 个月，当视交叉 V25 < 33%，且 27.5~28.5Gy 的体积很小（0.01~0.06cm³）时，未观察到视神经病变[50]。尽管研究表明 5×5Gy 或 3×7Gy 计划方案与低风险的 RION 和其他脑神经功能缺损有关，需要进一步的研究以更好地评估多分次 SRS 中视神经和视交叉的剂量 – 体积限制。

位于颞叶的脑转移瘤，应将海马勾画出来，以减少高剂量辐射对海马区神经认知功能的潜在不良反应。这种方法的原理已得到公认，但目前 SRS 治疗时保护海马的建议尚无足够的支持证据。

四、全身系统治疗联合脑照射

联合使用 WBRT 与化疗或全身药物的安全性方面的数据有限。Tsao 等[51] 对新诊断的多发性脑转移瘤使用 WBRT 治疗的疗效和毒性进行了系统评价。9 项完全公开发表的Ⅲ期临床试验的数据显示，WBRT 联合化疗与单独使用 WBRT 相比，毒性增加，并且增加多种化疗药物（包括顺铂、长春瑞滨、卡铂、吉西他滨、托泊替康和替莫唑胺）后，无生存获益[51-59]。一些Ⅱ/Ⅲ期试验评估了脑转移瘤患者联合 WBRT 与靶向药物或免疫疗法的应用情况[59-64]。一些评估表皮生长因子受体（epidermal growth factor receptor，EGFR）酪氨酸激酶抑制药（TKI）厄洛替尼或吉非替尼与 WBRT 联合使用的试验表明，联合治疗耐受性良好，但并未带来明显的生存获益[59-62]；然而，未对参与者进行 EGFR 突变检测，EGFR-TKI 在这些人群中的有益作用仍不确定。同样，尽管尚无基于大规模临床试验的可靠证据，但 WBRT 联合靶向药物 BRAF 和 MEK 抑制药或 CTLA-4 检查点抑制药的免疫疗法[63, 64] 并没有明显增加毒性。

随着 SRS 越来越多地用于治疗脑转移瘤患者，一些回顾性研究评估了 SRS 联合全身综合治疗的疗效和毒性[65-79]。对于人类表皮生长因子受体 2 阳性（HER2＋）的乳腺癌和 EGFR 突变型的非小细胞肺癌（NSCLC）患者，同时使用 SRS 和 TKI 治疗具有生存获益且低放射性坏死风险[65-68]。然而，剂量 – 体积参数与脑坏死的发生之间没有相关性的报道。一些回顾性研究表明，在 BRAF 突变的黑色素瘤患者中，BRAF/MEK 抑制药联合 SRS 能改善局部控制，虽然肿瘤内出血风险有所增加，但其安全性可以接受[69-72]。SRS 和检查点抑制药同时使用（检查点抑制药通常在 SRS 4 周内使用），与非同时使用相比，颅内控制有所改善，神经毒性类似[73-79]。值得注意的是，接受 SRS 和免疫治疗的患者，在治疗后的前 12 周，常规影像学检查可能会发现治疗病灶的短暂扩大，高达 50% 的病例会在几周内消失；这些改变被称为假性进展[74-79]（图 18–1）。免疫治疗后对影像学的正确解释，在患者的随访中起着至关重要的作用，最近，针对接受免疫治疗的神经肿瘤患者，提出了神经肿瘤免疫治疗反应评估（iRANO）标准[80]。iRANO 工作委员会建议，如果与初始影像相比，随访影像没有证实进展，在没有增加皮质类固醇剂量的情况下肿瘤稳定或缩小，应继续治疗。总的来说，SRS 与靶向药物或免疫疗法联合使用可改善肿瘤控制，而不会显著增加神经毒性。但是，由于缺乏大量的前瞻性研究，因此无法就联合治疗的安全性得出明确的结论。

再程放疗的有效性，且神经毒性可接受，但重复 SRS 后放射性坏死的风险仍未确定，目前尚无令人满意的模型来预测辐射引起毒性的风险。相比于单分次 SRS，尽管多分次 SRS 经常用于较大的复发性脑转移，但再程 SRS 的剂量耐受限制还没有临床建议。

五、再程照射

SRS 经常用于既往放疗后脑部进展的患者。少数研究报道了再程照射后发生神经毒性的风险[5, 81-85]。如 RTOG 90-05 研究[5]所示，在预先局部脑照射或 WBRT 之后，单分次 SRS 发生不可逆的严重神经毒性的风险，随着被照射病变体积的增加而增加（见上文）。据报道，接受单分次 SRS（15~20Gy）或多分次 SRS（7~8Gy/3 次）的患者中，有 13%~24% 出现 3 级或 4 级毒性的症状性放射坏死[81-85]。虽然回顾性研究证实了 SRS 用于

六、不确定性领域

关于脑转移瘤放疗后正常脑组织剂量耐受性的几个问题尚未确定。目前，预测单分次或多分次 SRS 后辐射诱发并发症风险的模型是有限的，应加以改进，如应纳入患者和治疗的特异性因素。另外，由于公认 LQ 模型高估了单分次 SRS 的效果，因此 LQ 是否适用于计算不同 SRS 计划的 BED 也是备受质疑的。

根据临床试验显示，仅接受 SRS 的患者相比于接受 SRS+WBRT 的患者在生存率、认知和生

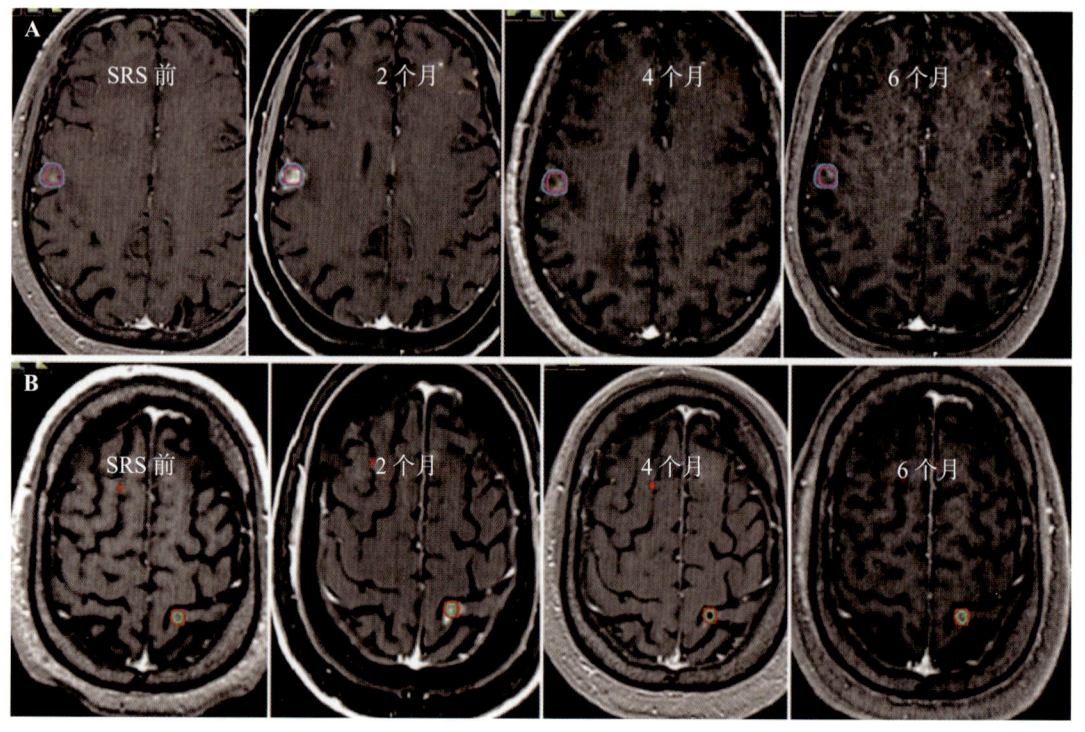

▲ 图 18-1　伴有脑转移的黑色素瘤（A）和非小细胞肺癌（B）患者的代表性轴向 T_1 加权 MRI 图像，均采用基于直线加速器（Linac）的，无框架，单次 SRS（剂量：22Gy；GTV 外扩 1mm 至 PTV），联合纳武利尤单抗治疗。在 SRS 后 2 个月内的 T_1 增强序列上出现病变暂时扩大（对比剂：钆），并在 6 个月内消失的现象被称为假性进展

活质量（quality of life，QOL）方面并无差异，因此，单独接受 SRS 已成为治疗局部脑转移瘤的首选方法。随着放射手术技术的广泛应用，单独接受 SRS 的脑转移瘤（5 个以上转移灶）患者越来越多。病例 2 中描述的 NSCLC 患者（10 个脑转移瘤）先接受了 SRS 治疗；随后，他又接受了 WBRT 作为进行性颅内疾病的抢救性治疗。一些研究表明，接受 SRS 治疗的患者中，有 5 个以上转移灶的患者与 1~4 个转移灶患者的生存率和安全性相似[86-89]。但是，前瞻性研究尚未评估此类患者认知功能下降的风险。需要模型来预测长期神经毒性的风险，包括转移的位置、数量和总体积。

如 III 期 RTOG 0614 试验和 II 期 RTOG 0933 试验所报道的那样，接受 WBRT 的患者联合应用美金刚和调强放疗（IMRT）对保留海马的认知功能有益处[90-93]。NRG 肿瘤 III 期试验 CC001 招募了 518 例患者，他们被随机分成两组：一组为接受 WBRT+ 美金刚，另一组为保护海马的 WBRT+ 美金刚（30Gy/10 次）[93]。主要终点是神经认知功能下降的时间。对存活的患者进行中位随访时间为 7.9 个月，保护海马的 WBRT+ 美金刚认知功能下降的风险显著降低（HR=0.74；95%CI 0.58~0.95；P=0.02）。这一差异可见于 4 个月时执行功能和 6 个月时学习记忆能力的下降较少。目前的研究结果提出了一个问题，即对于 5~10 个转移灶的患者，最佳的治疗方法是什么？根据脑转移瘤的位置、大小、数量和总体积，需要更多的数据来说明单独接受 SRS 或保护海马的 WBRT 的影响。在这方面，正在进行的试验（ClinicalTrials.gov：NCT01592968 和 NCT02353000）纳入 4~10 个或 15 个脑转移瘤的 WBRT 或 SRS 患者，其主要终点是肿瘤局部控制，认知功能或 QOL。

在 QUANTEC 指南中，关于多分次 SRS（每次照射 5~9Gy）后神经毒性的数据很少。在临床实践中，低分割方案通常作为单分次 SRS 的替代方案用于较大的脑转移瘤，目的是保持较高的局控率并避免放射毒性反应。但是，尚无前瞻性研究比较这些不同的方法。使用常见的剂量 - 体积参数，如 V12 用于单次 SRS，V18 用于 3 分次 SRS，这将有助于验证预测放疗后正常脑组织 / 结构毒性的生物等效剂量耐受限值的模型。

需要更多的数据，说明放疗联合全身综合治疗（靶向药物或免疫疗法），对剂量 - 体积结果的影响。具体而言，未来需要进行临床随机试验，以评估多分次 SRS 联合全身综合治疗相比于单次 SRS 联合全身综合治疗在放射诱发毒性、局部控制和脑转移患者的生活质量方面的优势。

最后，针对脑转移瘤的 SRS 研究应系统地报道 SRS 技术、处方剂量、治疗体积、病变部位、剂量参数、使用的全身性药物以及临床结果（局部控制或神经毒性），目的是开发适当的模型来预测辐射诱发的毒性并将大分割剂量转换为单次剂量。

七、结论与建议

单次 SRS 和多分次 SRS 是治疗脑转移瘤的有效方法，且长期神经毒性风险相对较低。目前，单独应用 SRS 是最多不超过 5 个脑转移瘤的患者的首选方法，与 SRS 联合 WBRT 相比，具有相同的生存率，且长期神经毒性的风险较低。对于单次和多分次 SRS，选择剂量和分次数的目的是有效控制肿瘤的生长并降低放射性脑坏死的风险。RTOG 指南推荐，对于 ≤ 20mm、21~30mm 和 31~40mm 的病灶，推荐的单次 SRS 剂量分别为 24Gy，18Gy 和 15Gy；随着肿瘤增大，向病灶安全地提供足够剂量的能力受限；具体来说，QUANTEC 关于脑组织剂量 - 体积毒性的数据表明，V12 > 5~10cm³ 时，神经毒性迅速增加。在实践中，按照 RTOG 的推荐剂量用单次 SRS 治疗大于 2.5~3cm 的病灶时，正常脑组织的被照射剂量都将超出其耐受限值。在这种情况下，通常采用 3 或 5 分次数的 SRS，目的是减少辐射诱发的毒性风险。基于同样的理由，多分次 SRS 通常用于术后较大的残腔、先前接受过照射的病灶或与重要器官组织（如视听器官或脑干 SRS）非常接近的病变。然而，尚未确定多分次 SRS 后的剂量 - 体积毒性，并且对于大病灶，其相对于单次 SRS 的优越性仍有待大量前瞻性研究证实。

SRS 经常用于多达 10 个脑转移瘤的患者，与 2～4 个转移灶的患者相比，其毒性没有显著增加，但是，由于缺乏随机临床研究，因此没有可靠的数据支持 SRS 更优于 WBRT。在应用 WBRT 时，应考虑采用 IMRT 计划进行海马保护并联合应用美金刚。

> **要 点**
> - 对于多达 5 个脑转移瘤的患者使用 SRS。
> - 对大的（最大尺寸超过 2～3cm）或紧邻关键组织结构（如视神经或脑干）的脑转移瘤，考虑用多分次 SRS 替代单次 SRS。
> - 多达 10 个脑转移瘤的特定患者考虑单独使用 SRS。
> - 对于 5～10 个以上转移灶的患者，WBRT 仍然是一种有效的策略。接受 WBRT 的患者使用美金刚和海马保护的 IMRT 计划限制了神经认知功能下降。
> - V12 是预测单次 SRS 后放射性坏死风险的重要因素。
> - 由于发生远处脑转移的风险高，仅接受 SRS 的患者必须进行严格的 MRI 随访。
> - 对于接受 SRS 和免疫疗法的患者，在治疗后的 12 周之内可能会出现照射病灶的短暂扩大，即所谓的假性进展。早期影像学检查结果应在最初怀疑影像学进展后的 3 个月内进行。

八、病例介绍

（一）病例 1

患者，72 岁，有乳腺癌病史，曾接受手术和化疗，2 年后出现左侧肢体功能障碍，提示脑转移。增强 MRI 显示有 5 处脑部病变：4 处＜ 2.0cm，1 处＞ 3.0cm。建议行 SRS 治疗，并使用厚度为 1.25mm 的热塑性面罩固定，进行 CT 扫描。将 CT 和 MR 图像融合后，勾画 GTV 和危及器官（organs at risk, OAR）。对所有病变没有进行 GTV 到 PTV 的外扩。SRS 计划是在 Varian TrueBeam STx 上采用容积调强治疗（volumetric modulated arc therapy, VMAT）进行实施。最大的病灶连续 3 天接受了 3×9Gy 的多分次 SRS；其他 4 个病灶接受剂量为 22Gy 的单次 SRS（图 18-2A）。治疗期间持续使用地塞米松，剂量为每天 4mg，然后在几天内逐渐停药。没有观察到与 SRS 相关的急性或长期毒性反应。在随后的随访中，MRI 显示所有治疗病变完全或部分缓解（图 18-2）。

（二）病例 2

一位 56 岁的 NSCLC 晚期患者因肝脏和肾上腺转移，首先接受了 6 周期含铂方案化疗。部分缓解后，CT 发现疾病进展（双肺多发小结节）。暂停化疗启用免疫疗法（纳武利尤单抗）。免疫治疗后的 6 个月，CT 和 MRI 检查发现 11 个 5～20mm 大小的脑部病灶。使用单个等中心动态共形弧（dynamic conformal arc, DCA）技术，所有病灶接受单次剂量为 22Gy 的无框架 SRS（图 18-3）。因颅外疾病保持稳定，因此继续进行免疫治疗。在 2 个月时进行了 MRI 检查，显示大多数病灶明显缩小，有些病灶完全消失（图 18-4）。在第 4 和 6 个月行 MRI 扫描显示颅内病灶稳定。在 9 个月时，CT 扫描显示颅外和颅内疾病进展，并在距离最初的 SRS 部位较远的地方出现多个且广泛的脑部病变。该患者在接受 WBRT 4 个月后死于颅内疾病进展。

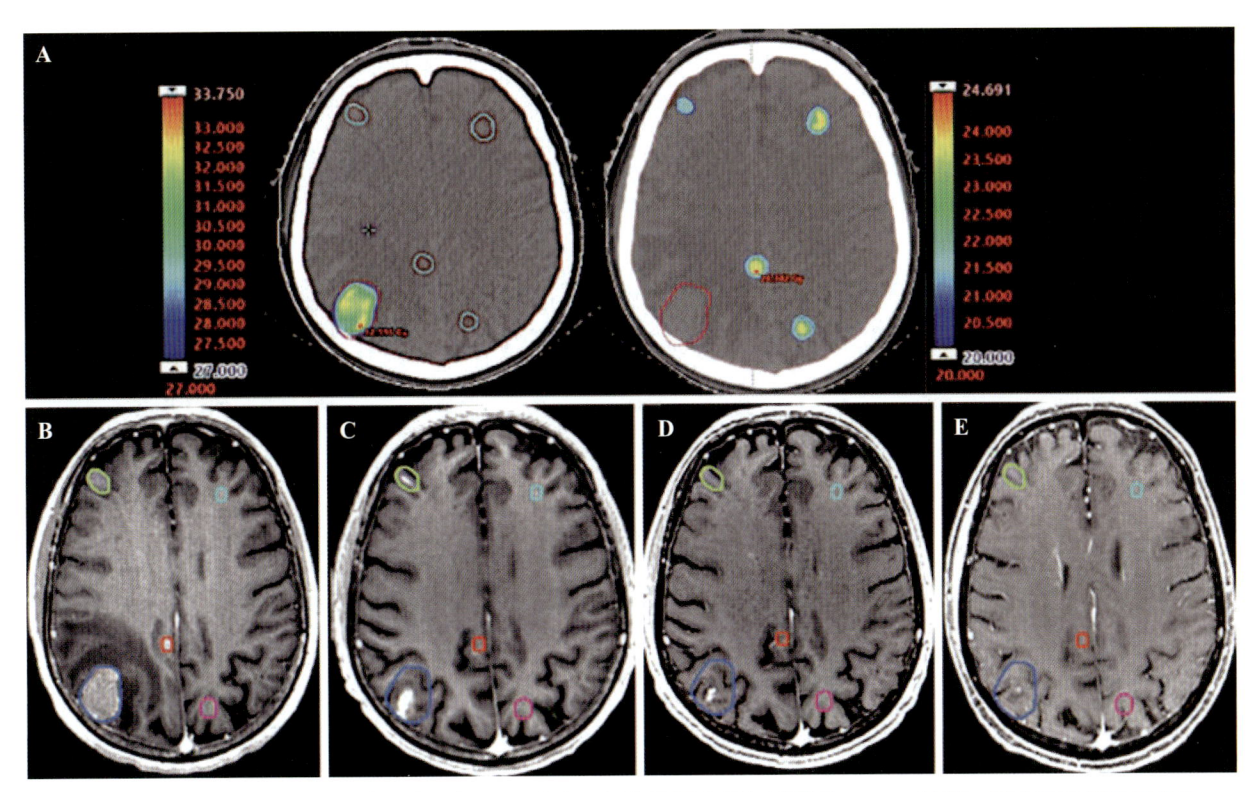

第 18 章 脑转移瘤治疗中的耐受剂量
Dose Tolerances in Brain Metastasis Management

▲ 图 18-2 存在 5 个脑转移瘤的患者行 SRS 治疗，制定基于直线加速器的 VMAT 计划；四个病灶接受了单分次的 SRS（22Gy）和一个病灶（蓝色轮廓）接受多分次 SRS（连续 3 天，9Gy/3 次）

图（A）中显示了多分次 SRS（左）和单次 SRS（右）的靶区体积 - 剂量分布。治疗前（B）和治疗后（C–E）MRI，T₁ 增强的横断面，分别在 2 个月（C），6 个月（D）和 12 个月（E）时的放射性反应

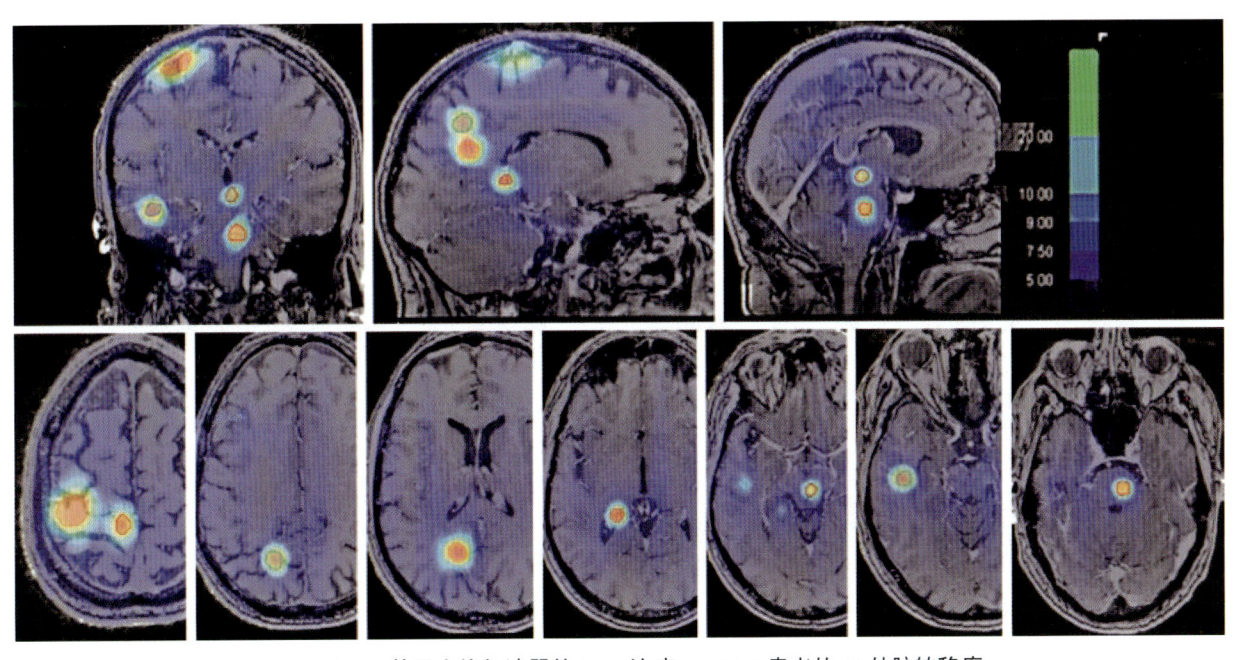

▲ 图 18-3 基于直线加速器的 SRS 治疗 NSCLC 患者的 11 处脑转移瘤

使用单个等中心动态共形弧技术，以单次剂量 22Gy 治疗所有靶区。经治疗的肿瘤总体积为 4.7cm³

249

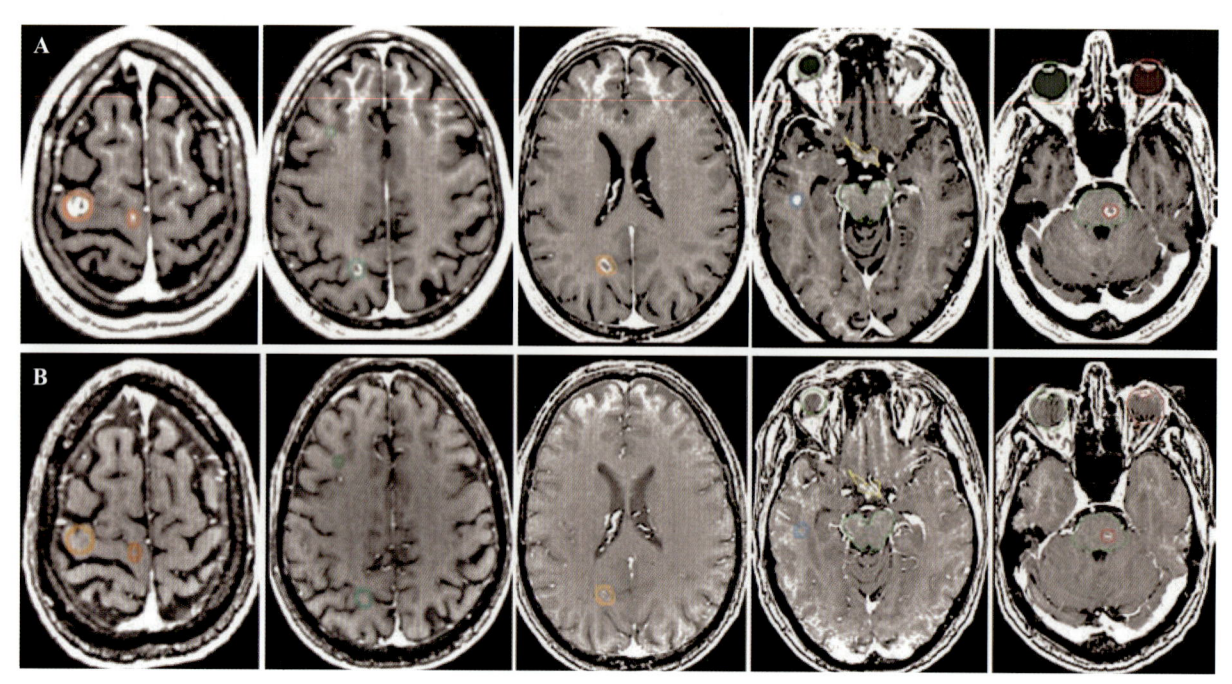

▲ 图 18-4　NSCLC 脑转移瘤对 SRS 的反应（A）在 SRS 之前，（B）在 SRS 之后

所有病灶均接受剂量为 22Gy 的单次 SRS（图 18-3）。SRS 后 2 个月的代表性轴向 T_1 增强 MRI 图像显示了所有治疗病变的完全或部分缓解

参考文献

[1] Aoyama H, Shirato H, Tago M, Nakagawa K, Toyoda T, Hatano K, et al. Stereotactic radiosurgery plus whole-brain radiation therapy vs stereotactic radiosurgery alone for treatment of brain metastases: a randomized controlled trial. JAMA. 2006;295(21):2483–91.

[2] Chang EL, Wefel JS, Hess KR, Allen PK, Lang FF, Kornguth DG, et al. Neurocognition in patients with brain metastases treated with radiosurgery or radiosurgery plus whole-brain irradiation: a randomised controlled trial. Lancet Oncol. 2009;10(11):1037–44.

[3] Kocher M, Soffietti R, Abacioglu U, Villà S, Fauchon F, Baumert BG, et al. Adjuvant whole-brain radiotherapy versus observation after radiosurgery or surgical resection of one to three cerebral metastases: results of the EORTC 22952-26001 study. J Clin Oncol. 2011;29(2):134–41.

[4] Brown PD, Jaeckle K, Ballman KV, Farace E, Cerhan JH, Anderson SK, et al. Effect of radiosurgery alone vs radiosurgery with whole brain radiation therapy on cognitive function in patients with 1–3 brain metastases: a randomized clinical trial. JAMA. 2016;316(4):401–9. Erratum in: JAMA. 2018;320(5):510.

[5] Shaw E, Scott C, Souhami L, Dinapoli R, Kline R, Loeffler J, et al. Single dose radiosurgical treatment of recurrent previously irradiated primary brain tumors and brain metastases: final report of RTOG protocol 90-05. Int J Radiat Oncol Biol Phys. 2000;47(2):291–8.

[6] Minniti G, Scaringi C, Paolini S, Lanzetta G, Romano A, Cicone F, et al. Single-fraction versus multifraction (3 × 9 Gy) stereotactic radiosurgery for large (>2 cm) brain metastases: a comparative analysis of local control and risk of radiation-induced brain necrosis. Int J Radiat Oncol Biol Phys. 2016;95: 1142–8.

[7] Minniti G, D'Angelillo RM, Scaringi C, Trodella LE, Clarke E, Matteucci P, et al. Fractionated stereotactic radiosurgery for patients with brain metastases. J Neuro-Oncol. 2014;117:295–301.

[8] Aoyama H, Shirato H, Onimaru R, Kagei K, Ikeda J, Ishii N, et al. Hypofractionated stereotactic radiotherapy alone without whole brain irradiation for patients with solitary and oligo brain metastasis using noninvasive fixation of the skull. Int J Radiat Oncol Biol Phys. 2003;56(3):793–800.

[9] Ernst-Stecken A, Ganslandt O, Lambrecht U, Sauer R, Grabenbauer G. Phase II trial of hypofractionated stereotactic radiotherapy for brain metastases: results and toxicity. Radiother Oncol. 2006;81(1):18–24.

[10] Murai T, Ogino H, Manabe Y, Iwabuchi M, Okumura T, Matsushita Y, et al. Fractionated stereotactic radiotherapy using CyberKnife for the treatment of large brain metastases:

[10] a dose escalation study. Clin Oncol (R Coll Radiol). 2014; 26(3):151–8.

[11] Kim JW, Park HR, Lee JM, Kim JW, Chung HT, Kim DG, et al. Fractionated stereotactic gamma knife radiosurgery for large brain metastases: a retrospective, single center study. PLoS One. 2016;11:e0163304.

[12] Lehrer EJ, Peterson JL, Zaorsky NG, Brown PD, Sahgal A, Chiang VL, et al. Single versus multifraction stereotactic radiosurgery for large brain metastases: an international meta-analysis of 24 trials. Int J Radiat Oncol Biol Phys. 2019;103(3):618–30.

[13] Fowler JF. 21 years of biologically effective dose. Br J Radiol. 2010;83(991):554–68.

[14] Kirkpatrick JP, Meyer JJ, Marks LB. The linearquadratic model is inappropriate to model high dose per fraction effects in radiosurgery. Semin Radiat Oncol. 2008;18(4):240–3.

[15] Joiner M. Quantifying cell kill and survival. In: Joiner M, Van der Kogel A, editors. Basic clinical radiobiology. 4th ed. London: Hodder Arnold; 2009. p. 102–19.

[16] Lawrence YR, Li XA, el Naqa I, Hahn CA, Marks LB, Merchant TE, et al. Radiation dose-volume effects in the brain. Int J Radiat Oncol Biol Phys. 2010;76(3 Suppl):S20–7.

[17] Marks LB, Yorke ED, Jackson A, Ten Haken RK, Constine LS, Eisbruch A, et al. Use of normal tissue complication probability models in the clinic. Int J Radiat Oncol Biol Phys. 2010;76(3 Suppl):S10–9.

[18] Mayo C, Martel MK, Marks LB, Flickinger J, Nam J, Kirkpatrick J. Radiation dose-volume effects of optic nerves and chiasm. Int J Radiat Oncol Biol Phys. 2010;76(3 Suppl):S28–35.

[19] Kirkpatrick JP, van der Kogel AJ, Schultheiss TE. Radiation dose-volume effects in the spinal cord. Int J Radiat Oncol Biol Phys. 2010;76(3 Suppl):S42–9.

[20] Kirkpatrick JP, Marks LB, Mayo CS, Lawrence YR, Bhandare N, Ryu S. Estimating normal tissue toxicity in radiosurgery of the CNS: application and limitations of QUANTEC. J Radiosurg SBRT. 2011;1:95–107.

[21] Blonigen BJ, Steinmetz RD, Levin L, Lamba MA, Warnick RE, Breneman JC. Irradiated volume as a predictor of brain radionecrosis after linear accelerator stereotactic radiosurgery. Int J Radiat Oncol Biol Phys. 2010;77(4):996–1001.

[22] Minniti G, Clarke E, Lanzetta G, Osti MF, Trasimeni G, Bozzao A, et al. Stereotactic radiosurgery for brain metastases: analysis of outcome and risk of brain radionecrosis. Radiat Oncol. 2011;6:48.

[23] Williams BJ, Suki D, Fox BD, Pelloski CE, Maldaun MV, Sawaya RE, et al. Stereotactic radiosurgery for metastatic brain tumors: a comprehensive review of complications. J Neurosurg. 2009;111(3):439–48.

[24] Chao ST, Ahluwalia MS, Barnett GH, Stevens GH, Murphy ES, Stockham AL, et al. Challenges with the diagnosis and treatment of cerebral radiation necrosis. Int J Radiat Oncol Biol Phys. 2013;87(3):449–57.

[25] Dequesada IM, Quisling RG, Yachnis A, Friedman WA. Can standard magnetic resonance imaging reliably distinguish recurrent tumor from radiation necrosis after radiosurgery for brain metastases? A radiographic-pathological study. Neurosurgery. 2008;63:898–904.

[26] Vellayappan B, Tan CL, Yong C, Khor LK, Koh WY, Yeo TT, et al. Diagnosis and management of radiation necrosis in patients with brain metastases. Front Oncol. 2018;8:395.

[27] Verma N, Cowperthwaite MC, Burnett MG, Markey MK. Differentiating tumor recurrence from treatment necrosis: a review of neuro-oncologic imaging strategies. Neuro-Oncology. 2013;15(5):515–34.

[28] Galldiks N, Stoffels G, Filss CP, Piroth MD, Sabel M, Ruge MI, et al. Role of O-(2-(18)F-fluoroethyl)- L-tyrosine PET for differentiation of local recurrent brain metastasis from radiation necrosis. J Nucl Med. 2012;53(9):1367–74.

[29] Terakawa Y, Tsuyuguchi N, Iwai Y, Yamanaka K, Higashiyama S, Takami T, et al. Diagnostic accuracy of 11C-methionine PET for differentiation of recurrent brain tumors from radiation necrosis after radiotherapy. J Nucl Med. 2008;49(5):694–9.

[30] Cicone F, Minniti G, Romano A, Papa A, Scaringi C, Tavanti F, et al. Accuracy of F-DOPA PET and perfusion-MRI for differentiating radionecrotic from progressive brain metastases after radiosurgery. Eur J Nucl Med Mol Imaging. 2015;42(1):103–11.

[31] Langen KJ, Galldiks N. Update on amino acid PET of brain tumours. Curr Opin Neurol. 2018;31(4):354–61.

[32] Andrews DW, Scott CB, Sperduto PW, Flanders AE, Gaspar LE, Schell MC, et al. Whole brain radiation therapy with or without stereotactic radiosurgery boost for patients with one to three brain metastases: phase III results of the RTOG 9508 randomised trial. Lancet. 2004;363(9422):1665–72.

[33] Korytko T, Radivoyevitch T, Colussi V, Wessels BW, Pillai K, Maciunas RJ, et al. 12 Gy gamma knife radiosurgical volume is a predictor for radiation necrosis in non-AVM intracranial tumors. Int J Radiat Oncol Biol Phys. 2006;64(2):419–24.

[34] Meeks SL, Buatti JM, Foote KD, Friedman WA, Bova FJ. Calculation of cranial nerve complication probability for acoustic neuroma radiosurgery. Int J Radiat Oncol Biol Phys. 2000;47(3):597–602.

[35] Foote KD, Friedman WA, Buatti JM, Meeks SL, Bova FJ, Kubilis PS. Analysis of risk factors associated with radiosurgery for vestibular schwannoma. J Neurosurg. 2001;95(3):440–9.

[36] Mayo C, Yorke E, Merchant TE. Radiation associated brainstem injury. Int J Radiat Oncol Biol Phys. 2010;76(3 Suppl):S36–41.

[37] Lin CS, Selch MT, Lee SP, Wu JK, Xiao F, Hong DS, et al. Accelerator-based stereotactic radiosurgery for brainstem metastases. Neurosurgery. 2012;70(4):953–8.

[38] Trifiletti DM, Lee CC, Kano H, Cohen J, JanopaulNaylor J, Alonso-Basanta M, et al. Stereotactic radiosurgery for brainstem metastases: an international cooperative study to define response and toxicity. Int J Radiat Oncol Biol Phys. 2016;96(2):280–8.

[39] Timmerman RD. An overview of hypofractionation and introduction to this issue of seminars in radiation oncology. Semin Radiat Oncol. 2008;18(4):215–22.

[40] Tishler RB, Loeffler JS, Lunsford LD, Duma C, Alexander E 3rd, Kooy HM, et al. Tolerance of cranial nerves of the cavernous sinus to radiosurgery. Int J Radiat Oncol Biol Phys. 1993;27(2):215–21.

[41] Leber KA, Berglöff J, Pendl G. Dose-response tolerance of the visual pathways and cranial nerves of the cavernous sinus to stereotactic radiosurgery. J Neurosurg. 1998;88(1):43–50.

[42] Stafford SL, Pollock BE, Leavitt JA, Foote RL, Brown PD, Link MJ, et al. A study on the radiation tolerance of the optic nerves and chiasm after stereotactic radiosurgery. Int J Radiat Oncol Biol Phys. 2003;55(5):1177–81.

[43] Leavitt JA, Stafford SL, Link MJ, Pollock BE. Longterm evaluation of radiation-induced optic neuropathy after single-fraction stereotactic radiosurgery. Int J Radiat Oncol Biol Phys. 2013;87(3):524–7.

[44] Pollock BE, Link MJ, Leavitt JA, Stafford SL. Dosevolume analysis of radiation-induced optic neuropathy after single-fraction stereotactic radiosurgery. Neurosurgery. 2014;75(4):456–60.

[45] Hiniker SM, Modlin LA, Choi CY, Atalar B, Seiger K, Binkley MS, et al. Dose-response modeling of the visual pathway tolerance to single-fraction and hypofractionated stereotactic radiosurgery. Semin Radiat Oncol. 2016;26(2):97–104.

[46] Adler JR Jr, Gibbs IC, Puataweepong P, Chang SD. Visual field preservation after multisession cyberknife radiosurgery for perioptic lesions. Neurosurgery. 2006;59(2):244–54.

[47] Killory BD, Kresl JJ, Wait SD, Ponce FA, Porter R, White WL. Hypofractionated CyberKnife radiosurgery for perichiasmatic pituitary adenomas: early results. Neurosurgery. 2009;64(2 Suppl): A19–25.

[48] Iwata H, Sato K, Tatewaki K, Yokota N, Inoue M, Baba Y, et al. Hypofractionated stereotactic radiotherapy with CyberKnife for nonfunctioning pituitary adenoma: high local control with low toxicity. NeuroOncology. 2011;13(8):916–22.

[49] Liao HI, Wang CC, Wei KC, Chang CN, Hsu YH, Lee ST, et al. Fractionated stereotactic radiosurgery using the Novalis system for the management of pituitary adenomas close to the optic apparatus. J Clin Neurosci. 2014;21(1):111–5.

[50] Minniti G, Esposito V, Clarke E, Scaringi C, Bozzao A, Falco T, et al. Fractionated stereotactic radiosurgery for patients with skull base metastases from systemic cancer involving the anterior visual pathway. Radiat Oncol. 2014;9:110.

[51] Tsao MN, Xu W, Wong RK, Lloyd N, Laperriere N, Sahgal A, et al. Whole brain radiotherapy for the treatment of newly diagnosed multiple brain metastases. Cochrane Database Syst Rev. 2018;1:CD003869.

[52] Guerrieri M, Wong K, Ryan G, Millward M, Quong G, Ball DL. A randomised phase III study of palliative radiation with concomitant carboplatin for brain metastases from non-small cell carcinoma of lung. Lung Cancer. 2004;46(1):107–11.

[53] Knisely J, Berkey B, Chakravarti A, Yung AWK, Curran WJ, Robins HI, et al. A phase III study of conventional radiation therapy plus thalidomide versus conventional radiation therapy for multiple brain metastases (RTOG 0118). Int J Radiat Oncol Biol Phys. 2008;71(1):79–86.

[54] Lee DH, Han J-Y, Kim HT, Yoon SJ, Pyo HR, Cho KH, et al. Primary chemotherapy for newly diagnosed nonsmall cell lung cancer patients with synchronous brain metastases compared with whole-brain radiotherapy administered first. Results of a randomized pilot study. Cancer. 2008;113(1):143–9.

[55] Mornex F, Thomas L, Mohr P, Hauschild A, Delaunay MM, Lesimple T, et al. A prospective randomized multicentre phase III trial of fotemustine plus whole brain irradiation versus fotemustine alone in cerebral metastases of malignant melanoma. Melanoma Res. 2003;13(1):97–103.

[56] Neuhaus T, Ko Y, Muller RP, Grabenbauer GG, Hedde JP, Schueller H, et al. A phase III trial of topotecan and whole brain radiation therapy for patients with CNS-metastases due to lung cancer. Br J Cancer. 2009;100(2):291–7.

[57] Postmus PE, Haaxma-Reiche H, Smit EF, Groen HJ, Karnicka H, Lewinski T, et al. Treatment of brain metastases of small-cell lung cancer: comparing teniposide and teniposide with whole-brain radiotherapy–a phase III study of the European Organization for the Research and Treatment of Cancer Lung Cancer Cooperative Group. J Clin Oncol. 2000;18(19):3400–8.

[58] Robinet G, Thomas P, Breton JL, Léna H, Gouva S, Dabouis G, et al. Results of a phase III study of early versus delayed whole brain radiotherapy with concurrent cisplatin and vinorelbine combination in inoperable brain metastasis of non-small-cell lung cancer: Groupe Français de Pneumo-Cancérologie (GFPC) Protocol 95-1. Ann Oncol. 2001;12(1):59–67.

[59] Sperduto PW, Wang M, Robins HI, Schell MC, Werner-Wasik M, Komaki R, et al. A phase 3 trial of whole brain radiation therapy and stereotactic radiosurgery alone versus WBRT and SRS with temozolomide or erlotinib for non-small cell lung cancer and 1–3 brain metastases: radiation Therapy Oncology Group 0320. Int J Radiat Oncol Biol Phys. 2013;85(5):1312–8.

[60] Ushio Y, Arita N, Hayakawa T, Mogami H, Hasegawa H, Bitoh S, et al. Chemotherapy of brain metastases from lung carcinoma: a controlled randomized study. Neurosurgery. 1991;28(2):201–5.

[61] Pesce GA, Klingbiel D, Ribi K, Zouhair A, von Moos R, Schlaeppi M, et al. Outcome, quality of life and cognitive function of patients with brain metastases from non-small cell lung cancer treated with whole brain radiotherapy combined with gefitinib or temozolomide. A randomised phase II trial of the Swiss Group for Clinical Cancer Research (SAKK 70/03). Eur J Cancer. 2012;48(3):377–84.

[62] Welsh JW, Komaki R, Amini A, Munsell MF, Unger W, Allen PK, et al. Phase II trial of erlotinib plus concurrent whole-brain radiation therapy for patients with brain metastases from non-small-cell lung cancer. J Clin Oncol. 2013;31(7):895–902.

[63] Jiang T, Su C, Li X, Zhao C, Zhou F, Ren S, et al. EGFR TKIs

plus WBRT demonstrated no survival benefit other than that of TKIs alone in patients with NSCLC and EGFR mutation and brain metastases. J Thorac Oncol. 2016;11(10):1718–28.

[64] Anker CJ, Grossmann KF, Atkins MB, Suneja G, Tarhini AA, Kirkwood JM. Avoiding severe toxicity from combined BRAF inhibitor and radiation treatment: consensus guidelines from the Eastern Cooperative Oncology Group (ECOG). Int J Radiat Oncol Biol Phys. 2016;95(2):632–46.

[65] Williams NL, Wuthrick EJ, Kim H, Palmer JD, Garg S, Eldredge-Hindy H, et al. Phase 1 study of ipilimumab combined with whole brain radiation therapy or radiosurgery for melanoma patients with brain metastases. Int J Radiat Oncol Biol Phys. 2017;99(1):22–30.

[66] Yang WC, Xiao F, Shih JY, Ho CC, Chen YF, Tseng HM, et al. Epidermal growth factor receptor mutation predicts favorable outcomes in non-small cell lung cancer patients with brain metastases treated with stereotactic radiosurgery. Radiother Oncol. 2018;126(2):368–74.

[67] Robin TP, Camidge DR, Stuhr K, Nath SK, Breeze RE, Pacheco JM, et al. Excellent outcomes with radiosurgery for multiple brain metastases in ALK and EGFR driven non-small cell lung cancer. J Thorac Oncol. 2018;13(5):715–20.

[68] Yomo S, Oda K. Impacts of EGFR-mutation status and EGFR-TKI on the efficacy of stereotactic radiosurgery for brain metastases from non-small cell lung adenocarcinoma: a retrospective analysis of 133 consecutive patients. Lung Cancer. 2018;119:120–6.

[69] Parsai S, Miller JA, Juloori A, Chao ST, Kotecha R, Mohammadi AM, et al. Stereotactic radiosurgery with concurrent lapatinib is associated with improved local control for HER2-positive breast cancer brain metastases. J Neurosurg. 2019;8:1–9.

[70] Ly D, Bagshaw HP, Anker CJ, Tward JD, Grossmann KF, Jensen RL, et al. Local control after stereotactic radiosurgery for brain metastases in patients with melanoma with and without BRAF mutation and treatment. J Neurosurg. 2015;123(2):395–401.

[71] Gallaher IS, Watanabe Y, DeFor TE, Dusenbery KE, Lee CK, Hunt MA, et al. BRAF mutation is associated with improved local control of melanoma brain metastases treated with gamma knife radiosurgery. Front Oncol. 2016;6:107.

[72] Xu Z, Lee CC, Ramesh A, Mueller AC, Schlesinger D, Cohen-Inbar O, et al. BRAF V600E mutation and BRAF kinase inhibitors in conjunction with stereotactic radiosurgery for intracranial melanoma metastases. J Neurosurg. 2017;126(3):726–34.

[73] Mastorakos P, Xu Z, Yu J, Hess J, Qian J, Chatrath A, et al. BRAF V600 mutation and BRAF kinase inhibitors in conjunction with stereotactic radiosurgery for intracranial melanoma metastases: a multicenter retrospective study. Neurosurgery. 2019;84(4):868–80.

[74] Mathew M, Tam M, Ott PA, Pavlick AC, Rush SC, Donahue BR, et al. Ipilimumab in melanoma with limited brain metastases treated with stereotactic radiosurgery. Melanoma Res. 2013;23(3):191–5.

[75] Kiess AP, Wolchok JD, Barker CA, Postow MA, Tabar V, Huse JT, et al. Stereotactic radiosurgery for melanoma brain metastases in patients receiving ipilimumab: safety profile and efficacy of combined treatment. Int J Radiat Oncol Biol Phys. 2015;92(2):368–75.

[76] Ahmed KA, Abuodeh YA, Echevarria MI, Arrington JA, Stallworth DG, Hogue C, et al. Clinical outcomes of melanoma brain metastases treated with stereotactic radiosurgery and anti-PD-1 therapy, anti-CTLA-4 therapy, BRAF/MEK inhibitors, BRAF inhibitor, or conventional chemotherapy. Ann Oncol. 2016;27(12):2288–94.

[77] Qian JM, Yu JB, Kluger HM, Chiang VL. Timing and type of immune checkpoint therapy affect the early radiographic response of melanoma brain metastases to stereotactic radiosurgery. Cancer. 2016;122(19):3051–8.

[78] Patel KR, Chowdhary M, Switchenko JM, Kudchadkar R, Lawson DH, Cassidy RJ, et al. BRAF inhibitor and stereotactic radiosurgery is associated with an increased risk of radiation necrosis. Melanoma Res. 2016;26(4):387–94.

[79] Chen L, Douglass J, Kleinberg L, Ye X, Marciscano AE, Forde PM, et al. Concurrent immune checkpoint inhibitors and stereotactic radiosurgery for brain metastases in non-small cell lung cancer, melanoma, and renal cell carcinoma. Int J Radiat Oncol Biol Phys. 2018;100(4):916–25.

[80] Minniti G, Anzellini D, Reverberi C, Cappellini GCA, Marchetti L, Bianciardi F, et al. Stereotactic radiosurgery combined with nivolumab or ipilimumab for patients with melanoma brain metastases: evaluation of brain control and toxicity. J Immunother Cancer. 2019;7(1):102.

[81] Okada H, Weller M, Huang R, Finocchiaro G, Gilbert MR, Wick W, et al. Immunotherapy response assessment in neuro-oncology: a report of the RANO working group. Lancet Oncol. 2015;16(15):e534–42.

[82] Minniti G, Scaringi C, Paolini S, Clarke E, Cicone F, Esposito V, et al. Repeated stereotactic radiosurgery for patients with progressive brain metastases. J Neuro-Oncol. 2016;126(1):91–7.

[83] McKay WH, McTyre ER, Okoukoni C, AlphonseSullivan NK, Ruiz J, Munley MT, et al. Repeat stereotactic radiosurgery as salvage therapy for locally recurrent brain metastases previously treated with radiosurgery. J Neurosurg. 2017;127(1):148–56.

[84] Koffer P, Chan J, Rava P, Gorovets D, Ebner D, Savir G, et al. Repeat stereotactic radiosurgery for locally recurrent brain metastases. World Neurosurg. 2017;104:589–93.

[85] Rana N, Pendyala P, Cleary RK, Luo G, Zhao Z, Chambless LB, et al. Long-term outcomes after salvage stereotactic radiosurgery (SRS) following infield failure of initial SRS for brain metastases. Front Oncol. 2017;7:279.

[86] Balermpas P, Stera S, Müller von der Grün J, Loutfi-Krauss B, Forster MT, Wagner M, et al. Repeated in-field radiosurgery for locally recurrent brain metastases: feasibility, results and survival in a heavily treated patient cohort. PLoS One.

[87] Yamamoto M, Serizawa T, Shuto T, Akabane A, Higuchi Y, Kawagishi J, et al. Stereotactic radiosurgery for patients with multiple brain metastases (JLGK0901): a multi-institutional prospective observational study. Lancet Oncol. 2014;15(4):387–95.

[88] Greto D, Scoccianti S, Compagnucci A, Arilli C, Casati M, Francolini G, et al. Gamma knife radiosurgery in the management of single and multiple brain metastases. Clin Neurol Neurosurg. 2016;141:43–7.

[89] Yamamoto M, Serizawa T, Higuchi Y, Sato Y, Kawagishi J, Yamanaka K, et al. A multi-institutional prospective observational study of stereotactic radiosurgery for patients with multiple brain metastases (JLGK0901 study update): irradiation-related complications and long-term maintenance of mini-mental state examination scores. Int J Radiat Oncol Biol Phys. 2017;99(1):31–40.

[90] Knoll MA, Oermann EK, Yang AI, Paydar I, Steinberger J, Collins B, et al. Survival of patients with multiple intracranial metastases treated with stereotactic radiosurgery: does the number of tumors matter? Am J Clin Oncol. 2018;41(5):425–31.

[91] Brown PD, Pugh S, Laack NN, Wefel JS, Khuntia D, Meyers C, et al. Memantine for the prevention of cognitive dysfunction in patients receiving whole-brain radiotherapy: a randomized, doubleblind, placebo-controlled trial. Neuro-Oncology. 2013;15(10):1429–37.

[92] Gondi V, Pugh SL, Tome WA, Caine C, Corn B, Kanner A, et al. Preservation of memory with conformal avoidance of the hippocampal neural stemcell compartment during whole-brain radiotherapy for brain metastases (RTOG 0933): a phase II multiinstitutional trial. J Clin Oncol. 2014;32(34):3810–6.

[93] Brown PD, Gondi V, Pugh S, Tome WA, Wefel JS, Armstrong TS, et al. For NRG Oncology. Hippocampal avoidance during whole-brain radiotherapy plus memantine for patients with brain metastases: Phase III trial NRG Oncology CC001. J Clin Oncol. 2020;38:1019–29.

第 19 章 放射外科计划的质量评估
Evaluation of the Quality of a Radiosurgery Plan

Evan M. Thomas　Richard A. Popple　John B. Fiveash　**著**

刘渊渊　张子健　**译**

邵其刚　**校**

一、背景

长期以来，放射外科已经成为替代 CNS 内组织侵入性切除或消融的一种安全、可行且具有成本效益的方法。放射外科的应用越来越广泛，作用持续增长。现在，对于肿瘤放疗医生和神经外科医生来说，熟悉放射外科的原理和实践是他们必须掌握的职业技能。

放射外科计划的质量评估不仅需要考虑治疗的临床疗效，同时也需要考虑诱发相关毒性的可能性。对放射外科计划进行一致性自评估，和计划间的对比评估是提高治疗质量的有效方法。

应用数值指标来评价放射外科计划质量，可以量化计划实现临床目标的能力。因为不同的临床情景可能有不同的临床目标，目前，已经建立了大量指数，在不同临床情况下，每一个指数都有其优缺点。设计放射外科计划的人员应该了解临床医生在特定计划中的目标，并选择一个最合适的指数，描述该临床目标的。

二、剂量-体积度量

用于放射外科计划评估的数值指数来自于剂量-体积度量。表 19-1 定义了本章考虑的数值指数中所使用的剂量体积度量。

表 19-1　本章中用于计划质量描述的各种度量和指数列表

度　量	描　述
TV	靶区体积为大体肿瘤区（GTV）或者计划靶区（PTV）而设定的实际靶区覆盖的体积
$TV_{<PI}$	受到小于处方剂量照射的靶体积
PIV	处方等剂量体积受到不小于处方剂量照射的体积
TV_{PIV}	受到处方剂量照射的靶区的体积
HTV_{PI}	受到不小于处方剂量照射的健康（非靶区）组织的体积
$PIV_{50\%}$	接受至少一半处方剂量的体积
V12Gy（cm³）	接受至少 12Gy 剂量的体积（cm³）
D_{Rx}	处方剂量
D_{max}	给定体积的最大剂量
D_{min}	给定体积的最小剂量
D_{mean}	给定体积的平均剂量
ID	积分剂量（一个结构接受的平均剂量与其体积的乘积）

（一）适形指数

适形指数被设计用于描述处方剂量与靶区重合的紧密程度。在一个绝对理想的计划中，处方剂量分布将刚好覆盖靶区，并且对于大多数适形指数，其理想值是 1。然而，计划者可能在一个度量中还想获得的其他方面的处方剂量覆盖信息，如靶区内的最大或最小剂量、处方等剂量与靶区的几何对齐程度及靶区附近重要器官的保护程度。Shaw 或 RTOG 适形指数是最简单的适形指数，其定义为受到处方剂量照射的组织体积与靶区体积的比值。图 19-1 说明了三种 RTOG 适形指数在理想值时未能反映出计划不适形的情形。正因为如此，人们又开发了大量的综合适形指数，用于衡量计划质量的其他指标。

1. Shaw/RTOG 适形指数

$$\text{RTOG CI} = \frac{\text{PIV}}{\text{TV}}$$

这是最简单和最常用的适形指数[2]，来源于 1993 年的 RTOG 放射外科指南。简单地说，就是处方剂量照射的体积除以靶区体积。如图 19-1 所示，它可能在图中的几种情况下错误地显示了良好的适形性，但是大多数现代治疗计划系统对这些错误都有很强的稳健性。其中一些错误情形的出现，促使提出了改进的适形指数定义，以解释靶区未覆盖的情况。靶区体积越大，计划者就越容易达到接近为 1 的适形指数。对于未覆盖的计划，该值 < 1，对于覆盖过度的计划，该值 > 1。

2. ICRU 适形指数

$$\text{ICRU CI} = \frac{\text{TV}}{\text{PIV}} = \text{RTOG CI}^{-1}$$

Shaw/RTOG 适形指数的倒数，最初是由 Dave Larson 博士提出的。它可以作为一种偏向喜好来使用，但没有特别的优势。对于覆盖不足的计划，此值 > 1，对于覆盖过度的计划，此值 < 1。

3. 辐射适形指数或治疗不足率

$$\text{RCI} = \frac{\text{TV}_{\text{PIV}}}{\text{TV}} \text{ 或者 } \text{RCI} = \frac{\text{TV}}{\text{TV}_{\text{PIV}}}$$

该指数首次由 Knös 等[3] 报道用于常规放疗，但 Paddick[4] 将其作为放射外科度量纳入了 Paddick 适形指数。该指数首次应用了受到处方

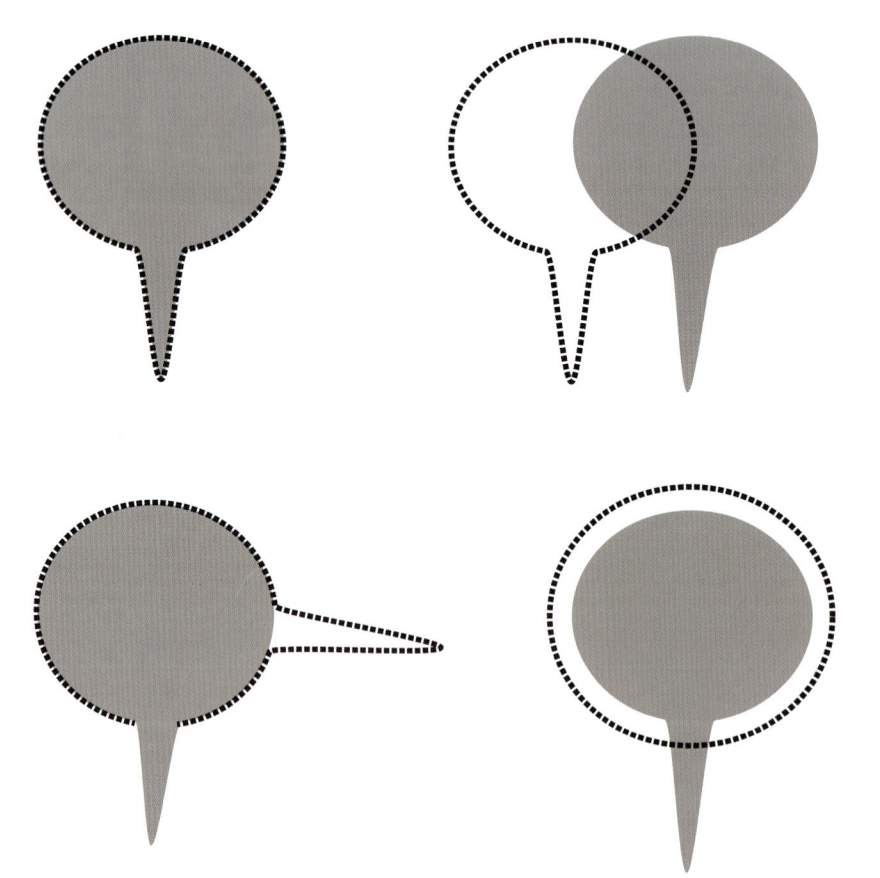

◀ **图 19-1** PV/TV=1 的四种可能性

经 Elsevier 许可转载，引自 Feuvret 等[1]

剂量照射的靶区的体积。最初，作者在会议记录[5]中将其描述为 TV_{PIV}/TV，但后来在出版物中报道为 TV/TV_{PIV} 以符合作者的偏好，即随着计划变得更加适形，度量朝着 1 的方向减少。后来 Paddick[4] 将其称为"治疗不足率"，Lomax[6] 将其简称为"适形指数"。

4. 过度治疗率或选择性指数或正常组织适形指数

$$健康组织适形指数: = \frac{TV_{PIV}}{PIV}$$

Paddick[4] 首先将这一指数描述为"过度治疗率"，是 Paddick 适形指数的一个组成部分。后来，Regis 等[7] 将其称为"选择性指数"。最后，Lomax 等[6] 将其更名为"正常组织适形指数"，通过计算靶区受处方等剂量照射的体积在全部处方等剂量体积的比例，来量化正常组织的受照射情况。因为计算受处方等剂量照射的靶体积仅是对正常组织受照射情况的间接评估，所以该指数在评估正常组织受照射时不是特别有效。

5. Paddick 适形指数

$$Paddick\ CI = \frac{TV_{PIV}^2}{TV \times PIV}$$

Ian Paddick[4] 在指出了 RTOG 适形指数的上述缺点后，于 2000 年提出了该适形指数。事实上，这是综合了他之前描述的相关度量、过度治疗率和治疗不足率的产物。Paddick 适形指数的理想值是 1，但总是小于 1，并且随计划质量提高而趋近于 1。如图 19-2 所示，它同时体现了靶区超覆盖、欠覆盖和（或）处方剂量与靶区的不重合情况。将这三者结合起来有一个缺点，即无法单独通过该值立即确定计划缺陷的来源。虽然大多数治疗计划系统在默认情况下不给出该指数值，但是其容易通过计算得到或通过编写脚本得到，而且非常有用。此外，该指数可以被当作 0~100 的质量评分，如一个 PCI=0.95 的计划可以被认为是 95% 的适形计划，这有助于新的计划者对该计划有更直观的了解。

6. 新适形指数（NCI）/ Nakamura's CI

$$NCI = \frac{TV \times PIV}{TV_{PIV}^2} = Paddick\ CI^{-1}$$

该指数是 Paddick 适形指数的倒数[8]。与 Paddick CI 相比，它没有实际的优势，只是一些计划者可能更喜欢他们的指数从大于 1 而不是小于 1 开始趋近于 1。

7. 几何适形指数

$$g = LUF + OHTF$$

$$LUF = \frac{TV_{<PI}}{TV}$$

$$HTOF = \frac{HTV_{PI}}{TV}$$

其中 LUF 表示病灶剂量不足体积比（或未受到处方等剂量照射的靶区体积比），HTOF 表示正常组织剂量过量体积比（接受处方剂量的非靶区组织体积与靶区组织的比值）。

几何适形指数是由 Saint-Anne，Lariboisiere，Tenon（SALT）[9] 小组设计的，目的是量化整体治疗质量，特别是接受放射外科治疗的动静脉畸形（arteriovenous malformations，AVM）队列。对于该指数，几何适形性在最小值时是最佳的，因为它是两个指数的总和，每个指数都反映了计划缺陷的一个方面。

8. 联合适形指数（COIN）

$$COIN = CN \times \prod_{i=1}^{N_{CO}}\left[1 - \frac{V_{COref,i}}{V_{COi}}\right]$$

N_{CO}：危及器官（CO）数量。

V_{COref}：接受参考剂量的危机器官体积。

V_{COi}：危及器官体积（图 19-3）。

Baltas 等[10] 将适形指数与一个附加指数结合起来，不仅可以评估处方剂量的适形性，还可以评估毗邻危及器官接受参考剂量照射的风险。它最初适用于近距离放射治疗，但同样适用于 EBRT 或 SRS。危及器官的参考剂量不需要与处方剂量相同。例如，视交叉脑膜瘤的放射外科治疗计划可以在计算适形指数时使用 14Gy 的处方剂

治疗计划	参数	RTOG PIV/TV	RCI TV$_{PIV}$/TV	HTCI/SI TV$_{PIV}$/PIV	Paddick CI $\frac{TV_{PIV} \times TV_{PIV}}{TV \times V_{RI}}$
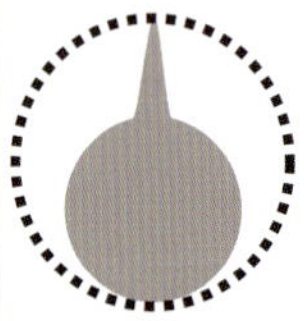	Tv = 5 cm³ PIV = 10 cm³ TV$_{PIV}$ = 5 cm³	2	1	0.50	0.50
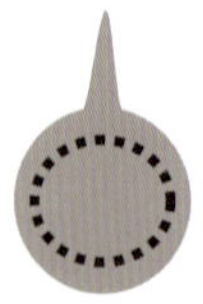	Tv = 5 cm³ PIV = 3 cm³ TV$_{PIV}$ = 3 cm³	0.60	0.60	1	0.60
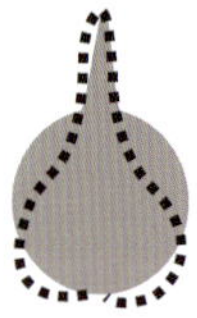	Tv = 5 cm³ PIV = 5 cm³ TV$_{PIV}$ = 4 cm³	1	0.80	0.80	0.64
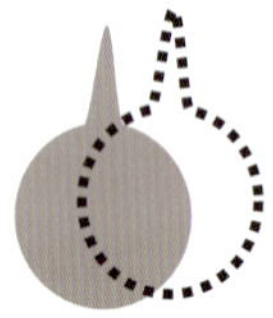	Tv = 5 cm³ PIV = 5 cm³ TV$_{PIV}$ = 2.5 cm³	1	0.50	0.50	0.25
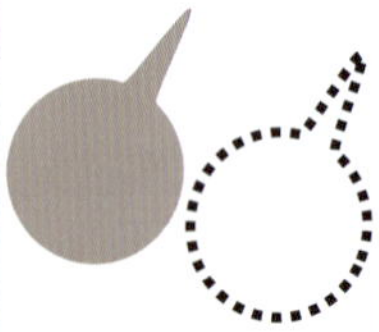	Tv = 5 cm³ PIV = 5 cm³ TV$_{PIV}$ = 0 cm³	1	0	0	0
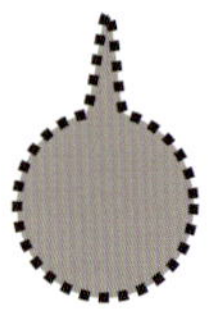	Tv = 5 cm³ PIV = 5 cm³ TV$_{PIV}$ = 5 cm³	1	1	1	1

▲ 图 19-2 以往的适形指数与 2000 年 Paddick 适形指数的比较

经 Elsevier 许可转载，引自 Feuvret 等[1]

量，在计算危及器官指数中使用 8Gy 的参考剂量。

（二）梯度指数

梯度指数通常测量靶区周围剂量衰减的一些方面，特别是处方等剂量与一半处方等剂量之间的陡度。更简单地说，梯度指数是中度等剂量体积紧密度的一种度量。

1. UF 梯度指数

$$CGIg = 100 - [100 \times (R_{Eff\ 50\%Rx} - R_{Eff,Rx}) - 0.3cm]$$

其中 R$_{Eff,\ 50\%Rx}$ 和 R$_{Eff,\ Rx}$ 分别是包含 PIV$_{50\%}$ 和 PIV 的球体的最小半径。UF 梯度指数是第一个

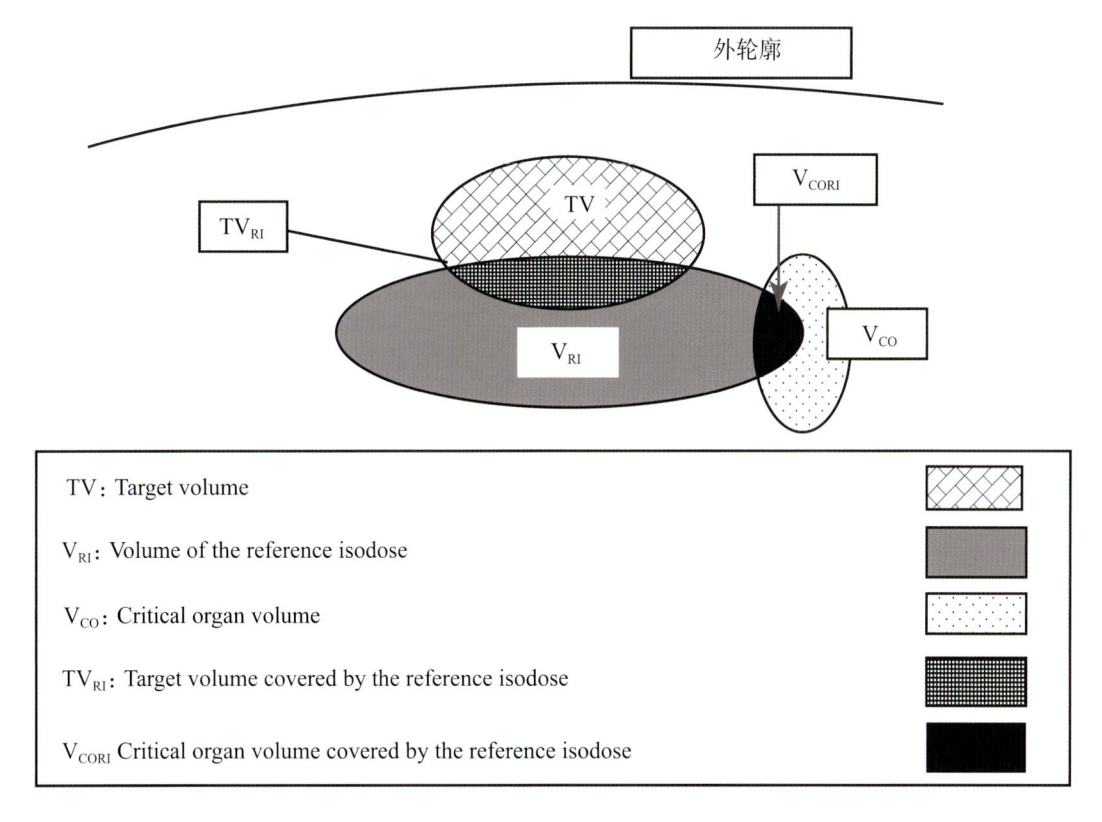

▲ 图 19-3 **COIN** 指数中使用的体积的图解

TV. 靶区体积；V_{RI}. 参考等剂量照射体积；V_{CO}. 重要器官体积；TV_{RI}. 参考等剂量覆盖的靶区体积；V_{CORI}. 参考等剂量覆盖的重要器官体积。经 Elsevier 许可转载，引自 Feuvret 等[1]

评价处方等剂量线与半处方等剂量线衰减陡度的梯度指数。其主要缺点是在某些治疗计划系统中难以计算有效等剂量曲线半径，并且它假设了在所有方向上都是各向同性衰减的。

2. Paddick/ 剂量梯度指数

$$\text{Paddick GI} = \frac{\text{PIV}_{50\%}}{\text{PIV}}$$

Paddick GI 可能是最常用的梯度指数。Paddick 于 2006 年[11]提出了一种简化剂量衰减度量计算的方法。他发现在日常使用中，计算等剂量体积的有效半径过于烦琐。Paddick GI 很容易计算，但在计划间的比较中并不是很有效。如果两个计划具有相同的 $\text{PIV}_{50\%}$，因为 PIV 是分母，适形性较差的计划将虚假地显示出较好的梯度。相反，即使 $\text{PIV}_{50\%}$ 相同，提高计划的适形性也会错误地显示更差的梯度指数。这种效应如图 19-4 所示。因此，不应使用此通用梯度指数比较适形性不同的计划。

3. R50% 或衰减指数（FI）

$$\text{FI} = \frac{\text{PIV}_{50\%}}{\text{TV}}$$

在 RTOG0915 研究中，R50% 首次被广泛用于计划质量的度量，该研究比较了医学上不能手术的非小细胞肺癌患者的 SBRT 计划。与 Paddick 梯度指数相比，它的优势是不依赖于给定计划的适形性质量。

（三）覆盖范围

最小覆盖范围

$$\text{Coverage} = \frac{D_{\min}}{D_{Rx}}$$

覆盖范围是最初的 RTOG 放射外科指南中的另一个量化指数。显然，靶区中的最小剂量应尽可能的接近处方剂量。

参数	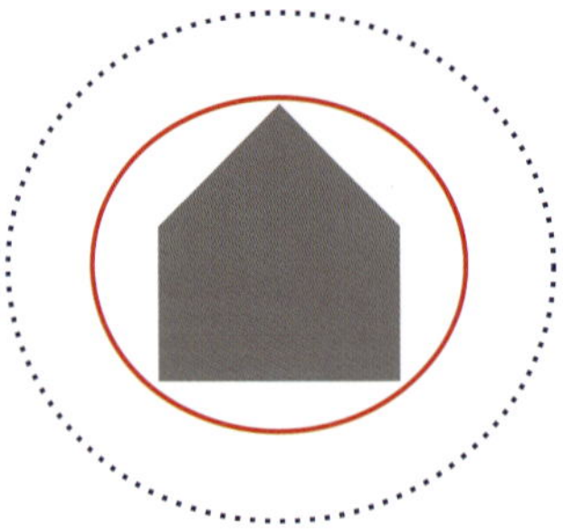 TV=1.5　　PIV=2.25　　PIV$_{50\%}$=9.0	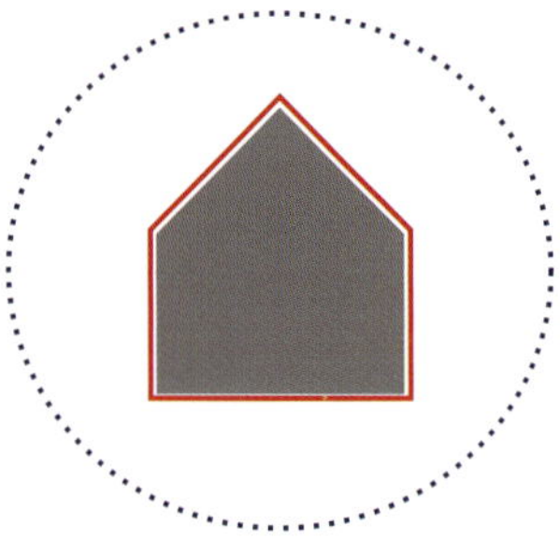 TV=1.5　　PIV=1.55　　PIV$_{50\%}$=9.0
RTOG CI	1.5	1.03
Paddick CI	0.67	0.97
Paddick GI	4	5.81
R50%	6	6

▲ 图 19-4　具有相同 PIV$_{50\%}$ 但不同适形指数的剂量分布的梯度指数

红色实线表示处方剂量，蓝色虚线表示处方剂量的一半。请注意，虽然右边的计划是一个更适形的计划，虽然具有相同的 PIV$_{50\%}$，但它的 Paddick GI 更差

（四）均匀性

1. 均匀性（RTOG）

$$\text{Homogeneity} = \frac{D_{\max}}{D_{\text{Rx}}}$$

RTOG 定义的均匀性指数是最大剂量与处方剂量的比值。按照惯例，如果 > 2，则视为轻微违反协议；如果 > 5，则视为严重违反协议。某些中心试图通过保持靶区最大剂量在处方剂量的 120% 以内来作为这一指数的限量。这是可以做到的，但代价是牺牲了计划的剂量梯度或剂量跌落。对于转移瘤，根本没有理由这么做。

2. 能量指数（YOMO）

$$EI = \frac{ID}{TV \times D_{\text{Rx}}}$$

能量指数[12]是评估靶区内部非均匀性程度的另一个指数。这个指数包含了靶区的整体剂量，并且对靶区剂量不足或过量非常敏感。

（五）其他有用的指数

1. AUC-DVH 指数

$$AUC_{100\%-50\%} = \int_{Rx_{50\%}}^{Rx_{100\%}} V_{\text{structure}} \delta \text{dose}$$

AUC-DVH 指数不仅可以量化特定剂量体积与处方等剂量体积的比值，而且可以量化两者之

间的所有剂量体积。这有助于进一步描述给定放射外科计划的剂量跌落性能。在图 19-5 所示的例子中，使用了 50% 等剂量体积和处方等剂量体积[13]，相比评估临床总剂量的 R50% 或梯度指数来说，在比较不同计划时是一个更可靠的衰减度量，也可用于 DVH 曲线上的任意两点。

2. 效率指数

$$\eta_{50\%} = \frac{\text{Useful Energy}}{\text{Total Energy}} = \frac{\text{Integral Dose}_{TV}}{\text{Integral Dose}_{50\%PIV}} = \frac{\int_{D_{\min}}^{D_{\max}} TV \delta dose}{\int_{PIV_{50\%}}^{D_{\max}} V \delta dose}$$

$$G\eta_{12Gy} = \frac{\text{Integral Dose}_{TV1} + \text{Integral Dose}_{TV2}}{\text{Global Integral Dose}_{12Gy}}$$

$$OAR \eta_{50\%} = \frac{\text{Integral Dose}_{OAR}}{\text{Integral Dose}_{50\%PIV}}$$

效率指数是最近提出的一个指数，尚未广泛应用，但其独特之处在于，它试图获得并量化所有"有益"剂量与"有害"剂量的比例。它将适形性、梯度和平均剂量合并为一个指数[14]。我们可以看到该度量的理论效用，它包括评价计划质量的三个最有意义的方面。然而，仍然需要一些工作来验证该指数与之前建立的计划质量和临床疗效/毒性结果的关系。

3. 12Gy 等剂量体积（V12Gy）

接受 12Gy 剂量照射的组织体积是最常见的脑放射性坏死预测因子。最初在动静脉畸形的伽马刀放射外科中研究[15]，后来在治疗良性和恶性肿瘤中也发现 V12Gy 的放射性坏死相关[16]，同时对于直线加速器的 SRS 也一样[17]。值得注意的是，当给定位置的 V12Gy 超过 10~15cm³ 时，毒性发生的可能性更高。某些研究人员在计算 V12Gy 时将靶区排除在外。这个指数的主要问题是，它与靶体积大小密切相关，靶区体积是已知的放射毒性预测因子。图 19-6 显示了治疗多发性脑转移瘤时，对于 18Gy 的处方剂量，无论在直线加速器还是伽马刀平台上，V12Gy 与靶体积呈直接线性关系。在治疗计划可用之前，根据靶体积或靶直径，可以临床上更容易做出处方决策。

使用 V12Gy 的第二个问题是，错误的在多发性脑转移瘤计划中使用。最常用的基于 V12Gy 的毒性模型是治疗单一靶区的（如 AVM）。对于一个多发性脑转移瘤的完整计划，不应该简单地由单一靶区模型推算得到由 V12Gy 预估放射性坏死可能性。考虑图 19-7 中包含 10 个转移瘤的病例。最大的转移灶位于左侧小脑，最大直径约 16mm，体积为 2.6cm³。所有肿瘤的总靶体积为 5.3cm³，但单次放射外科计划的总 V12Gy 为 16cm³。与单个肿瘤总靶体积相同的患者相

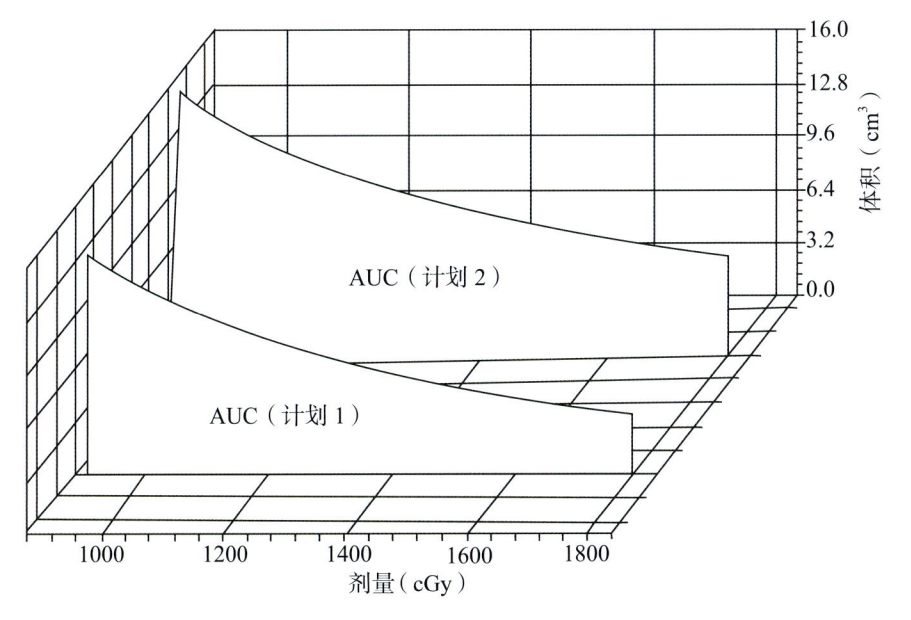

◀ 图 19-5　图示为两个放射外科计划 DVH 曲线中描绘为 9Gy（50%）和 18Gy（100%）区域

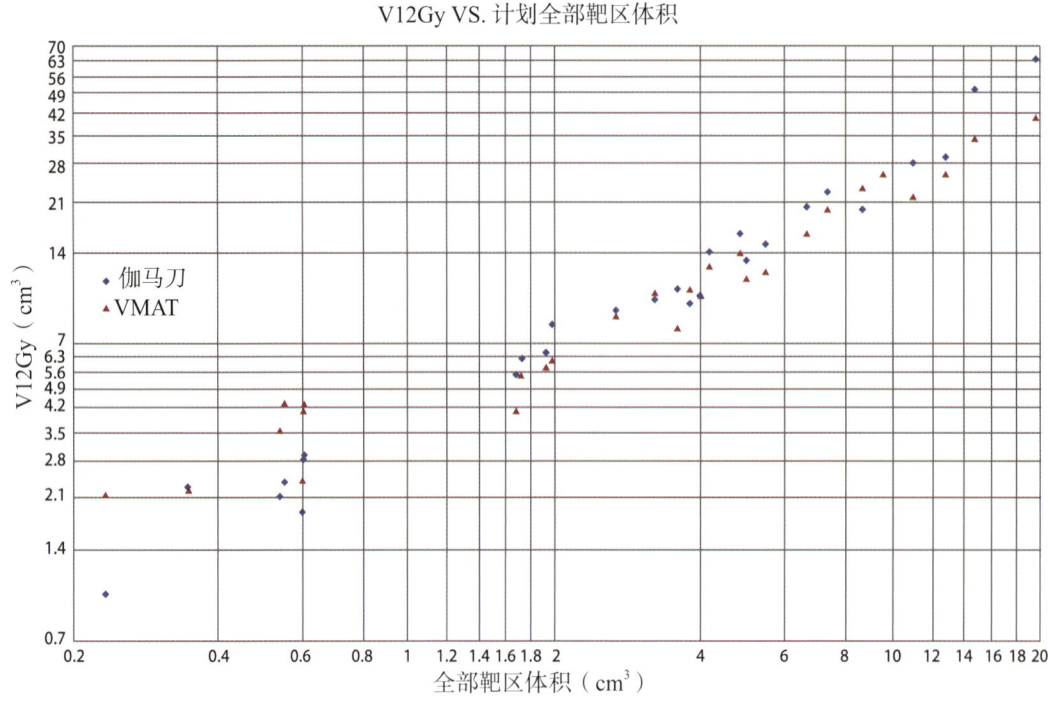

▲ 图 19-6 多发脑转移瘤伽马刀和直线加速器 SRS 计划中 V12Gy 与靶区总体积的比较

比，该患者发生放射性损伤的风险较低。该患者有一个高的 V12Gy，但不需要减少剂量或降低分割。

三、病例介绍

器官规避是治疗计划设计的目标之一

（一）病例 1

放射治疗计划设计的主要目标通常可以归类为三维适形性或器官规避。适形是脑转移瘤的治疗的首要目标，即肿瘤周围的所有组织都有同样的风险。但是，如果肿瘤非常接近一个敏感结构，那么与在邻近的关键结构上的高剂量相比，在所有方向上的适形性就变成次要的了。例如，在脑放射外科中，这些邻近关键结构可能是视觉神经结构或脑干。如果器官规避是计划质量的主要决定因素，那么先前关注适形性和梯度指数的指标可能会受到影响。图 19-8 显示了一例第四脑室的肾细胞转移瘤（靶区为洋红色）。这名患者既往

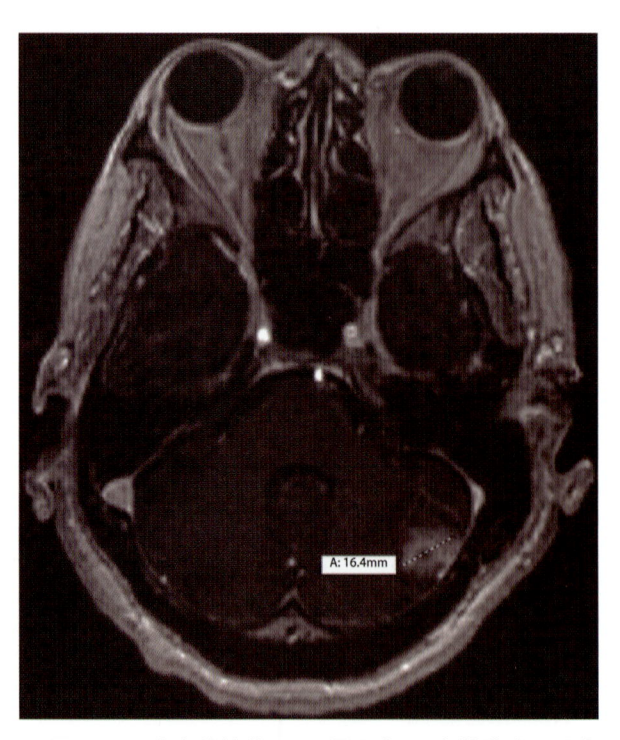

▲ 图 19-7 患者的轴位 MRI 层面有 10 个转移瘤，最大的位于左侧小脑，长 16.4mm 共有 10 个转移瘤（其他未显示）导致放射外科计划中的高 V12Gy，但所有肿瘤均 < 2cm。将毒性的单靶区 V12Gy 毒性模型外推到多靶区计划时应谨慎。这种情况下单次放射外科应该是安全的，尽管总的 V12Gy 很高

进行了全脑放疗，并对第四脑室中不断增长的肿块给予了 5 分次共 30Gy（黄色等剂量线）的处方剂量。虽然 RTOG 适形指数仍为 1.3，但梯度指数较差，为 8.3。强行规避器官通常对梯度指数不利。在这种情况下，剂量梯度的水平（3Gy/5 次，15Gy 的等剂量线显示为绿色）可能比较小的体积接受到 25～30Gy 照射的临床相关性更小。

（二）病例 2

患者女，68 岁，表现为间歇性的右侧面部感觉麻木。MR 影像显示一个 1.8cm 的环形增强病灶，刚好位于脑桥 - 脊髓交界处。胸部 CT 显示左侧乳房一个肿块和左侧腋窝一个淋巴结。淋巴结切除组织活检示转移性乳腺癌。患者的受体状态还没有确定。转诊医生给她地塞米松片 4mg，口服，每日 3 次后，症状有所缓解。她的 PFS 评分良好且没有其他主要的并发症（图 19-9）。

问题：
1. 这种病例该怎么处理？
2. 这种病灶的合理剂量分割方案是什么？
3. 这是一个适形还是器官规避计划？
4. 评价这种病例的相关计划质量指数是什么？

病灶明显不可手术切除且短时间内可能有生命危险，急需处理。考虑到它的大小，病灶可选单次或分次放射外科。对于这种患者，更谨慎决定对病灶进行分次放射外科治疗。选择 25

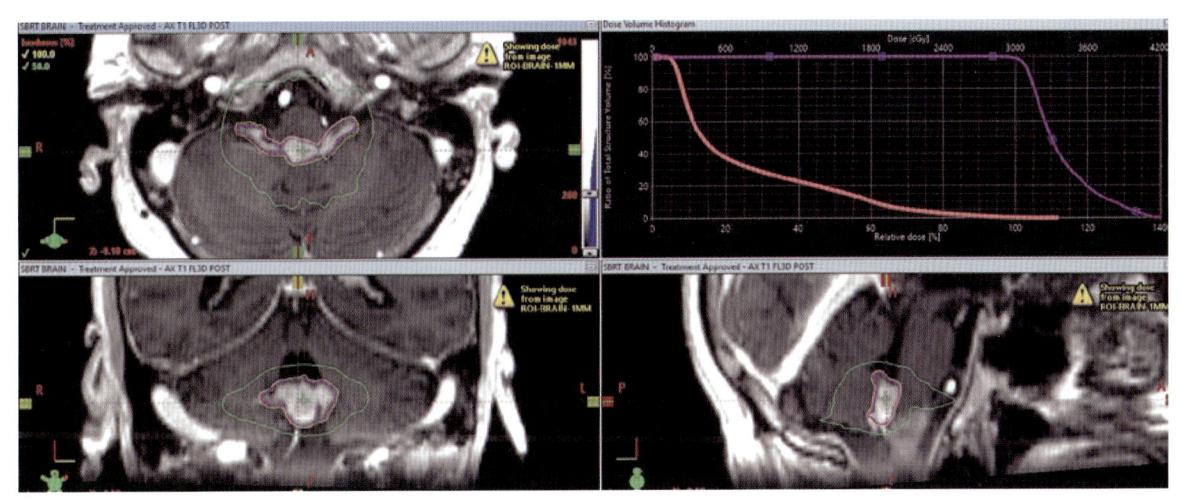

▲ 图 19-8 第四脑室转移瘤的器官规避治疗计划，分 5 次照射 30Gy
这个计划优先考虑在高等剂量水平下保护脑干而不是适形和剂量梯度

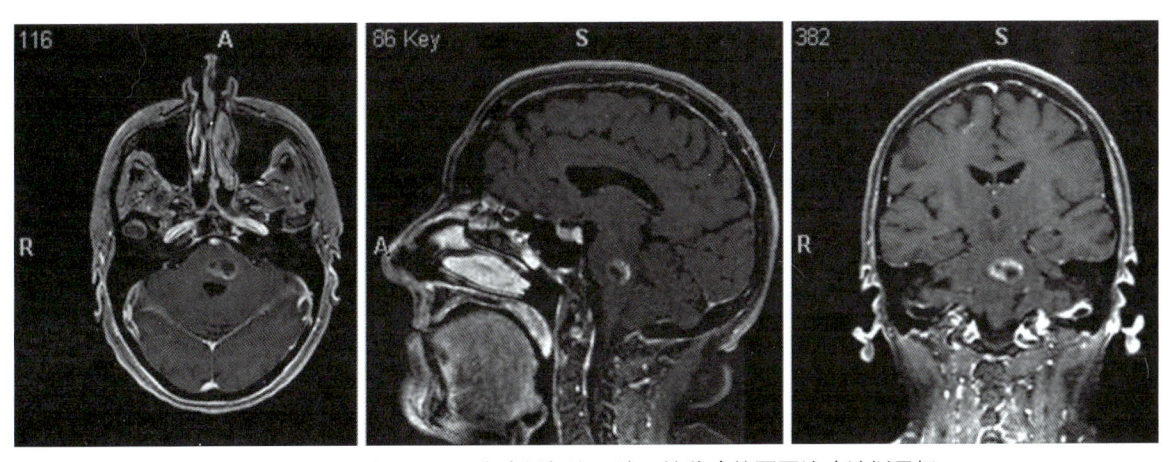

▲ 图 19-9 与图 19-8 中病例相比，脑干转移瘤的不同治疗计划目标

Gy/5fx 的剂量方案，并规定 100% 的处方剂量输送到 99% 的靶区体积。其他合理剂量方案包括 15～18Gy/1fx、24～27Gy/3fx 和 25～30Gy/5fx。对于基于机架的直线加速器，发展出了一种多个非共面弧的计划。由于病灶被重要的危及器官（脑干）包围，在各个方向上组织都同样重要。因此，目标是最大限度地减少处方在各个方向上的剂量跌落，使之成为一个适形计划。将本例的计划目标与图 19-8 所示的目标进行对比，尽管这两个计划都受到脑干的剂量限制。该患者的相关计划质量指数包括一个或多个适形指数，一个梯度测量和一个放射性坏死风险的替代指数。该计划的等剂量曲线如下所示。因为 V12Gy 是单次治疗放射性坏死最常见的替代指数；我们选用了 V18Gy 作为评审五个分次计划的指数（图 19-10）。

$$TV = 2.53 \, cc$$

$$PIV = 2.67 \, cc$$

$$PIV_{50\%} = 8.71$$

$$TV_{100\%} = 2.51$$

$$D_{max} = 34.4 \, Gy$$

$$D_{min} = 23.5 \, Gy$$

$$\text{Brainstem } D_{0.1cm^3} = 25.5 \, Gy$$

$$\text{Brainstem } V18_{Gy} = 2.6 \, cm^3$$

$$\text{RTOG CI} = \frac{PIV}{TV} = 1.06$$

$$\text{Paddick CI} = \frac{TV_{PIV}^2}{TV \times PIV} = 0.93$$

$$\text{Paddick GI} = \frac{PIV_{50\%}}{PIV} = 3.26$$

$$FI = \frac{PIV_{50\%}}{TV} = 3.44$$

$$\text{Coverage} = \frac{D_{min}}{D_{Rx}} = 94\%$$

$$\text{Homogeneity} = \frac{D_{max}}{D_{Rx}} = 1.37$$

$$EI = \frac{ID}{TV \times D_{Rx}} = 1.14$$

$$OAR\,\eta_{50\%} = \frac{\text{Integral Dose}_{OAR}}{\text{Integral Dose}_{50\%PIV}} = \frac{\text{Integral Dose}_{Brainstem}}{\text{Integral Dose}_{50\%PIV}} = 1.55$$

四、建议

尽管有大量关于放射外科计划质量评价指数的文献，但是目前仍缺乏将任何临床结果与计划质量指数相关联的数据。如图 19-11 所示，可达到的适形性随靶区体积的不同而变化，小肿瘤的适形指数高于大肿瘤。这在直线加速器和伽马刀平台上都可以观察到。肿瘤较大且适形指数良好的计划可能具有较高的 V12Gy 体积，并

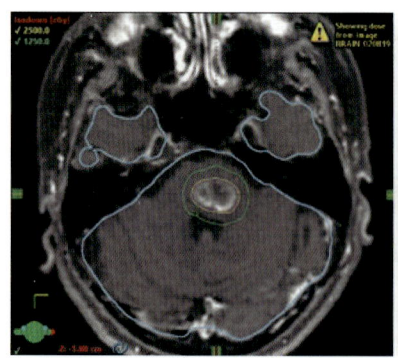

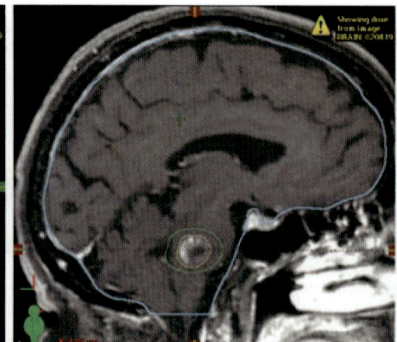

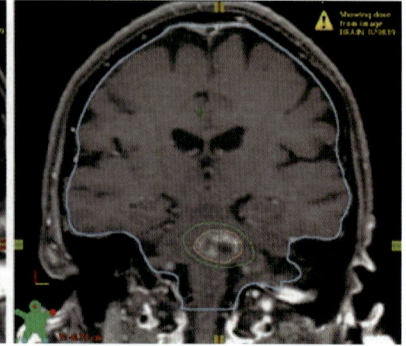

▲ 图 19-10 由于靶区周围几乎都是敏感组织，放射外科计划的首要目标是适形性处方等剂量以黄色显示。绿线代表 50% 的处方剂量

表现出较高的辐射损伤风险。相反，RTOG 适形指数＞2 的非常小的肿瘤通常治疗起来非常安全。

作者建议在评估一个放射治疗计划时，临床医生首先通过相关的轴向层面序列评估计划的等剂量曲线，然后是处方剂量和靶区之间的一致，从处方剂量到一半处方剂量或可能与附近重要结构相关的任何临床上重要的危及器官剂量的剂量跌落速度，最后是低剂量的溢出。

在我们的临床实践中，通过回顾一个放射外科计划，我们在相关影像上显示了 100%（处方）和 50% 处方等剂量曲线。我们没有为处方指定一个预定义的等剂量线，而是按照最大程度覆盖靶区的线开处方。对于 VMAT 治疗的单个等中心多靶区计划，部分靶区通常获得 130%～160% 的额外处方剂量。这种规范化方案不同于通常伽马刀的习惯，即预先选择 50% 等剂量体积来接受处方剂量。然后评估以下指数。

- RTOG 适形性。
- R50%（＜4 用于 TV＞2cm，＜5～6 用于 $0.5＜TV＜2.0cm^3$，＜7～10 用于 $TV＜0.5cm^3$）。
- V12Gy［（相对于单次，对于分次放射外科计划为 V66%），如果 V12＞10cm³ 邻近体积，考虑分次放射外科治疗］。
- 正常脑组织的平均剂量（合理可行尽可能低，但是如果单次不＜3Gy 则考虑重新计划）。
- 计划的均匀性通常认为对完整转移瘤的治疗没有益处，并可能对其他指数有害。

> **要 点**
> - 执行良好的放射外科是 CNS 疾病（恶性肿瘤和良性疾病）治疗的重要和有效组成部分。
> - 许多计划的质量指数可用于评估放射外科计划设计的好坏。
> - 掌握计划质量指数的相关知识对高质量放射外科的设计和实施至关重要。

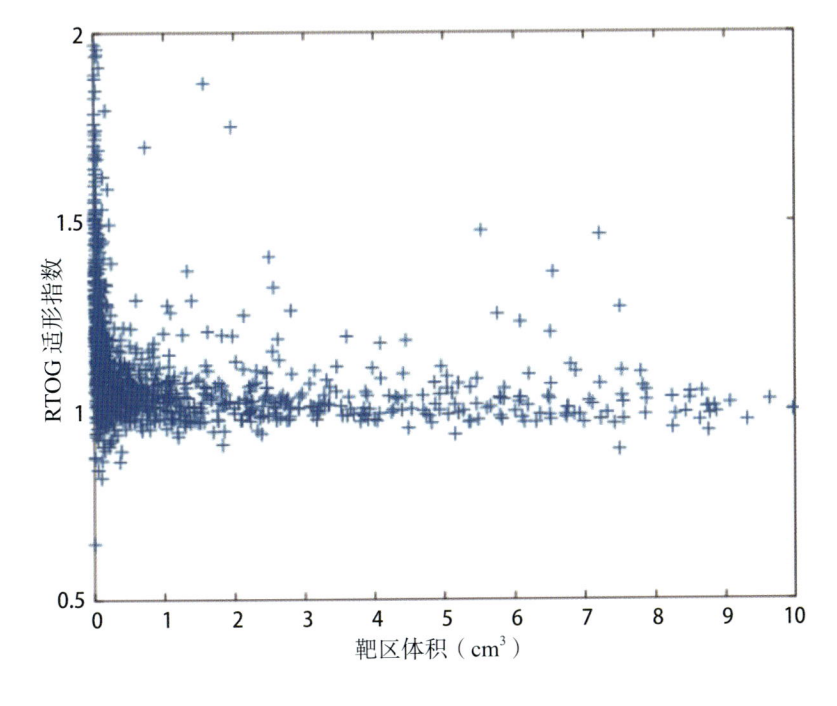

◀ 图 19-11 多发转移瘤直线加速器 SRS 计划中治疗的靶区肿瘤体积与 RTOG 适形指数的比较

对于非常小的肿瘤，可达到的适形性将高于较大的肿瘤。值得注意的是，在这张图上超过 1cm³ 的异常值通常表示肿瘤几何上接近并且不可避免地有剂量溢出的情况（引自 R.Popple）

参考文献

[1] Feuvret L, Noël G, Mazeron J-J, Bey P. Conformity index: a review. Int J Radiat Oncol Biol Phys. 2006;64(2):333–42.

[2] Shaw E, Kline R, Gillin M, Souhami L, Hirschfeld A, Dinapoli R, et al. Radiation Therapy Oncology Group: radiosurgery quality assurance guidelines. Int J Radiat Oncol Biol Phys. 1993;27(5):1231–9.

[3] Knöös T, Kristensen I, Nilsson P. Volumetric and dosimetric evaluation of radiation treatment plans: radiation conformity index. Int J Radiat Oncol Biol Phys. 1998;42(5):1169–76.

[4] Paddick I. A simple scoring ratio to index the conformity of radiosurgical treatment plans. J Neurosurg. 2000;93(Suppl 3):219–22.

[5] Knoos T, Kristensen I, Nilsson P, editors. Results from clinical practice of 3D conformal radiotherapy at Lund University Hospital. Proceedings of the twelfth international conference on the use of computers in radiation therapy. Madison: Medical Physics Publishing; 1997.

[6] Lomax NJ, Scheib SG. Quantifying the degree of conformity in radiosurgery treatment planning. Int J Radiat Oncol Biol Phys. 2003;55(5):1409–19.

[7] Régis J, Hayashi M, Porcheron D, Delsanti C, Muracciole X, Peragut JC. Impact of the model C and automatic positioning system on gamma knife radiosurgery: an evaluation in vestibular schwannomas. J Neurosurg. 2002;97(Supplement 5):588–91.

[8] Nakamura JL, Verhey LJ, Smith V, Petti PL, Lamborn KR, Larson DA, et al. Dose conformity of gamma knife radiosurgery and risk factors for complications. Int J Radiat Oncol Biol Phys. 2001;51(5):1313–9.

[9] Lefkopoulos D, Dejean C, El-Balaa H, Platoni K, Grandjean P, Foulquier J-N, et al. Determination of dose-volumes parameters to characterise the conformity of stereotactic treatment plans. In: The use of computers in radiation therapy. Heidelburg, Germany: Springer; 2000. p. 356–8.

[10] Baltas D, Kolotas C, Geramani K, Mould RF, Ioannidis G, Kekchidi M, et al. A conformal index (COIN) to evaluate implant quality and dose specification in brachytherapy. Int J Radiat Oncol Biol Phys. 1998;40(2):515–24.

[11] Paddick I, Lippitz B. A simple dose gradient measurement tool to complement the conformity index. J Neurosurg. 2006;105(Supplement):194–201.

[12] Yomo S, Tamura M, Carron R, Porcheron D, Régis J. A quantitative comparison of radiosurgical treatment parameters in vestibular schwannomas: the Leksell Gamma Knife Perfexion versus Model 4C. Acta Neurochir. 2010;152(1):47–55.

[13] Thomas EM, Popple RA, Wu X, Clark GM, Markert JM, Guthrie BL, et al. Comparison of plan quality and delivery time between volumetric arc therapy (RapidArc) and Gamma Knife radiosurgery for multiple cranial metastases. Neurosurgery. 2014;75(4):409–18.

[14] Dimitriadis A, Paddick I. A novel index for assessing treatment plan quality in stereotactic radiosurgery. J Neurosurg. 2018;129(Suppl1):118–24.

[15] Flickinger JC, Lunsford LD, Kondziolka D, Maitz AH, Epstein AH, Simons SR, et al. Radiosurgery and brain tolerance: an analysis of neurodiagnostic imaging changes after gamma knife radiosurgery for arteriovenous malformations. Int J Radiat Oncol Biol Phys. 1992;23(1):19–26.

[16] Korytko T, Radivoyevitch T, Colussi V, Wessels BW, Pillai K, Maciunas RJ, et al. 12 Gy gamma knife radiosurgical volume is a predictor for radiation necrosis in non-AVM intracranial tumors. Int J Radiat Oncol Biol Phys. 2006;64(2):419–24.

[17] Blonigen BJ, Steinmetz RD, Levin L, Lamba MA, Warnick RE, Breneman JC. Irradiated volume as a predictor of brain radionecrosis after linear accelerator stereotactic radiosurgery. Int J Radiat Oncol Biol Phys. 2010;77(4):996–1001.

第 20 章 无头架放射外科的图像引导技术（包括体表成像）
Image Guidance for Frameless Radiosurgery Including Surface Mapping

Guang Li　Yoshiya Yamada　Åse Ballangrud　著
王翰宇　译
唐　杜　校

随着近期图像引导放疗（image-guided radiotherapy，IGRT）和体表引导放疗（surface-guided radiotherapy，SGRT）的出现，放射治疗精度得到了显著提高[1-3]。这对于那些要求高精度单次高剂量的计划肿瘤结构（planning tumor volume，PTV）以及要求 PTV 外剂量急剧跌落的颅内放射治疗计划至关重要。通过仔细的校准和完善的步骤，IGRT 使分次间患者摆位精度可达亚毫米，SGRT 可实时监测治疗期间患者的运动。

尽管基于头架的 SRS 为脑转移患者提供了高精度的治疗，但该技术在临床实施和工作流程中存在一定的局限性。例如，使用侵入式头架要求从定位、计划制作到照射的整个过程在 1 天内完成。这种对时间的要求成为在一次摆位下能治疗的肿瘤数目的限制因素。此外，基于头架的有创技术不能用于治疗低分割放疗（SRT）的患者。接下来，我们通过一个临床病例来讨论基于头架技术的局限性和无头架 SRS 以及 SRT 技术的优势；描述应用无头架 SRS/SRT 详细的 IGRT/SGRT 技术，包括系统需求、校准和治疗流程以及涉及的不确定性，然后提供建议和未来展望。

一、病例介绍

病例：需要单次分割放疗和低分割放疗的一名患者。

一名 66 岁女性，大细胞神经内分泌肺癌，有 8 个脑转移病灶。治疗前的 MRI 成像如图 20-1 所示。体检未扪及病灶，患者无神经系统症状。患者担心全脑放射治疗对神经认知功能的潜在影响，选择立体定向放射治疗。虽然患者有其他部位的颅外转移，但颅内是病灶活跃的唯一的部位。处方剂量和每个病灶的剂量分割是根据病灶的体积、位置和与其他准备治疗的病灶的邻近程度来确定的。放射治疗肿瘤医生给予的处方为：其中 2 个病灶为 1800cGy/1 次，4 个病灶为 2100 cGy /1 次，2 个病灶为 900cGy/3 次。治疗方案包括用一个单次的 SRS 计划治疗 6 个病灶以及一个单独的 SRT 计划分 3 次治疗另外 2 个病灶。在治疗过程中采用无头架固定结合图像引导患者摆位和光学体表监测的方法以辅助摆位。单分次的计划作为大分割计划的第一次的部分一同执行照射。其余分次每日照射，并在 3 天完成治疗。在治疗后 26 个月的最后一次随访中，患者的颅内病灶稳定，并没有明显的放疗相关的不良反应。

无头架固定和图像引导的摆位为需要不同分次治疗病灶的患者进行安全的颅内照射提供了一个灵活的解决方案。然而，如果患者在 SRS 计划中使用有创头架进行治疗，那么患者将在两套独

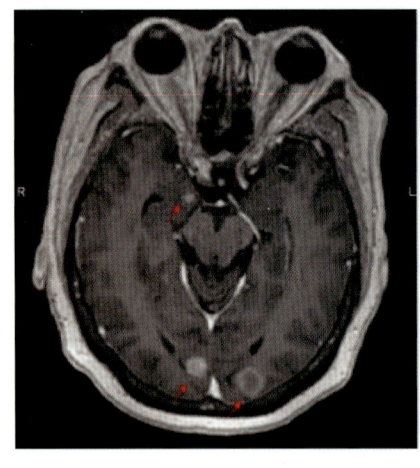

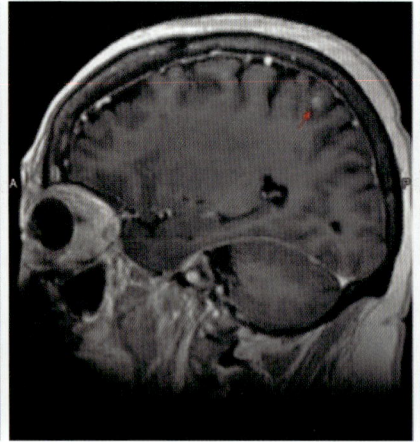

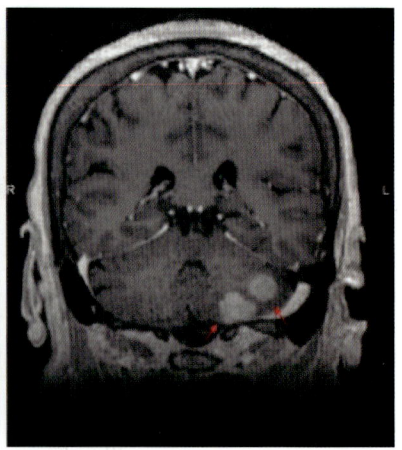

▲ 图 20-1 预处理 MR 影像显示 8 个转移病灶中的 6 个

立的流程中进行定位、计划和治疗：一套是基于有创头架的，另一套是基于无创头部面罩的。此外，这两种治疗将依次执行，增加了总体治疗次数。相比之下，无头架固定不仅为患者提供了舒适和方便，而且还为临床治疗提供了更多的选择，且治疗次数可能更少。

近年来，更有效的全身治疗方法对多发性脑转移的患者来说变得尤为重要。例如，免疫检查点抑制药在黑色素瘤脑转移和非小细胞肺癌脑转移患者中表现出良好的颅内疗效[4, 5]。脑转移的治疗越来越个体化，这取决于患者的身体状态、原发肿瘤类型和基因类型。有几项研究结果表明，与全脑放疗相比，转移病灶的局部放疗更能改善这些患者的认知功能[6-8]。全脑放疗已不再是所有多发性脑转移患者的标准治疗方法。需要新的治疗计划和照射技术来满足这些新的临床需求。无创固定系统的使用，加上图像引导摆位和运动监测，定制满足新的临床标准的 SRS 和 SRT 治疗可以更加灵活。

二、背景和动机

传统的基于有创头架的 SRS 已经成为使用直线加速器（linear accelerator，LINAC）治疗脑转移病变的标准治疗方式，该技术可提供高几何精度（≤ 1.0mm）[9-11]。实施立体定向技术需要神经外科医生先在计算机断层扫描（computed tomography，CT）定位之前用四颗外科螺钉将头架固定在患者的颅骨内，这是一个复杂的临床过程。头架可作为头部固定及治疗时患者立体定位的外部基准参照系统。CT 定位之后，患者的治疗计划设计完成，由放射治疗肿瘤医生审核和批准，并通过物理师二次核查，在此期间，患者需要在放射肿瘤科等待。立体定向技术要求治疗前对定位和治疗过程中使用的有创头架和参考头架以及直线加速器进行质控（quality assurance，QA）工作。墙上的激光灯用于进行立体定向的摆位，在治疗前，必须使用温斯顿－卢茨（Winston-Lutz）试验来验证激光等中心与加速器兆伏辐射等中心是否一致[12, 13]。从定位到治疗的时间通常是 4～6h，这对患者来说是漫长的。如果使用传统的计划技术且每个病灶都有一个等中心时，治疗计划时间、执行 QA 所需的时间和治疗时间随着病灶数目的增加而增加。每增加一个病灶，计划设计和治疗的总时间增加 1～1.5h。因此，临床工作人员压力很大，时间紧迫，必须及时创建、批准、验证和治疗。

除了上述缺点，有创头架立体定向系统还缺乏灵活性。对于放射治疗前已接受手术切除转移病灶的患者，安装有创头架是一件有挑战的事情。有时，考虑到患者的解剖结构和要治疗的病灶位置，很难将有创头架放置到一个最终能够进行立体定向治疗的位置。由于改进的系统治疗方法延长了许多癌症患者的寿命，因此需要一个灵活的系统来提供重复的头颅放射外科，通常是针对多发的头颅转移瘤。过去，无创固定设备已经得到应用[14-19]，但在没有使用自动床、图像引导摆位和运动监测的情况下，放射外科的准确性仍然不够。早期的研究已经报道了一种无头架方法[20, 21]，这种方法能使分次治疗更加精确。

随着颅脑放射外科逐渐成为多发性脑转移患者的标准治疗方法，进而需要一种无头架固定和定位系统来保证与有创头架系统相同的高几何精度。这种无头架固定系统也可以用于高精度分次治疗。由于无头架固定系统在治疗过程中可能不能提供与基于头架固定系统相同水平的固定效果，所以在治疗过程中患者的运动监测对于无头架头颅放射外科是至关重要的。直线加速器上的放射治疗计划将包括多个床和机架角度，这使运动监测的方法选择更加复杂。由于存在多个床角，安装在加速器机架上的影像板成像（on-board imaging，OBI）系统无法避免与床和患者的碰撞。因此，在颅脑放射外科[22]中，经常使用一种独立安装在地板上的非共面 X 线成像系统。这种 X 线系统在人为确定的时间点提供亚毫米精度的骨性配准验证，但不能用于持续监测。另外，基于视频的光学表面成像（optical surface imaging，OSI）系统可以提供实时成像（帧率为 3～4Hz）。这些系统使用三个安装在天花板上的摄像头，在任何时候至少有两个摄像头不会被机架挡住，且能定位患者的面部表面区域。OSI 监测系统使用患者面部的一个未覆盖的开放区域作为替代推断肿瘤的位置，利用头部的刚性解剖结构，提供体表和辐照靶区之间的固定关系。如果使用封闭的面罩进行固定，不能监测到皮肤表面，因此 OSI 系统就不能使用。运动监测是通过将实时 OSI 影像与参考体表进行匹配来实现的，该参考体表可以从计划 CT 的外轮廓获得，也可以在对患者使用锥形束计算机断层扫描（cone-beam computed tomography，CBCT）确定治疗位置后获取。配备图像引导技术的直线加速器如图 20-2 所示。

三、图像引导无头架式放射治疗

（一）选择固定和监控系统

由于有创头架的立体定向系统必须提供准确的患者定位和固定，患者在治疗过程中的活动是很受限的。综合考虑以下因素十分重要：6 维床对精确定位与 CBCT 摆位的实用性；运动监控系统（治疗期间连续运动监测门控治疗或周期性验证）的有效性；选择一个患者固定系统以提供充分的运动限制并与运动监控系统配合使用。

某些固定系统通过使用口含器复现模拟定位的位置，而其他系统使用扩展床用于调整倾斜/翻转[18, 23]。强烈推荐使用自动的 6 维床辅助患者摆位，提高准确性和缩短摆位时间。另外，旋转可调的扩展床可用于手动减少 OSI 实时引导的旋转误差。如果仅针对 CBCT 与 CT 配准所确定的三维平移进行移床，则任何残余的旋转误差都可能影响运动监测精度。当残余的旋转误差很大时，平移和旋转运动可能会混合在一起，导致误差难以解释。因此，传统的三维患者摆位不能为 SRS 治疗提供足够的准确性。

为精确摆位去设置适当的平移和旋转的临床容差十分重要。例如，如果计划是一个靶区且等中心放置在靶区内部，残余旋转误差对照射剂量的准确性的影响可能很小。然而，如果某个等中心与容积旋转调强治疗（volumetric-modulated arc therapy，VMAT）计划一起用于治疗分布在脑内的多个病灶时，一个小的残余旋转误差可能会造成远离等中心的病灶的摆位误差很大。这将在"不确定性和未来方向"一节中更详细地讨论。

带有 3 个摄像头的 OSI 系统是无头架 SRS 治疗期间进行运动监控的理想选择（图 20-2）。OSI 系统需要对患者的面部进行映射，因此应该使用带有开放面部的固定系统[24]，见图 20-3。如果无法使用自动六维床或旋转可调的扩展床，

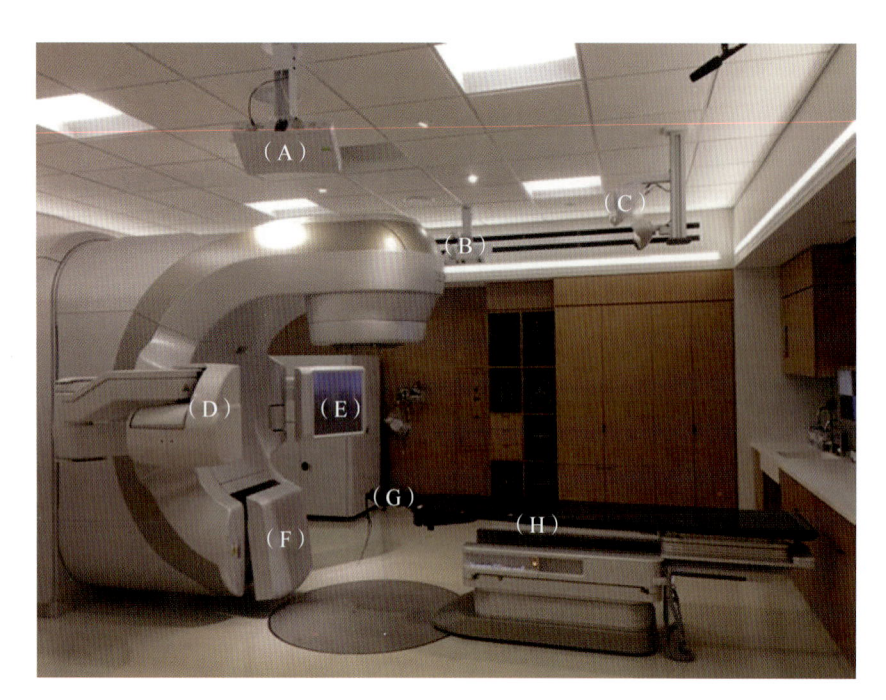

◀ 图 20-2 线性加速器（直线加速器）和图像引导技术，包括（A～C）安装摄像系统的光学表面成像（OSI）(D, E) 锥束计算机断层扫描（CBCT）的千伏（kV）成像系统，(F) 兆伏（MV）电子成像探测器（EPID）和（G）机械床外延在（H）调整患者位置的六维（6D）自动床

那么选择一个能在治疗时精确地重现模拟定位时的头部位置的固定系统是很重要的。在没有六维床的情况下，患者的治疗摆位可能需要相当长的时间才能达到预期的准确性。

一些头部固定系统会通过扩展床来手动校正旋转[23, 24]。这些系统利用一个开放式面罩和一个定制的头部支撑，形成一个"蛤壳"对患者头部位置进行固定，并有一个扩展板，提供倾斜和翻转的手动调整功能。当与 OSI 系统一起使用时，通过将计划 CT 的外轮廓与 OSI 体表进行匹配，首先纠正头部旋转（< 0.5°），然后纠正床平移移位（< 0.5mm），它将显著缩短摆位时间[18, 23]。当患者的位置在这个范围内时，可以由自动床来进一步校正。当采集 CBCT 后，所有基于 CBCT 与 CT 配准的旋转和平移移动都通过六维床进行调整，在这个最终的治疗位置获得新的 OSI 系统参考影像，用于治疗期间的运动监测。

（二）无头架图像引导放射外科流程的描述

在 CT 定位阶段，负责定位的技师要为患者定制一个固定的系统。在图 20-3 所示的例子中，头模从后脑勺一直覆盖到头顶，并从侧面包裹到耳朵。在模具硬化后，将热塑开放式面罩敷在患者面部，并锁定在扩展床板上，完成蛤壳式组装。前额和下巴大致水平对齐的头部固定可使皮肤表面可见面积更大，从而改善 OSI 监测的信噪比。

使用定位 CT 的外轮廓和计划等中心作为参考，定义一个感兴趣区域（region of interest，ROI），该区域通常覆盖面罩的开口区域（不包括唇/嘴），然后就可以基于 OSI 进行摆位。

去除有创头架后，无头架放射外科的定位 - 治疗日程安排可以遵循与其他图像引导治疗计划相同的流程。计划技术可以是 VMAT、动态适形旋转（dynamic conformal arc，DCA）技术或多静态野技术[25]。

图像引导放射外科所需的直线加速器的 QA 包括：CBCT 成像系统和兆伏（MV）治疗野之间的等中心一致性测试及验证 OSI 系统等中心的每日校准。采用两级校准过程连同 OSI-MV 射野等中心一致性检查作为每月校准项目，可实现比一级校准更高的精度[26]。每天早上，放射治疗师进行 QA，然后由物理师进行检查。

在治疗时，患者被固定在六维床附加的扩展床上的头模和开放式面罩中。采用 OSI 系统引导调整扩展床上的倾斜和翻转。这可以确保将患者

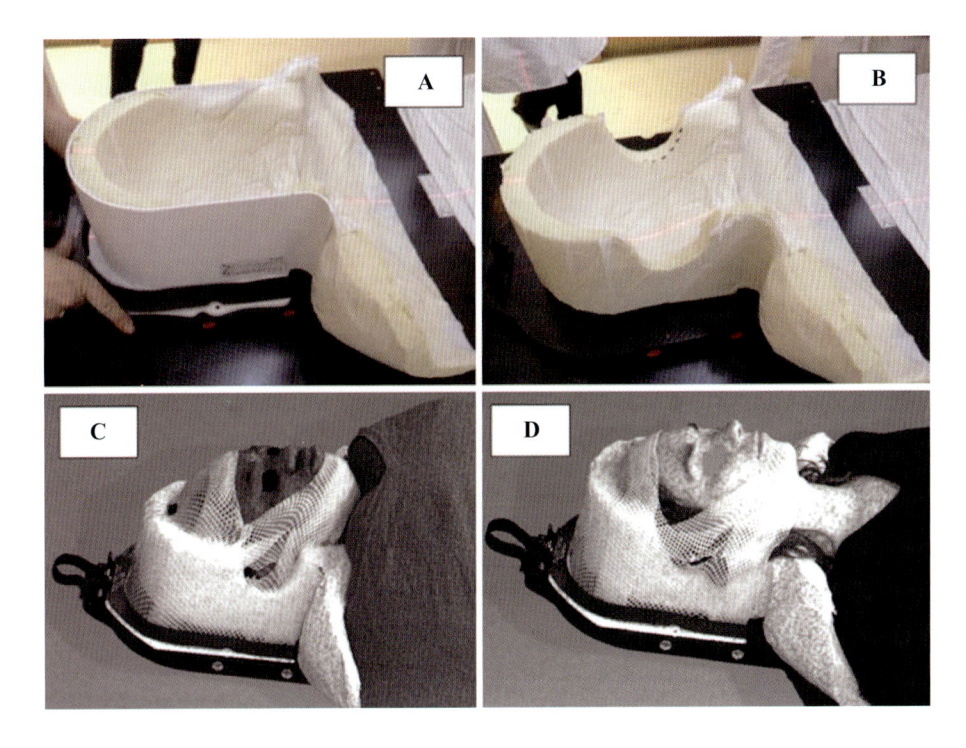

第 20 章　无头架放射外科的图像引导技术（包括体表成像）
Image Guidance for Frameless Radiosurgery Including Surface Mapping

◀ 图 20-3　一种无头架立体定向放射治疗（SRS）固定系统，包括定制的头模和允许采用的光学表面成像（OSI）系统对面部实时运动监测的开放式面罩
图片由 Dr.Li 提供，发表于 J App Clin Med Phys [23]

摆位至自动床可调的范围内。整个过程在治疗室内不超过 1min。在采集 CBCT 后，由治疗师进行骨性配准，由物理师进行验证，并由主管医生批准，然后 OSI 进行持续监控。初始 OSI 引导的摆位和最终 CBCT 配准之间的差异通常＜ 2mm。一旦基于 CBCT 移床，采集一个新的 OSI 参考影像，来确定治疗位置，ROI 自动映射到新的参考图像中去。新的 ROI 通过抓取静态影像，用于不同床角度的位置验证，并在治疗期间使用实时差量（real-time delta，RTD）进行运动监测。静态影像比 RTD 影像具有更大的射野视图（field of view，FOV），而 RTD 影像只重建 ROI 区域的影像，因此具有更高的帧率以用于连续运动监测。如果患者的运动超过了设定的临床容差，通过一个与直线加速器连接的运动管理接口（motion management interface，MMI）控制停止出束，直到运动回到容差范围内。

如果在某一治疗床角度的静态 OSI 图像与基于 CBCT 的初始参考体表之间的偏差＞ 1.0mm，区分患者运动误差和床角度相关的误差的一个简单方法是将床移回零位，并重新获取静态 OSI 验证影像。如果静态 OSI 验证影像与治疗前影像一致，则患者没有移动，偏移是由于摄像系统的技术层面的因素造成的。床在零位时，OSI 验证影像之间存在的任何差异都表明患者已经移动，需要采集新的 CBCT 来重新确定患者位置。通过使用六维床（最大限度地减少初始头部的旋转）和使用二级（3D）校准替代一级（2D）平板校准，患者运动的误报提示的频率已经显著降低。根据我们的临床经验，使用上述固定、摆位和监测技术，只有不到 2% 的患者在治疗过程中移动达1.0mm 及以上。

总之，OSI 系统允许通过初始体表匹配来实现室内快速的患者摆位；在通过 CBCT 摆位后，建立一个新的 OSI 参考影像进行运动监测；在每个床角度验证患者的位置；治疗中以 3～4Hz 的帧率实现 OSI 实时运动监测。灵活的开放式固定系统[24]、结合用于校正 CBCT 六维移位的自动床以及用于运动监测的 OSI 系统，提供了头颅放射外科[23] 所需的几何精度，包括单个等中心[25] 的多病灶治疗。虽然新的无头架固定系统保证了良好的患者固定，但如果要避免延长治疗，需要患者的良好配合[24]。此外，为捕捉在治疗[25] 期间移动的异常值，实时运动监测是很有必要的。

四、图像引导放射治疗中的几何不确定性

无头架SRS治疗中可能存在的几何不确定性包括：成像系统的不确定性、运动监测的不确定性及操作人员的变动。下面讨论调试和校准成像系统的流程，而临床工作人员的培训和资格认证则在本节的最后讨论。

（一）OSI系统的调试、校准和QA

OSI系统最初是为乳腺癌治疗开发的，其中，皮肤是一个很好的靶区替代物[27-29]。之后该系统被改进，为无头架放射外科提供足够的空间和时间精度，并开发了QA程序，以保证足够的精度[18]。为了确保系统满足无头架SRS的要求，OSI系统的调试、每月校准和常规的每日QA至关重要。近年来，两级平板校准方法、先进摄像机优化（advance camera optimization，ACO）技术和OSI-MV等中心一致性检查项目的开发和临床应用极大地减少了患者运动中的误报数据，促进了无头架SRS治疗的顺利开展[26, 30, 31]。

1. 系统特性描述与调试

在临床应用前必须确定OSI系统的特有精度和帧率。使用高精度平台控制装载的头部模体运动是确定空间精度的最佳方法，如图20-4A所示。由于该平台只能在某一水平方向上增加0.1mm的运动，所以实验要在0°和90°的床角度上进行以覆盖两个水平维度，而第三个垂直维度可以由床控制。对于该平台的准确性[27]已有报道。对运动的监测是通过运行RTD将实时抓取的体表与初始摆位时抓取的参考影像进行比较来完成。结果如图20-4B和C所示。

通常放射外科的计划包含非共面野，因此评估OSI系统的床角依赖性是很重要的。在OSI调试过程中，强烈建议包括床角关联测试，以确保系统在所有床角提供相似的运动检测精度。在系统标定后，可进行头模实验，以在0°床角条件下抓取的影像为参照，以10°为间隔，从0°旋转到±90°，检查模体影像在各角度下的匹配情况。通过将一级平板校准改为两级平板校准（见下文），与床角有关的误差降低到0.5~1.0mm。

应在调试中包含OSI的RTD基线漂移的测试项目以证明实时成像系统的稳定性。对于采用低散热的LED作为光源进行斑点投射的新高清（HD）相机系统，在最初的5~10min内，垂直方向的漂移幅度已减小到-0.3mm水平。综上所述，上述两个调试测试可提供新OSI系统的基准误差，作为评价无头架SRS治疗的临床误差参考。

2. OSI校准流程

根据临床使用目的的准确性要求，有三种方法可用来校准OSI系统。前两种方法使用一个有圆形黑色点阵和十字准线（表示校准板的中心）的1m×1m校准平板。通过将机架上由光投射的十字准线对准板中心，将平板精确地放置在直线加速器的等中心，这样就可以确定OSI等中心。根据天花板上的两个相机与平板表面上的一个点（如黑点的中心）之间的三角正弦规律为三维表面影像重建提供必要的数据。这两种方法的区别是是否需要改变板的位置。与一级校准不同，二级校准是真正的3D校准，提供了接近实际临床成像条件的校准条件，正如患者的皮肤表面位于深度肿瘤的等中心上方。因此，推荐使用两级校准程序。

第三种校准方法是通过使用一个大立方形模体（15cm×15cm×15cm）来微调OSI等中心位置，该体模具有一个大的表面，并包含5个内部放射显影的标记。由于OSI旋转变换有一个更精确的旋转中心，通过最小化OSI等中心与兆伏（MV）放射等中心的偏差，OSI系统的不确定性变得不那么依赖床角。如果不进行校准，除了床移动和OSI部分视图的不确定性外，OSI等中心的偏差将在床旋转时放大，即存在所谓的床角依赖关系。

3. 系统QA和年度预防性维护（PM）

日常QA包括每日一致性检查和每月校准。每日QA由治疗师进行，并由物理师进行验证。

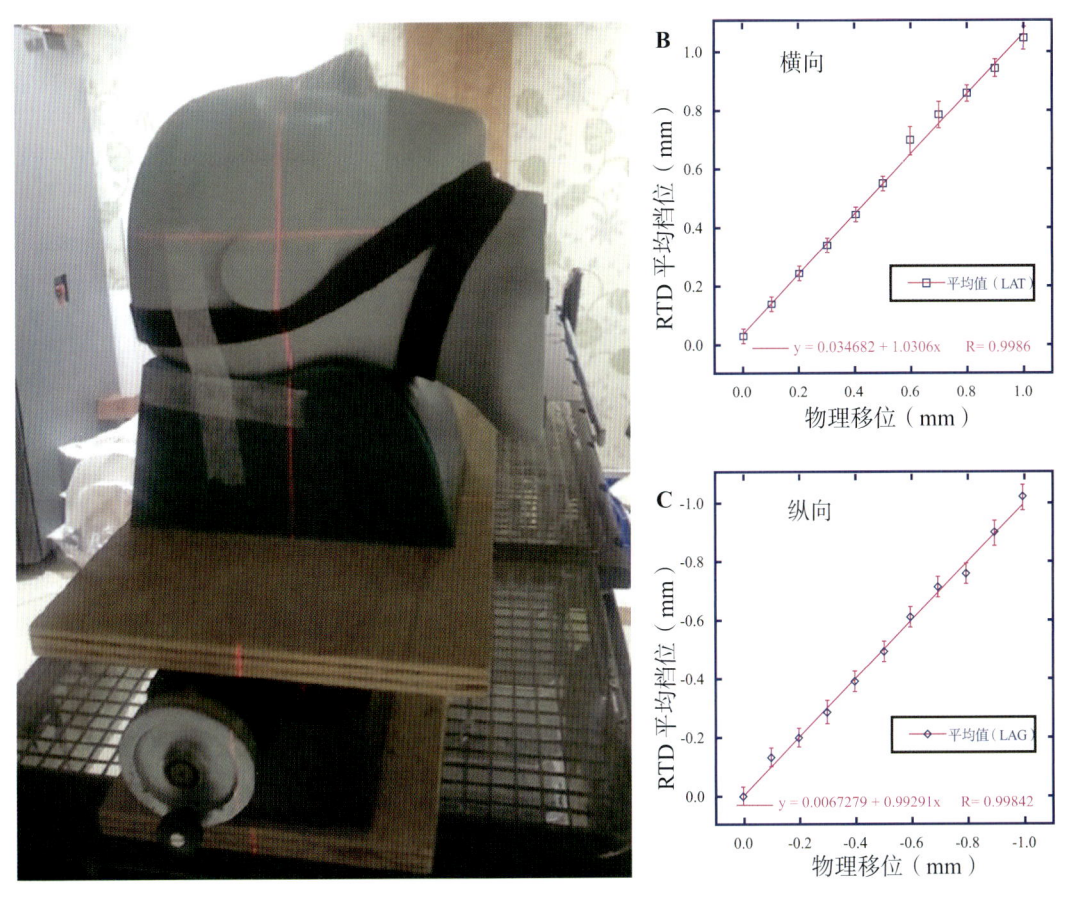

▲ 图 20-4 建立头部模型实验，以确定光学表面成像（optical surface imaging，OSI）系统使用实时误差（RTD）检测模式的运动检测能力（由 Dr. Li 提供，发表于 Med Phys [18]）

如果每日 QA 始终符合要求，则可将校准周期延长至每季度或每半年 1 次。根据服务合同，每年应由供应商的工程师进行预防性维护（preventive maintenance，PM）服务。PM 服务后或系统升级后，需要对系统进行重新校准。当每日 QA 失败时，可能是由于校准文件损坏或安装在天花板上的 OSI 摄像机的物理移动造成的，这种情况则需要做一个专门的校准。

（二）X 线成像的 QA

必须检查成像等中心和射野等中心的一致性，并在严格的容差范围内对图像引导下摆位的患者进行放射外科。CBCT 是放射外科患者摆位的临床标准，将 CBCT 与计划 CT 影像基于颅骨进行配准。CBCT 是在治疗室使用影像板（on-board imager，OBI）获取的，OBI 带有垂直于兆伏（MV）治疗射野的千伏（kV）射束。将 kV 和 MV 等中心对齐对于准确的 IGRT 治疗至关重要，因为这种不确定性对临床用户是显而易见的。根据 AAPM（美国医学物理学家协会）TG104 [32] 和 TG142 [33] 的指南，直线加速器的 QA 过程中，验证和（或）调整 kV CBCT 和 MV 治疗等中心必须由物理师执行。每天早上由治疗师进行等中心一致性检查，并在治疗开始前由物理师进行检查。

一旦固定系统和摆位流程确立，必须按照从定位到治疗的精确临床流程执行端到端测试，以证明治疗的准确性。可以用在中心插入放射胶片的仿真头部模体确定几何和剂量的准确性。由治疗师对模体进行 CT 扫描，由物理师勾画、设计计划及核查，并模拟真实治疗过程，由治疗师摆位和"治疗"，由物理师分析胶片。几何精度必须在 1mm 以内。所有用于无头架头颅放射治疗的直线加速器都要完成端到端的测试。

（三）OSI 实时运动监测系统中的不确定性

1. 计划 CT 的外轮廓

已有研究探讨了光学体表是否可以用于脑内靶区相关的运动跟踪[34]。人们提出了"如果患者面部感兴趣区域内有细微的变化是否有关系？"这一疑问。例如，如果患者眨眼或做鬼脸怎么办？眨眼效应可以忽略，因为眼睑厚度较薄，面积相对于 ROI 较小；睁开的眼睛往往会在影像中产生空洞，这对匹配没有帮助。由于面罩会硬化（24h 后收缩约 1mm），紧致的面罩使患者很难不用力就使面部皮肤发生移动。

在某些情况下，计划 CT 的外轮廓不能很好地反映等中心位置。一些患者从定位到治疗的这段时间内会出现面部肿胀，这使得 OSI 预匹配不可靠。通过在 CBCT 配准前在面罩上画一个临时的 ROI 可以直观地识别并避免这种情况。在对患者使用 CBCT 将骨骼配准确定位置后，需要抓取一个新的 OSI 参考体表用于运动监测。

2. 用于运动监测的 OSI 分辨率和帧率

由于患者的运动是十分随机的，因此在治疗过程中进行持续监测以捕捉可能的患者运动是很重要的。对于 OSI 系统，帧率受图像抓取速度和图像重建速度的影响。图像抓取过程包括数据保存的时间小于 50ms，而图像重建的时间则要长得多，这取决于 ROI 的大小和 OSI 的空间分辨率。对于临床的 SRS 流程，应使用最高的分辨率为 SRS 治疗提供最佳的空间分辨率，并且在面罩的开放区域内的 ROI 尺寸应尽可能大。在这种情况下，帧率为 3~4 秒/帧，成像相关的延迟为 250ms。理想情况下，应该使用自动控制射束功能，但考虑到头部固定的严格限制，手动控制射束也足够了。

OSI 系统通过运动管理接口（motion management interface，MMI）与直线加速器通信，一旦 RTD 超过设定的容差范围，自动控制射束功能就被触发。当 MMI 为 OSI 射野启用门控时，不管 OSI 是否将被用于 SGRT，整个治疗日都将"被预订"在 OSI 工作站中，以免去该 OSI 工作站的重新准备过程。

五、员工培训和资格认证

图像引导无头架 SRS 的高精度需求推进了包括医生、物理师、治疗师和护士的培训项目。图像引导 SRS 的过程虽然类似于非 SRS 治疗，但每个人都理解 SRS 需要更高精度这一点很重要。因为从基于头架到无头架的 SRS 的大多数变化都与使用 IGRT 和 SGRT 技术有关，所以对医生、物理师和治疗师的培训主要集中在技术变化和更新上。对于物理师的培训重点是 IGRT 患者摆位和 SGRT 运动监测以及它们的容差范围，还包括所需的 SRS 每日 QA，体表 ROI 准备，DICOM 和现场参考体表以及对 OSI 假阳性数据和患者运动情况的处理。SRS 物理师应在 SRS 治疗中充当一名监督者。

为了执行员工培训和资格认证，可以建立一个由经验丰富的医生、物理师、治疗师和护士组成的资格认证委员会。应制定培训计划，包括所有人员都能遵循的初始培训和定期培训计划，以在临床中保证无头架放射外科的质量。

六、建议和未来展望

总之，使用 IGRT 和 SGRT 开发无头架 SRS 流程需要做好以下工作以确保 SRS 精度，如认真选择固定系统、制定详细的定位、计划和治疗流程、仔细进行成像系统的日常 QA 工作。此外，还需要对所有相关人员进行培训。

一个详细的临床工作流程是成功实施无头架 SRS/SRT 计划的必要条件。一个完整的端到端空转测试必须要所有相关人员一起完成，以解决从开始到结束过程中可能出现的问题。例如，在 CT 定位之前进行头部固定时，为了确保 OSI 系统进行最佳的运动监测，将患者的面部和前额进行水平放置是很重要的，因为三个安装在天花板上的摄像头位于患者前下方。为了加快患者的摆位，在患者进入治疗室之前，应根据固定装置上的标记及等中心的位移提示获取治疗床的位置。患者在头模中固定后，可将床直接移动到治疗位置。在 OSI 引导下，首先要最小化旋转移位，然后再最小化平移移位。在采集 CBCT 图像时，应继续进行 RTD 运动监测，以便在 CBCT 采集和配准时对患者进行监测。同时，摄像机系统可以预热和保持稳定（基线漂移至稳定水平），为治疗做好准备。在治疗结束时，建议使用 OSI 对在零位床的头部位置进行最后检查。这些是工作流程中的关键步骤示例，可以对流程进行优化，以确保 SRS 治疗的顺利进行。对某些患者来说，使用完全相同的工作流程、固定、计划类型和摆位以及运动监测，采用低分割治疗方式可能更适合，这与靶区的位置和大小、先前的脑部放射疗程或同步系统治疗有关的。这样做可使 PTV 边缘从 3mm 减少到 2mm。IGRT/SGRT 提供了灵活的解决方案，如果需要快速患者轮转，通过该方案也可以制定当日无头架 SRS/SRT 的工作流程。

使用 CBCT 的图像引导摆位和使用 OSI 的体表引导实时运动监测为无头架放射治疗提供了足够的几何精度。这为在同一疗程中对某些病灶进行单分次治疗，对其他病灶进行低分割治疗提供了可能性。随着灵活性的增加，可以根据脑部病灶的数量、病灶的体积、所有病灶相对于其他病灶和危及器官的位置定制治疗方案。治疗计划时间是目前实现快速定位到执行多病灶 VMAT SRS 治疗的限制因素。更好的剂量计算算法可以简化计划过程[25]，更好的优化算法可以缩短计划时间并生成更好的计划；连续 MRI 上追踪新的和治疗过的靶区的更好工具对于再次治疗来说可以进一步显著改善直线加速器的 SRS 计划。

> **要 点**
> - 使用 IGRT 和 SGRT 的无头架 SRS 流程的设计需要做好以下工作确保 SRS 精度：仔细选择固定系统、制定详细的模拟定位、计划和治疗流程、完成成像系统的每日 QA，此外还需要对所有相关人员进行培训。
> - 端对端的完整空转测试必须由所有相关人员参与完成以排除流程中自始至终可能出现的问题。
> - 利用 CBCT 的图像引导摆位和 OSI 体表引导的实时运动监控可以为无头架 SRS 提供足够的几何精度，减少无头架放射外科相关的不确定性。
> - 仔细的调试和持续的 QA 对于 OSI 系统的恰当使用至关重要。
> - 强烈建议对使用 OSI 系统的人员进行培训和认证。

参考文献

[1] Chen GT, Sharp GC, Mori S. A review of imageguided radiotherapy [published online ahead of print 2009/01/01]. Radiol Phys Technol. 2009;2(1):1–12.

[2] Jaffray DA. Image-guided radiotherapy: from current concept to future perspectives. Nat Rev Clin Oncol. 2012;9(12):688–99.

[3] Li G, Mageras G, Dong L, Mohan R. Image-guided radiation therapy. In: Khan FM, Gerbi BJ, editors. Treatment planning in radiation oncology. 4th ed. Philadelphia: Lippincott Williams & Wilkins; 2016. p. 229–58.

[4] Murphy B, Walker J, Bassale S, et al. Concurrent radiosurgery and immune checkpoint inhibition: improving regional intracranial control for patients with metastatic melanoma [published online ahead of print 2018/12/18]. Am J Clin Oncol. 2019;42(3):253–7.

[5] Kamath SD, Kumthekar PU. Immune checkpoint inhibitors for the treatment of central nervous system (CNS) metastatic

[6] Kirkpatrick JP, Wang Z, Sampson JH, et al. Defining the optimal planning target volume in image-guided stereotactic radiosurgery of brain metastases: results of a randomized trial. Int J Radiat Oncol Biol Phys. 2015;91(1):100–8.

[7] Savitz ST, Chen RC, Sher DJ. Cost-effectiveness analysis of neurocognitive-sparing treatments for brain metastases. Cancer. 2015;121(23):4231–9.

[8] Brown PD, Jaeckle K, Ballman KV, et al. Effect of radiosurgery alone vs radiosurgery with whole brain radiation therapy on cognitive function in patients with 1 to 3 brain metastases: a randomized clinical trial. JAMA. 2016;316(4):401–9.

[9] Palta JR, Liu C, Li JG. Current external beam radiation therapy quality assurance guidance: does it meet the challenges of emerging image-guided technologies? Int J Radiat Oncol Biol Phys. 2008;71(1 Suppl):S13–7.

[10] Friedman WA. Linear accelerator radiosurgery. In: Chin LS, Regine WF, editors. Principles and practice of stereotactic radiosurgery. New York: Springer; 2008. p. 129–40.

[11] Schell MC, Bova FJ, Larson DA, et al. Stereotactic radiosurgery. AAPM Report No. 54. 1995. https://www.aapm.org/pubs/reports/RPT_54.pdf.

[12] Winston KR, Lutz W. Linear accelerator as a neurosurgical tool for stereotactic radiosurgery. Neurosurgery. 1988;22(3):454–64.

[13] Lutz W, Winston KR, Maleki N. A system for stereotactic radiosurgery with a linear accelerator. Int J Radiat Oncol Biol Phys. 1988;14(2):373–81.

[14] Bova FJ, Buatti JM, Friedman WA, Mendenhall WM, Yang CC, Liu C. The University of Florida frameless high-precision stereotactic radiotherapy system. Int J Radiat Oncol Biol Phys. 1997;38(4):875–82.

[15] Ryken TC, Meeks SL, Pennington EC, et al. Initial clinical experience with frameless stereotactic radiosurgery: analysis of accuracy and feasibility. Int J Radiat Oncol Biol Phys. 2001;51(4):1152–8.

[16] Kamath R, Ryken TC, Meeks SL, Pennington EC, Ritchie J, Buatti JM. Initial clinical experience with frameless radiosurgery for patients with intracranial metastases. Int J Radiat Oncol Biol Phys. 2005;61(5):1467–72.

[17] Das S, Isiah R, Rajesh B, et al. Accuracy of relocation, evaluation of geometric uncertainties and clinical target volume (CTV) to planning target volume (PTV) margin in fractionated stereotactic radiotherapy for intracranial tumors using relocatable Gill-ThomasCosman (GTC) frame. J Appl Clin Med Phys. 2010;12(2):3260.

[18] Li G, Ballangrud A, Kuo LC, et al. Motion monitoring for cranial frameless stereotactic radiosurgery using video-based three-dimensional optical surface imaging. Med Phys. 2011;38(7):3981–94.

[19] Tachibana H, Uchida Y, Shiizuka H. Technical note: determination of the optimized image processing and template matching techniques for a patient intrafraction motion monitoring system. Med Phys. 2012;39(2):755–64.

[20] Shirato H, Suzuki K, Nishioka T, et al. Precise positioning of intracranial small tumors to the linear accelerator's isocenter, using a stereotactic radiotherapy computed tomography system (SRT-CT). Radiother Oncol. 1994;32(2):180–3.

[21] Willner J, Flentje M, Bratengeier K. CT simulation in stereotactic brain radiotherapy–analysis of isocenter reproducibility with mask fixation. Radiother Oncol. 1997;45(1):83–8.

[22] Lewis BC, Snyder WJ, Kim S, Kim T. Monitoring frequency of intra-fraction patient motion using the ExacTrac system for LINAC-based SRS treatments. J Appl Clin Med Phys. 2018;19(3):58–63.

[23] Li G, Ballangrud A, Chan M, et al. Clinical experience with two frameless stereotactic radiosurgery (fSRS) systems using optical surface imaging for motion monitoring. J Appl Clin Med Phys. 2015;16(4):5416.

[24] Li G, Lovelock DM, Mechalakos J, et al. Migration from full-head mask to "open-face" mask for immobilization of patients with head and neck cancer. J Appl Clin Med Phys. 2013;14(5):243–54.

[25] Ballangrud A, Kuo LC, Happersett L, et al. Institutional experience with SRS VMAT planning for multiple cranial metastases. J Appl Clin Med Phys. 2018;19(2):176–83.

[26] Paxton AB, Manger RP, Pawlicki T, Kim GY. Evaluation of a surface imaging system's isocenter calibration methods. J Appl Clin Med Phys. 2017;18(2):85–91.

[27] Bert C, Metheany KG, Doppke K, Chen GT. A phantom evaluation of a stereo-vision surface imaging system for radiotherapy patient setup. Med Phys. 2005;32(9):2753–62.

[28] Djajaputra D, Li S. Real-time 3D surface-imageguided beam setup in radiotherapy of breast cancer. Med Phys. 2005;32(1):65–75.

[29] Bert C, Metheany KG, Doppke KP, Taghian AG, Powell SN, Chen GT. Clinical experience with a 3D surface patient setup system for alignment of partialbreast irradiation patients. Int J Radiat Oncol Biol Phys. 2006;64(4):1265–74.

[30] Hoisak JDP, Pawlicki T. The role of optical surface imaging systems in radiation therapy. Semin Radiat Oncol. 2018;28(3):185–93.

[31] Covington EL, Fiveash JB, Wu X, et al. Optical surface guidance for submillimeter monitoring of patient position during frameless stereotactic radiotherapy. J Appl Clin Med Phys. 2019;20(6):91–8.

[32] Yin F, Wong J, Balter J, et al. The role of in-room kV x-ray imaging for patient setup and target localization. AAPM Task Group Report No. 104. 2009. https://www.aapm.org/pubs/reports/detail.asp?docid=104.

[33] Klein EE, Hanley J, Bayouth J, et al. Task Group 142 report: quality assurance of medical accelerators. Med Phys. 2009;36(9):4197–212.

[34] Cervino LI, Pawlicki T, Lawson JD, Jiang SB. Frameless and mask-less cranial stereotactic radiosurgery: a feasibility study. Phys Med Biol. 2010;55(7):1863–73.

第21章 放射外科治疗的安全程序和检查清单
Safety Procedures and Checklists for Radiosurgery

Richard A. Popple 著
王翰宇 译
吕知平 校

一、概述

当实施准确时，放射外科治疗被认为是一种安全的治疗方法，有着低水平的不良反应[1,2]发生率。然而，由于每次实施的高剂量，其投照的误差仍可能带来严重的后果。

放射外科治疗中的投照误差可大致分为剂量学误差、几何误差和机器误差。当投照剂量和处方剂量有临床意义上的重大不一致时，就会出现剂量学误差。"临床意义重大"的定义没有明确说明，但报道的事件中通常是指超过规定的阈值。例如美国核管理委员会对医疗事件的定义[3]。剂量学误差的例子包括佛罗里达州[4]一台用于放疗手术的直线加速器的刻度误差和法国图卢兹输出因子的测量误差[5-7]。佛罗里达事件中的误差是刻度机器输出时的误差引起的。最初的机器刻度没有被独立检查，直到1年后RPC的例行审查期间（现在改名为IROC休斯顿）才发现误差。错误的机器刻度导致了77名患者实际照射剂量超出50%。在法国的事件中，治疗计划系统调试时小野（MLC＜3cm²）的输出因子是通过使用不适合测量小野的探测器测量的。结果导致145名患者接受了过量治疗。调试完1年后，当厂家对多个医院使用的输出因子进行相互比较时，才发现这个误差。厂家发现了这一差异并通知了医院。在接受听神经瘤治疗的32例患者中，有31%的患者在12个月[5]时有三叉神经病变。相比之下，尽管过失投照剂量超出61.2%（平均剂量31.5Gy），但33名接受脑转移治疗的患者在事故发生3年后没有发病，且生存率与文献[7]中报道的相似。

当剂量被投照到错误的位置时，就会出现几何误差。作用位置错误是所有医学领域[8]都会面临的问题。几何误差会导致靶区剂量不足和正常组织过量。靶区剂量不足可导致疗效欠佳；但是，在放射外科中，对正常组织的超量照射，会对其造成灾难性的后果。在美国核管理委员会公布的与伽马刀放射外科相关的不良事故的回顾中，2/3的事故（15例中的10例）都是由坐标错误导致的[9]，如预期的靶区目标是左三叉神经，却对右三叉神经进行了治疗。同样，在对2005—2010年核管理委员会（Nuclear Regulatory Commission，NRC）辐射事故报道通知数据库的审查中，超过一半（13个中的7个）与放射治疗相关的事故，涉及治疗部位的错误[10]。

当治疗机器没有按预期运行时，就会发生机器误差。机器误差可由设计缺陷或设备配置不当造成。在一个众所周知的例子中，装有锥筒装置的直线加速器的次级准直器设置得太大，导致在锥筒以外也受到完全剂量照射。三名患者严重受伤，至少一人处于接近植物人的状态[11]。法国也发生过类似的事故，患者患上了一种食管气管瘘，术后出血死亡[6]。

本章将回顾降低风险的重要概念：安全文

化、人因工程学、失效模式和影响分析。然后总结专业指导文件中的重点建议。

二、减少风险的概念

（一）安全文化

减少错误的基石是安全文化。强大的安全文化促进团队成员之间的信任和协作，鼓励报告错误，并使用错误报告来改进治疗流程[12]。建立和维护安全文化除了价值观的声明外，还需要具体的行动。其中重要的行动包括建立质量委员会和使用事件学习系统。

一个专门的质量委员会是一个多学科的团队，由医生、物理师、剂量师、放射治疗技师、护士、IT专业人员和任何其他涉及放射治疗流程的专业人员组成。委员会的职责是制定和实施安全措施，传播安全及质量信息，并与医院或卫生系统内其他安全委员会保持联系。委员会应定期开会，审查政策和流程，调查事故和险些发生的事故。委员会应有迅速调查严重事故的流程，通常在24h内进行调查。质量委员会负责定期向临床领导报告过失、趋势和安全措施。

建立事件学习系统及事件报告的政策和流程，是安全文化的关键要素，也是质量委员会收集、调查和在事件发生时采取行动的必要条件。虽然医院可以自行建立内部系统，但也有现成的几个多机构系统可用。参与一个既定的，多机构事故学习系统的优势有两个。首先，数据库和报告工具已经开发出来了，其次，参与多机构系统可以让个体医院从别处的过失中吸取教训。现有系统中的其中一个系统是RO-ILS：放射肿瘤学事件学习系统®（www.astro.org/Patient-Care-and-Research/Patient-Safety/RO-ILS），该系统由ASTRO和美国医学物理师协会（American Association of Physicists in Medicine，AAPM）开发。RO-ILS数据库结构的框架是基于"放射肿瘤学事件学习数据库结构的共识"，该建议是AAPM工作小组为预防放射肿瘤学[13]中的过失而开发的。其他事件学习系统包括放射肿瘤学安全教育信息系统（ROSEIS，roseis.estro.org）[14]和放射科学评估中心的放射治疗事件报告和分析系统（www.cars-pso.org）。

（二）人因工程学

放射外科治疗中的许多过失可归因于人为过失[4, 10, 15, 16]。然而，在导致过失的一系列事件中，人为过失往往是最终的原因，但不是根本原因。不良事件通常是系统和流程造成的不良环境的产物——那种人们会犯错或未能阻止错误发生的环境[17]。为了将过失的可能性降到最低，放射外科系统和流程必须设计得使过失难以产生[17]。AAPM的TG100指出，缺乏标准化流程、培训不足、通信不畅、硬件和软件故障、资源不足、设计规范不足和调试不足是过失的重要来源[15]。人因工程学是流程和系统设计的方法学，对人为错误具有鲁棒性。它已被应用于许多行业，如航空，以提高安全性和可靠性，但最近才应用于医疗保健行业[18]。人因工程学的一个基本原则是流程和系统的设计应该考虑人的表现和行为。因此，人为过失是系统设计缺陷，而不是失败的根本原因。有一系列可用的策略来减轻用户的过失。然而，它们并不都是同等有效的。策略（也称为干预措施）和相对有效性如图21-1所示。最低效率的干预措施是教育、培训、规则和政策。这些方法要求操作者在执行任务时高度可靠，也就是说，无误地调用完成任务所需的所有信息。尽管教育、培训、规则和政策是防过失流程的必要组成部分，但它们单独来看却不足以解决安全问题。例如，在过失事件数据库中，84%的事件都是未能遵循策略和流程引起的[4]。检查清单和双重检查更有效，因为它们建立在教育、培训、规则和政策的基础上，为用户提供回顾上的帮助。检查清单应用于医疗保健已被证明可减少不良事故发生[19, 20]，并被专业指南文件强烈推荐应[4]用于放射外科。

检查清单的使用是放射外科降低风险的一个重要组成部分。然而，不应该使用检查清单来代替更有效的风险降低策略。检查清单的弱点在于它们仍然依赖于人类的行为。组织必须有领导来开发和实施检查清单，并保持警惕以确保它们得到使用。组织必须主导开发和实施"检查清单"，并保持警惕以确保它们的施行。因此，如图 21-1 所示，简单化和标准化、自动化和数字化以及强制功能在减轻复杂系统中的风险方面更为有效。因为这些策略是系统固有的，它们不依赖人类行为来降低风险。简单化和标准化通过减少出错的机会来降低风险。此外，简单化和标准化最大限度地提高了使用检查清单的有效性，因为检查清单可以有更少的项目，从而更好地针对流程。比简单化和标准化更有效是软件和自动化。记录和验证系统是自动化在放射治疗中的应用实例。这些系统消除了将处理参数输入机器控制系统时的人为过失（前提是记录和验证系统中的参数是正

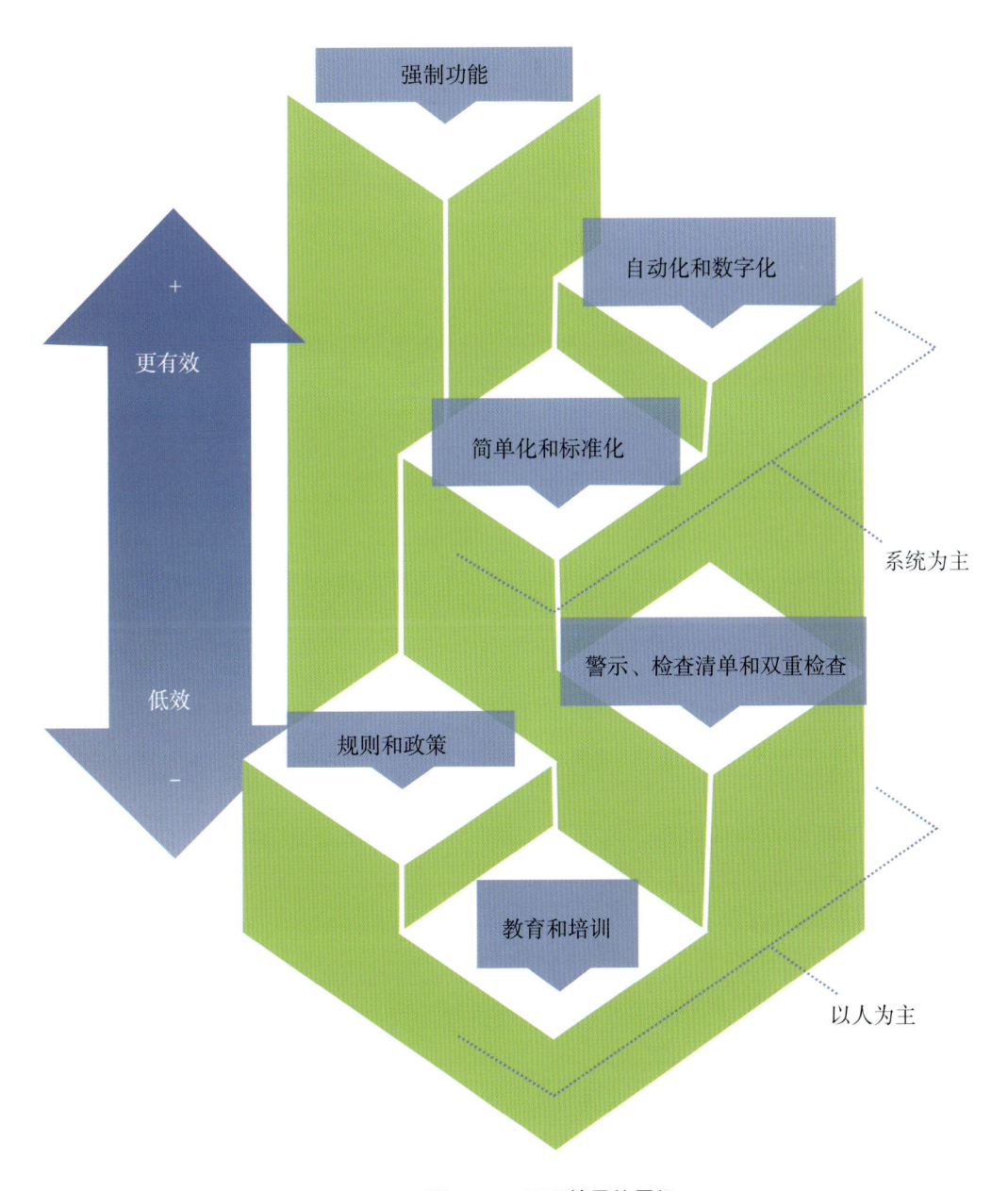

▲ 图 21-1 干预效果的层级

经 Healthcare Quarterly 许可转载，引自 Cafazzo 和 St Cyr[18]。除法律另有的规定外，不得再复制、分布和传播

确的）。最后，最有效的干预是强制功能。强制功能是指流程中任务被设计成使用户不可能过失地执行该任务。强制功能的一个例子是无处不在的门联锁，它防止机器在门打开时产生辐射。

三、病例介绍

（一）病例 1

1. 人因工程在锥筒尺寸选择中的应用

某患者，对靠近脑干的单个 4.7mm 直径的转移病灶照射 20Gy。治疗计划使用直径为 5mm 锥筒的直线加速器进行治疗。治疗小组的一名成员误读了治疗计划，装了一个 15mm 的锥筒。另一名成员由于被医生询问每日日程安排而分散了注意力，尽管接受了培训，却没有独立验证锥筒的大小。致使患者正常大脑的非预期体积接受了大剂量照射，包括脑干的一部分接受了全部处方剂量。

这个例子说明了图 21-1 所示的层次结构。该系统依靠受过专业培训的操作员来安装正确尺寸的锥筒，并依靠受过专业培训第二名团队成员来验证锥筒尺寸与治疗计划是否匹配。正规的政策和流程会在一定程度上减少这类过失的概率，因为第一个团队成员可能记得让第二个团队成员检查锥筒的大小。然而，政策和流程仍然受用户是否能回顾或者可能遗忘的影响，特别是当其他事情造成干扰时，一个需要确认锥筒尺寸的检查清单将会大大降低这个错误发生的概率。然而，防止这种错误的最有效方法是自动联锁，如果连接在机器上的锥筒与治疗计划中要求的锥筒不匹配，就会阻止治疗。

2. 失效模式和影响分析

失效模式和影响分析（failure modes and effects analysis，FMEA）是一种系统化的技术，用于评估潜在失效和失效对流程的影响。AAPM 任务组 100[15] 对 FMEA 在放疗过程中的应用进行了彻底的研究和描述。FMEA 是一个多学科的流程，应该由一个团队来进行。对于放射外科，FMEA 团队应该由放射肿瘤医生、医学物理师、治疗技师，和一个定位技师组成。其他成员，如剂量师、护士和神经外科医生，应根据计划和治疗流程的细节情况而定。简单地说，一个流程的 FMEA 包括四个步骤。

① 创建一个流程图。
② 失效模式的识别。
③ 对每种失效模式的发生率、严重程度、可探测性打分。
④ 制定预防措施，将风险降到最低。

第一步是开发详细的流程图，然后评估流程中可能出现的故障事件。通过过程（故障树分析）评估故障事件的传播，以确定故障事件对结果的影响。基于故障树分析，团队成员将每个失效模式分配三个类别的分数。

- 发生率（用 O 表示）是指故障事件发生的可能性。从 1（不太可能发生故障事件，< 0.01%）到 10（超过 5% 的次数）。

- 严重性（用 S 表示）是指如果发生故障事件但仍就未被发现，其结果的严重性。从 1（临床常规的最小干扰）到 10（灾难性）不等。

- 可检测性（用 D 表示）是指未能及时检测到故障事件以防止事故发生的可能性。范围从 1（非常容易被检测到，< 0.01% 的故障事件在整个治疗过程中未被检测到）到 10（非常难以检测：超过 20% 的故障事件在整个治疗过程中持续存在）。

OSD 乘积称为风险优先系数（risk priority number，RPN），它是每个故障模式对患者造成的相对风险的度量。高 RPN 值表明可能发生的故障事件难以检测，并对患者造成严重后果。FMEA 流程的最后一步是对 RPN 值进行排序，并设计一个质量管理程序来降低失效风险。通常情况下，特定故障事件的严重程度无法降低，因此风险缓解的重点是降低故障事件发生率和提高检测的可能性。文献中已经有一些关于 FMEA 应用于放射外科的描述[21-24]。与 AAPM TG100 的报道一起，这些报道在进行 FMEA 时可以作为指导；然而，它们不能代替本单位流程的 FMEA，因为失效模式和相应的风险优先级数值强烈依赖于所考虑流程的细节。

(二)病例 2

1. 放射治疗的 FMEA 分析

意大利诺瓦拉皮埃蒙特大学医院将 FMEA[21] 应用于放射外科上。该医院有几年使用带有锥筒和头架固定的直线加速器的放射外科经验。医院成立了一个 FMEA 工作组，目的是提高流程质量，防止错误发生。该小组由 8 名放射肿瘤医生、2 名住院医师、3 名医学物理师、4 名放射技师和 1 名护士组成。

该 FMEA 工作组确定了放射外科流程中的 73 个步骤和 116 种可能的失效模式。其中风险优先值范围为 1~180，平均值为 14。严重程度范围为 1~9，平均值为 3.4，该严重程度范围表明有一些故障事件将是灾难性的（团队将近乎致命损伤的事件定义为 9）。发生率范围为 1~4，平均值为 1.5。可检测性范围为 1~5，平均值为 1.6。表明错误并不经常发生（该小组将可检测性定义为 2 是指一万个事件中只有有一个错误会发生），并且很容易检测到（团队将可检测性定义为 2 是指事件几乎总是检测到）。该工作组将风险优先值 125 作为采取纠正措施的阈值。确定了两种超过阈值的失效模式：使用错误的准直器大小进行治疗和定位中设置了错误的等中心坐标。

准直器大小不正确的影响可能是严重的，特别是实际的准直器偏大，这个过失的严重程度评分为 9（近乎致命的伤害）。尽管治疗流程要求准直器的大小需要由技师、物理师和医生进行检查，但是二次检查并不能充分可靠地使可检测性降到最低。因此，安装带有记录和验证系统接口的条形码阅读器将提高可检测性，从而使可检测性评分降到最低评分（1）。

等中心坐标不正确的影响与准直器大小不正确的影响一样具有灾难性，因此也被授予 9 级的严重程度评分。同样与准直器大小核查相似，治疗流程依赖于双重检查以验证等中心坐标是否正确。该团队使用表面成像系统对患者体位进行了第二次独立检查。在定位框架上设置等中心后，表面成像系统将患者的面部图像与从治疗计划系统获得的渲染图进行比较。新的流程建立了一个 1mm 的阈值来检查定位框架上的坐标。

从这个病例研究中可以得出几点总结。首先，该机构有一个启动 FMEA 流程的持续质量改进程序。其次，该机构致力于根据 FMEA 分析的结果进行改进。具有最高风险优先值的两种失效模式不仅需要流程更改，还需要大量的财务投资来降低风险。最后，请注意，这两种流程改进都依赖于将流程向上移动到有效性层级。准直器的改变从第二次检查的策略转变为强制功能：如果准直器的条形码与治疗计划不匹配，治疗无法继续进行。表面成像系统使用软件和自动化来确保正确的等中心放置。

2. 检查清单及其设计

检查清单只是一个有组织的项目列表，提示用户考虑或完成每个项目。清单是一种有效的风险缓解战略，因为它们建立在教育、培训、政策和流程的基础上，为用户提供回顾上的帮助（图 21-2）。与直接引用流程相比，清单的一个优点是以列表形式组织的指令比以段落形式[25]的指令更容易理解。因此，检查清单的使用是放射外科中的一个关键因素，ASTRO 和 AAPM 都强烈推荐使用[4, 26]。ASTRO 建议 SRS 前检查清单内容至少包括以下几点。

① 患者身份核实。

② 医生和物理师对患者治疗前的治疗计划进行审核和批准。

③ 确认患者的摆位和靶区的重新定位是准确的。

④ 验证所选的投照射野 / 弧与待治疗的患者是否匹配。

除此之外，检查清单的编制需要了解特定的治疗过程。FMEA 分析可以用来指导检查清单的

```
病史
患者 Jane Doe，89 岁，女性，回到诊所评估右侧面部疼痛。3 年前，
患者主要集中在三叉神经第二支位置出现右侧面部疼痛。她……
```

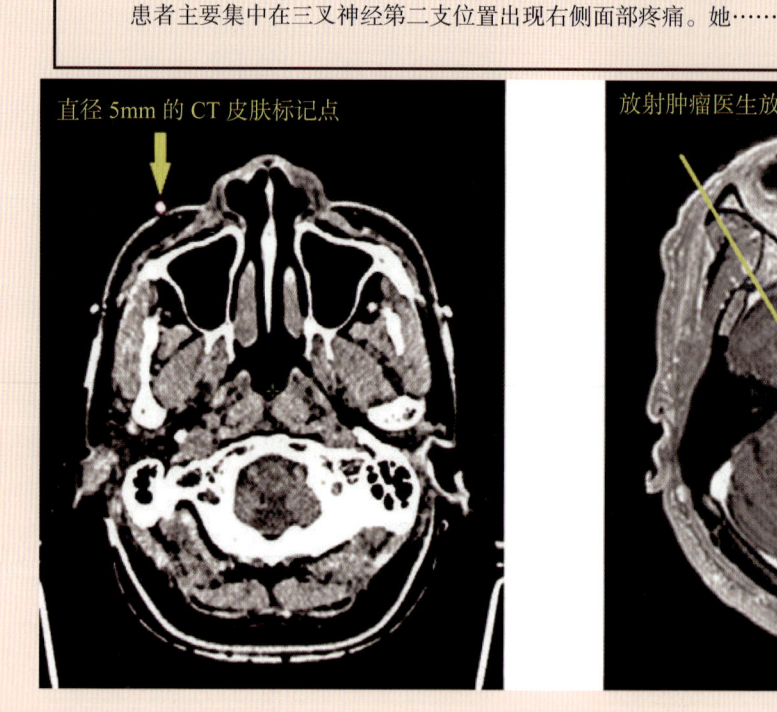

直径 5mm 的 CT 皮肤标记点 | 放射肿瘤医生放置的等中心位置

☑ EHR 中参考注释的偏侧性（圈一）　　　　　　　　　　　　　　　（右）　左
☑ 偏侧性标记的位置（圈一）　　　　　　　　　　　　　　　　　　（右）　左
☑ 医生放置的等中心位置（圈一）　　　　　　　　　　　　　　　　（右）　左
☑ 参考注释中的偏侧性，侧向标记位置和等中心一致

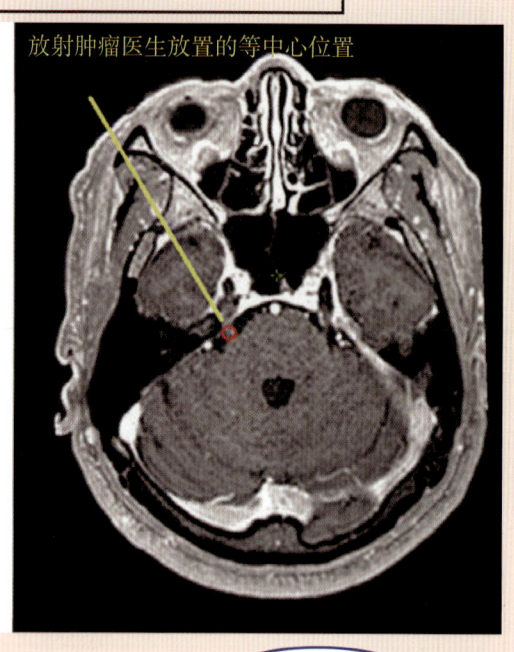

▲ 图 21-2　右侧三叉神经痛患者的侧位治疗计划清单，以及相关部分的神经外科门诊记录和相关影像

制定。使用检查清单可以减少错误的发生，提高错误的可检测性，从而减少已识别的故障模式的风险优先评定值。值得注意的是，检查清单不应该被用作流程改进的替代品。清单依赖于人的行为，因此不如以系统为重点的干预有效。例如，检查清单规定技师检查安装到机器上的锥筒是否正确，不能代替软件验证安装到照射系统上的锥筒是否与治疗计划中的锥筒相匹配。

美国医学物理师协会在医学物理实践指南 4.a 中为检查清单的开发、实施、使用和维护安全检查提供了广泛的实践指导[26]。

清单不是万能的，应该恰当使用。检查清单如果被过度使用，将导致用户在完成检查清单时负担过重，从而阻碍而不是帮助提高医疗的质量。此外，检查清单的过度使用可能导致医务人员依赖于检查清单，从而干扰专业判断。因此，检查列表应该包含有限数量的条目，这些条目应集中在高风险的步骤上，对于这些步骤，过失的后果是严重的。医院应将定期审查检查清单作为持续质量改进流程的一部分。

（三）病例 3

使用检查清单来化解偏侧性错误

某患者，右侧三叉神经需要接受 90Gy 的放射治疗。医学物理师将 MRI 和 CT 图像导入治疗计划系统，并制定了对侧（左侧）三叉神经的治疗计划。放射肿瘤医生审查并批准了该治疗计划。在神经外科医生、放射肿瘤医生和医学物理

师在场的情况下，对左侧三叉神经进行了照射。神经外科医生在放疗后准备手术记录时发现这个错误。患者不得不进行第二次放射外科来治疗右侧三叉神经，由于治疗错误导致左侧面部麻木。

左右位置错误是治疗三叉神经痛最常见的错误之一，治疗流程应考虑到这一点。当对三叉神经放射外科进行成像时，应要求患者指出疼痛的一侧并在该侧放置标志物。在制定治疗计划时，应检查标志物的位置、放射肿瘤医生指定的等中心位置和神经外科医生指定的侧位是否一致。治疗计划检查清单的示例部分如图21-2所示。在治疗时，再次要求患者指向疼痛的一侧，这应与治疗计划的偏侧性一致，并经神经外科医生和放射肿瘤科医生确认。这一步应该包括在治疗前检查清单中。

四、主要建议

专业指导文献[4, 27, 28]对放射外科项目的质量和安全的组成部分进行了广泛的讨论。本文对这些因素进行了总结，但强烈建议读者直接查阅相关文献。

立体定向放射外科需要团队成员接受适当的培训，并具有SRS特有的资格证书。一个SRS团队至少应由放射肿瘤医生、医学物理师、剂量师、神经外科医生和放射技师组成。团队成员必须有适当的认证或许可，并且经过充分的针对SRS的培训（无论是作为正式培训还是继续教育的一部分），团队成员应该有明确定义的角色和职责。

SRS项目需要比常规放射治疗更多的资源投入。对SRS项目所要求的人员水平的指导是有限的，所以医院有责任评估人员需求，并确保员工有足够的时间来完成他们的任务。同样，设备需求将取决于项目目标。磁共振成像是进行放射外科的先决条件。如果对动静脉畸形（arterio-venous malformations，AVM）进行治疗，血管造影将是必要的。在过去，头架被用于患者的固定，而现在无框架固定系统正变得越来越普遍。治疗计划系统必须能够支持小野的精确剂量计算。计划系统的这种固有性能专门用于立体定向放射外科，但应该认真评估。当使用通用放射治疗计划系统而非立体定向放射外科专用的计划系统时，需要特别谨慎。除了剂量计算，治疗计划系统必须有能力导入和配准多模态影像，以便用于靶区的勾画。特别是在动静脉畸形的放射外科中，并不是所有的治疗计划系统都能够使用双平面血管造影来设计放射外科计划。照射系统应设计成符合立体定向放射外科的规范和安全系统。当使用图像引导进行定位时，成像系统等中心和治疗投照等中心之间的重合度应符合SRS规范（通常＜1mm）。如果一个基于头架的系统用于固定和定位，强烈建议尽可能使用图像引导系统来验证患者的位置。使用锥筒的治疗系统应该具备验证锥筒已经正确安装上去的能力。在为放射外科选择设备时，也应考虑相应的质量保证设备。由于严格的机械容差和小野剂量测量的挑战，用于常规放射治疗的QA设备不足以执行放射外科的QA。所需要的设备应包括用于评价治疗成像系统的模体、用于常规温斯顿-卢茨测试的工具和软件、适用于小野测量的探测器。如果需要应用调强技术，应有患者特有的QA设备。

设备验收和调试是放射外科流程的两个组成部分。验收是指与厂家一起验证设备在规定的规格范围内运行。设备规范由厂家和客户在采购流程中制定，应满足或超过放射外科系统专业指导文件中的建议[4, 29]。调试是收集临床使用配置系统所需的测量值，然后测试系统以确保配置正确的过程。最常见的是测量辐射束特征数据，用于调试计划系统。由于小野的存在，这个任务对于放射外科[30]是特别具有挑战性的，负责光束数据的收集以及计划系统的配置的医学物理师应专门为调试放疗计划系统进行培训和装备。除了光束数据收集和处理计划系统的配置外，调试还包括放射外科治疗过程中所需的所有系统的整合和配置。这些系统包括定位系统[31]、放射肿瘤信息系统（radiation oncology information system，ROIS）、图像配准系统[32]、CT模拟定位和图像引导系统[33, 34]。端到端测试是放射外科系统调试[28]的最后一个重要步骤，独立的端到端测试尤其重要。M.D 安德森医院的剂量测量实验室（M.D. Anderson Dosimetry Laboratory，MDADL）可以提供一个拟人化的头部模体，头部模体内包含胶片和点剂量计。使用该模体的医院可以使用M.D 安德森医院标准的放射外科计划和投照流程，包括定位，然后将模体返回给 M.D 安德森医院的剂量测量实验室。M.D 安德森医院的剂量测量实验室会根据医院提供的治疗计划数据对测量的剂量分布进行评估，并向医院提供一份结果报告，报告摘要见图 21-3。

为减少放射外科实践过程的错误，一个健全的质量保证程序是必要的。描述一个完整的质量保证程序超出了本章的范围，所以鼓励读者查阅相关文献[4, 12, 27-29, 32, 34, 35]。然而，这里总结了几个重要项目。第一，一个放射外科项目必须建立并保持一种安全文化，在这种文化中，所有的团队成员都有权质疑，如果有任何关于治疗安全性的问题，必要时，停止手术。这样的安全文化需要团队成员之间的信任和沟通。一些团队成员认为他们必须服从他人或者在表达担忧时担心受到惩罚，这种社会等级问题应特别注意。第二，在治疗开始前应该进行暂停。暂停最少要包括确认正确的患者和正确的部位。暂停还可以包括对其他安全检查列表的验证。第三，应为治疗流程的所有方面制定标准政策和程序，包括质量保证。政策和程序应在适当的时候包含检查清单。第四，定期进行同行评审和独立审计。同行评审包括内部评审和外部评审。独立审计包括由外部机构对机器校准的年度评估，如 IROC-Houston 或 M.D. Anderson 认可剂量学实验室。最后，验收测试、调试和质量保证活动应该被完整地记录下来。

持续的质量改进对放射外科项目至关重要，是质量保证程序的扩展。应定期审查和更新政策和流程，以反映任何实践变化。应考虑使用统计过程控制等工具对 QA 测试结果进行定量监测[36-41]。

程序说明：

对含有直径 1.9cm 的球形靶的拟人头部模体进行成像和辐照，在靶区中心附近放置两片热释光计量片以获取剂量信息。两张正交的辐射自显影胶片提供侧向剂量分布和评估投照剂量分布。结果汇总如下，详细报告见附表。

热释光计量计的典型计量学精度为 ±3%，胶片和密度计系统的空间精度为 ±1mm

热释光计量计和胶片的结果总结：

	比例	标准；（图中有2处）	可接受；（图中有2处）
靶区中心计量（热释光计量计/机构）	1.03	0.95～1.05	是

胶片平面	伽马指数*	标准；（图中有2处）	可接受；（图中有2处）
冠状面	99%	≥ 85%	是
矢状面	99%	≥ 85%	是

*. 满足伽马指数标准 5% 和 3mm 的百分比
上表中列出的模体辐照结果符合 IROC 休斯顿制定的标准

▲ 图 21-3 报告摘录，总结 IROC 休斯顿 /M.D 安德森剂量测量实验室 SRS 头模照射模体和通过目标中心的剂量分布如 22 章的图 22-2 所示

五、未来及展望

如图 21-1 所示，以系统为中心的干预措施在减少错误方面最有效。不幸的是，与对人类行为的控制相比，个别机构对系统的控制要少得多。机构可以简化和标准化其流程，但自动化和强制功能经常需要工程专业知识和设备厂家的软件/硬件。例如，将固定在直线加速器上的锥筒与治疗计划进行自动比较，就需要传感器硬件来检测锥筒已经安装，同时需要软件来检查锥筒是否与方案匹配。如果一个投照系统没有被设计来做这样的比较，用户就很难建立一个独立的自动核查系统。因此他们必须依靠核对表。医疗保健提供者必须与行业合作，以促进改善患者安全。

跨机构的标准化和简化将进一步减少错误。在治疗计划系统中，标准化的其中一个成熟领域就是在治疗计划系统中的束流建模。许多放射外科中的剂量过量与输出因子的测量错误有关。然而，输出因子在同一型号的治疗机器之间并没有显著的差别。在治疗计划系统中标准化射野数据和输出因子会改变测量错误的影响。在目前的模式下，调试期间的测量误差将直接转移到患者的治疗中去。对于一个拥有标准化射野数据的系统，调试期间的测量误差将导致计划系统和测量之间的不匹配。这将引发调试的物理师去调查之前过程的不一致性。重要的是要理解，这种类型的标准化不是一个全面的解决方案，而且也可能失败。负责调试放射外科治疗系统的物理师仍然需要专业判断和警惕，因为测量和治疗计划系统之间的不一致表明可能存在实际的问题，而不是测量误差。

投照系统质量保证的另一改进方面是标准化和自动化。设备的验收和容差是有标准的[4, 29]，但实施的细节是现场特定的。验收的自动化具有很大的潜力，因为治疗照射可以依赖于所做的适当测试和规范。例如，如果机器的输出超出容差范围，医院应该实施程序确保治疗不会发生。厂家[42-45]和多个机构[46]正在努力开发标准化和自动化的 QA 工具。

> **要点 – 建议**
> - 发展和培育安全文化。
> - 实施事故学习系统。
> - 成立专门的质量委员会。
> - 确保放射外科治疗团队成员有相应的培训和证书。
> - 为放射外科治疗项目提供充足的资源。
> - 根据失效模式和影响分析（failure modes and effects analysis，FMEA）和人因工程学（human factors engineering，HFE）制定程序和检查清单。
> - 定期获得独立的项目评审。

参考文献

[1] Suh JH. Stereotactic radiosurgery for the management of brain metastases. N Engl J Med. 2010;362(12):1119–27.

[2] Combs SE, Welzel T, Schulz-Ertner D, Huber PE, Debus J. Differences in clinical results after LINAC-based single-dose radiosurgery versus fractionated stereotactic radiotherapy for patients with vestibular schwannomas. Int J Radiat Oncol Biol Phys. 2010;76(1):193–200.

[3] NRC regulations: title 10, code of federal regulations. Sect. 35.3045.

[4] Solberg TD, Balter JM, Benedict SH, Fraass BA, Kavanagh B, Miyamoto C, et al. Quality and safety considerations in stereotactic radiosurgery and stereotactic body radiation therapy: executive summary. Pract Radiat Oncol. 2012;2(1):2–9.

[5] Gourmelon P, Bey E, De Revel T, Lazorthes Y, Lotteries J, Lataillade JJ. The French radiation accident experience: emerging concepts in radiation burn and ARS therapies and in

brain radiopathology. Radioprotection. 2008;43(5):23–6.

[6] Derreumaux S, Etard C, Huet C, Trompier F, Clairand I, Bottollier-Depois JF, et al. Lessons from recent accidents in radiation therapy in France. Radiat Prot Dosim. 2008;131(1):130–5.

[7] Borius PY, Debono B, Latorzeff I, Lotterie JA, Plas JY, Cassol E, et al. Dosimetric stereotactic radiosurgical accident: study of 33 patients treated for brain metastases. Neurochirurgie. 2010;56(5):368–73.

[8] Stahel PF, Sabel AL, Victoroff MS, Varnell J, Lembitz A, Boyle DJ, et al. Wrong-site and wrong-patient procedures in the universal protocol era: analysis of a prospective database of physician self-reported occurrences. Arch Surg. 2010;145(10):978–84.

[9] Information notice 2000–22: medical misadministrations caused by human errors involving Gamma stereotactic radiosurgery (Gamma knife) 2000.

[10] Solberg TD, Medin PM. Quality and safety in stereotactic radiosurgery and stereotactic body radiation therapy: can more be done? J Radiosurg SBRT. 2011;1(1):13–9.

[11] Bogdanich WR, Rebelo K. A pinpoint beam strays invisibly, harming instead of healing. The New York Times. 2010. https://www.nytimes.com/2010/12/29/health/29radiation.html. Accessed 27 May 2019.

[12] (ASTRO). Safety is no accident: a framework for quality radiation oncology and care. 2012. https://www.astro.org/uploadedFiles/_MAIN_SITE/Daily_Practice/Accreditation/Content_Pieces/SafetyisnoAccident.pdf. Accessed 27 May 2019.

[13] Ford EC, Fong de Los Santos L, Pawlicki T, Sutlief S, Dunscombe P. Consensus recommendations for incident learning database structures in radiation oncology. Med Phys. 2012;39(12):7272–90.

[14] Cunningham J, Coffey M, Knoos T, Holmberg O. Radiation Oncology Safety Information System (ROSIS)–profiles of participants and the first 1074 incident reports. Radiother Oncol. 2010;97(3):601–7.

[15] Huq MS, Fraass BA, Dunscombe PB, Gibbons JP Jr, Ibbott GS, Mundt AJ, et al. The report of Task Group 100 of the AAPM: application of risk analysis methods to radiation therapy quality management. Med Phys. 2016;43(7):4209.

[16] British Institute of Radiology, the Institute of Physics and Engineering in Medicine, the National Patient Safety Agency, the Society and College of Radiographers and the Royal College of Radiologists. Towards safer radiotherapy. 2008.

[17] Institute of Medicine (US) Committee on Quality of Health Care in America. In: Linda TK, Janet MC, Molla SD, editors. To err is human: building a safer health system. Washington, DC: The National Academies Press; 2000.

[18] Cafazzo JA, St-Cyr O. From discovery to design: the evolution of human factors in healthcare. Healthc Q. 2012;15(April (Special Issue)):24–9.

[19] Pronovost P, Needham D, Berenholtz S, Sinopoli D, Chu H, Cosgrove S, et al. An intervention to decrease catheter-related bloodstream infections in the ICU. N Engl J Med. 2006;355(26):2725–32.

[20] Hales BM, Pronovost PJ. The checklist–a tool for error management and performance improvement. J Crit Care. 2006;21(3):231–5.

[21] Masini L, Donis L, Loi G, Mones E, Molina E, Bolchini C, et al. Application of failure mode and effects analysis to intracranial stereotactic radiation surgery by linear accelerator. Pract Radiat Oncol. 2014;4(6):392–7.

[22] Manger RP, Paxton AB, Pawlicki T, Kim GY. Failure mode and effects analysis and fault tree analysis of surface image guided cranial radiosurgery. Med Phys. 2015;42(5):2449–61.

[23] Teixeira FC, de Almeida CE, Saiful HM. Failure mode and effects analysis based risk profile assessment for stereotactic radiosurgery programs at three cancer centers in Brazil. Med Phys. 2016;43(1):171.

[24] Xu AY, Bhatnagar J, Bednarz G, Flickinger J, Arai Y, Vacsulka J, et al. Failure modes and effects analysis (FMEA) for Gamma knife radiosurgery. J Appl Clin Med Phys. 2017;18(6):152–68.

[25] Morrow DG, Leirer VO, Andrassy JM, Hier CM, Menard WE. The influence of list format and category headers on age differences in understanding medication instructions. Exp Aging Res. 1998;24(3):231–56.

[26] Fong de Los Santos LE, Evans S, Ford EC, Gaiser JE, Hayden SE, Huffman KE, et al. Medical Physics Practice Guideline 4.a: development, implementation, use and maintenance of safety checklists. J Appl Clin Med Phys. 2015;16(3):5431.

[27] Seung SK, Larson DA, Galvin JM, Mehta MP, Potters L, Schultz CJ, et al. American College of Radiology (ACR) and American Society for Radiation Oncology (ASTRO) Practice Guideline for the Performance of Stereotactic Radiosurgery (SRS). Am J Clin Oncol. 2013;36(3):310–5.

[28] Halvorsen PH, Cirino E, Das IJ, Garrett JA, Yang J, Yin FF, et al. AAPM-RSS medical physics practice guideline 9.a. for SRS-SBRT. J Appl Clin Med Phys. 2017;18(5):10–21.

[29] Klein EE, Hanley J, Bayouth J, Yin FF, Simon W, Dresser S, et al. Task Group 142 report: quality assurance of medical accelerators. Med Phys. 2009;36(9):4197–212.

[30] Palmans H, Andreo P, Huq MS, Seuntjens J, Christaki KE, Meghzifene A. Dosimetry of small static fields used in external photon beam radiotherapy: summary of TRS-483, the IAEA-AAPM international Code of Practice for reference and relative dose determination. Med Phys. 2018;45(11):e1123–45.

[31] Lightstone AW, Benedict SH, Bova FJ, Solberg TD, Stern RL. Intracranial stereotactic positioning systems: report of the American Association of Physicists in Medicine Radiation Therapy Committee Task Group No. 68. Med Phys. 2005;32(7Part1):2380–98.

[32] Brock KK, Mutic S, McNutt TR, Li H, Kessler ML. Use of image registration and fusion algorithms and techniques in radiotherapy: report of the AAPM Radiation Therapy Committee Task Group No. 132. Med Phys. 2017;44(7):

e43–76.

[33] Langen KM, Willoughby TR, Meeks SL, Santhanam A, Cunningham A, Levine L, et al. Observations on real-time prostate gland motion using electromagnetic tracking. Int J Radiat Oncol Biol Phys. 2008;71(4):1084–90.

[34] Bissonnette JP, Balter PA, Dong L, Langen KM, Lovelock DM, Miften M, et al. Quality assurance for image-guided radiation therapy utilizing CT-based technologies: a report of the AAPM TG-179. Med Phys. 2012;39(4):1946–63.

[35] Willoughby T, Lehmann J, Bencomo JA, Jani SK, Santanam L, Sethi A, et al. Quality assurance for nonradiographic radiotherapy localization and positioning systems: report of Task Group 147. Med Phys. 2012;39(4):1728–47.

[36] Pawlicki T, Whitaker M, Boyer AL. Statistical process control for radiotherapy quality assurance. Med Phys. 2005;32(9):2777–86.

[37] Palaniswaamy G, Scott Brame R, Yaddanapudi S, Rangaraj D, Mutic S. A statistical approach to IMRT patient-specific QA. Med Phys. 2012;39(12):7560–70.

[38] Letourneau D, Wang A, Amin MN, Pearce J, McNiven A, Keller H, et al. Multileaf collimator performance monitoring and improvement using semiautomated quality control testing and statistical process control. Med Phys. 2014;41(12):121713.

[39] Chung JB, Kim JS, Ha SW, Ye SJ. Statistical analysis of IMRT dosimetry quality assurance measurements for local delivery guideline. Radiat Oncol. 2011;6:27.

[40] Breen SL, Moseley DJ, Zhang B, Sharpe MB. Statistical process control for IMRT dosimetric verification. Med Phys. 2008;35(10):4417–25.

[41] Able CM, Baydush AH, Nguyen C, Gersh J, Ndlovu A, Rebo I, et al. A model for preemptive maintenance of medical linear accelerators-predictive maintenance. Radiat Oncol. 2016;11:36.

[42] Barnes MP, Pomare D, Menk FW, Moraro B, Greer PB. Evaluation of the TrueBeam machine performance check (MPC): OBI X-ray tube alignment procedure. J Appl Clin Med Phys. 2018;19(6):68–78.

[43] Barnes MP, Greer PB. Evaluation of the TrueBeam machine performance check (MPC) beam constancy checks for flattened and flattening filterfree (FFF) photon beams. J Appl Clin Med Phys. 2017;18(1):139–50.

[44] Barnes MP, Greer PB. Evaluation of the TrueBeam machine performance check (MPC) geometric checks for daily IGRT geometric accuracy quality assurance. J Appl Clin Med Phys. 2017;18(3):200–6.

[45] Barnes MP, Greer PB. Evaluation of the TrueBeam machine performance check (MPC): mechanical and collimation checks. J Appl Clin Med Phys. 2017;18(3):56–66.

[46] Eckhause T, Al-Hallaq H, Ritter T, DeMarco J, Farrey K, Pawlicki T, et al. Automating linear accelerator quality assurance. Med Phys. 2015;42(10):6074–83.

第22章 小野放疗的质量保证
Quality Assurance for Small Fields

Richaed A.Popple 著
王翰宇 译
杨晓喻 校

一、概述

小野剂量测量具有挑战性。放射外科的几起放疗事故均与错误的测量方式有关，如法国的一家医院在对治疗计划系统进行调试时，错误地使用Farmer电离室测量小野（＜3cm²）的输出因子，厂商在一年后对比不同医院的输出因子，最终发现了这个错误，结果显示[1]，有145名放疗患者的剂量超量；在美国密苏里州一家医院的计划系统调试中也发生了类似的错误[2]；伽马刀治疗计划系统中4mm的射野输出因子长期都被低估了9%[3]。

不当的小野剂量测量会产生严重的后果，因此开展放射外科治疗的单位必须配备合适的小野测量设备，并对从事SRS调试和质量保证工作的物理师进行专业培训。目前已有一些可供参考的小野剂量学方面的文献，包括国际辐射单位和测量委员会（International Commission on Radiation Units，ICRU）的91号报告[4]、国际原子能机构（International Atomic Energy Agency，IAEA）的483号报告[5]以及美国医学物理学家协会（American Associate of Physicists in Medicine，AAPM）针对483号报告的总结[6]，物理师在开展放射外科技术前应全面并深入地阅读这些文献。本章主要内容为小野剂量学关键概念的概述。

目前并没有特别明确的小野定义，较为普遍的观点是若射束中心轴上的感兴趣点满足以下三个条件中任意一个即可认为是小野：①侧向带电粒子失衡；②准直器对初级射线源存在部分遮挡，从探测器视角无法看到完整的射线源；③探测器响应随射野尺寸变化。

当次级电子的射程大于射野尺寸的一半时就会出现带电粒子失衡现象。根据蒙特卡洛模拟，次级电子的射程 r_{LCPE} 与射线质有关，定义射线质为 %dd（10，10）x，两者关系如下：

$$r_{LCPE}(\text{cm}) = 0.07797\%dd(10,10)_X - 4.112$$

射线质也可以用 $TPR_{20,10}$ 来表述。对于能量为6～10MV的射束，带电粒子失衡的射野尺寸小于2～3cm。

初级射线源尺寸有限，导致了准直器对初级放射源的部分遮挡。初级放射源的尺寸定义为电子束打靶后产生的韧致辐射在出射靶平面的半高宽。一个孔径足够小的准直器能够遮挡有限尺寸的初级射线源的外围，导致射束中心轴上的输出比同样准直器尺寸的理想点源小。当射野尺寸和射线源尺寸相当或者小于射线源尺寸时，这种现象更加明显。因此，有限的射野尺寸会造成准直器对初级射线源的部分遮挡，亦能导致带电粒子失衡。

在小野测量中，造成探测器响应变化的主要原因就是体积平均效应。如果在灵敏体积内剂量分布不均匀，探测器响应将会是探测器形状和剂量分布的卷积。此外，探测器对带电粒子通量的扰动会导致布拉格-格雷空腔理论无效。因此，当探测器边缘至射野边缘的尺寸大于 r_{LCPE} 时，比较适合小野测量。造成探测器响应变化的另一个原因是小野的能谱变化。与大野相比，小野中的模体散射较少，同时直线加速器机头内的低能量散射会因准直器尺寸变小而减少，因此，小野光谱更硬（拥有更多的高能光子）。光谱硬化会改变探测器材料的质能吸收系数和阻止本领比，这种效应对于硅基二极管探测器和具有电极为高原子序数材料的电离室特别明显。

二、相对剂量学

配置计划系统通常需要相对于刻度条件下的输出（输出因子）、射束中心轴百分深度剂量和特定深度的侧向剂量曲线。对于使用固定准直器（锥筒）的 SRS 技术，必须测量每个准直器的输出；对于使用多叶准直器的 SRS 技术，必须配置计划系统特定射野尺寸的输出因子、百分深度剂量和侧向剂量曲线，这些特定射野可以通过 MLC 准直，也可以不通过 MLC 准直。

直线加速器的标准剂量刻度指南规定的测量尺寸为 10cm 方野。其他类型的机器，如伽马刀或射波刀，不能产生 10cm 的射野。因此，人们开发了多种方法将直线加速器的标准剂量刻度指南推广到非标准射野。对于特定的机器类型，参考射野被定义为特定机器参考（machine-specific reference，MSR）射野，MSR 射野通常是指该机器能够形成的最大射野。其输出因子（$\Omega_{Q_{\text{clin}},Q_{\text{msr}}}^{f_{\text{clin}},f_{\text{msr}}}$），是感兴趣射野的水中吸收剂量与 MSR 射野的水中吸收剂量的比值。

输出因子是在特定的源皮距和深度处测量的，测量深度通常为 5cm 或 10cm，这样可以消除电子污染的影响。输出因子可通过测量并代入以下公式获得。

$$\Omega_{Q_{\text{clin}},Q_{\text{msr}}}^{f_{\text{clin}},f_{\text{msr}}} = k_{Q_{\text{clin}},Q_{\text{msr}}}^{f_{\text{clin}},f_{\text{msr}}} \frac{M_{Q_{\text{clin}}}^{f_{\text{clin}}}}{M_{Q_{\text{msr}}}^{f_{\text{msr}}}}$$

其中 $M_{Q_{\text{clin}}}^{f_{\text{clin}}}$ 是感兴趣射野中的探测器测量信号，$M_{Q_{\text{msr}}}^{f_{\text{msr}}}$ 是机器参考射野中的探测器测量信号，$k_{Q_{\text{clin}},Q_{\text{msr}}}^{f_{\text{clin}},f_{\text{msr}}}$ 是输出修正因子，大野的输出修正因子近似是 1。输出修正因子取决于探测器的设计、射线质和射野大小。实验测量特定探测器的修正因子需要使用其他已知修正因子的探测器，同时修正因子也可以用蒙特卡罗模拟计算。国际原子能机构 TRS-483 号报告提供了许多探测器的[5]修正因子，若未列出，则应当搜索文献找到对应探测器的修正因子，已发表的文献报道了大多数适用于小野剂量测定的商用探测器的修正因子[7-11]。

探测器方向对输出因子测量有影响，首选的方向取决于探测器的类型和设计。射野中电缆的长度应尽量小，以限制漏电流信号。应特别注意，必须将探测器定位在射束中心轴上，可以通过沿着与射束中心轴垂直的两个侧向轴扫描侧向剂量曲线，并将探测器置于信号最大的位置。因为输出因子与小野的尺寸关系较大，测量输出因子前应先测量射束侧向剂量曲线来确认射野的尺寸，这个过程对于尺寸可变的准直器（如 MLC）尤其重要。

百分深度剂量和侧向剂量曲线

在小野百分深度剂量（percent depth dose，PDD）的测量中，射野尺寸和能谱随深度变化，这会对 PDD 的测量精度产生影响。由于射野的横向尺寸随着深度的增加而增加，体积平均效应的程度也随之增大。这个问题在微型电离室中最为明显。例如，对于体积为 0.007cm³ 的球体，在 6MV 射野中，5mm² MLC 定义射野的体积平均效应修正从深度 2cm 到深度 20cm 减少了约 1%。二极管探测器材料中使用了高原子序数材料，能谱随深度的变化对测量的 PDD 有较大影响。带有高原子序数材料电极的电离室也具有随深度变化的[12]响应。在测量 PDD 时，探测器轴应平行于射束中心轴，以减小射野随深度增加造成的影响。正式测量前首先对射束进行扫描，以确保探测器在所有感兴趣的深度都与射束中心轴对齐。

一些计划系统要求测量组织体模比（tissuephantom ratios，TPR）而不是百分深度剂量。大野中PDD转换为TPR的方法在小野中并不准确[13]。虽然有其他方法将PDD转化为TPR[14-16]，但这些方法在小野中的准确性有待验证。因此，当需要TPR时，建议直接测量[4]。

测量侧向剂量曲线可以不用考虑能量依赖性，因为能谱在侧向不会发生显著变化。体积平均效应会造成射野的半影模糊，使用高分辨率探测器能够减少这种模糊效应。扫描侧向剂量曲线时选择合适的探测器方向以优化空间分辨率，同时保证体积平均效应最小。在选择探测器方向时，特别是选择微型电离室的方向，应评估来自探测器外的干扰信号（如杆效应）。

三、探测器类型

（一）电离室

使用标准电离室（如Farmer电离室）测量小野与放射外科的误差存在相关性[1]。虽然微型电离室（体积小于约0.02cm³）的设计初衷是用于小野测量，但使用该微型电离室测量小于2cm²的方野时，响应会降低15%。例如，一个体积为0.015cm³的商用电离室，测量1.5cm×1.5cm、1.0cm×1.0cm和0.5cm×0.5cm射野的输出因子[17]，对应的输出修正因子$k_{Q_{clin},Q_{10\times10}}^{f_{clin},f_{10\times10}}$分别为1.005、1.025和1.128。由于电离室存在较大的体积平均效应和能量依赖性，因此应避免使用电离室进行小野测量。

由于微型电离室的修正因子$k_{Q_{clin},Q_{10\times10}}^{f_{clin},f_{10\times10}}$和其他探测器的一样，都和探测器结构设计相关，因此修正因子应对应特定的电离室型号，而设计相似或者体积相似的微型电离室采用同一修正因子也是不合适的。测量输出因子时，微型电离室的方向应该垂直于束轴，这样可以减少灵敏体积外辐照信号的干扰。

射束扫描时，灵敏体积小的探测器对灵敏体积外的辐射更敏感。为了减少这种影响，测量侧向剂量曲线时，电离室应平行于射束轴，尽量减少电缆受辐射的长度。尽管微型电离室是为小野设计的，但其尺寸通常有几毫米，会导致半影模糊。对于百分深度剂量的测量，野大小随深度的变化导致体积平均效应的变化。此外，有效测量点位置并不确定，特别是当探测器平行于束轴时，这种现象更加明显[12]。

（二）二极管

二极管探测器由一个硅p-n结组成，辐射在p-n结中产生电子空穴对。常见灵敏体积的截面面积为1mm²，厚度为1μm到几百微米。因为硅的原子序数（Z=14）高于水，所以二极管的辐射响应具有显著的能量依赖性，对低能光子存在过响应。虽然探测器的屏蔽设计能够过滤低能粒子，减轻能量依赖性，但是过响应现象并未消除，由于屏蔽二极管使用的高原子序数材料对辐射通量分布的扰动增加，导致屏蔽二极管相对于未屏蔽二极管在小野内产生过度响应。例如，某个商用屏蔽二极管，对于1.5cm²、1.0cm²和0.5cm²的方野，其修正因子$k_{Q_{clin},Q_{10\times10}}^{f_{clin},f_{10\times10}}$分别为1.005、0.995和0.968，然而屏蔽二极管的修正因子分别是0.983、0.966和0.933。由于高原子序数的屏蔽材料会产生扰动，市面上有多种专为小野设计的非屏蔽二极管，因此在小野剂量测定中应避免使用屏蔽二极管。

针对小野设计的非屏蔽二极管（立体定向二极管）主要应用于测量侧向剂量曲线。小灵敏体积能够实现高分辨测量，减小半影的模糊现象。这些探测器测量的相对侧向剂量曲线与蒙特卡罗计算结果几乎完全相同。因为光子能谱不会随侧向距离增加而产生显著变化，所以可以不用考虑二极管响应的能量依赖性。二极管具有圆盘状的灵敏体积，测量时圆盘平面应垂直于束轴[19]，即探测器杆平行于射束中心轴。然而，正确的摆位方向不一定都是上述情况，制造商通常会对探测器灵敏体积的方向进行标记，应参考厂家提供的文件，以确认探测器的推荐摆位方式。

在测量百分深度剂量时，二极管的能量依赖性是一个值得关注的问题。然而，响应随深度的变化并不显著，因此无屏蔽二极管适合测量小野的 PDD [18]。二极管的摆位方向应与侧向扫描时的方向相同，探测器的灵敏体积截面垂直于束轴。将探测器的最小尺寸置于射束方向，通常是几微米，这样测量的 PDD 结果空间分辨率高，可以忽略体积平均效应。

（三）钻石探测器

商用钻石探测器由一层用化学气相沉积法生产的人造钻石组成。灵敏体积的尺寸与二极管类似，直径约 2mm、厚度约 1μm。钻石几乎和水等效，原子序数 Z=6，而水的有效原子序数 Z=7.4，因此具有最小的能量依赖性。钻石探测器在小野内存在过响应，类似于无屏蔽二极管。对于直径为 2cm、1.08cm 和 0.76cm 的射野，商用合成钻石探测器的修正因子 $k_{Q_{clin},Q_{10 \times 10}}^{f_{clin},f_{10 \times 10}}$ 分别为 0.991、0.986 和 0.975，屏蔽二极管的修正因子分别为 0.994、0.983 和 0.964。由于钻石探测器比二极管大，体积平均效应在 1cm 以内的射野中不可忽略，刚好在一定程度上能够补偿过度响应现象。已有研究对极小射野（＜ 8mm）应使用的修正因子存在分歧[20]。

钻石探测器非常适合测量侧向剂量曲线和百分深度剂量曲线。与二极管类似，灵敏体积应该垂直于束轴。钻石探测器比二极管稍大一些，直径约为 2mm，而立体定向野二极管的直径约为 1mm。当扫描侧向剂量曲线时，立体定向二极管将有更好的分辨率和较小的模糊半影。

（四）塑料闪烁体

塑料闪烁体探测器由连接在光纤上的小型有机塑料闪烁体组成。在闪烁体中产生的光通过光纤耦合到光电探测器上。近水等效性、体积小是塑料闪烁体探测器的优点，闪烁体探测器的修正因子非常接近于 1[21]，唯一对修正因子有显著影响的是体积平均效应。商用闪烁体探测器直径约为 1mm，长 1～3mm，对于长度＞ 1mm 的探测器，其长轴方向应与束轴平行。辐射除了在探测器内产生闪烁光，也可在周围产生切伦科夫光，切伦科夫光的数量与射野中光纤的数量成正比，对探测器输出光的贡献取决于辐照条件，必须进行校正。人们已经研究了几种方法来去除切伦科夫背景[22]，但只有一种方法用于商用探测器，即光谱识别。闪烁谱相对较窄，而切伦科夫谱较宽。为了确定闪烁体接收到的剂量，将光信号在两个具有不同光学过滤的光电探测器之间分离。一个探测器通过闪烁光谱中的波长，而另一个探测器只通过比闪烁光谱长的波长。因此，第一个探测器（S_{Blue}）的信号主要是闪烁光，而第二个探测器（S_{Green}）的信号主要是切伦科夫光。闪烁体中的剂量由以下公式给出：

$$D = k_{gain} \times (s_{Blue} - k_{CLR} \times s_{Green})$$

对射野内不同长度的光纤进行已知剂量的辐照，可以确定常数 k_{CLR} 和 k_{gain}。通过对切伦科夫本地进行仔细校正，塑料闪烁体探测器非常适合测量输出因子、百分深度剂量和侧向剂量曲线[23]。

（五）辐射自显影胶片

辐射自显影胶片是一种薄膜材料，暴露于电离辐射后可以不用进一步显影就会变色。商用的医用放射性胶片由有机分子组成，暴露在电离辐射下会引发聚合反应，使薄膜变成蓝色。放射性胶片的优点包括近水等效性、能量依赖性小[24]和空间分辨率高。

基于透射模式的红 – 绿 – 蓝（red-green-blue，RGB）扫描仪是目前最常用的评估辐射自显影胶片光密度的方法，与卤化银射线照相胶片相似，最敏感的通道（通常是红色通道）用于确定吸收剂量。但这种方法有几个局限性：第一，胶片上聚合物厚度的变化导致了空间响应的变化[25]；第二，扫描信号强度与扫描位置距中心的横向距离存在依赖性，这种影响在距离＜ 5cm 的情况下是很小的，但当扫描位置接近扫描区域边缘时，可能会导致剂量高估。对小野而言，如果扫描的胶片放置在扫描床同样的位置上，这种依赖性较小。多通道法可以弱化上述局限性，在该方法中，所有三个颜色通道都用来确定剂量[26]。

辐射自显影胶片适用于测量输出因子、百分深度剂量和侧向剂量曲线。然而，由于胶片和扫描仪的特性，它可能有很大的不确定性，因此需要严谨的处理标准[27]。辐射自显影胶片的另一个缺点是并非"实时"的剂量计。

四、病例介绍

（一）病例1

1. 直线加速器小野的调试

利用 $0.125cm^3$ 电离室测量了射野 $\geq 3cm$ 的直线加速器 10 MV 无均整射束的输出因子。对于 VMAT 计划，治疗计划系统只需要次级准直器铅门的输出因子。为了确定 2cm 射野的输出因子，使用 3 种探测器：$0.007cm^3$ 的微型电离室、直径为 1mm 的立体定向二极管和直径为 2.2mm 的人造钻石探测器。探测器被放置在三维扫描水箱中，深度为 10cm 和源皮距（SSD）为 90cm。探测器在射野内横向和径向进行扫描，放置在信号最大的点进行输出因子测量。测量方野为 4cm×4cm、3cm×3cm、2cm×2cm，矩形野为 2cm×Y 和 X×2cm，一直扫描到 40cm 的最大射野。读数都参考 4cm×4cm 的射野，基于之前用 $0.125cm^3$ 电离室测量的 4cm×4cm 输出因子获得相对于 10cm×10cm 的输出因子。对于 >1.5cm×1.5cm 的射野，三个探测器的输出修正因子都较小（<0.8%）[5, 10]。

表 22-1 对每个探测器的测量结果进行了比较。治疗计划系统可以外延到更小的射野。同一模型直线加速器在 SSD 为 95cm 和深度 5cm 测量的数据用于检查治疗计划系统的计算，见表 22-2。

2. 治疗计划系统调试和端到端测试

除了输入正确的小野测量值到治疗计划系统（treatment planning system，TPS），还要通过反复验证治疗计划系统对小野的计算精度。AAPM 医学物理实践指南 5.a（MPPG 5）就剂量计算算法的调试和质量保证提供了广泛的指导；但是，MPPG 5 明确地将小野排除在报告之外[29]。尽管 MPPG 5 排除了小野，临床实践仍应遵循其中的剂量计算算法调试、验证和常规 QA 的工作流程。基本验证测试应包括验证治疗计划系统的计算数据与输入数据在可接受的容差范围内。在可实现的情况下，对于没有包含在调试数据集中的射野，应额外测量其输出因子、百分深度剂量和侧向剂量曲线，以便与计划系统计算结果进行比较。

端到端测试是调试和放疗项目持续质量控制的关键组成部分。端到端测试范围比评估小野的准确性内容要广泛得多。然而，剂量测量的准确性是端到端测试的一个重要组成部分。端到端测试包括模体成像、创建与实际患者类似的治疗计划、将治疗计划投射到模体并评估产生的剂量分布。端到端测试可以用简单的水等效塑料模体或

表 22-1 SSD 为 90cm 深度为 10cm 处使用三种探测器以及使用治疗计划系统计算的输出因子

X	Y	微型电离室	立体定向二极管	钻 石	治疗计划系统计算
3	3	0.887	0.886	0.888	0.888
2	2	0.832	0.835	0.837	0.835
2	5	0.875	0.878	0.878	0.877
5	2	0.870	0.870	0.871	0.869

表 22-2 SSD 为 95cm 深度为 5cm 处使用治疗计划系统计算的以及 Wen 等报道的输出因子

X	Y	治疗计划系统计算	Wen 等[28]
3	3	0.926	0.925
2	2	0.880	0.880
1	1	0.737	0.731
2	5	0.915	0.916
5	2	0.906	0.908
1	5	0.815	0.821
5	1	0.808	0.800

类人模体来完成。市面上可以买到各种各样的模体，可以用各种探测器（包括胶片）来测量。一个具有价值的端到端测试是使用由外单位提供和评估的模体，并对投射准确性进行独立审核。安德森剂量测量实验室提供了一个包含直径为 20mm 目标靶区的头部模体，以及用于测试锥筒输出的模体。有公司提供 3D 打印的模体，其中包含一个聚合物凝胶剂量计，也可以用于端到端测试。

（二）病例 2

端到端的 VMAT 立体定向系统测试

对 VMAT 立体定向系统进行了两个终端到终端测试。第一个测试是在内部完成的，第二个测试使用了外部测量仪器。

内部测试使用的是商用丙烯酸树脂。如图 22-1 所示，模体放置在无框架系统中。模体有两个可互换的插入。第一种包含一个直径为 20mm 的靶区，具有足够的对比度，可以在 CT 图像上进行识别。第二个装有一个通道，用于在靶区球体的中心位置放置体积为 $0.007cm^3$ 的微型电离室。用靶区球体插入物进行了 CT 扫描。将 CT 导入治疗计划系统，将 20mm 球体作为计划靶区体积（planning target volume，PTV）。另外一个直径为 5mm 的球形体积与 PTV 呈同心轮廓，以控制电离室位置周围剂量分布的均匀性。采用逆向调强计划，按照标准的临床方案制定治疗计划。5mm 中心体积的目的是控制靶区球体中心部分的剂量均匀性。计划完成后，将治疗计划传输到直线加速器。使用与患者相同的图像引导方案定位插入电离室的模体。模体被对准至将腔室的有效测量点放置在靶区球体的中心。实施治疗计划，电离室的腔室剂量为 21.05Gy，治疗计划系统计算的腔室剂量为 20.73Gy。

在内部终端到终端测试之后，使用得克萨斯大学 M.D. 安德森剂量测量实验室（http：//rpc.mdanderson.org/mdadl）（MDADL）提供的类人立体定向放射外科头部模体进行外部测试。模体设计目的是为了高度精确的测试定位和治疗颅内靶区的能力。模体有两个可互换的插件，影像插件用于定义治疗体积，剂量测定插件包括辐射自显影胶片和 TLD。MDADL 的指南是将模体成像、计划和治疗作为实际患者，目标靶区中最大剂量为 30Gy（匹配插入的辐射自显影胶片的量程）。

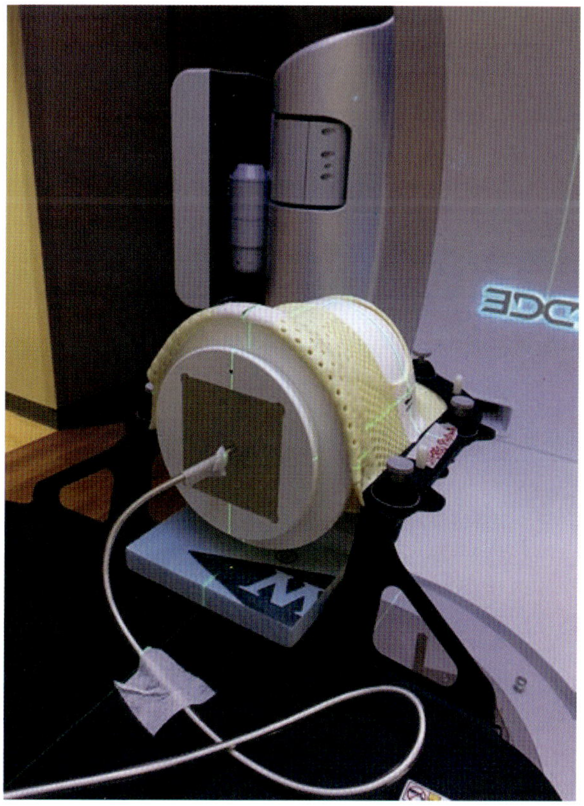

▲ 图 22-1 无支架定位系统的模体及插入靶区体积中心的微型电离室

模体被固定在无框架系统的个体化面罩中，并获取了 CT 影像。对球型靶区进行勾画，并使用逆向计划系统为处方剂量为 20Gy 的 PTV 设计治疗计划。优化和剂量计算后，调整计划归一，最大剂量为 30Gy（调整 1.5%）。与实际患者治疗一样，对计划进行了质量保证测量。在模体上执行该计划，模体在加速器上使用与患者相同的图像引导流程定位。将模体寄回 MDADL，分析胶片和 TLD 的剂量，并与治疗计划进行比较。TLD 结果比治疗计划系统计算值高 3%，剖面如图 22-2 所示。

五、特定患者的质量保证

调强放疗计划需要进行剂量测量，以验证剂量投射精度[30]。然而，目前缺少关于特定患者小范围调强剂量分布的验证指南。辐射自显影胶片具有水等效性，能量依赖小，适合用于特定患者

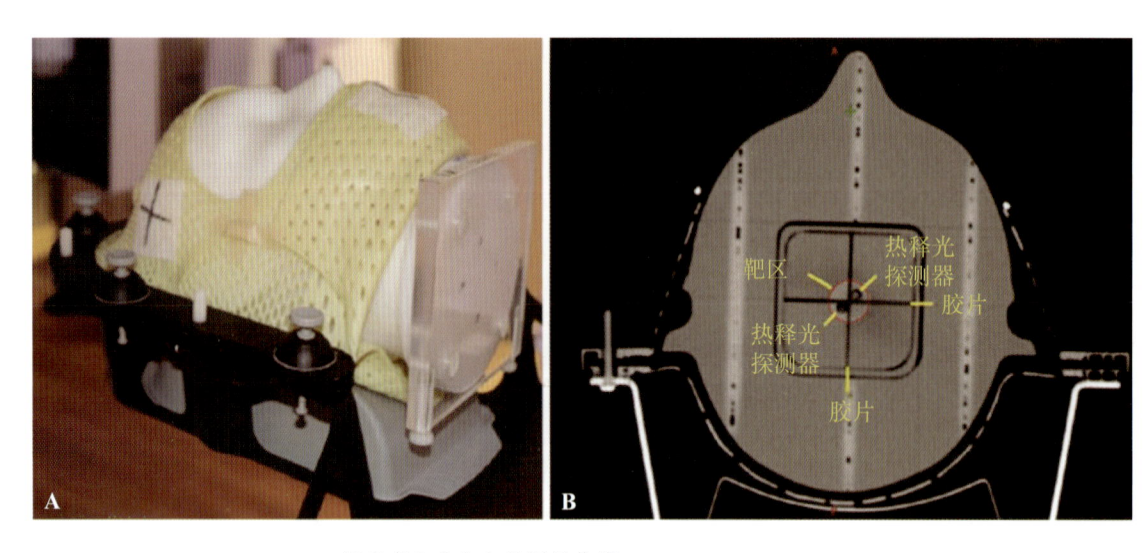

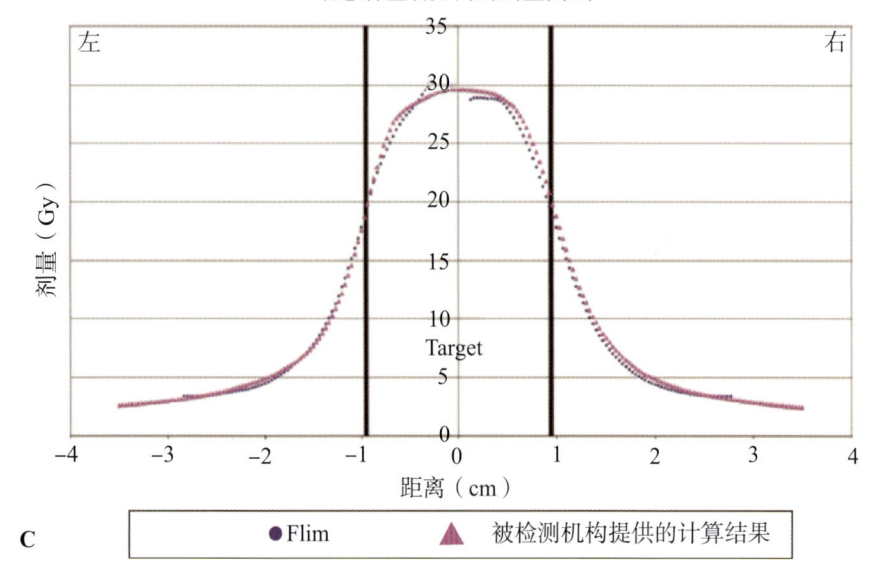

▲ 图 22-2 **A.** 放置于无支架定位系统中的 **SRS** 头部模体，由位于休士顿的 **MD** 安德森剂量实验室 **IROC** 提供；**B.** 显示 CT 图像，包括靶区、热释光探测器以及放置于冠状面和矢状面的胶片；**C.** 报道示例，显示了中心靶区的剂量曲线，总结报道见 **21** 章图 **21–3**
蓝色圆点为胶片测量结果，红色三角为被检测机构提供的计算结果

的 QA。经过仔细的刻度，它可以用于绝对剂量测定[31]。然而，放射自显影胶片费时费力，需要严格遵守精心设计的处理程序。因此，有必要使用其他类型的探测器实时测量剂量分布，但在使用前应当仔细评估它们的适用性。调强计划的射野尺寸没有明确定义，不能使用测量的输出因子，可以定义剂量分布的尺寸为 50% 等剂量体积的直径（最大剂量为 100%），以此来评估给定的探测器尺寸是否合适。除了应当评估探测器响应对于剂量分布尺寸的依赖性以外，还应评价响应对射束方向的依赖。微型电离室适用于尺寸 > 15mm 的剂量分布。塑料闪烁体探测器适用于测量放射外科的剂量分布[32, 33]。如果探测器尺寸与剂量分布尺寸相当，则必须考虑体积平均效应。

六、未来及展望

治疗计划系统数据的标准化将减少小野测量误差影响患者疗效的可能性。治疗计划系统的厂家能够通过对比不同机构间的调试数据，找到异常值，从而发现放射外科的治疗事故。然而，标准化的射野数据并非都是正确的，如伽马刀最小尺寸的准直器输出存在变化。负责调试计划系统的物理师需要独立地验证系统是否按照预期运行，计算结果是否与独立的测量结果匹配。此外，用户间共享数据、对调试后的计划系统进行多机构评估也很重要。

实验测量仍然是特定患者调强放疗计划质量保证的标准。然而，系统层面测试、独立的患者计划剂量计算以及数据完整性测试，可能在未来取代特定患者计划的 QA。

> **要 点**
> - 对于输出因子的测量，需要选择合适的探测器，其小野修正因子应 < 5%。
> - 对于输出因子的测量，建议使用两个或两个以上不同探测器测量，并对比结果。
> - 对于百分深度剂量曲线和侧向剂量曲线的测量，建议使用专属立体定向野的二极管探测器、合成钻石探测器或者塑料闪烁晶体探测器。
> - 在用于临床使用之前，与厂家的、文献报道的或者其他用户的参考数据进行对比，验证自己的数据。
> - 在用于临床使用之前，进行独立的端对端测试，例如使用 MD 安德森剂量实验室的 SRS 头部体模。

参考文献

[1] Derreumaux S, Etard C, Huet C, Trompier F, Clairand I, Bottollier-Depois JF, et al. Lessons from recent accidents in radiation therapy in France. Radiat Prot Dosim. 2008;131(1):130–5.

[2] Bogdanich WR, Rebecca R. Radiation errors reported in Missouri. New York Times. February 25, 2010.

[3] Goetsch S. 4-mm Gamma Knife helmet factor. Int J Radiat Oncol Biol Phys. 2002;54(1):300; author reply 301.

[4] International Commission on Radiation Units and Measurements. Prescribing, recording, and reporting of stereotactic treatments with small photon beams. Oxford: Oxford University Press; 2017.

[5] International Atomic Energy Agency. Dosimetry of small static fields used in external beam radiotherapy: an IAEA–AAPM international code of practice for reference and relative dose determination. Technical Report Series No. 483. Vienna; 2017.

[6] Palmans H, Andreo P, Huq MS, Seuntjens J, Christaki KE, Meghzifene A. Dosimetry of small static fields used in external photon beam radiotherapy: summary of TRS-483, the IAEA-AAPM international Code of Practice for reference and relative dose determination. Med Phys. 2018;45(11):e1123–45.

[7] Veselsky T, Novotny J Jr, Pastykova V, Koniarova I. Determination of small field synthetic single-crystal diamond detector correction factors for CyberKnife, Leksell Gamma Knife Perfexion and linear accelerator. Phys Med. 2017; 44:66–71.

[8] Huet C, Moignier C, Barraux V, Loiseau C, SebeMercier K, Batalla A, et al. Study of commercial detector responses in non-equilibrium small photon fields of a 1000MU/min CyberKnife system. Phys Med. 2016;32(6):818–25.

[9] Francescon P, Kilby W, Satariano N. Monte Carlo simulated correction factors for output factor measurement with the CyberKnife system-results for new detectors and correction factor dependence on measurement distance and detector orientation. Phys Med Biol. 2014;59(6):N11–7.

[10] Papaconstadopoulos P, Tessier F, Seuntjens J. On the correction, perturbation and modification of small field detectors in relative dosimetry. Phys Med Biol. 2014; 59(19):5937–52.

[11] Garnier N, Amblard R, Villeneuve R, Haykal R, Ortholan C, Colin P, et al. Detectors assessment for stereotactic radiosurgery with cones. J Appl Clin Med Phys. 2018;19(6): 88–98.

[12] Tessier F, Kawrakow I. Effective point of measurement of thimble ion chambers in megavoltage photon beams. Med Phys. 2010;37(1):96–107.

[13] Ding GX, Krauss R. An empirical formula to obtain tissue-phantom ratios from percentage depth-dose curves for small fields. Phys Med Biol. 2013;58(14):4781–9.

[14] Bjarngard BE, Zhu TC, Ceberg C. Tissue-phantom ratios from percentage depth doses. Med Phys. 1996;23(5):629–34.

[15] Xiao Y, Altschuler MD, Bjarngard BE. Quality assurance of central axis dose data for photon beams by means of a functional representation of the tissue phantom ratio. Phys Med Biol. 1998;43(8):2195–206.

[16] Sauer OA. Determination of the quality index (Q) for photon beams at arbitrary field sizes. Med Phys. 2009;36(9):4168–72.

[17] Francescon P, Cora S, Satariano N. Calculation of k(Q(clin), Q(msr)) (f(clin), f(msr)) for several small detectors and for two linear accelerators using Monte Carlo simulations. Med Phys. 2011;38(12):6513–27.

[18] Tyler M, Liu PZ, Chan KW, Ralston A, McKenzie DR, Downes S, et al. Characterization of small-field stereotactic radiosurgery beams with modern detectors. Phys Med Biol. 2013;58(21):7595–608.

[19] Beddar AS, Mason DJ, O'Brien PF. Absorbed dose perturbation caused by diodes for small field photon dosimetry. Med Phys. 1994;21(7):1075–9.

[20] O'Brien DJ, Leon-Vintro L, McClean B. Small field detector correction factors kQclin,Qmsr (fclin,fmsr) for silicon-diode and diamond detectors with circular 6 MV fields derived using both empirical and numerical methods. Med Phys. 2016;43(1):411.

[21] Wang LL, Beddar S. Study of the response of plastic scintillation detectors in small-field 6 MV photon beams by Monte Carlo simulations. Med Phys. 2011;38(3):1596–9.

[22] Liu PZ, Suchowerska N, Lambert J, Abolfathi P, McKenzie DR. Plastic scintillation dosimetry: comparison of three solutions for the Cerenkov challenge. Phys Med Biol. 2011;56(18):5805–21.

[23] Gagnon JC, Theriault D, Guillot M, Archambault L, Beddar S, Gingras L, et al. Dosimetric performance and array assessment of plastic scintillation detectors for stereotactic radiosurgery quality assurance. Med Phys. 2012;39(1):429–36.

[24] Butson MJ, Cheung T, Yu PK. Weak energy dependence of EBT gafchromic film dose response in the 50 kVp-10 MVp X-ray range. Appl Radiat Isot. 2006;64(1):60–2.

[25] Hartmann B, Martisikova M, Jakel O. Homogeneity of Gafchromic EBT2 film. Med Phys. 2010;37(4):1753–6.

[26] Micke A, Lewis DF, Yu X. Multichannel film dosimetry with nonuniformity correction. Med Phys. 2011;38(5):2523–34.

[27] Paelinck L, De Neve W, De Wagter C. Precautions and strategies in using a commercial flatbed scanner for radiochromic film dosimetry. Phys Med Biol. 2007;52(1): 231–42.

[28] Wen N, Li H, Song K, Chin-Snyder K, Qin Y, Kim J, et al. Characteristics of a novel treatment system for linear accelerator-based stereotactic radiosurgery. J Appl Clin Med Phys. 2015;16(4):5313.

[29] Smilowitz JB, Das IJ, Feygelman V, Fraass BA, Kry SF, Marshall IR, et al. AAPM medical physics practice guideline 5.a.: commissioning and QA of treatment planning dose calculations – megavoltage photon and electron beams. J Appl Clin Med Phys. 2015;16(5):14–34.

[30] Halvorsen PH, Cirino E, Das IJ, Garrett JA, Yang J, Yin FF, et al. AAPM-RSS medical physics practice guideline 9.a. for SRS-SBRT. J Appl Clin Med Phys. 2017;18(5):10–21.

[31] Devic S, Tomic N, Lewis D. Reference radiochromic film dosimetry: review of technical aspects. Phys Med. 2016;32(4):541–56.

[32] Dimitriadis A, Patallo IS, Billas I, Duane S, Nisbet A, Clark CH. Characterisation of a plastic scintillation detector to be used in a multicentre stereotactic radiosurgery dosimetry audit. Radiat Phys Chem. 2017;140:373–8.

[33] Qin Y, Gardner SJ, Kim J, Huang Y, Wen N, Doemer A, et al. Technical note: evaluation of plastic scintillator detector for small field stereotactic patient-specific quality assurance. Med Phys. 2017;44(10):5509–16.

第 23 章 保护海马的全脑放疗技术
Techniques of Whole Brain Radiation Therapy Including Hippocampal Avoidance

Sean S. Mahase　Diana A.R.Julie　Jonathan Knisely　著
梁　瞻　译
李书舟　校

一、病例介绍

（一）病例 1

男性，65 岁，有高血压病史，1 年前因右侧结肠腺癌ⅢB 期行结肠癌切除术，术后给以希罗达和奥沙利铂辅助化疗，因癫痫发作送到急诊室。影像显示右侧额叶有大片出血灶，同时还有 20 多个大小不一的小病灶。大部分病灶是血管源性，但在脑干内有两个点状转移瘤。手术切除占位效应病灶，病理显示转移性腺癌，结肠癌来源。

全身影像显示肺和肝多处转移，鉴于患者全身广泛转移，颅内病变不适合 SRS（放射外科）或手术切除。WBRT（全脑放射治疗）能最大限度地减轻病灶发展或使这些脑转移瘤消退，延缓病情进展，可作为姑息治疗的合适选择。

（二）病例 2

女性，32 岁，在哺乳时触摸到右乳房的肿块，检查后初步诊断为三阳浸润性导管癌ⅢB 期。基因检测无治疗靶点。在接受阿霉素、环磷酰胺、紫杉醇和曲妥珠单抗的新辅助化疗后进行了右侧乳腺切除术，术后辅以帕妥株单抗和曲妥株单抗治疗。两年后，影像显示多个小的脑部和肺部转移灶，因此接受了拉帕替尼和卡培他滨的治疗，同时对脑转移瘤进行了 SRS 治疗。6 个月后，复查影像显示肺部转移灶完全缓解，但出现几个新的实质性脑转移瘤，以及颅后窝的局限性软脑膜疾病。行腰椎穿刺在脑脊液中没有检测到癌细胞。将治疗方案改为曲妥珠单抗 - 美坦新，脑转移瘤（包括局灶性软脑膜病变）并再次给予 SRS 治疗。随访影像显示颅后窝、内耳道和左顶叶沿脑回的软脑膜强化进展，而颅外病变稳定。患者目前没有任何症状。

尽管进行了多种方案的全身治疗和多次 SRS，但脑膜病变的存在使 CNS 疾病仍难以控制，需行 WBRT 才能够减缓疾病的进一步发展，考虑到她一般情况较好，年龄小，颅外病变控制良好，应该尽量减少 WBRT 的长期后遗症。

（三）病例 3

男性，55 岁，40 包 / 年吸烟史，持续咳嗽，一般情况良好。经过全面检查（包括脑部 MRI），诊断右肺局限性小细胞肺癌（small cell lung cancer，SCLC），ⅡB 期，$T_3N_0M_0$。行同步放化疗（顺铂和依托泊苷）治疗完成后，复查显示肺部病灶完全缓解，MRI 显示无脑转移迹象。

对同步放化疗后完全或部分缓解的局限期小细胞肺癌的标准治疗方法是预防性全脑照射（prophylactic cranial irradiation，PCI）；因此，该患者可作为预防性 WBRT 的合适人选。然而，考虑到他年轻，一般情况良好，且对治疗完全有效，应该尽量减少放疗后的神经认知后遗症，可以考虑选择 NRG 肿瘤学会 CC003（HA-WBRT 同时辅以美金刚）试验方法。或者，选择继续观察，如果他最终在整体表现良好的情况下非功能区出现了有限数目的转移，可以考虑采用 SRS 和 WBRT 作为补救方案。

二、概述

全脑放疗（whole brain radiation，WBRT）用于脑转移瘤、白血病[1]、生殖细胞肿瘤和多中心 CNS 淋巴瘤[2]，并可作为儿童恶性肿瘤（包括髓母细胞瘤）全脑全脊髓放射治疗的一部分[3]。脑转移瘤是成人中最常见的颅内肿瘤[4]，几乎 1/3 的癌症患者都会发生脑转移，其中高达 50% 的人因此疾病死亡[5]。癌症患者的脑转移发生率上升与全身药物的研发进展是大致同步的，这些药物可以增加全身无进展生存期，并可能在某些情况下提高总生存获益。然而，这些药物中的大多数通过血脑屏障的能力有限[6]。另外，目前只有 10% 的癌症患者因为有症状表现才被确诊出脑转移瘤，但随着常规影像检查手段的普及，这一诊出比例在持续上升[5]。脑转移瘤需要使用皮质类固醇和其他对症支持治疗[7]。由于手术切除只适用于特定情况，而大多数化疗药物无法进入 CNS，且新的靶向药物和免疫疗法的疗效还正在研究当中，因此最终有效的治疗方案的选择是有限的。WBRT 由此成为脑转移瘤的初始治疗标准，并且是多发性病灶、复发性转移和（或）脑膜病变的主要治疗方式，因此精确的放疗计划设计和治疗对于控制肿瘤生长和缓解症状至关重要。在越来越有效的全身疗法的帮助下，接受 WBRT 治疗的患者生存期得到延长，所以研究并采取措施将放射毒性降至最低需要重点关注。

三、早期探索

放疗作为一种癌症治疗方式，可以迅速缓解症状，与手术切除和全身治疗相比具有某些方面的天然优势[8, 9]。它可以对诸如脑部等化疗药物难以渗透的部位实施有效治疗，并且不受血管供应、肝和肾功能以及其他全身性药物的影响，加上其非侵入的特性，使其能够应用于一般状态差或肾、肝功能受损的患者。如果需要治疗脊柱等部位的病灶，或者必须加快治疗进程，也可以根据实际情况灵活地调整治疗方案。

Lenz 和 Fried 于 1931 年最早记录了使用脑照射的系列方法，他们治疗的三名有症状脑病变的晚期转移性乳腺癌患者。颅内压增高引起相关症状：前两名患者表现为头痛，第三名患者表现为呕吐和惊厥。结果显示施行放疗可以在几个月内暂时缓解每位患者的症状，在出现症状后的生存期分别为 11、18 和 20 个月。此外，几例继发于乳腺癌的有症状的脑转移瘤晚期患者接受了脑照射，症状得到有效缓解并持续数周至数月[10]。1948 年，Richmond 报道 8 例接受放疗的脑转移瘤患者的症状得到持续性改善（4 例原发乳腺癌，3 例原发肺癌，1 例原发肾癌）。考虑到脑转移瘤的浸润性，他强调了放疗照射的靶区范围应大于 X 线和临床检查所显示的病灶范围的重要性[11]。

纪念斯隆·凯特琳癌症中心（Memorial-Sloan Kettering Cancer Center，MSKCC）于 1954 年发布的单中心研究结果表明，在 38 例有症状的脑转移瘤患者中，有 24 例因接受脑照射使症状得到改善（23 例原发性肺癌患者中的 15 例，7 例原发性乳腺癌患者中的 4 例，1 例前列腺癌，1 例内皮瘤，1 例畸胎瘤，1 例食管癌和 1 例白血病）。结果表明，放疗敏感的患者平均生存时间为 8.2 个月，不敏感的患者和未完成治疗的患者的平均生存时间为 4.6 个月。著者认为，无论肿瘤的组织学特征或其在脑内位置如何，脑照射似乎都能有效缓解神经系统症状。此外，虽然干预前出现症状的持续时间不影响脑照射的症状缓解能力，但症状出现时间越短的患者，功能恢复越快。作者得出结论，认为 WBRT 对于多发性脑转移瘤和术后残留肿瘤等总体预后较差的患者，具有缓解症状的能力[8]。

随后，Chu 等报道了在 MSKCC 接受 WBRT 治疗的 158 例患者中，有 77.8% 的患者症状得到了持续缓解（持续定义为 1 个月以上）。对放疗敏感的患者症状得到控制的持续时间为平均 4.7 个月，平均生存时间为 6.6 个月，而不敏感的患者平均生存时间为 2.3 个月，其中 86% 的 64 例乳腺癌患者和 83.3% 的 54 例肺癌患者对 WBRT 敏感。17 例因症状复发而接受第二次 WBRT，其中 12 例为放疗敏感，症状平均控制时间为 4.6 个月，平均生存期为 8.1 个月，而不敏感患者的平均生存期为 1.4 个月，该类患者大多数死于非 CNS 的病因[12]。

四、WBRT 临床实验评估

早期 RTOG（放疗肿瘤学组）随机试验验证结果表明，对于原发疾病控制良好和一般情况好的患者，WBRT 可作为一种有效的治疗方法，但这些研究报道同时也表明许多患者在完成治疗后也仅存活了几个月[13]。Patchell 等随后进行了一项试验，该试验将具有影像学证据的单个脑转移瘤的患者随机分为单独行 WBRT 或手术切除后行术后 WBRT。结果表明手术联合术后 WBRT 可将总生存期提高至 40 周，而单独行 WBRT 则可将总生存期提高至 15 周[14]。Patchell 等将 95 例行脑转移切除术的患者随机分为观察组或术后 WBRT 组进行随访。尽管结果显示两组患者的总体生存率无显著差异，但复发率从观察组的 46% 降至术后 WBRT 组的 10%。WBRT 还降低了新发的脑转移病灶和由神经系统原因引起的死亡率，从此将术后 WBRT 确立为脑转移瘤的治疗标准[15]。

五、技术、剂量及分次数的演变

（一）千伏时代

Lenz 和 Fried 试验了两种放疗方式，第一种使用带 0.5mm 的铜滤光片的 200 千伏（kV）X 线，源皮距设置为 50cm；第二种使用镭源，源皮距设置为 2~3cm。治疗时间的长短取决于病灶上方皮肤出现红斑的时间，分别将 1 个、2 个、2 个以上的"标准红斑剂量"视为低剂量、中剂量、高剂量。报道称接受了中剂量放射治疗的患者大多数都出现了症状缓解[10]。在接下来的几十年中，WBRT 技术根据以上所取得的结果开始缓慢发展。

在 20 世纪 40 年代，用于放疗的光子能量范围为 180~250kV。考虑到可能发生多处转移，许多医生选择使用简单的 AP-PA 位或对穿侧野照射整个大脑，到了 20 世纪 60 年代，WBRT 的治疗已基本上只使用两个对穿侧野照射，射野平均大小为 14cm×20cm（图 23-1 和图 23-2）。射野下界设置为起于眶上脊和外耳道、终止于枕骨大孔形成的平面，而前界，上界和后界分别定义为距前额、颅骨顶点和枕骨 2cm 处。在治疗过程中经常会使用到组织补偿物，X 线半值层一般为 2.0mm 铜，但由于设备的光子输出较低，导致其靶皮距一般只有 50~70cm。一些医生使用铅块来保护眼睛和射野下界以下的正常组织免受照射[8,12,16]。

按照惯例，医生一般以小剂量开始治疗，避免因治疗过程中引起的水肿进一步加重颅内压。分次数的选择还取决于患者的状态，在最初的 3~4 天使用 50~100cGy/ 次，然后在无任何恶化迹象或症状（头痛，呕吐和视盘水肿）的情况下以 50cGy 的增量逐渐增加至 350~400cGy/ 次[12]。虽然一些研究报道表明使用 2000cGy 或更小剂量就可有效缓解实体瘤原发灶的转移，但大多数放射医师一般在 3 周内给予 3000cGy 剂量的治疗，因为有报道称患者接受较低剂量治疗时更易复发[17]。Chao 等指出在他们的 14 例治疗失败案列

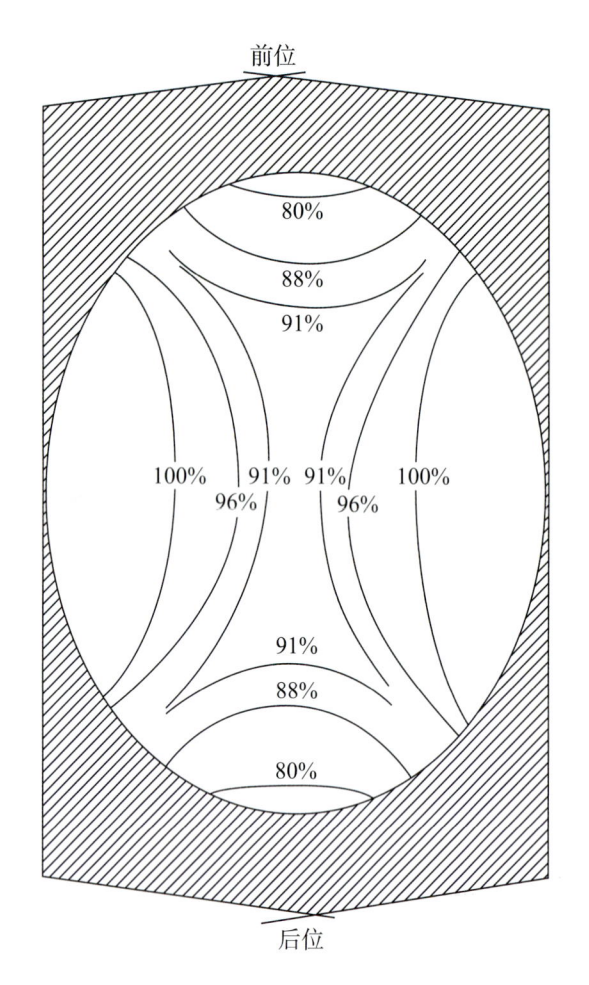

▲ 图 23-1 使用 2.0mm Cu HVL 和 70cm TSD 的 250kV X 线形成的 WBRT 射野等剂量线分布（引自 Chao 等[8]）。在该分布图中，低能量 X 线的散射和被骨吸收的影响被忽略

在所述的治疗方案中，头部周围与头皮接触的区域使用了组织补偿物（灰色）。经 John Wiley and Sons 许可转载，引自 Chao 等[8]

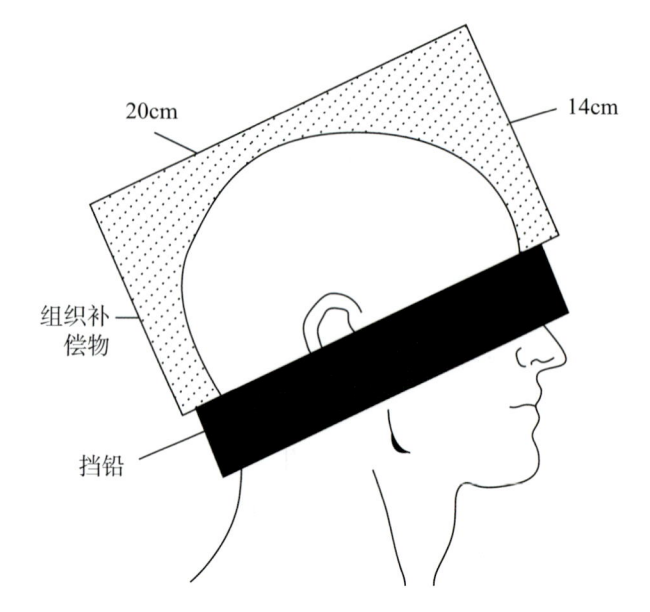

▲ 图 23-2 如图 23-1 所述的平行对穿侧野 WBRT 示意图

经 John Wiley and Sons 许可转载，引自 Chu 和 Hilaris[12]

中有 9 例接受的总剂量低于 3000cGy。相反，如果将总剂量增加到超过 3000cGy，则会增加湿性脱皮和永久性脱发的发生概率，但在病症缓解的持续时间上却没有明显的改善[8]。Chu 等报道，接受至少 2750cGy 剂量的患者其缓解率更高，其中没有肺癌患者和仅有 11% 的乳腺癌患者在接受低于该阈值剂量时，可以获得 5 个月或 6 个月的持续性缓解[12]。

（二）二维放疗计划设计时代

20 世纪 60 年代，在放疗计划设计过程中引入了透视引导成像技术，以辅助计划布野和挡块设计。然而，WBRT 通常是在没有模拟引导的情况下施行的，如上所述，在临床上一般使用外部标志物辅助设计照射范围，但通常不能覆盖大脑最下层的部分。

随着临床医生对筛骨区域的髓母细胞瘤或白血病等疾病的颅底复发，以及 WBRT 射野设计不合理（没有完全包围筛骨的）导致的晶体毒性的了解更加深入，射野设计受到了更多的关注[3]。为避免遗漏眼球之间后侧下方延伸的部分脑组织，颅顶照射一般采用包括眶后间隙在内的两个平行对穿侧野，其下界为从眶上嵴延伸至乳突尖端，包括第一、二颈椎，射野上界和后界向头皮上方和后方往外延伸 1~2cm。同时使用面罩固定，方便放疗医师在面罩上描绘出界标[1,3]。另外一种固定方式是在额头上拉一条胶带贴在治疗床的两侧进行固定。使用这种布野方法可以确保晶体接受的剂量≤处方剂量的 10%，使晶体接受的总剂量保持在 400cGy 以下[3]。另外，建议将射束的中心轴设置在外侧眼角而非其他位置，这样可以在避免调整治疗床或机架位置的情况下最大程度地减少对对侧眼睛的不必要散射[18]。

(三)三维放疗计划设计时代

研究人员们越来越担心上述计划设计方法不能完全覆盖靶区(特别是颞叶和额下区域),从而导致治疗失败[19]。一些研究将额下区的高失败率归因于不合理的眼部挡块定位[20, 21]。CT 的出现和广泛使用为射野设置和屏蔽设计提供了更精确的空间定位,产生了比现有的二维(2D)方法更全面的三维(3D)计算机辅助放疗计划设计方法。计划 CT 数据可以生成影像,称为数字重建放射影像(digitally reconstructed radiograph,DRR),其作用类似于透视模拟器中使用的传统 X 线片,可验证治疗期间的射束位置准确度[22-24]。现代放疗计划设计软件已经可以将 CT 影像生成的解剖结构轮廓、准直器边界、自定义挡块和十字叉丝投影到 DRR 上,并创建适当缩放的物理或虚拟胶片,用于模拟和验证射野设计的合理性[25]。

Gripp 等对 5 例原发性脑癌患者和 15 例脑转移瘤患者进行了分别基于 CT 和基于放射平片设计放疗计划的前瞻性研究。他们使用面罩固定患者头部,并使用不同的扫描层厚,厚度 3~5mm。基于 CT 的计划方案将靶区遗漏从 8% 降低到 0.6%,额下区的不完全覆盖率从 10% 减少到 1%,同时将同侧晶状体的暴露率从 3% 减少到 0%,对侧晶状体的暴露率从 22% 减少到 11%[21]。Mah 等的研究表明,基于 CT 的 3D 模拟可通过更好地定位危及器官和靶区结构,提高了射野和屏蔽设计的准确性,并且比 2D 模拟所需的时间要短得多,这在治疗儿科患者时是一个特别重要的考虑因素[26]。Andic 等对 30 例患者的 2D 和 3D 的 WBRT 进行剂量学比较,2D 和 3D 计划的射野中心和角度均相同。在 3D 计划中,脑接收的最小剂量平均值明显提高[27]。所有患者均接收了至少 95% 的处方剂量,相比于 2D 计划,剂量均匀性得到改善,晶体也保护得更好。

六、当代 WBRT 实践

(一)放疗计划设计、剂量和分次数

对于仰卧位 WBRT 计划,患者的模拟定位一般使用头部支架和热塑面罩进行固定,制作面罩大约需要 15min,将用于定位的放射显像标记放置在面罩上,而不是放在患者的皮肤上。对于计划 CT,建议使用从头顶到上段颈椎的最大层厚为 3~5mm 的 CT 平扫。在布野时可以对平行对穿侧野沿中心轴旋转微调,通常在其前斜方向上旋转两到三度,形成共面的前野边界,使射线不会散射到对侧晶体。在临床中一般采用等中心治疗技术,即患者的中线与矢状线对齐。中心轴可以由眼角外侧(图 23-3A 和 B)确定,这一点并不需要着重强调,因为通过调整治疗床和机架角度,也可避免射线散射进入对侧眼,且仍能覆盖整个颅骨,特别是筛骨(图 23-3C 和 D)。这种可调整性很重要,因为患者在模拟定位时摆位并不总是对称的。射野铅门一般要打开至包围整个大脑,并从颅骨向外延伸几厘米,射野的下界一般置于第一或第二颈椎的末端。布野完成后设计屏蔽物保护大脑以外的正常组织。MRI 图像的解剖信息也可以通过图像配准算法转换到 CT 计划图像中,虽然这一步对于 WBRT 计划并不是必需的。

患者躺在治疗床上后,需验证治疗前摆位的准确性,以保证放疗精确度。这一过程一般是通过检查 MV 或 kV 放射胶片来确认等中心位置和挡块定位的准确性来完成的。光学体表引导放疗(使用允许追踪面部特征的开放式面罩)可以通过在每次治疗过程中光学监测患者的位置来完善这一过程[28, 29]。

目前,WBRT 或 PCI 有一系列公认的处方剂量和分割方案,包括 50Gray(Gy)/20 次、40Gy/20 次、40Gy/15 次、37.5Gy/15 次、36Gy/18 次、30Gy/(10 或 15 次)、25Gy/10 次、24Gy/12 次、20Gy/5 次、8Gy/1 次[13]。RTOG 已经临床

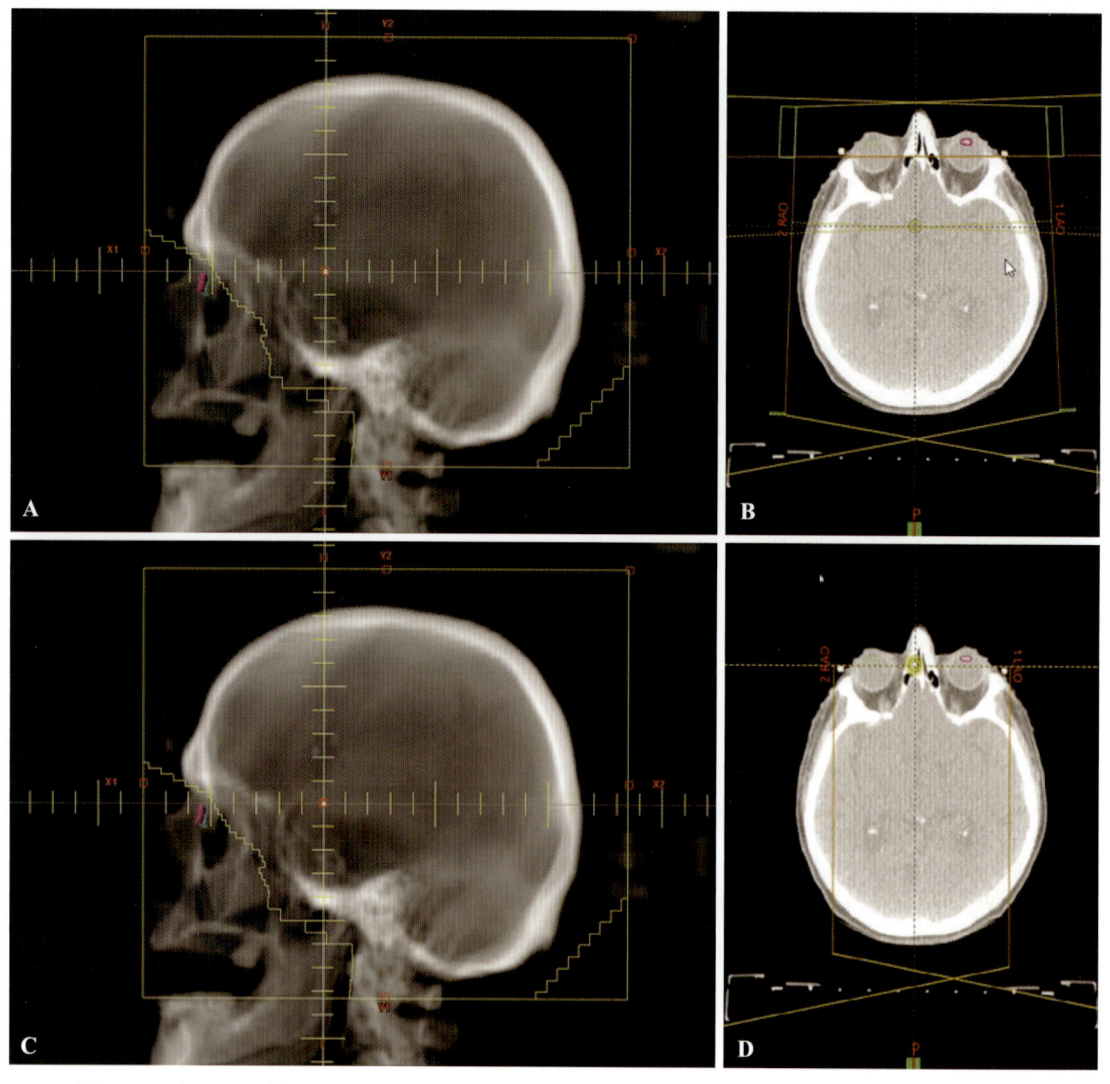

▲ 图 23-3 加 MLC 的 WBRT 计划（A）加入了 MLC 的 WBRT 计划左（侧）前斜野 DRR，晶体在图中是彩色的；（B）位于额骨眶水平面的 WBRT 射野示意图，等中心位置由固定面罩上的放射显像标记确定。旋转机架以确保前野边界是共面的，且不会散射到对侧晶体中；（C）左侧 DRR，显示了放置在额骨外侧上的 X 线显像标记位置，射野区域未显示；（D）位于额骨眶水平面的 WBRT 射野示意图，等中心设置在两标志物的正中间，该图显示了后野的散射，需防止晶体被意外照射

评估了其中几种方案[30]。然而，迄今为止，还没有哪种 WBRT 分割方案显示在症状缓解的频率、进展时间或总体生存率方面有显著提升。研究人员还研究了改变分割方案的效果。其中一项评估 WBRT 的研究显示，以 2Gy/ 次，3 次 / 天，治疗一周总剂量达 30～36Gy，45% 的患者在治疗 6 个月后症状持续缓解，没有明显的不良反应[31]。然而，尽管改变分割方案可以快速完成治疗，但在 1 天内进行多次治疗会增大医疗人员的负担，而且还会加速不良反应的出现，因

为数据不足，无法证明其是否优于传统分割方式。一项 Cochrane 分析显示，与常规的 30Gy/10 次或 20Gy/5 次的放疗方案相比，采用非常规分割放疗方案不会改善总体生存率或症状[32]。因此，大多数医生在制定 WBRT 方案时都会遵循他们各自的机构指南，在美国，30Gy/10 次是最常用的分割方案[33]。

常规的 2D 或 3D WBRT 计划一般采用平行对穿侧野的布野方式，这种方式的剂量不均匀性会高达 +/-20%[34, 35]，据我们所知，目前尚无关

于这种剂量不均匀性对 WBRT 治疗产生的影响的具体数据。但是有研究报道称，脑部的剂量热点区域、以及在体积较大的靶区使用＞3Gy/次的分割方案，可能都与放射毒性增加有某种联系[36, 37]。因此，放疗专家一直在努力减小 WBRT 的剂量不均匀性。WBRT 计划通常使用 6 MV 光子，但 10MV 光子可以改善剂量均匀性，减少热点，并在不影响靶区覆盖率的情况下累积剂量更低[38]（图 23-4）。我们机构的研究人员回顾性对常规 WBRT 重新分别设计了 6MV 和 10MV 光子能量的计划方案，并对这些方案开展了剂量学分析，结果表明，10MV 计划显著提高了 98% 处方剂量的靶区体积，减少了 105% 处方剂量的靶区体积，降低了最大剂量，改善了计划的剂量均匀性（未发表的数据）。另外，野中野技术也被证明可以提高剂量均匀性和减少热点[34]。

在三维适形放射治疗中，每个射野的孔径与其射束的目标投影一致，在整个射野内形成均匀的辐射强度。相反，如果使用调强放射治疗（intensity-modulated radiotherapy，IMRT），在某

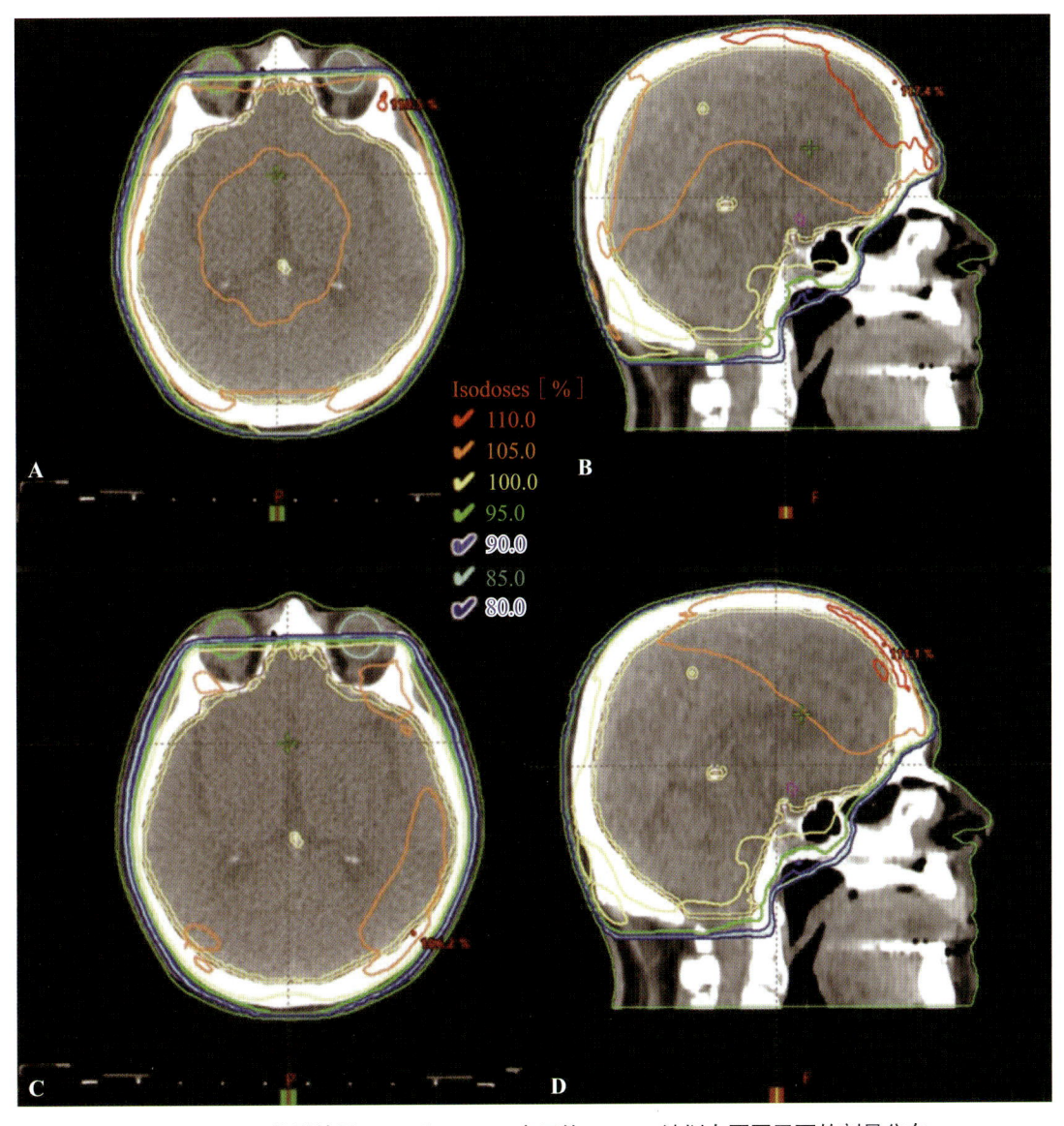

▲ 图 23-4 分别使用 6MV 和 10MV 光子的 WBRT 计划在不同平面的剂量分布
A. 使用 6MV 光子的 WBRT 在等中心水平面剂量分布；B. 使用 6MV 光子的 WBRT 在等中心矢状面剂量分布；C. 使用 10MV 光子的 WBRT 在等中心水平面剂量分布；D. 使用 10MV 光子的 WBRT 在等中心矢状面剂量分布

个单野中指向危及器官的辐射束部分可以设法阻挡掉，然后通过其他射野补偿对应靶区的剂量。这一过程可以通过使用动态 MLC 技术来实现，动态意味着 MLC 叶片在治疗过程中一直处于运动状态，或者可以使用相对静态或步进式的分段 MLC 技术，即在每个单独的射束和机架角度将 MLC 叶片在不同的位置和时间点固定住[39]。

IMRT 技术也可以显著降低 WBRT 的剂量不均匀性。Yu 等对 10 例患者开展了使用 6MV 光子的 3DRT 计划和 IMRT 计划的剂量学评估，处方剂量为 30 Gy/10 次。他们的报道显示，IMRT 计划的剂量均匀性明显更好，脑部接受＞ 105% 剂量的平均体积百分比从 3DRT 的 29.3% 降至 IMRT 的 0.03%。平均最大剂量从 3DRT 的 113% 降至 IMRT 的 105%，而接受至少 98% 处方剂量的平均体积分别为 99.5%（3DRT）和 100%（IMRT）。对于常规的 WBRT 计划，一般会在上额叶和中额叶等区域出现剂量热点，而用 IMRT 技术可以消除这些热点。尽管 IMRT 需要增加大约三倍的机器跳数来执行计划，但却是在没有牺牲靶区覆盖的情况下实现了这些改进。作者预测，IMRT 计划设计比常规计划设计只需多花 20～25min，而且因为靶区勾画和计划优化需要更长的时间，IMRT 的计划质控可能也需要花更长的时间[36]。这些减少剂量不均匀性的临床意义，尤其是对主要负责认知功能的额叶的临床意义目前尚不清楚，需要进一步研究。

容积旋转调强放疗（volumetric modulated arc therapy，VMAT）是 IMRT 的一种特殊形式，在旋转调强放疗过程中，机架围绕着患者旋转，同时治疗机不断出束，潜在地改善了剂量分布的均匀性。通过使用动态拉弧技术，VMAT 可以比 IMRT 更快地结束治疗。缩短治疗时间可以改善患者的舒适度，减少治疗过程中患者的运动次数。研究表明将 VMAT 用于 WBRT 表现出极好的靶区覆盖率和剂量均匀性，且毒性发生率也低于历史性对照组。据报道，VMAT-WBRT 的治疗时间仅为 3～4min[35]。但是，与其他任何 IMRT 技术一样，VMAT 计划确实增加了治疗计划设计和质控方面的工作量。

下一节将讨论海马保护性全脑放疗技术。

（二）肿瘤组织学

随着对放射生物学的进一步了解，放疗医生如今在选择 WBRT 方案时会更多地考虑肿瘤对射线的相对敏感性。有研究显示，提高剂量可改善黑色素瘤脑转移瘤的姑息治疗疗效[40]，而另一项研究表明，尽管放射毒性会有所增加，但使用分次大剂量（≥ 500cGy）可改善治疗效果[41]。Rades 等通过回顾性分析证明使用更大剂量可使肾癌脑转移的 6 个月局部控制率从 21%（30Gy/10 次）提高到 57%（40Gy/20 次或 45Gy/15 次），总体 1 年生存率从 13% 提升到 47%[42]。

（三）WBRT + SRS 推量

为了改善临床疗效，研究人员开始探索 WBRT 后使用 SRS（放射外科）推量对肿瘤的作用。一项早期研究发现行 WBRT 至 35Gy，然后对单一脑转移瘤施行 15Gy 的 SRS 推量，其结果与单独 WBRT 相比没有区别[43]。在一项对 27 例多发性脑转移瘤患者的前瞻性试验中，将患者随机分为单独 WBRT（14 例）和 WBRT+SRS（13 例），其结果显示 WBRT+SRS 组一年局部控制率为 100%，而单独 WBRT 组为 8%。局部失控的中位时间 WBRT 组 6 个月，WBRT+SRS 组 36 个月，且与肿瘤组织学或肿瘤数目无关，但与颅外病变的程度有关。此外，WBRT+SRS 组没有观察到发病率增加[44]。

RTOG 9508 号报道就此进行了迄今为止规模最大的试验，将 1～3 个脑转移瘤的患者随机分为接受 WBRT+SRS 治疗组（167 例）和只接受 WBRT 治疗组（164 例）。与 WBRT 组的 4.9 个月中位生存期相比，WBRT+SRS 组的中位生存期有显著改善，达到了 6.5 个月。WBRT+SRS 组在 6 个月时 KPS 评分稳定或有改善，局部控制率和完全缓解率均有提高。值得注意的是，在接受

WBRT+SRS治疗组的多发性脑转移瘤患者中，没有观察到生存获益，但这些患者的一般状况有所改善，类固醇依赖性降低[45]。因此，WBRT+SRS加量对脑单发转移瘤患者是有益的。然而，目前还不清楚SRS或手术是否能获得更好的结果，或者手术后再行WBRT和SRS是否能够改善疗效。最近一项Cochrane分析报道称，WBRT+SRS与单独WBRT相比，1年期的脑部整体发病控制风险比为0.39，该结果表明WBRT+SRS治疗效果更好[32]。

WBRT和SRS一般按先后顺序依次施行，也可以在直线加速器上用VMAT技术同步施行[36,39]。某团队评估了行WBRT 20Gy/5次，同时行SRS同步推量（SIB）20Gy/5次，将40Gy剂量分5次照射到转移瘤中心。执行两个旋转拉弧所需的平均跳数和平均"出束"时间分别为1600 MU和180s[46]。Borghetti等分别用螺旋IMRT技术和VMAT技术设计SRS和SIB计划并对其进行剂量学和技术分析比较。对于研究的10个病例中的每一例，都计算和优化了4种计划，并实际实施了其中一种：使用螺旋IMRT技术或VMAT技术行WBRT（30Gy/10次）+SRS推量（15Gy/1次），以及WBRT+SIB（45Gy/10次）。他们的报道称，螺旋IMRT计划取得了比VMAT计划更好的靶区覆盖率。基于VMAT的SIB计划、基于VMAT的SRS计划、基于螺旋IMRT的SIB计划、基于螺旋IMRT的SRS计划的平均治疗时间分别为210s、467s、440s和1598s[47]。

（四）术后WBRT

术后WBRT的目的是治疗手术后的残留肿瘤，同时控制颅内其余部分的显微和肉眼可见病灶。除了前面提到的Patchell的研究外，还有几个III期实验评估了术后WBRT的有效性[15]。Muacevic等将64名单发脑转移瘤患者（肿瘤直径≤3cm，KPS≥70，颅外病变稳定）随机分为两组，一组行伽马刀SRS，另一组行手术切除加术后WBRT。WBRT在肿瘤切除后14天内施行，分割方案为40Gy/20次。行SRS的肿瘤边缘剂量平均为21Gy，对于黑色素瘤等辐射不敏感肿瘤为20～27Gy，对于乳腺癌等辐射敏感肿瘤为14～20Gy。虽然在1年的局部控制率、放疗后6个月的生活质量（quality of life, QOL）、中位生存期（WBRT组9.5个月和SRS组10.3个月）或神经系统疾病导致的死亡率等评估指标方面没有明显差异，但SRS组的1年颅内远处控制率更差（3% vs. 25.8%）[48]。

Kocher等研究了359例有1～3个脑转移瘤、颅外病变稳定、一般情况良好的患者的预后情况，这些患者中有199例先期接受了SRS，160例接受了手术切除，并随机分为WRBT组和观察组，虽然WRBT组和观察组的总体生存率相似（10.9个月 vs. 10.7个月），但是行WBRT降低了原发灶（手术组：59%～27%；SRS组：31%～19%）和颅内转移灶（手术组：42%～23%；SRS组：48%～33%）的2年复发率[49]。Brown等随机选择多例接受了脑转移瘤手术切除的患者（瘤腔直径＜5cm），行术后SRS（12～20Gy/1次）或术后WBRT（30Gy/10次或37.5Gy/15次）。与WBRT组相比，SRS组颅内进展时间更短（6.4个月 vs. 27.5个月），6个月瘤床控制率更低（80.4% vs. 87.1%）。虽然接受SRS的患者的颅内局部和远处控制率都较差，但两组间脑膜疾病的发生率没有差别。值得注意的是，SRS组中20%的患者后来接受了WBRT，作为挽救疗法的一部分[50]。但这项试验的重点是在SRS组中提高认知无恶化条件下的生存率，这一点将在下文中详细讨论。

（五）再程WBRT

在行WBRT首次疗程后肿瘤增长或出现新的脑转移瘤的患者可以考虑行再程WBRT[12]。Wong等回顾性分析了86例患者在行首次WBRT至30Gy后再次接受WBRT至中位剂量20Gy的进展性脑转移的预后情况，其中27%的患者出现了神经症状缓解，45%的患者出现部分缓解，

脑转移瘤放射治疗学：基于病例的研究
Radiotherapy in Managing Brain Metastases: A Case-Based Approach

29% 的患者症状稳定或恶化。多因素分析表明有无颅外转移是影响预后的主要因素[51]。另一项研究的 17 名患者行中位剂量为 35Gy 的首次 WBRT 后出现神经症状及放射证据的新的或进展性脑转移，再程 WBRT 中位剂量为 21.6Gy，在有完整随访资料的 10 名患者中有 8 名显示症状完全或部分缓解。该组在行再程 WBRT 后的中位总生存期为 5.2 个月，其中颅外疾病稳定患者的中位生存期为 19.8 个月，颅外疾病进展的患者的中位生存期为 2.5 个月。再程 WBRT 的不良反应均为急性反应，但严重程度仅为 1~2 级，包括乏力（35.5%）、头痛（23.5%）、恶心呕吐（23.5%）、共济失调（5.9%）、皮肤刺激（5.9%）和头晕（5.9%）[52]。因此，对于预期生存期有限的患者，可以安全地给予 20Gy 的剂量，从而有效地缓解症状或减少类固醇依赖。

七、危及器官的保护

由于传统认为脑转移瘤患者的预后效果有限，所以 WBRT 的后遗症在很大程度上被忽视。然而，小部分患者（特别是年轻患者），转移数量少，一般情况好，原发灶位置好，生存期较长。随着诊断模式的进步，转移性病变的及早发现，以及全身综合治疗方法的改善，脑转移瘤患者的总体生存期正在延长。因此，研究人员现在越来越重视如何将治疗的后遗症影响降至最低。

（一）海马体

以往研究表明，WBRT 会导致神经认知和记忆力下降[36, 53-57]。在接受 WBRT 治疗的患者中，很难区分放疗和化疗、手术对颅内疾病进展产生的影响。然而，对接受了 WBRT 的患者在随后进行严格的神经认知测试时，约 50% 的患者表现出显著异常，一些研究报道更表明患者接受 WBRT 后痴呆症的发生率为 11%~52%[36, 55, 57]。海马齿状回区的颗粒细胞与新记忆的形成有关。据推测，该部位受照射导致的干细胞损伤会造成记忆损伤和认知能力下降。有证据表明海马体受照射与认知功能（如回忆）下降之间存在剂量 - 反应关系[53, 54, 56]。

为了验证这一点，放疗专家尽量在 WBRT 治疗期间减少对海马体的辐射剂量，为了降低神经认知后遗症的发生率，减轻其严重程度（图 23-5）。近年来，已开发出相应的 IMRT 技术来保护海马，即所谓的海马回避保护性 WBRT（HA-IMRT）。通过这项技术，可以在不影响靶区覆盖率或剂量均匀性的情况下，使海马神经干细胞平均接受的剂量减少至少 80%[53]。目前有多种 HA-WBRT 计划设计方法，包括螺旋断层放疗、IMRT 和 VMAT。通过对这些技术进行剂量学比较发现，螺旋断层放疗能最大程度降低海马的平均剂量、中位数剂量和最大剂量，还可以通过减少热点来提高靶区的剂量均匀性，并且不影响靶区的覆盖率，可能是 HA-WBRT 的最佳方式，如果没有条件使用螺旋断层放疗，可以退而求其次用 VMAT，IMRT 作为最后备选[58, 59]。如前所述，我们的既往研究表明，在常规 WBRT 治疗计划中，使用 10MV 的光子可以比 6MV 的光子减少

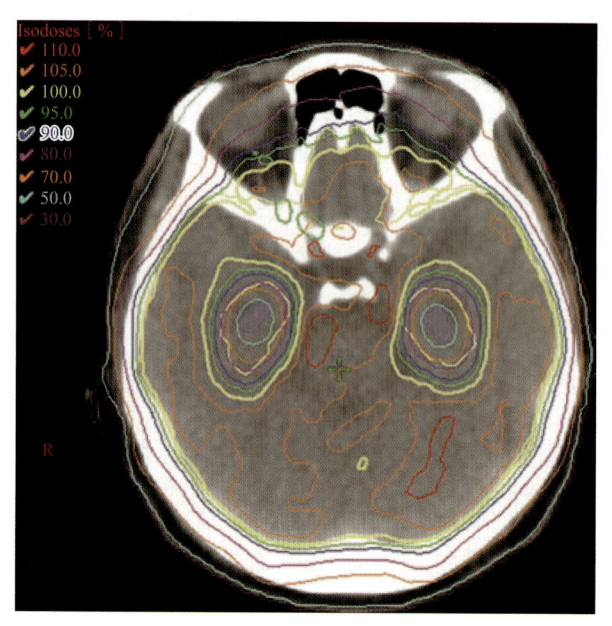

▲ 图 23-5 使用 6 MV 光子的保护海马的 WBRT 水平面剂量分布

对海马的照射剂量。

RTOG 0933 项目是一项Ⅱ期国际性、多机构试验，旨在评估 HA-WBRT 对神经认知的影响。患者脑转移瘤距离海马区≥5mm，处方为 30Gy/10 次。在 MRI 图像上勾画海马，外扩 5mm 形成海马体保护结构。PTV 为脑实质（不包括海马保护结构）。海马区的最大点剂量不超过 16Gy，100% 海马区不超过 9Gy。根据霍普金斯语言学习测试 – 修订版（HVLT-R DR）中的方法进行评估，发现患者的短期记忆平均相对下降了 7%，历史对照为 30%。作者认为，与常规 WBRT 相比，HA-WBRT 可观察到患者显著保存记忆功能、生活质量显著提升[53]。其他前瞻性试验所得结果与该试验一致，Tsai 等对 40 名患者行预防性或治疗性 HA-WBRT，评估包括记忆、执行功能、信息处理速度、注意力跨度在内的神经认知功能，并在随访 4 个月时报道神经认知功能稳定。海马区 D0、D10、D50 和 D80 分别低于 12.6Gy、8.81Gy、7.45Gy 和 5.83Gy，反映了不同的神经认知能力保存状态[56]。

我们用 RTOG 0933 中定义的靶区、保护结构和剂量限制条件，分别使用 6MV 和 10MV 的光子束为 20 名 WBRT 患者设计了基于 VMAT 的 HA-WBRT 方案。10MV 光子的计划更容易满足预先定义的剂量限制，但海马的最低和最高剂量指标更差，6MV 光子的计划在靶区覆盖率和剂量均匀性等指标上表现更优（未公布数据）。据此，我们建议使用 6MV 光子能量设计基于 VMAT 的 HA-WBRT 计划。

降低海马区剂量会增加该区域疾病进展的风险。但是，已发表的文献表明海马区内或附近的脑转移率很低。对颅内转移瘤患者的大规模研究显示，海马区 5mm 范围内的转移率低于 3%[53, 60-62]。迄今为止，使用 HA-WBRT 技术开展的相关研究显示海马区的治疗失败率较低，并且没有证据表明孤立的海马区内有复发[53, 63, 64]。HA-WBRT 与海马区内或附近新的脑转移瘤的显著发展无关，只有不到 5% 的患者在该区域的病情程度变差（RTOG 00933）[53]。

（二）美金刚

美金刚是一种 N- 甲基 –D- 天冬氨酸（NMDA）受体拮抗药，用于治疗与阿尔茨海默病相关的痴呆症[56]。两个Ⅲ期安慰剂对照随机试验证实了美金刚在血管性痴呆治疗中的耐受性和有效性[57, 65]。美金刚还可能在放射治疗后起到神经保护作用，延缓神经认知功能衰退，减少对记忆、执行功能和反应速度的损伤[57]。RTOG 0614 是一项双盲、随机、安慰剂对照试验，对接受 WBRT 的患者行 37.5Gy/15 次治疗，评估美金刚相对于安慰剂的神经保护作用。试验采用多种经过验证的评估工具对神经认知功能展开评估。口服美金刚（剂量方案逐步递增）与 WBRT 同时辅助使用，共 24 周。

与安慰剂组的患者相比，美金刚组患者认知功能衰退出现的时间明显延迟，认知功能衰竭的可能性更小，患者执行功能、反应速度和认知延迟也显著改善。与安慰剂组相比，美金刚组延迟回忆下降趋势明显放缓（P=0.059）。作者将结果未能达到显著水平归因于低依顺性和由此导致的有限统计功效。作者报道，美金刚耐受性良好，不同试验组患者出现的 3 级或 4 级不良反应无差异。值得注意的是，在 RTOG 0614 的入组患者中，80% 的患者在完成 WBRT 后的 6 个月内出现了神经认知功能衰退，这凸显了减轻该患者群体与治疗相关的后遗症的重要性[56]。

两项基于 RTOG 0933 和 RTOG 0614 试验结果的 NRG 肿瘤学试验正在进一步评估 HA-WBRT 和美金刚在神经认知功能方面的保护作用。NRG CC003（NCT02635009）是接受 PCI 的小细胞肺癌患者的Ⅱ期或Ⅲ期试验，这些患者将被随机分为 HA-WBRT 组或常规 WBRT 组。该试验的Ⅱ期部分，研究人员将评估颅内复发，而Ⅲ期部分将使用 HVLT-R DR 设备评估认知功能衰退。NRG CC001（NCT02360215）是一项针对脑转移瘤患者接受 WBRT 和美金刚治疗（按照 RTOG0614

给药）的Ⅱ期临床试验，患者被随机分为HA-WBRT组和常规WBRT组[66]。该项研究发现，患者在接受HA-WBRT+美金刚治疗后认知功能丧失的风险明显低于常规WBRT+美金刚，HA-WBRT+美金刚组被观察到在放疗后4个月时有更好的执行功能（23.3% vs. 40.4%，P=0.01）；在6个月时有更好的学习和记忆能力（11.5% vs. 24.7%，P=0.049；16.4% vs. 33.3%，P=0.02）。试验组之间在总生存期（overall survival，OS）、颅内无进展生存期（progress-free survival，PFS）或毒性等方面没有显著差异。6个月后，综合分析所有数据，发现接受HA-WBRT+美金刚治疗的患者，更不容易疲劳（P=0.04），记忆事物的难度较小（P=0.01），说话较不困难（P=0.049），日常活动对神经症状的干扰更少（P=0.008），认知症状较少（P=0.01）。该项实验的研究结论是，HA-WBRT+美金刚更好地保留了认知功能、减轻了患者的症状，而在颅内PFS和OS方面没有差别，应该被考虑纳入海马区周围无转移、一般情况良好的脑转移瘤患者接受WBRT的标准治疗方法。

（三）腮腺

腮腺和其他唾液腺对辐射特别敏感，有证据表明，即使是相对较低的剂量也会使其功能受损[67-70]。腮腺受到照射会导致口干症，并最终引起口腔卫生不良、龋齿、口腔感染、口腔不适、吞咽困难和营养不良等一系列问题[68,70,71]。严重的口干症会显著降低生活质量[69,70]。口干症一般发生在放疗后1~2周内，并在治疗结束后持续6~12个月[70,72]。常用的腮腺剂量限制是平均剂量<24~26Gy，至少一个腮腺平均剂量<20Gy，V15<66%[69,70,73,74]。

腮腺在常规WBRT的照射范围内，如果不采取措施规避，很容易超出其剂量限制。关于WBRT患者的腮腺受照射剂量和毒性关系的文献有限，而且在设计WBRT计划时，惯例上并没有将腮腺勾画为OAR[68-71,75]。相对于骨骼来讲，腮腺的体积和位置是变化的。现在随着3D计划设计的广泛应用，腮腺与射野的相对位置被可视化，腮腺接受的剂量也更容易被计算出来[69,70,76]。

几位研究人员评估了接受常规WBRT治疗的患者腮腺的受照射剂量，发现约1/3的患者平均腮腺剂量超过了20Gy[69,70,72]。据我们了解，目前还没有研究专门评估WBRT的腮腺剂量-体积直方图与后续的唾液分泌功能或口干症状之间的关系。但有一项评估WBRT后口干症的前瞻性试验已经完成，结果尚未发表（NCT02682199）。

幸运的是，有几种简单的治疗技术已经被证明可以减少腮腺的辐射剂量，达到减少毒性的目的。常规的WBRT通常将射野下界设置在C_1或C_2的下缘。一些研究人员已经证明，如果把射野下界回缩至C_1的下缘，或者只把脑实质作为照射范围，腮腺剂量将会降低[67,74,76]。当然，必须根据临床情况判断是否需要照射上颈椎，例如脑膜病变。已发表的文献还表明，将准直器旋转到70°或110°，或者在不影响脑部靶区覆盖的情况下微调MLC规避腮腺，可以显著降低腮腺剂量[74,77,78]。根据我们的经验，在常规的WBRT计划设计中使用10MV而非6MV的光子能量，可以减少腮腺接受的剂量（图23-6）。我们回顾性为WBRT患者重新设计了6MV和10MV计划，结果显示10MV计划的腮腺平均和最大剂量均显著降低（未发表的数据）。增加射野也可以降低腮腺剂量，Park等证明增加一个上前野，可以在不影响脑部靶区覆盖率的前提下使腮腺剂量显著降低[79]，在同一研究中，还使用了四野盒式方法设计WBRT计划，并将患者的头部倾斜40°，计划采用野中野技术来最大程度地减少热点，并使用动态楔形板补偿颅骨凸出区域的剂量。通过这种方法，腮腺平均剂量、V5、V10、V15和V20等指标均得到了明显改善[79]。

一些研究人员还评估了通过优化IMRT计划减少腮腺剂量的可行性。在两项类似的研究中，Pokhrel等和Sood等回顾性分析了HA-WBRT在

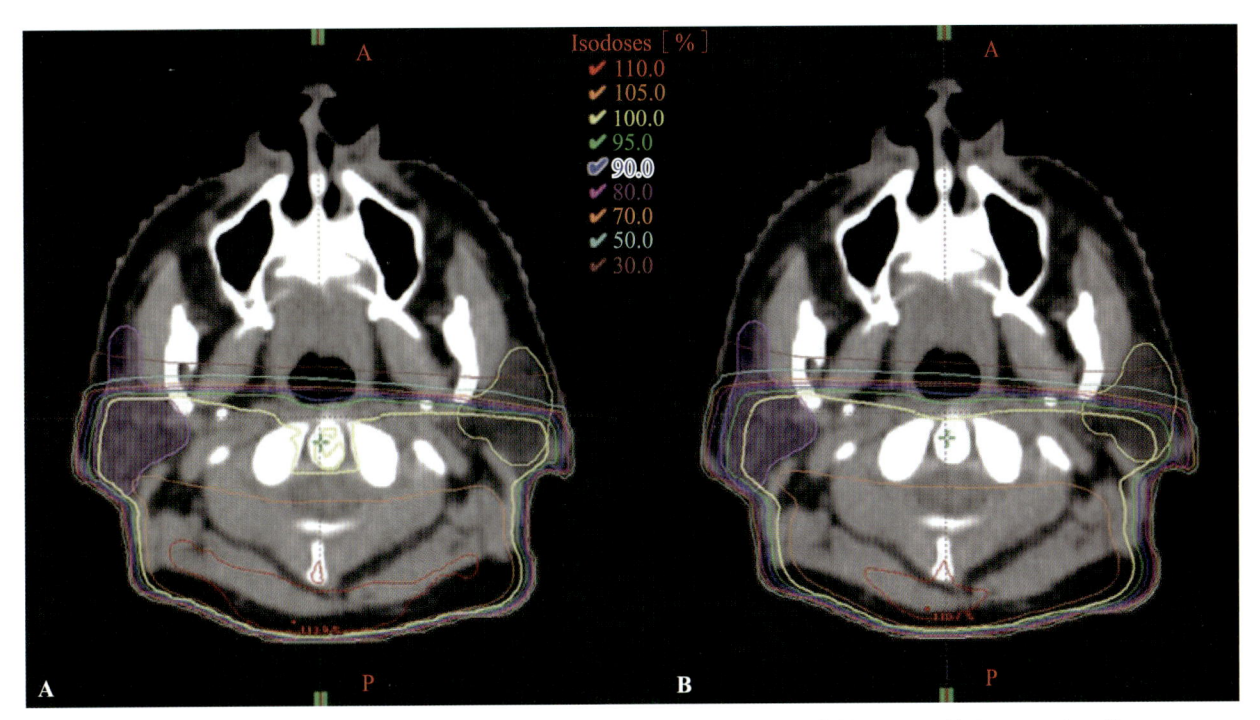

▲ 图 23-6 使用 10MV 光子的 WBRT 相较于 6MV 光子，可以减少腮腺剂量（A）使用 6MV 光子的 WBRT 在腮腺水平面的剂量分布，几乎所有受照射的腮腺都被黄色的 100% 等剂量线覆盖；（B）使用 10MV 光子的 WBRT 在腮腺水平面的剂量分布，腮腺的表浅部分未受到 100% 剂量照射

减少腮腺剂量方面的可行性。上述研究表明，接受 HA-WBRT 的患者腮腺平均剂量、最大剂量和 V15 显著降低，且没有影响靶区覆盖率[80, 81]。北卡罗来纳大学教堂山分校开展的一项评估常规 WBRT 与腮腺保护性 WBRT 的随机试验目前正在招募患者（NCT03595878）。

（四）头皮保护

对于常规 WBRT，整个头皮（包括毛囊）都是被包括在照射范围内的。毛囊对辐射非常敏感，耐受量低至 1 次 2~3Gy[82, 83]。不幸的是，几乎所有接受常规 WBRT 的患者都经历了几乎完全脱发，脱发是患者生活质量下降的一个重要原因[80-85]。放疗引起的脱发持续时间是剂量依赖性的，并且可以通过保护头皮来缩短[80-83, 85]。头发一般在放疗结束后的 2~4 个月再生。不幸的是，在分次放疗中，关于暂时性脱发的剂量-反应关系的证据有限[82, 83]。

尽管先验知识有限，研究人员们仍在减少 WBRT 的头皮剂量方面做了不少工作，并取得了不同程度的成功。根据经验，在常规的 WBRT 治疗方案中，使用 10MV 而非 6MV 光子能量可以显著降低头皮的平均和最大辐射剂量（未发表的数据）。随着放疗技术的进步（如 IMRT 的应用），保护头皮的可行性越来越高[82-84]。有证据表明，利用 IMRT 技术将头皮平均剂量限制在 16~18Gy，可以缩短暂时性脱发的病程，并降低永久性脱发的风险[81, 84]。几位研究人员发现 IMRT-WBRT 技术的模拟结果和实际测量都显示能显著减少头皮剂量。不幸的是，这些报道的头皮剂量的减少部分可能还不足以推动脱发的显著改善[82, 83]。一项头皮保护性 IMRT-WBRT 试验因无效而停止，因为没有观察到脱发的显著改善[83]。一些研究还根据 RTOG 0933 评估了 HA-WBRT 的头皮保护效果，并证明了平均头皮剂量、最大头皮剂量及头皮 V24 和 V30 都有显著降低[80, 81, 85]。

八、不确定性问题及展望

（一）去全脑放疗

QUARTZ 试验是一项Ⅲ期、多机构研究，将 538 名不适合接受手术切除或 SRS 的非小细胞肺癌脑转移患者随机分为最佳支持治疗（optimal supportive care，OSC）+WBRT 组（20Gy/5 次）或单独 OSC 组。两组在严重不良反应发生率、总生存率或生活质量方面没有差异[7]。虽然该试验表明，对于不能切除或行放疗的脑转移肺癌患者，OSC 是一种不逊于 WBRT 的治疗选择，但重要的是要考虑到，试验组的大部分患者预后非常差，两组患者的中位生存期都在 2 个月以下。因此，尽管 WBRT 可以为包括 60 岁以下、一般情况良好、颅外病变控制良好的患者带来生存获益[86, 87]，但 SRS 更适合作为先期治疗方案，WBRT 可作为挽救疗法，因为这类患者生存时间可能会很长，不得不考虑 WBRT 的诸多后遗症。

（二）预防性颅脑照射在小细胞肺癌治疗中的作用

预防性颅脑照射（prophylactic cranial irradiation，PCI）需要对表现出较高嗜神经性的原发恶性肿瘤患者行 WBRT，如 SCLC[88]。对小细胞肺癌患者脑转移的影像学诊断之前行 PCI 一直是一个受到持续争议的话题。早期研究表明，PCI 可以降低发生脑转移的概率，提高接受全身治疗但没有发生脑转移的患者的无病生存期和总体生存期[89]。Slotman 等将对系统治疗有效的 283 名广泛期小细胞肺癌患者随机分为两组，一组为观察组，另一组为 PCI。1 年后脑转移发生率从观察组的 40.4% 下降到 PCI 组的 14.6%，平均中位生存期从观察组的 5.4 个月提高到 PCI 组的 6.7 个月。但没有足够的证据表明患者在接受化疗或 PCI 前没有脑转移。该试验还尝试了不同的 PCI 分割方案：20Gy/5 次或 8 次、24Gy/12 次、25Gy/10 次、30Gy/10 次或 12 次[90]。这些研究得到了最近一项 Meta 分析的支持，该分析认为 SCLC 患者在完成 PCI 之后观察到显著的生存获益，合并相对风险为 0.92[91]。然而一项类似的日本的Ⅲ期临床试验并没有获得相同结果，该试验将化疗敏感的广泛期 SCLC 患者随机分为 PCI 组（25Gy/10 次）和观察组，患者化疗后 MRI 显示无脑转移迹象，该试验并未观察到生存获益[92]。对此的解释为，两项试验在评价标准和患者选择、PCI 分割方案、化疗药物，以及患者遗传学和人口统计学等方面存在差异（不同程度上）。相关的研究仍在阐明 PCI 在小细胞肺癌中的作用和益处，PCI 联合 HA-WBRT 和美金刚治疗可能会降低发病率，但目前尚未在临床试验中得到证明。

（三）减少治疗相关的后遗症

随着 WBRT 患者预后的改善，研究人员更多地将注意力转向治疗的不良反应。如何降低重要器官的辐射剂量，以降低毒性和改善生活质量一直是研究的重点。使用 10MV 能量光子，或使用 IMRT 技术和 VMAT 技术设计 HA-WBRT 计划，已经被证明可以降低对海马的照射剂量。越来越多的证据表明，HA-WBRT 相对于常规 WBRT 可以减少神经认知衰退。此外，有初步的证据表明美金刚具有神经保护作用。Ⅲ期研究评估美金刚的疗效并确定其最佳剂量和给药时间将大有裨益。上面提到的正在进行的 NRG 试验将进一步加深我们对 HA-WBRT、美金刚及其组合在缓解 WBRT 引起的神经认知功能衰退的作用的理解。

许多复杂的技术都可以用来降低 CNS 外高危器官（如头皮和腮腺）的潜在发病率，但不能忘记控制脑转移才是治疗的首要目标。未来的试验需要证明这些剂量学方面的进展能够在临床上显著改善 WBRT 患者的预后。

第 23 章 保护海马的全脑放疗技术
Techniques of Whole Brain Radiation Therapy Including Hippocampal Avoidance

> **要　点**
>
> - 以下几类患者可以将 WBRT 作为首选治疗方法，如脑膜病变患者、脑转移瘤发生在大脑功能区的患者，多发脑转移瘤患者、转移瘤太大而无法切除或行 SRS 的患者。
> - 行 WBRT 应考虑使用皮质类固醇和抗癫痫药物，以帮助患者迅速缓解症状，并有可能改善神经功能。
> - 常规 WBRT 需要分 10 次，每次 300cGy，总剂量为 3000cGy。
> - 最常见的 WBRT 计划一般设计两个对穿侧野，在前斜方向上稍微偏离轴线旋转 2°～3°，形成合理的共面野边界，规避散射到晶体的剂量。射野下界通常设置在第一或第二颈椎的下端，后界和上界各向外扩 2cm。
> - 相比于 6MV 光子，选择用 10MV 光子设计 WBRT 计划，能在不影响靶区覆盖率的情况下改善颅内的剂量均匀性，并能更好的保护腮腺。
> - 常规 WBRT 常见的不良反应包括神经认知功能下降、口干症和脱发。
> - 先进的放疗技术可以设计出海马回避保护性 WBRT，已被证明安全，并可减少神经认知后遗症。
> - 在设计海马回避保护性 WBRT 计划时，用 6MV 光子比用 10MV 光子可以更好地保护海马。
> - 先进的计划设计技术也被证明可以减少腮腺和头皮的辐射剂量，但口干症和脱发能否有效缓解还需要临床检验。

参考文献

[1] Hustu H, Aur R, Verzosa M, Simone J, Pinkel D. Prevention of central nervous system leukemia by irradiation. Cancer. 1973;32(3):585–97.

[2] Jenkin D. The radiation treatment of medulloblastoma. J Neurooncol. 1996;29(1):45–54.

[3] Uozumi A, Yamaura A, Makino H, Miyoshi T, Arimizu N. A newly designed radiation port for medulloblastoma to prevent metastasis to the cribriform plate region. Childs Nerv Syst. 1990;6(8):451–5.

[4] Gavrilovic I, Posner J. Brain metastases: epidemiology and pathophysiology. J Neurooncol. 2005;75(1):5–14.

[5] Halperin E, Wazer D, Perez C, Brady L. Perez & Brady's principles and practice of radiation oncology. 6th ed. Philadelphia: Lippincott Williams & Wilkins; 2013.

[6] Steeg P, Camphausen K, Smith Q. Brain metastases as preventive and therapeutic targets. Nat Rev Cancer. 2011;11(5):352–63.

[7] Mulvenna P, Nankivell M, Barton R, Faivre-Finn C, Wilson P, McColl E, et al. Dexamethasone and supportive care with or without whole brain radiotherapy in treating patients with non-small cell lung cancer with brain metastases unsuitable for resection or stereotactic radiotherapy (QUARTZ): results from a phase 3, non-inferiority, randomised trial. Lancet. 2016;388(10055):2004–14.

[8] Chao J, Phillips R, Nickson J. Roentgen-ray therapy of cerebral metastases. Cancer. 1954;7(4):682–9.

[9] Order S, Hellmän S, Von Essen C, Kligerman M. Improvement in quality of survival following whole-brain irradiation for brain metastasis. Radiology. 1968;91(1):149–53.

[10] Lenz M, Freid J. Metastases to the skeleton, brain and spinal cord from cancer of the breast and the effect of radiotherapy. Ann Surg. 1931;93(1):278–93.

[11] Jackson Richmond J. Cerebral tumours. J Fac Radiol. 1949;1(1):23–7.

[12] Chu F, Hilaris B. Value of radiation therapy in the management of intracranial metastases. Cancer. 1961;14(3):577–81.

[13] Borgelt B, Gelber R, Kramer S, Brady L, Chang C, Davis L, et al. The palliation of brain metastases: final results of the first two studies by the radiation therapy oncology group. Int J Radiat Oncol Biol Phys. 1980;6(1):1–9.

[14] Patchell R, Tibbs P, Walsh J, Dempsey R, Maruyama Y, Kryscio R, et al. A randomized trial of surgery in the treatment of single metastases to the brain. N Engl J Med. 1990;322(8):494–500.

[15] Patchell R, Tibbs P, Regine W, Dempsey R, Mohiuddin M, Kryscio R, et al. Postoperative radiotherapy in the treatment of single metastases to the brain. JAMA. 1998;280(17):1485–9.

[16] Merriam G, Focht E. A clinical study of radiation cataracts and

the relationship to dose. Am J Roentgenol Radium Therapy, Nucl Med. 1957;77(5):759–85.

[17] Holmes G, Schulz M. Therapeutic Radiology. 1st ed. Philadelphia: Lea & Febiger; 1950.

[18] Woo S, Donaldson S, Heck R, Nielson K, Shostak C. Minimizing and measuring lens dose when giving cranial irradiation. Radiother Oncol. 1989;16(3):183–8.

[19] Dhellemmes P, Demaille M, Lejeune J, Baranzelli M, Combelles G, Torrealba G. Cerebellar medulloblastoma: results of multidisciplinary treatment. Report of 120 cases. Surg Neurol. 1986;25(3):290–4.

[20] Jereb B, Sundaresan N, Horten B, Reid A, Galicich J. Supratentorial recurrences in medulloblastoma. Cancer. 1981;47(4):806–9.

[21] Gripp S, Doeker R, Glag M, Vogelsang P, Bannach B, Doll T, et al. The role of CT simulation in wholebrain irradiation. Int J Radiat Oncol Biol Phys. 1999;45(4):1081–8.

[22] Cheng C, Chin L, Kijewski P. A coordinate transfer of anatomical information from CT to treatment simulation. Int J Radiat Oncol Biol Phys. 1987;13(10):1559–69.

[23] Goitein M, Abrams M, Rowell D, Pollari H, Wiles J. Multi-dimensional treatment planning: II. Beam's eye-view, back projection, and projection through CT sections. Int J Radiat Oncol Biol Phys. 1983;9(6):789–97.

[24] Mohan R, Barest G, Brewster L, Chui C, Kutcher G, Laughlin J, et al. A comprehensive three-dimensional radiation treatment planning system. Int J Radiat Oncol Biol Phys. 1988;15(2):481–95.

[25] Sherouse G, Novins K, Chaney E. Computation of digitally reconstructed radiographs for use in radiotherapy treatment design. Int J Radiat Oncol Biol Phys. 1990;18(3):651–8.

[26] Mah K, Danjoux C, Manship S, Makhani N, Cardoso M, Sixel K. Computed tomographic simulation of craniospinal fields in pediatric patients: improved treatment accuracy and patient comfort. Int J Radiat Oncol Biol Phys. 1998;41(5):997–1003.

[27] Andic F, Ors Y, Niang U, Kuzhan A, Dirier A. Dosimetric comparison of conventional helmet-field whole-brain irradiation with threedimensional conformal radiotherapy: dose homogeneity and retro-orbital area coverage. Br J Radiol. 2009;82(974):118–22.

[28] Freislederer P, Reiner M, Hoischen W, Quanz A, Heinz C, Walter F, et al. Characteristics of gated treatment using an optical surface imaging and gating system on an Elekta linac. Radiat Oncol. 2015;10(1):68.

[29] Pham N, Reddy P, Murphy J, Sanghvi P, Hattangadi J, Kim G, et al. Frameless, real time, surface imaging guided radiosurgery: clinical outcomes for brain metastases. Int J Radiat Oncol Biol Phys. 2015;93(3):E105.

[30] Mehta M, Khuntia D. Current strategies in whole-brain radiation therapy for brain metastases. Neurosurgery. 2005;57(Supplement):S4-33–44.

[31] Biti G, Santoni R, Ponticelli P, Magrini S, Mungar V. Multiple daily fractionation in cerebral metastases. In: Proceedings of the third European conference on clinical oncology and cancer nursing. Stockholm: Federation of European Cancer Societies; 1985.

[32] Tsao M, Xu W, Wong R, Lloyd N, Laperriere N, Sahgal A, et al. Whole brain radiotherapy for the treatment of newly diagnosed multiple brain metastases. Cochrane Database Syst Rev. 2018;1:CD003869.

[33] Coia L, Hanks G, Martz K, Steinfeld A, Diamond J, Kramer S. Practice patterns of palliative care for the United States 1984—1985. Int J Radiat Oncol Biol Phys. 1988;14(6):1261–9.

[34] Lo SS, Sahgal A, Ma L, Chang EL. Advances in radiation therapy of brain metastasis. In: Kim DG, Lunsford LD, editors. Current and future management of brain metastasis. Basel: Karger; 2012.

[35] Andrevska A, Knight KA, Sale CA. The feasibility and benefits of using volumetric arc therapy in patients with brain metastases: a systematic review. J Med Radiat Sci. 2014;61(4):267–76.

[36] Yu J, Shiao S, Knisely J. A dosimetric evaluation of conventional helmet field irradiation versus two-field intensity-modulated radiotherapy technique. Int J Radiat Oncol Biol Phys. 2007;68(2):621–31.

[37] Lee A, Foo W, Chappell R, Fowler J, Sze W, Poon Y, et al. Effect of time, dose, and fractionation on temporal lobe necrosis following radiotherapy for nasopharyngeal carcinoma. Int J Radiat Oncol Biol Phys. 1998;40(1):35–42.

[38] Zhang I, Yamamoto M, Knisely JPS. Multiple brain metastases. In: Chang EL, Brown PD, Lo SS, Sahgal A, Suh JH, editors. Adult CNS radiation oncology. Cham: Springer International Publishing; 2018.

[39] Jin J, Wen N, Ren L, Glide-Hurst C, Chetty I. Advances in treatment techniques arc-based and other intensity modulated therapies. Cancer J. 2011;17(3):166–76.

[40] Konefal J, Emami B, Pilepich M. Analysis of dose fractionation in the palliation of metastases from malignant melanoma. Cancer. 1988;61(2):243–6.

[41] Katz H. The relative effectiveness of radiation therapy, corticosteroids, and surgery in the management of melanoma metastatic to the central nervous system. Int J Radiat Oncol Biol Phys. 1981;7(7):897–906.

[42] Rades D, Heisterkamp C, Schild S. Do patients receiving whole-brain radiotherapy for brain metastases from renal cell carcinoma benefit from escalation of the radiation dose? Int J Radiat Oncol Biol Phys. 2010;78(2):398–403.

[43] Hoskin P, Crow J, Ford H. The influence of extent and local management on the outcome of radiotherapy for brain metastases. Int J Radiat Oncol Biol Phys. 1990;19(1):111–5.

[44] Kondziolka D, Patel A, Lunsford L, Kassam A, Flickinger J. Stereotactic radiosurgery plus whole brain radiotherapy versus radiotherapy alone for patients with multiple brain metastases. Int J Radiat Oncol Biol Phys. 1999;45(2):427–34.

[45] Andrews D, Scott C, Sperduto P, Flanders A, Gaspar L, Schell M, et al. Whole brain radiation therapy with or without

stereotactic radiosurgery boost for patients with one to three brain metastases: phase III results of the RTOG 9508 randomised trial. Lancet. 2004;363(9422):1665–72.

[46] Lagerwaard F, van der Hoorn E, Verbakel W, Haasbeek C, Slotman B, Senan S. Whole-brain radiotherapy with simultaneous integrated boost to multiple brain metastases using volumetric modulated arc therapy. Int J Radiat Oncol Biol Phys. 2009;75(1):253–9.

[47] Borghetti P, Pedretti S, Spiazzi L, Avitabile R, Urpis M, Foscarini F, et al. Whole brain radiotherapy with adjuvant or concomitant boost in brain metastasis: dosimetric comparison between helical and volumetric IMRT technique. Radiat Oncol. 2016;11(1):59.

[48] Muacevic A, Wowra B, Siefert A, Tonn J, Steiger H, Kreth F. Microsurgery plus whole brain irradiation versus Gamma Knife surgery alone for treatment of single metastases to the brain: a randomized controlled multicentre phase III trial. J Neurooncol. 2008 May;87(3):299–307.

[49] Kocher M, Soffietti R, Abacioglu U, Villà S, Fauchon F, Baumert B, et al. Adjuvant whole-brain radiotherapy versus observation after radiosurgery or surgical resection of one to three cerebral metastases: results of the EORTC 22952-26001 study. J Clin Oncol. 2011;29(2):134–41.

[50] Brown P, Ballman K, Cerhan J, Anderson S, Carrero X, Whitton A, et al. Postoperative stereotactic radiosurgery compared with whole brain radiotherapy for resected metastatic brain disease (NCCTG N107C/ CEC·3): a multicentre, randomised, controlled, phase 3 trial. Lancet Oncol. 2017;18(8):1049–60.

[51] Wong W, Schild S, Sawyer T, Shaw E. Analysis of outcome in patients reirradiated for brain metastases. Int J Radiat Oncol Biol Phys. 1996;34(3):585–90.

[52] Son C, Loeffler J, Oh K, Shih H. Outcomes after whole brain reirradiation in patients with brain metastases. Int J Radiat Oncol Biol Phys. 2010;78(3):S170–1.

[53] Gondi V, Pugh S, Tome WA, et al. Preservation of memory with conformal avoidance of the hippocampal neural stem-cell compartment during whole-brain radiotherapy for brain metastases (RTOG 0933): a phase II multi-institutional trial. J Clin Oncol. 2014;32(34):3810–6.

[54] Gondi V, Hermann BP, Mehta MP, Tome WA. Hippocampal dosimetry predicts neurocognitive function impairment after fractionated stereotactic radiotherapy for benign or low-grade adult brain tumors. Int J Radiat Oncol Biol Phys. 2013;85(2):348–54.

[55] Tsai PF, Yang CC, Huang TY, et al. Hippocampal dosimetry correlates with the change in neurocognitive function after hippocampal sparing during whole brain radiotherapy: a prospective study. Radiat Oncol. 2015;10:253.

[56] Brown PD, Pugh S, Laack NN, et al. Memantine for the prevention of cognitive dysfunction in patients receiving whole-brain radiotherapy: a randomized, double-blind, placebo-controlled trial. NeuroOncology. 2013;15(10):1429–37.

[57] Gondi V, Tolakanahalli R, Mehta MP, et al. Hippocampal-sparing whole-brain radiotherapy: a "how-to" technique using helical tomotherapy and linear accelerator-based intensity-modulated radiotherapy. Int J Radiat Oncol Biol Phys. 2010;78(4):1244–52.

[58] Rong Y, Evans J, Xu-Welliver M, et al. Dosimetric evaluation of intensity-modulated radiotherapy, volumetric modulated arc therapy, and helical tomotherapy for hippocampal-avoidance whole brain radiotherapy. PLoS One. 2015;10(4):e0126222.

[59] Ghia A, Tome WA, Thomas S, et al. Distribution of brain metastases in relation to the hippocampus: implications for neurocognitive functional preservation. Int J Radiat Oncol Biol Phys. 2007;68(4):971–7.

[60] Marsh JC, Gielda BT, Herskovic AM, Abrams RA. Cognitive sparing during the administration of whole brain radiotherapy and prophylactic cranial irradiation: current concepts and approaches. J Oncol. 2010;2010:198208.

[61] Zhao R, Kong W, Shang J, Zhe H, Wang YY. Hippocampal-sparing whole brain radiotherapy for lung cancer. Clin Lung Cancer. 2017;18(2):127–31.

[62] Oehlke O, Wucherpfennig D, Fels F, et al. Whole brain irradiation with hippocampal sparing and dose escalation on multiple brain metastases: local tumour control and survival. Strahlenther Onkol. 2015;191(6):461–9.

[63] Lin SY, Yang CC, Wu YM, et al. Evaluating the impact of hippocampal sparing during whole brain radiotherapy on neurocognitive functions: a preliminary report of a prospective phase II study. Biom J. 2015;38(5):439–49.

[64] Orgogozo JM, Rigaud AS, Stoffler A, et al. Efficacy and safety of memantine in patients with mild to moderate vascular dementia: a randomized, placebo-controlled trial (MMM 300). Stroke. 2002;33:1834–9.

[65] Wilcock G, Mobius HJ, Stoffler A, et al. A doubleblind, placebo-controlled multicentre study of memantine in mild to moderate vascular dementia (MMM500). Int Clin Psychopharmacol. 2002;17:297–305.

[66] Brown PD, Gondi V, Pugh S, Tome WA, Wefel JS, Armstrong TS, et al. for NRG Oncology. Hippocampal avoidance during whole-brain radiotherapy plus memantine for patients with brain metastases: Phase III trial NRG Oncology CC001. J Clin Oncol. 2020;38:1019–29.

[67] Wu CC, Wuu YR, Jani A, et al. Whole-brain irradiation field design: a comparison of parotid dose. Med Dosim. 2017;42(2):145–9.

[68] Trignani M, Genovesi D, Vinciguerra A, et al. Parotid glands in whole-brain radiotherapy: 2D versus 3D technique for no sparing or sparing. Radiol Med. 2015;120(3):324–8.

[69] Noh OK, Chun M, Nam SS, et al. Parotid gland as a risk organ in whole brain radiotherapy. Radiother Oncol. 2011;98(2):223–6.

[70] Park J, Yea JW. Whole brain radiotherapy using fourfield box technique with tilting baseplate for parotid sparing. Radiat Oncol J. 2019;37(1):22–9.

[71] Burlage FR, Coppes RP, Meertens H, Stokman MA, Vissink A. Parotid and submandibular/sublingual salivary flow during

high dose radiotherapy. Radiother Oncol. 2001;61(3):271–4.
[72] Eisbruch A, Ten Haken RK, Kim HM, Marsh LH, Ship JA. Dose, volume, and function relationships in parotid salivary glands following conformal and intensity-modulated irradiation of head and neck cancer. Int J Radiat Oncol Biol Phys. 1999;45(3):577–87.
[73] Deasy JO, Moiseenko V, Marks L, Chao KSC, Nam J, Eisbruch A. Radiotherapy dose-volume effects on salivary gland function. Int J Radiat Oncol Biol Phys. 2010;76(3 Suppl):S58–63.
[74] Cho O, Chun M, Park SH, et al. Parotid gland sparing effect by computed tomography-based modified lower field margin in whole brain radiotherapy. Radiat Oncol J. 2013;31(1):12–7.
[75] Roesink JM, Terhaard CH, Moerland MA, van Iersel F, Battermann JJ. CT-based parotid gland location: implications for preservation of parotid function. Radiother Oncol. 2000;55(2):131–3.
[76] Fiorentino A, Caivano R, Chiumento C, et al. Technique of whole brain radiotherapy: conformity index and parotid glands. Clin Oncol (R Coll Radiol). 2012;24(9):e140–1.
[77] Fiorentino A, Chiumento C, Caivano R, et al. Whole brain radiotherapy: are parotid glands organs at risk? Radiother Oncol. 2012;103(1):130–1.
[78] Loos G, Paulon R, Verrelle P, et al. Whole brain radiotherapy for brain metastases: the technique of irradiation influences the dose to parotid glands. Cancer Radiother. 2012;16(2):136–9.
[79] Park J, Park JW, Yea JW. Non-coplanar whole brain radiotherapy is an effective modality for parotid sparing. Yeungnam Univ J Med. 2019;36(1):36–42.
[80] Pokhrel D, Sood S, Lominska C, et al. Potential for reduced radiation-induced toxicity using intensity modulated arc therapy for whole-brain radiotherapy with hippocampal sparing. J Appl Clin Med Phys. 2015;16(5):131–41.
[81] Sood S, Pokhrel D, McClinton C, et al. Volumetric modulated arc therapy (VMAT) for whole brain radiotherapy: not only for hippocampal sparing, but also for reduction of dose to organs at risk. Med Dosim. 2017;42(4):375–83.
[82] Roberge D, Parker W, Niazi TM, Olivares M. Treating the contents and not the container: dosimetric study of hair-sparing whole brain intensity modulated radiation therapy. Technol Cancer Res Treat. 2005;4(5):567–70.
[83] De Puysseleyr A, Van De Velde J, Speleers B, et al. Hair-sparing whole brain radiotherapy with volumetric arc therapy in patients treated for brain metastases: dosimetric and clinical results of a phase II trial. Radiat Oncol. 2014;9:170.
[84] Kao J, Darakchiev B, Conboy L, et al. Tumor directed, scalp sparing intensity modulated whole brain radiotherapy for brain metastases. Technol Cancer Res Treat. 2015;14(5):547–55.
[85] Mahadevan A, Sampson C, LaRosa S, et al. Dosimetric analysis of the alopecia preventing effect of hippocampus sparing whole brain radiation therapy. Radiat Oncol. 2015;10:245.
[86] Sperduto P, Kased N, Roberge D, Xu Z, Shanley R, Luo X, et al. Summary report on the graded prognostic assessment: an accurate and facile diagnosisspecific tool to estimate survival for patients with brain metastases. J Clin Oncol. 2012;30(4):419–25.
[87] Gaspar L, Scott C, Rotman M, Asbell S, Phillips T, Wasserman T, et al. Recursive partitioning analysis (RPA) of prognostic factors in three radiation therapy oncology group (RTOG) brain metastases trials. Int J Radiat Oncol Biol Phys. 1997;37(4):745–51.
[88] Arriagada R, Le Chevalier T, Borie F, Riviere A, Chomy P, Monnet I, et al. Prophylactic cranial irradiation for patients with small-cell lung cancer in complete remission. J Natl Cancer Inst. 1995;87(3):183–90.
[89] Aupérin A, Arriagada R, Pignon J, Le Péchoux C, Gregor A, Stephens R, et al. Prophylactic cranial irradiation for patients with small-cell lung cancer in complete remission. N Engl J Med. 1999;341(7):476–84.
[90] Slotman B, Faivre-Finn C, Kramer G, Rankin E, Snee M, Hatton M, et al. Prophylactic cranial irradiation in extensive small-cell lung cancer. N Engl J Med. 2007;357(7):664–72.
[91] Zhang W, Jiang W, Luan L, Wang L, Zheng X, Wang G. Prophylactic cranial irradiation for patients with small-cell lung cancer: a systematic review of the literature with meta-analysis. BMC Cancer. 2014;14(1):793.
[92] Takahashi T, Yamanaka T, Seto T, Harada H, Nokihara H, Saka H, et al. Prophylactic cranial irradiation versus observation in patients with extensive-disease smallcell lung cancer: a multicentre, randomised, openlabel, phase 3 trial. Lancet Oncol. 2017;18(5):663–71.